KU-335-462

Pathology in Surgical Practice

Pathology in Surgical Practice

Edited on behalf of
The Royal College of Surgeons of England and the Royal College of Pathologists, London by

G. J. Hadfield, CBE, TD, MS, FRCS

Formerly, Vice-President and Chairman of the Court of Examiners, Royal College of Surgeons of England; Surgeon, Stoke Mandeville Hospital, Aylesbury, Bucks

M. Hobsley, TD, PhD, MChir, FRCS

Director, Department of Surgical Studies, The Middlesex Hospital Medical School, London

B. C. Morson, VRD, DM, FRCS, FRCP, FRCPath

Pathologist and Director of the Research Department, St Mark's Hospital, City Road, London; Honorary Treasurer, Royal College of Pathologists and Civilian Consultant in Pathology to the Royal Navy

With a Foreword by

Professor Sir Geoffrey Slaney, KBE, MSc, ChM, PRCS
President of the Royal College of Surgeons of England; Barling Professor of Surgery, University of Birmingham, at Queen Elizabeth Hospital and

Professor Barbara Clayton, CBE, MD, FRCP, PRCPath
President of the Royal College of Pathologists, London

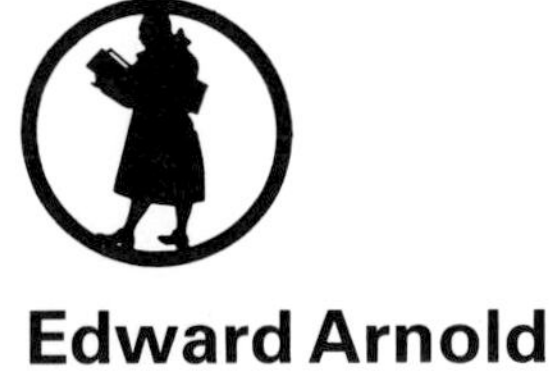

Edward Arnold

First published in Great Britain 1985
by Edward Arnold (Publishers) Ltd
41 Bedford Square
London WC1 3DQ

Edward Arnold (Australia) Pty Ltd
80 Waverly Road
Caulfield East 3145
PO Box 234
Melbourne

Edward Arnold
3 East Read Street
Baltimore, Maryland 21202, U.S.A.

British Library Cataloguing in Publication Data

Pathology in surgical practice.
1. Pathology, Surgical
I. Hadfield, G. J. II. Hobsley, Michael
III. Morson, B. C. IV. Royal College of Surgeons of England V. Royal College of Pathologists
617′.07 RD57

ISBN 0–7131–4471–8

Text set in 10/11 pt Times
Printed in Great Britain at The Bath Press, Avon

Contributors

G. J. Hadfield, CBE, TD, MS, FRCS,
Surgeon,
Stoke Mandeville Hospital,
Aylesbury,
Bucks, HP21 7LR.

M. Hobsley, TD, PhD, MChir, FRCS,
Professor of Surgery,
The Middlesex Hospital Medical School,
London, W1N 8AA.

B. C. Morson, VRD, DM, FRCS, FRCP, FRCPath,
Histopathologist,
St Mark's Hospital,
City Road,
London, EC1V 2PS.

A. Levene, MB, PhD, FRCS, FRCPath,
Head of Department of Surgical Pathology,
The Royal Marsden Hospital,
London, SW3 6JJ.

A. C. Thackray, MD, FRCS, FRCPath,
Emeritus Professor of Morbid Histology
University of London.
Formerly Consultant Pathologist to
The Middlesex Hospital, Mortimer Street,
London, W1N 8AA.

Sir Paul Bramley, MB, ChB, BDS, FRCS, FDSRCS, FRACDS,
Professor of Dental Surgery,
University of Sheffield,
Sheffield, S10 2TN.

C. J. Smith, BDS, PhD, LDSRCS, FRCPath,
Professor of Oral Pathology,
University of Sheffield,
Sheffield, S10 2TN.

R. M. Kirk, MS, FRCS,
Surgeon,
The Royal Free Hospital,
Hampstead,
London, NW3 2QG.

J. E. McLaughlin, BSc, MB, BS, FRCPath,
Histopathologist,
The Royal Free Hospital,
Hampstead,
London, NW3 2QG.

J. B. McFarland, MD, ChM, FRCS, FRCSEd,
Surgeon,
The Royal Liverpool Hospital and
Clinical Lecturer in Surgery,
University of Liverpool,
PO Box 147,
Liverpool, L69 3BX.

D. W. Day, MB, BChir, MRCPath,
Senior Lecturer in Pathology,
University of Liverpool,
Duncan Building,
PO Box 147,
Liverpool, L69 3BX.

N. V. Addison, FRCS, FACS,
Surgeon,
The Bradford Royal Infirmary,
Bradford,
West Yorks, BD9 6RJ.

G. I. Horsfield, MD(Lond.), FRCPath,
Pathologist,
The Royal Infirmary,
Bradford,
West Yorks, BD9 6RJ.

D. A. Macfarlane, MCh, FRCS, FRCS(Ed)
Surgeon,
St Stephen's Hospital,
London, SW10 9TH.

J. N. Harcourt-Webster, MD, MA, BChir, FRCPath,
Histopathologist,
St Stephen's Hospital,
London, SW10 9TH.

R. J. Nicholls, MChir, FRCS,
Surgeon,
St Thomas' and St Mark's Hospital,
London, EC1V 2PS.

J. Alexander-Williams, MD, FRCS, FACS,
Surgeon,
The General Hospital,
Birmingham, B4 6NH.

H. Thompson, MD, FRCPath,
Histopathologist,
The General Hospital,
Birmingham, BT4 6NH.

M. M. Henry, MB, BS, FRCS,
Surgeon,
The Central Middlesex Hospital and St Mark's Hospital,
London, EC1V 2PS.

J. L. Dawson, MS, FRCS,
Surgeon,
King's College Hospital,
London, SE5 9RS.

K. J. Arulambalam, MB, MRCPath,
Histopathologist,
Farnborough Hospital,
Orpington,
Kent, BR6 8ND.

W. S. Shand, MA, MD, FRCS(Ed), FRCS(Eng),
Surgeon,
St Bartholomew's Hospital,
London, EC1A 7BE.

A. G. Stansfeld, MA, MB, BChir, FRCPath,
Consulting Histopathologist,
St Bartholomew's Hospital,
West Smithfield,
London, EC1A 7BE.

J. S. Malpas, MB, BS, BSc, DPhil, FRCP, FRCR,
Professor of Medical Oncology,
and Honorary Consulting Physician,
The Hospital for Sick Children,
Great Ormond Street and
St Bartholomew's Hospital,
West Smithfield,
London, EC1A 7BE.

J. S. H. Wade, MC, TD, MA, FRCS,
Consulting Surgeon,
University Hospital of Wales,
Cardiff, CF4 4XN.

E. D. Williams, MD, FRCP, FRCPath,
Professor of Pathology,
Welsh National School of Medicine,
Cardiff, CF4 4XN.

P. D. M. Ellis, MA, FRCS,
Otolaryngologist,
Addenbrooke's Hospital,
Cambridge, CB2 2QQ.

D. G. D. Wight, MA, MB, BChir, MRCPath,
Histopathologist,
Addenbrooke's Hospital,
Cambridge, CB2 2QQ.

Jason Brice, MB, FRCS,
Neurosurgeon,
Wessex Neurological Centre,
Southampton SO9 4XY.

J. S. Garfield, MA, MChir, FRCP, FRCS,
Neurosurgeon,
Wessex Regional Neurological Centre,
Southampton, SO9 4XY.

R. O. Weller, BSc, MD, PhD, FRCPath,
Professor of Neuropathology,
University of Southampton Medical School,
Southampton General Hospital,
Southampton, SO9 5NH.

P. S. Boulter, FRCS(Ed), HonFRACS, FRCS,
Surgeon,
Royal Surrey County Hospital,
Guildford, Surrey, GU2 5XX.

N. M. Gibbs, MRCP, FRCPath,
Histopathologist,
Royal Surrey County Hospital,
Guildford, Surrey, GU2 5XX.

B. T. Jackson, MS, FRCS,
Surgeon,
St Thomas' Hospital,
London, SE1 7EH.

J. R. Tighe, BSc, MD, FRCP, FRCP(Ed), FRCPath,
Histopathologist,
St Thomas's Hospital Medical School,
London, SE1 7EH.

R. M. Greenhalgh, MA, MB, BChir, FRCS,
Professor of Surgery,
Charing Cross Hospital,
London, W6 8RF.

N. Woolf, MD, PhD, FRCPath,
Professor of Pathology,
Middlesex Hospital,
London, W1N 8AA.

D. Negus, MA, DM, MCh, LRCP, FRCS,
Surgeon,
Lewisham Hospital,
London, SE13 6LH.
Teacher in Surgery to the United Dental and Medical Schools of Guy's and St Thomas's,
London, SE13 6LH.

S. J. Machin, MB, MRCPath,
Haematologist,
Middlesex Hospital,
London W1N 8AA.

M. F. Sturridge, MS, FRCS,
Cardiothoracic Surgeon
Middlesex Hospital,
Mortimer Street,
London W1N 8AA.
Surgeon to the London Chest Hospital, London, E2 9JX and Honorary Consultant Thoracic Surgeon, National Hospital for Nervous Diseases, London WC1N 3BG.

C. P. Chilton, MB, BS, FRCS,
Urologist,
Derbyshire Royal Infirmary,
Derby, DE1 2QY.

K. M. Cameron, MB, ChBEd, FRCPath,
Histopathologist,
Institute of Urology,
London WC2H 8JE.

W. J. Highman, MB, ChB, FRCPath,
Cytopathologist,
St Paul's Hospital,
London, WC2H 9AE.

M. C. Parkinson, BSc, MD, MRCPath,
Cytologist,
St Paul's Hospital,
London, WC2H 9AE.

P. B. Clark, MD, MChir, FRCS,
Urologist,
General Infirmary and
St James's University Hospital,
Leeds, LS1 3CX,

C. K. Anderson, MB, FRCPath,
Reader in Pathology,
University of Leeds;
Histopathologist,
General Infirmary,
Leeds, LS1 3EX.

J. P. Williams, RD, MChir, FRCS,
Urologist,
St Paul's Hospital,
London, WC2H 9AE.

R. C. B. Pugh, MD, FRCS, FRCPath,
Consulting Pathologist to St Peter's Hospital and the Institute of Urology,
London, WC2H 8JE.

R. L. Hurt, FRCS,
Thoracic Surgeon,
North Middlesex Hospital,
London, N18 1QX.

W. F. Whimster, MD, FRCP, FRCPath,
Reader in Histopathology,
King's College Hospital Medical School,
London, SE5 8RX.

M. Bates, FRCS, FACS,
Thoracic Surgeon,
North Middlesex Hospital,
London, N18 1QX.

K. J. Jarvis, MB, BS, MRCPath,
Histopathologist,
North Middlesex Hospital,
London, N18 1QX.

T. L. Kennedy, MD, MS, FRCS,
Surgeon,
Royal Victoria Hospital,
Belfast, BT12 6BA.

K. D. Buchanan, MD, FRCP(Glas),
FRCP(Edin), FRCP(Lond),
Professor of Metabolic Medicine,
Queen's University; Physician,
Royal Victoria and City Hospitals,
Belfast, BT12 6BA.

E. F. McKeown, MD, FRCP(Lond),
FRCPath,
Professor of Pathology,
Queen's University of Belfast,
Belfast, BT7 1NN.

P. M. Yeoman, MD, FRCS,
Orthopaedic Surgeon,
The Royal United Hospital,
Bath, BA1 3NG.

A. W. F. Lettin, MS, FRCS,
Orthopaedic Surgeon, Royal
National Orthopaedic Hospital and
St Bartholomew's Hospital,
London, EC1A 7BE.

A. N. Henry, MCh, FRCS, FRCSI,
Orthopaedic Surgeon,
Guy's Hospital,
London, SE1 9RT.

P. D. Byers, PhD, MD, FRCPath,
Reader in Morbid Anatomy and Head of the
Department, Institute of Orthopaedics,
London, W1N 6AD.

L. Spitz, PhD, FRCS,
Professor of Paediatric Surgery,
Institute of Child Health,
London, WC1N 1EH.

J. R. Pincott, MB, BS, MRCPath,
Senior Lecturer in Histopathology,
Institute of Child Health,
London, WC1N 1EH.

J. D. Atwell, FRCS,
Paediatric and Neonatal Surgeon,
Wessex Regional Centre for Paediatric Surgery
and Southampton General Hospital,
Southampton, SO9 4XY.

A. G. MacIver, MD, MRCPath,
Senior Lecturer, Morbid Anatomy and
Experimental Pathology, University of
Southampton and Southampton General
Hospital,
Southampton, SO9 4XY.

M. R. B. Keighley, MS, FRCS,
Professor of Surgery,
The General Hospital,
Steelhouse Lane, Birmingham, B4 6NH.

D. W. Burdon, MB, FRCPath,
Senior Lecturer in Medical Microbiology,
University of Birmingham and Microbiologist,
The General Hospital,
Birmingham, B4 6NH.

B. Zederfeldt, MD
Professor of Surgery,
Malmo General Hospital,
Malmo, 21401, Sweden.

F. Rank, MD, PhD,
Chief Pathologist,
Institute of Pathology,
University of Copenhagen,
Herlev Hospital,
DK-2730
Herlev, Denmark.

R. J. Cooling, MB, ChB, FRCS,
Ophthalmic Surgeon,
Moorfields Eye Hospital,
London EC1V 2PS.

A. Garner, MD, PhD, MRCP, FRCPath,
Professor and Director of Pathology,
Institute of Ophthalmology,
University of London,
London EC1V 9AD

D. Lowe, MB, BS, MIBiol, MRCPath,
Histopathologist,
St Bartholomew's Hospital,
West Smithfield,
London, EC1A 7BE.

M. D. Cameron, MA, MB, BChir, FRCS,
FRCOG,
Gynaecologist,
Department of Obstetrics and Gynaecology,
St Thomas' Hospital,
London, SE1 7EH.

P. J. Guillou, BSc, MD, FRCS,
Senior Lecturer in Surgery,
University of Leeds,
and Surgeon
St James's University Hospital,
Leeds,
LS9 7TF.

P. R. Millard, MD, MRCPath,
Histopathologist,
John Radcliffe Hospital,
Oxford,
OX3 9DU.

O. N. Tubbs, MB, BChir, FRCS,
Orthopaedic Surgeon,
General Hospital and Royal Orthopaedic
Hospital, Birmingham; Honorary Lecturer in
Surgery, University of Birmingham.
Birmingham, B15 2TJ.

H. B. Stoner, MD, BSc, FRCS, FRCPath,
Honorary Pathologist, Hope Hospital, Salford.
Formerly, Honorary Professor of Surgical Science,
University of Manchester, and Director,
MRC Trauma Unit,
University of Manchester, M13 9PT.

Foreword

Many notable books have already been written, the majority of them by individual surgeons or pathologists, on various aspects of surgical pathology.

The uniqueness of this particular book, 'Pathology in Surgical Practice', lies in the fact that it represents a combined approach, for each chapter has been written by a surgeon and a pathologist working in unison. This is especially timely because the disciplines of surgery and pathology are now so inextricably linked that they really constitute a therapeutic team. It is on the basis of the pathologist's expertise and advice that the surgeon has to plan the management of an individual patient and attempt to formulate a prognosis.

The close inter-relationship between surgery and pathology constitutes the philosophical 'raison d'être' of this book. The various subject headings cover a wide field and deal in detail with clinical presentations, their related pathological aspects and the manner in which they influence both diagnosis and treatment. Each chapter has been written by two acknowledged experts so the style and format varies; this adds to the appeal of the work and the editors have sensibly not imposed rigid conformity on their contributors.

We are confident that this book will be of interest not only to young surgeons, pathologists, oncologists and radiologists but equally to the established specialist, and we are particularly happy that it is to be published under the combined aegis of our respective Colleges.

Geoffrey Slaney **Barbara Clayton**

Preface

This book is an attempt to bring together the two disciplines of surgery and pathology, demonstrating their interdependence. Each contribution is the work of a team of at least one surgeon and one pathologist. Coverage of the topics is not intended to be encyclopaedic: nevertheless, the authors have assembled the material that they consider important for the total care of the patient. The editors have deliberately avoided imposing a uniformity of style and format: each presentation represents the authors' views on the handling of the clinical problems covered in that particular section.

While this book will be of use to the trainee surgeon, pathologist and oncologist, we hope that it will also be of interest to established practitioners in these subjects. To facilitate reading we have omitted references from the text, but each chapter has a reading list from which a detailed bibliography can be compiled.

1985

G J H
M H
B C M

Contents

The Surgeon and the Pathologist: an editorial introduction

G. J. Hadfield, M. Hobsley and B. C. Morson

The best guide to the natural history of a disease, its response to treatment and the likelihood of complications is usually the morbid antomy and histopathology (macroscopic and microscopic appearances) of the tissues affected. Of course, there are exceptions and other types of laboratory tests such as those in haematology, microbiology or chemical pathology may be more important in particular cases. Examples of such cases are referred to in appropriate sections of this book. Nevertheless, in the overwhelming majority of clinical situations it is histopathological information which has special importance for surgeons. The aims of this book are primarily to show why a knowledge of histopathology is valuable, how to make use of a histopathology department, and how best to benefit from what the histopathologist has to contribute to clinical management. It must be remembered that the pathologist is a consultant who is asked to advise on the diagnosis and pathogenesis of disease in a patient, not just on the histological changes in a piece of tissue.

Surgeons require detailed knowledge of the naked-eye appearances (morbid anatomy) of disease in surgical specimens and at autopsy because these are relevant to what they encounter during clinical and endoscopic examination, in the images produced by various techniques such as radiology, as well as in the operating room. Without such knowledge they are not properly equipped to appreciate the planning of surgical procedures, the potential for spread of disease and the value of staging, particularly in the field of oncology. Although they do not require detailed knowledge of microscopic pathology, which can only be acquired by years of full-time training, it is essential that they should understand the implications and limitations of microscopic interpretation and diagnosis, especially in biopsy reports.

Formal consultation with the histopathology department begins with filling in a request form and ends with the receipt of a definitive report, but along the way there are many hurdles which cannot be successfully surmounted without co-operation as well as understanding between surgeon and pathologist if both are to extract the maximum amount of useful information for diagnosis and management of the patient. The co-operation will only be effective if there is *sustained commitment by both parties to communicate with each other* at every opportunity. This communication is vital, otherwise a histopathology department will dengenerate to the level of a postal service with loss of its valuable contribution to patient care. Let us now examine the whole process in detail.

Filling in forms

This is often regarded as a bore and so the information written on the form may be sketchy, incomplete and sometimes indecipherable. The task is often delegated to a very junior member of staff or a nurse, who may not be familiar with the problem or cannot spell the more technical words; this can be hilarious for the pathologist but hinders him in his task of interpretation.

Apart from the obvious details of surnames and forename, age, sex, hospital number, ward or outpatient clinic, date and the name of the consultant, it is to the clinical summary that the pathologist looks for information. For example, he needs to know exactly from where the biopsy was taken and to be given a brief, but pertinent, summary of the clinical circumstances. Personal contact between pathologist and surgeon may be necessary at this stage. Endoscopic appearances should always be described. If the request is for examination of an operation specimen then the type of operation should be stated along with details of the surgical anatomy of the procedure. Often a simple diagram in support of clinical information is immensely valuable to the reporting pathologist. The trouble taken over filling in forms will be amply repaid by a better service from the pathologist.

Essentially, the pathologist wishes to know what problems face the surgeon and what questions are being asked, for example about completeness of excision, likelyhood of recurrence or necessity for further therapy. The reply may be brief, but represents the end point of skilled work by his technical staff and long experience of gross and microscopical features of a disease in the context of the clinical information which is provided.

Taking and handling biopsies

There is considerable skill in taking a biopsy of sufficient size and quality from the right place. A biopsy is, after all, often only a tiny sample of a large surface area of disease or volume of tissue. The pathologist needs to know how representative the sample is and he can only appreciate this by looking at the microscopic slide in the context of information given on the request form.

Specimens should be sent directly to the pathology department with as little interference as possible. In particular specimens should not be divided, part being taken for some other purpose, without consultation with the pathologist, as unlike blood samples, tissue is not homogenous, and the pathologist is the best person to advise on what tissues can safely be sampled and used for other purposes.

It should be remembered that human tissues are easily crushed by handling and this can produce what the pathologist calls "crushing artefact". If diathermy is used for biopsy then "heat artefact" can occur. Both types of artefact can make interpretation difficult and sometimes impossible. But the commonest artefact seen in the laboratory must certainly be the result of delay in fixation. It cannot be emphasized too strongly that immediate fixation in the right fluid is vital. Buffered 10 per cent formaldehyde solution is the best available for routine purposes but there are others more suitable for special purposes, such as glutaraldehyde for electron micrscopy. It is the responsibility of the laboratory to see that containers contain fresh buffered formaldehyde but surgeons should be aware that buffered formaldehyde solution loses its quality in weeks rather than months. From time to time every pathologist comes across the biopsy which is not floating freely in the fixative and may be stuck to the side of the container or even in the cap, so that it is not fixed. Containers should be labelled carefully (not their caps, which may become interchanged!) and make sure that the information given on them corresponds accurately with that written on the request form.

Apart from the obvious example of frozen section diagnosis, some technical procedures carried out in histopathology departments can only be made on fresh tissue. This is particularly applicable to immunocytochemical and histochemical methods which have growing importance in diagnostic histopathology. It is worth remembering that if in doubt about whether to fix or not to fix in formaldehyde solution it is nearly always safe to place a surgical specimen or a biopsy temporarily in a small, empty and sealed container in the 4°C compartment of a refrigerator, but not at 0° when ice crystals form which disrupt the tissue when thawed. If in doubt, the pathologist or a senior member of his technical staff should be consulted.

It should be appreciated by pathologists that the person taking the biopsy is usually preoccupied with the patient (who is often conscious) and observing clinical signs. He may need to be so absorbed in these problems that he cannot give sufficient attention to what actually happens to a biopsy after he has taken it. This is where junior medical staff in attendance, and nurses in particular, have an important role. It is generally true that nursing staff receive little or no instruction in laboratory methods and this is a pity because they can play a crucial part in making sure that the biopsy specimen goes into the right container, correctly labelled. Moreover, there is a special role for nurse endoscopy assistants in the process of orientating biopsies correctly.

The technical staff of the laboratory are the next to receive the specimen and it is they who begin the complicated and lengthy process which eventually results in the microscopic slides presented to the histopathologist. It would be in the interests of all involved if surgeon, nurse, laboratory technician and pathologist met regularly to discuss the whole chain of events because the quality of the ultimate product depends on the way they interact. Perhaps if medical, nursing and laboratory staff were taught this before qualification many of these problems would not arise.

Handling surgical specimens

In an ideal world all surgical specimens would be delivered *directly* to the laboratory (preferably situated in the neighbourhood of the operating room) where they can be observed in the fresh state by both the surgeon and the pathologist. This is seldom practicable and it is also often unnecessary. Because pathologists have the main responsibility for the preparation and fixation of surgical specimens in formaldehyde solution in such a way that the anatomy is preserved and gross lesions clearly demonstrated, it can be argued that they should receive all specimens in the laboratory fresh and untouched by operating room staff. In some instances, and particularly when the surgical anatomy is complex or the surgeon has some special point to make, it may be desirable for him to open and prepare the specimen either in the operating room or the laboratory. Either way, these problems must be solved by mutual agreement. What must be avoided is that state of affairs, unfortunately all too common, in which specimens are partially examined and fixed in the operating room and then received in the laboratory in such a distorted and decolourized state that for the pathologist the surgical anatomy and pathology are largely obscured.

Careful preparation of major surgical specimens, whether by surgeon or pathologist, is essential for colour as well as for black and white photography. Colour photography is ideal but the introduction of Polaroid photography has made it easy and cheap for *all* well prepared surgical specimens to be photographed in black and white. Prints can be issued as a component of the final report by the pathologist. They are a better and more permanent record of the gross appearances than long and detailed macroscopic descriptions, although this is not to deny the value of descriptive morbid anatomy which is a skill all surgeons and pathologists should assiduously cultivate. Black and white photographs of well-prepared surgical specimens can usefully be duplicated for additional reports to attending physicians and family doctors. Moreover, the polaroid method includes a negative which can be used for making lantern slides for teaching purposes and can be stored for use in research and publication. Colour photography has obvious value for teaching purposes.

It is opportune at this point to return again to the issue of filling in forms. It is quite insufficient to label an operation specimen as 'breast', 'parotid', 'colon' or 'kidney'. Detail, which need not be lengthy, is required which informs the pathologist of the anatomical extent of the operation specimen and identifies, with thread markers, such anatomical or other features which may have special importance in the surgical pathology. Examples which come to mind are limits of surgical excision, the position of the axillary gland dissection in a mastectomy specimen, the renal vein in a removed kidney and the point of ligature of the main blood supply in a colon resection. Diagrams illustrating these points can be especially valuable. The surgeon asks a question on the form. The pathologist answers this and also gives other information or opinions that he may derive from his examination. Commonly, where there is a lump the question is, what is this lump? But there may be many other questions such as, are the axillary lymph nodes invaded?

A careful description of the morbid anatomy of a surgical specimen is a discipline which should be cultivated by every surgeon and pathologist. This is not achieved without knowledge of the anatomy, and particularly the surgical anatomy, of the part. It is by education and experience that we learn to concentrate on those features which have greatest clinical importance. Careful morbid anatomical observation is also essential in the selection of blocks of tissue for microscopic examination which are most likely to reveal the necessary detail for microscopic diagnosis. The selection of appropriate blocks of tissue is no random decision but is based on knowledge and experience of the pathology.

This section began with a plea for a more idealistic approach to the methodology of handling surgical specimens. Regrettably the practice in most hospital laboratories falls far short of this ideal. All too often specimens are received fixed in such a way that the morbid anatomy is obscured and part of the specimen (e.g. the inside of an unopened stomach) has not had sufficient access to the fixative and the tissues are autolysed. The practice of stuffing specimens into bottles of inadequate capacity so that the fixative overflows is still deplorably common. Sometimes specimens are cut by the surgeon and then fixed, even further obscuring the detail of the pathology.

Technical methods in histopathology

Buffered 10 per cent formaldehyde (formalin) solution is the most widely used fixative for biopsies and excision specimens. No fixative will be wholly effective unless it is fresh and used in sufficient volume. Containers should be of sufficient size to accommodate a specimen easily and large resections, such as gastrectomies, colectomies and pneumonectomies, need to be floated in large tanks of formaldehyde. These can be sited only in the laboratory as strict safety regulations on their use must be monitored by trained technical staff.

Surgeons should appreciate the considerable skill involved in processing tissues for microscopical examination. Although great improvements are being made in processing and staining machines, the histology technician remains very much a craftsman on whom the pathologist is dependent. The quality of his product directly influences the ability of the pathologist to make an accurate and confident diagnosis. There are many variables in tissue processing, embedding and sectioning which have to be adjusted for the type, size and consistency of the tissues received. The successful operation of a microtome for cutting even undistorted wax-embedded sections requires long training and experience.

This book is not the place for a detailed description of technical skills, but surgeons in training can greatly benefit from visiting the laboratory and becoming acquainted with its scientific staff. They can provide information on fixing and handling of specimens and on the length of time which must elapse before a result may be available.

The relationship between pathologist and technician is essentially the same as that of surgeon and theatre nurse; all four are completely interdependent in the process of patient care.

The special technique of making frozen sections is used for certain immunocytochemical and histochemical techniques as well as for rapid diagnosis. Its place will be described in the appropriate chapters. It should be realized, however, that the procedure is open to misuse—it demands an instant and dogmatic diagnosis by a pathologist which may be undesirable, impossible or unwarranted. Just as operative surgery should not be undertaken precipitately, pathological diagnosis requires reflection and consideration. Whenever possible frozen section requests should be booked in advance, to ensure the availability of the pathologist and technical staff and should not be overused, especially in smaller laboratories, as the procedure inevitably interrupts routine processing and reporting.

It is important for surgeons to understand the advantages of cytological diagnosis, and its limitations. Exfoliated cells from body fluids (e.g. ascites, pleural effusions) or from mucosal surfaces (brush biopsies of stomach or bronchus) require special techniques of fixation and staining. Cytopathologists may be technician screeners, medical cytopathologists or histopathologists with an interest in cytology. Their diagnosis may be acted upon directly (as with aspiration breast cytology preceding mastectomy without frozen section) or in combination with biopsy. Cytology has the advantage over histology that a greater field is sampled but by corollary has the disadvantage that identification of a specific site may necessitate subsequent biopsy.

The special techniques of histochemistry, immunocytochemistry and electron microscopy are essential for the investigation of the growing number of different types of endocrine tumour of the gastrointestinal tract. Electron microscopy may allow the classification of connective tissue tumours and of apparently undifferentiated neoplasms. Familiarity with such techniques is unnecessary but knowledge of their existence is surgically useful, so that tissue may be provided in suitable cases.

Tissues for research

There is a growing practice among those engaged in research of soliciting pieces of fresh tissue from surgical specimens before the pathologist has been consulted. This is not only discourteous to the pathologist but can seriously impair his ability to give an accurate report. For his part, the pathologist should be as cooperative as possible in making himself available to supervise the provision of fresh tissue and seeing that adequate histology is taken of the removed portion.

Writing a histopathology report

A properly constructed histopathological report should first include, preferably with accompanying black and white photographs, a gross description of the anatomy of the specimen with measurements and detail of the position, size and appearances of any pathology relative to the normal parts. This is followed by a section on microscopic features. Sometimes the diagnosis is obvious from the gross examination alone, but the microscopic features still have importance in the detection of detail which may be important in, for example, future surgical management and prognosis. In the absence of photographic documentation line drawings can be a useful way of communicating information. Long, highly descriptive pathological reports have the reputation of being the least valuable to surgeons but pathologists require proper training and experience in order to achieve relevance and brevity. Reports written by juniors in training should be edited (and if necessary rewritten) by their seniors to ensure that the final report is accurate, authoritative and brief.

The histological grading and staging of cancer has particular importance for the surgeon and he should communicate his requirements on the request form. Grading and staging have influence on choice of treatment, whether by surgery, radiotherapy, chemotherapy or a combination of such therapies. They are also important in the long-term management and prognosis of cancer patients. The individual pathologist may not have had sufficient experience of staging and grading of a particular cancer in which case it is the responsibility of the surgeon to make his requirements absolutely clear.

Before finishing this section, and writing as a pathologist, it is my experience that surgeons appreciate accurate and relevant surgical pathology reports accompanied by photographs of the pathology they have removed. This is not necessarily because of any 'trophy hunting' satisfaction which they may derive from having successfully performed a difficult surgical procedure, but rather the need to document the results of their efforts in such a way as to communicate them to attending physicians and family doctors, further their skill by studying the result of their work and last, but not least, to use reports for the education of students, both undergraduate and postgraduate.

Further comments on communication

Increasing work-load, the introduction of new laboratory techniques and specialization within histopathology are current trends which are making it increasingly difficult for pathologists to leave their laboratories and spend time in the clinical arena. Add to this the natural pre-occupation of the surgeon with bedside problems and operating room techniques and there is a real danger that communication between surgeon and pathologist will become relegated to little more than a postal service from the laboratory. This is bad practice into which it is easy to slide unless effort is put into personal two-way contact. How are we to achieve this?

Biopsy reports must be read as expressions of opinion based on knowledge and experience of appearances seen under the microscope. These opinions are essentially *subjective and interpretative*, unlike the objective reports given, for example, in chemical pathology and haematology. Microscopic diagnosis is a discipline acquired by long experience of pattern recognition; the more experienced the histopathologist the greater is his capacity to 'read' the meaning of histological and cytological changes in the context of particular clinical situations. It is possible to give a confident and positive diagnosis in many instances; in others this is more difficult and then equivocating expressions such as 'compatible with' or 'consistent with' are commonly used. Specialization within histopathology is rapidly advancing and there is an increasing range of clinical situations in which such a specialist opinion should be sought in the interests of patient care. Surgeons must learn to understand the limits of histopathological diagnosis and interpretation. Yet the pathologist is often in a position to give useful negative reports just by saying that the appearances are not consistent with any one of a number of options put to him by his clinical colleagues. Personal consultation and discussion can often clarify a clinical problem in ways which the written report cannot hope to achieve.

Regular visits by the surgeon to the histopathologist and his technical staff should be matched by the presence of the pathologist at the bedside or in the operating room where he can use his knowledge of disease in the context of the whole clinical situation. He is also, after all, qualified to examine patients and should avoid losing his clinical skills, acquired during many years of training. For this reason, among others, histopathology can never be practised successfully by non-medical scientists. It is essentially a clinical discipline.

Of course, there is always the telephone but this has its disadvantages whether they be the frustration of the "engaged" tone or difficulties and delays in contacting the appropriate person. Communication is greatly enhanced by regular meetings at which the special problems of the week or month can be discussed in depth. These are not only a valuable aid to patient care, but are important for teaching and research. Improved communication within hospitals is a neglected subject which deserves more attention and capital investment because the technology is available whereby instant communication can be achieved. So far, such methods have been restricted to contact, independent of the telephone system, between operating room and laboratory, but there is no reason why modern communications systems, even including television, could not be installed between the out-patient clinic, the hospital wards and the laboratory. This costs money but would be a considerable advance in making the team approach to patient care more of a reality.

Value of a pathology museum

"Pots" are still important, although for ease of storage and ready availability surgical or autopsy specimens sealed in plastic bags can be valuable for teaching purposes. However, these do not have the lasting qualities of "pots". A comprehensive museum of specimens offers the student of surgical pathology the opportunity not only to observe disease but to correlate the appearances with those seen in the living patient, whether at the bedside, the operating room or during an endoscopic examination. But there is a method in reading pots which must be followed closely and methodically if the maximum benefit is to be gained from the experience.

The first and the most essential observation is recognition of the anatomy of the part displayed in the "pot". An illustrated text-book of anatomy will help the observer to recognize detail which may be vital to full understanding of the pathological changes. Secondly, the student has to learn how to describe, both by word of mouth and in writing, those changes which depart from the norm. This is a difficult and time-consuming discipline which can be learnt only by reference to one or more illustrated text-books of morbid anatomy while observing the specimen. Thirdly, the observer has to understand the significance of the morbid anatomical changes in terms of the history of the patient's disease, including clinical signs and symptoms, surgical treatment and prognosis. The only way to achieve this is again by "reading up the pot" with the aid of text-books of surgery and medicine. In most museums the description of the specimen is too brief but it does act as a guide for more detailed study of a particular specimen. Thus the study of "pots" can only be really fruitful in conjunction with the reading of appropriate books. Describing a 'pot' to an examiner must be based on this method of study.

Observing a specimen in a 'pot' is like looking at part of a patient in the same way that we study X-rays. If it is examined in the way described above, not only is it possible to identify the disease with the naked-eye but also to say how the pathologist can help with the care of the patient.

The purpose of this book is to define a clinical situation in each chapter and show how knowledge of the histopathology of disease helps to establish the diagnosis, explain the signs and symptoms, and influence treatment and prognosis. The questions asked of the pathologist are formulated, and guidance given about the provision of appropriate material for study and the ways in which a pathologist's report influences the management of the patient.

The histopathologist may be regarded as a collector of information, including clinical, radiological or other laboratory data, which he integrates with his own observations; but he is also contributing evidence to the surgeons' collection of evidence who takes the ultimate decision and responsibility. The observations made by the histopathologist principally involve the discipline of pattern recognition of macroscopic and microscopic appearances, which are largely subjective, but can be objective (e.g. the dissection of all lymph nodes from a cancer operation specimen to count the numbers involved), aided by a variety of special techniques appropriate to the tissue under examination. The haematologist, microbiologist and chemical pathologist play their important parts, but this book is essentially about histopathology and its contribution to surgical practice.

1

The Breast

G J Hadfield and A Levene

Introduction

The methods of arriving at a diagnosis have already been described generally in the Introduction. In this chapter we have tried to classify the clinical circumstances in which patients with breast disease present to a surgeon, and to correlate these clinical entities with the underlying surgical pathology. Many of these modes of presentation are a paraphrase of the patient's own words or a clinical description. They therefore do not absolutely fit with the pathological appearances and so necessitate overlap and cross referencing. These clinical entities are as follows and will be discussed in this order: A breast lump, carcinoma of the breast, lumps that can be mistaken for cancer, breast lumps other than carcinoma, papillary lesions of the breast, the large breast, breast augmentation, pain in the breast and diseases of the nipple and skin of the breast.

A breast lump

Clinical examination

In the clinic

This produces a working or clinical diagnosis which is finalized by pathological examination. It is our practice to perform a simple needle puncture and aspiration of all breast lumps. This differentiates solid lumps from cysts and at the same time provides material for cytological examination on the fluid obtained. At the first visit a Tru-cut needle biopsy is performed on all discrete solid lumps. This can give the surgeon and his patient a pre-operative diagnosis and a chance to discuss and plan the form of treatment. To perform a Tru-cut biopsy requires operative skill. At least two samples should be obtained from different sites in the tumour mass and it must be remembered that while a positive gives a tissue diagnosis, a negative has no significance.

Needle biopsy This has two connotations—obtaining thin worm-like cores of tissue by, for example, the Tru-cut method, or fine needle aspiration in which detachable cells are sucked out. The former is a small biopsy and is processed as such to produce sections. The latter serves to obtain a cytological specimen. The second technique is certainly an inferior diagnostic method, the former is only inferior to open biopsy in the information yielded 1. because of the disadvantages inherent in all biopsies when the surgeon does not see or handle the tissue; and 2. the inevitably more limited information from the smaller tissue volume available for study. The terms suspicious, suggestive of, and strongly suggestive of have no place in a tissue biopsy report, but are commonplace in a cytology report. Depending on the surgeon's approach to management of the various sorts of breast cancers, he may be content or not with the laconic statement "carcinoma cells present" or even "malignant cells present". This is usually the most that can be obtained from the study of a fine needle aspirate. From the Tru-cut biopsy we should be able to distinguish carcinoma from sarcoma, primary tumour from metastasis, and perhaps three or four different sorts of breast carcinoma. The Tru-cut method is no way of distinguishing innocent from malignant papillary changes and sclerosing adenosis from similar looking carcinoma, for in both these instances an *architectural* dimension is to be assessed and the most generous biopsy material available should be provided. One valuable use of Tru-cut procedure is in studying the effect of treatment, usually radiotherapy, on the carcinoma left *in situ*. The lump may not have resolved after radiotherapy and a Tru-cut biopsy is an elegant method of demonstrating that it is either a tumour graveyard or that it contains effete or actively growing cells. The tissue column is quite adequate for the histochemical and immunochemical studies of the research worker.

Needle biopsies stick to the rubber washer lining the cap of a universal container. To prevent this the specimen should either be shaken in the fixative, which should *not* be more than an inch from the mouth of the container, or placed on a card which must be submerged in the fluid.

In hospital excisional biopsy and frozen section of a breast lump

This was formerly the main method of making a tissue diagnosis when the commonest method of management of carcinoma was total mastectomy and has, in the practice of some surgeons, had some of its role taken over by Tru-cut biopsy which does not involve an operation and can be done at the patient's first visit. Others prefer to use the excision and frozen section method for their patients (*see* Fig. 1.1).
Lump excision and pathological examination is a valuable method when Tru-cut biopsy fails or is inapplicable to the lesion. A pathologist may not be able to give an instant diagnosis at frozen section and a rapid paraffin section may be needed for the purpose of definitive surgery. Indeed, some would argue that with the increased use of needle biopsy, the use and value of frozen section in these patients is diminished.

Frozen section This is only valuable when it answers the question whether or not the surgeon should proceed to further adequate local surgery, otherwise, local excision and the result of paraffin sections must be awaited. Generally speaking the indications for frozen section are: 1. to ascertain that a piece of tissue selected for study is indeed relevant to the clinical diagnosis and is not neighbouring tissue of a similar consistency, e.g. in the case of a small lump in the breast and occasionally in the investigation of a mammographic abnormality; and 2. as a diagnostic procedure on a swelling when the surgeon considers that for certain malignancies a definitive radical procedure should be carried out immediately. The most important use of rapid cryostat section technique should be as a guide to some major surgery, or abstention from it. Therefore it has little place in the management of pigmented cutaneous lesions suspected of being melanoma, when assessment of type and depth of invasion may modify management.

Where the differential diagnosis in paraffin section is likely to be difficult, it is highly inadvisable to subject the tissue preliminary to study as cryostat section material. Should this be done there may be bad consequences: 1. the wrong diagnosis; 2. the destruction of a biopsy, or the best

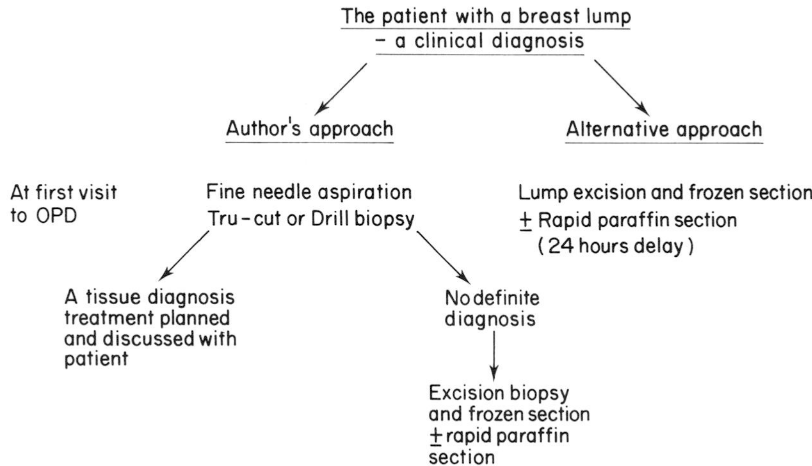

Fig. 1.1 Methods of tissue diagnosis.

part of it, by trimming away on a freezing microtome leaving inadequate material for paraffin processing; 3. the degree of distortion permanently induced in the tissue by the freezing process may be critical when the cytology of the paraffin section comes to be assessed.

A 100 per cent correlation between the results of cryostat section and paraffin section studies on the fixed material should not be expected beyond *no* overdiagnosis of carcinoma. Papillary intraduct and intracystic tumours are most safely diagnosed as innocent or malignant on paraffin section. If suspected, the tissue should not be sent for frozen section. A symptomatic duct papilloma may be tiny and is best discovered, not by slitting up the duct system with fine scissors which may dislodge or destroy the object of the search, but by multiple parallel slicing through the fixed specimen.

The distinction of papillary carcinoma from the common duct papilloma may be among the more difficult in pathology and require considerable judgement and experience from the microscopist. It is usually simple and consists of demonstrating a persistent myoepithelial layer, that is two cell types are present, but papilloma and intraduct papillary carcinoma share many features, and may co-exist in the same specimen. To quote McDivitt, Stewart and Berg, "It must be acknowledged that there is a zone of altered cell growth where the diagnosis of carcinoma versus atypical papillomatosis is a question of occult distinction and must be accepted or rejected on the grounds of faith, or lack of it, in the pathologist."

2. *The Second Stage* in the diagnosis is the examination of the pathology of the fresh specimen.
3. *The Third Stage* is when the definitive pathological report is available for making a diagnosis and formulating a plan of management.

The pathologist first examines and cuts up the lump to decide his strategy on how best to deal with it. For example, to swab what appears to be a suppurative lesion, select for electron microscopic study tissue from an uncommon lesion, or retain a portion for oestrogen assay.

Handling and presentation The handling and presentation of a specimen are of vital importance to the pathologist. Apart from the name and age of the patient, the sex must be stated. The symptomatology must be outlined, e.g. the relationship to menstrual cycle, pregnancy, rapidity of onset and so on. No relevant past history should be omitted, for example "removal of mole on leg". In the last example it should be remembered that an achromic melanoma will simulate a polygonal cell carcinoma of the breast and in a pigmented metastasis the pigment may go unnoticed in haemorrhage within the tumour. If the lump is an obvious clinical carcinoma the request for oestrogen assay should be included (when the specimen is sent fresh).

It is always safe to send the specimen fresh to the pathologist, with an indication from the surgeon of any noteworthy feature along the lines of "I am concerned about ... marked with a black silk suture". Otherwise, one clean cut should be made through the specimen (with a scalpel for a small specimen, larger ones demand an amputation knife) then *submerge* it in at least five times its volume of formalin and in a container in which it may move freely. A specimen rammed into a jar with inadequate fixative will steadily undergo autolysis, thus preventing critical examination of cytological detail.

Special Procedures When a specimen needs to be examined fresh, but delay is inevitable, it may be refrigerated for up to 12 hours before final study.

The fresh gross specimen often alerts the pathologist to the correct diagnosis because of a characteristic appearance. The following brief descriptions are no more than a guide to essentials.

The "lesion" may be normal mammary tissue. This varies in appearance with the type of breast containing more or less adipose tissue, and with the age of the subject. The surgeon and the pathologist must be familiar with the wide variation manifested naked eye. The pathologist must be scrupulous in his opinion. If the excised tissue appears to be normal or show no significant abnormality this should be clearly stated. To credit an occasional slightly dilated duct or enlarged mammary lobule with being the pathological basis of the clinical presentation is misleading. It is a disservice to both patient and surgeon to find *some* abnormality always.

An unequivocal segmental induration of the breast may on excision have the appearances of a normal mammary gland. Presumably its palpability was the result of a disturbed tissue tension. It is in these cases that the surgeon and pathologist excise the fresh specimen in vain for a discrete lump. The excised breast may contain unduly prominent and large pale tan-coloured nodules—lobular hyperplasia, puckered foci with microcystic change—sclerosing adenosis, multiple small cysts in a hard area of breast which is ill-defined—florid cystic mastopathy, or combinations of these changes. Multiple cysts with soft greenish-yellow contents may be found in cystic disease as well as in duct ectasia. Small bright yellow areas, xanthomatous foci, are due to the aggregation of lipophages. When the pathology is that of malignancy we must consider various types of carcinoma together with other malignant mammary tumours.

Throughout this chapter the naked eye appearance has been described under each entity. Many lesions like an obvious florid breast cancer have characteristic and highly suggestive appearances. There are so many chances of mistakes by false negatives and positives, that we consider that a histopathological opinion is mandatory, whether this is based on lump excision and frozen section, rapid paraffin section or needle biopsy of a suspicious lump. All the restrictions of a sampling biopsy discussed elsewhere in this chapter are relevant to a negative or positive decision.

Carcinoma of the breast

Appearance

Tubular adenocarcinoma of the breast is small and scirrhous and microscopically consists of gaping, somewhat angulated tubules scattered in a fibroblastic stroma. There is an association with the presence of psammoma bodies, amyloid in the stroma and the co-existence of other patterns of primary breast carcinoma. Though lymph node metastases may occur, death from tubular carcinoma is unlikely.

Sclerosing adenosis by contrast has a lobular architecture, the periphery of tubular carcinoma is infiltrating, with a loose reactive stroma compared with the hyaline of sclerosing adenosis and the presence of two layers in the tubules of the latter. *Medullary carcinoma* with lymphoid stroma is sharply defined, firm and tan-coloured. *Mucoid (colloid) carcinoma* is distinctly gelatinous, papillary carcinoma is warty on section, perhaps intracystic. Advanced intraductal carcinoma is the classical comedo carcinoma with worm-like yellowish threads expressable from its cut surface while its earlier phase when it exhibits cartwheel or cribriform epithelial patterns microscopically may be indistinguishable from benign epithelial proliferations. There are *no* gross features of *in situ* lobular carcinoma. The common poorly differentiated adeno- or polygonal cell carcinoma with more or less hyalinizing fibrous stroma (particularly in its middle) is a hard greyish ill-defined mass possibly with a stellate depressed configuration on section, gritty to the knife and speckled with yellow foci of elastosis (*not* of focal necrosis). Very like a mammary carcinoma naked eye is granular cell myoblastoma and the microscopic appearance with cells perhaps growing in columns in a densely collagenous stroma is another trap for the unwary. However, the "pure" type of carcinoma, so useful for clinical analysis is the exception.

The rare carcinomas of the breast

Sweat gland carcinoma, adenoid cystic carcinoma and metaplastic varieties such as squamous (in whole or in part), spindle cell and others lack characteristic naked eye appearances. Adenoid cystic carcinoma does not metastasize to axillary lymph nodes. The growth pattern is sometimes seen in parts of an otherwise intraduct and infiltrating carcinoma. It occurs preferentially in the region of the nipple and areolar. Inflammatory carcinoma is of high grade malignancy. Biopsy, the only material the pathologist ever sees, reveals oedema, fibrin deposition and an inflammatory exudate. The superficial capillaries and the lymphatics are plugged by tumour cells. The histological appearances merely serve to confirm the clinical impression of this "erysipeloid" variant of breast cancer.

The various sarcomas in so far as any have naked eye characteristics in their more usual sites of presentation in the limbs or skeleton, retain these when they occur in the breast; liposarcoma variants being the best recognized though among the least common of the sarcomas of the breast.

Secondary deposits from remote sites are spherical usually. The commonest source of metastases is mammary carcinoma, the deposits varying in appearance but commonly maintaining the naked eye appearances of primary carcinoma. Metastatic melanoma is not always pigmented. Other metastases may carry their hallmarks with them, for example haemorrhagic appearances in chorion-carcinoma.

Management

Staging

What does staging mean and why is it done? All forms of staging depend on a code of initials and numbers based on the clinical and pathological assessment of where the cancer is and what it involves locally, and generally how extensive it is.

After answering these questions treatment can be planned, as all treatment is based on the stage of the disease.

Furthermore, staging is essential in discussing the patient's management by the therapeutic team of clinician and pathologist, at all stages and for follow-up and evaluation of various forms of treatment and their comparative results.

Clinical classification

The surgeon, in trying to treat breast cancer, recognizes three main entities:

1. Local disease, which may be clinically definable or a microfocus demonstrable on mammography, both confirmed by histological examination.
2. When the disease is no longer locally confined.
3. Metastatic disease with treated or untreated local disease.

This is the basis of the tumour, node and metastases, T N and M classification which is described as follows:

*T*umour, *N*odes, *M*etastases

The TNM system of stage classification of mammary carcinoma is, of course, based on the observation that in general the bigger the tumour and the greater the extent of its spread at the time of presentation, the worse the prognosis. This pre-treatment classification is given in Table 1.1.

Mammary carcinoma is associated with a variety of physical signs depending on its type, size and growth rate. Several histological varieties of infiltrating carcinoma are described, but mixed growth patterns are common, and sharp distinction for the purpose of statistical study of the differential effects of treatment is inherently impossible. What follows is a series of generalizations about infiltrating carcinoma.

Well-defined tumours grossly, corresponding to a pushing margin microscopically, are always a minority in any series, carry a relatively good prognosis and are the three distinctive histological patterns of medullary carcinoma with lymphoid sarcoma, colloid (mucoid) carcinoma and intracystic papillary carcinoma.

Ill-defined tumours grossly and microscopically form the remainder, the 90 per cent of breast carcinomas. The breast tumour then freshly cut has a depressed greyish white appearance in which are yellow specks of fibro-elastosis and radiating fibrous strands deforming the surrounding parenchyma is the type.

Histological grading

A great number of methods have been tried to link histological grading with prognosis and in some cases, treatment. Present opinion does not support the absolute claims once made.

Histological tumour grading was founded primarily on the degree of cell differentiation and growth activity as shown by mitosis. Doubtless, this is significant but it is now felt that the state of the stroma, the presence of lymphoid aggregations to the tumour margin, and the histological picture of the rest of the breast are complementary in defining the high risk patients and tumour grade. When the histopathologist can combine this and

Table 1.1 Pre-treatment classification.

	Pre-invasive carcinoma (i.e. in situ) non-infiltrating intraductal or Paget's disease of the nipple with no demonstrable tumour.	
T 1	a tumour 2cm or less	
T 2	a tumour more than 2cm but less than 5cm	(a) Without fixation fascia/muscle (b) With fixation fascia/muscle
T 3		
T 4	Extension to chest wall/skin	(a) Chest wall (b) Skin oedema/infiltration or ulceration (c) Both
N 1	Mobile axillary	(a) Not considered metastatic (b) Considered metastatic (c) Both
N 2	Fixed axillary	
N 3	Supraclavicular/oedema arm	
M 0 or M 1	By site if relevant	

other indices in a single, simple, clinically usable system, then their contribution will be enhanced.

The aim of a classification of breast cancer must be to link the pathological and clinical data. Fresh clinico-pathological discoveries lead inevitably to discarding an old classification and creating a new one. Much of the impetus and classifications have been American in origin. Recently Azzopardi and his colleagues have re-examined the problem and classified primary breast carcinoma into the following groups:

1. Lobular carcinoma which may be *in situ* or invasive.
2. Duct carcinoma *in situ* or invasive, or of some special types.
3. Invasive carcinoma ductal or lobular.
4. Mixed intra-duct and intra-lobular growths in the same tumour mass.
5. Carcinoma in a pre-existing tumour, e.g. carcinoma in a fibroadenoma or cystosarcoma phylloides.
6. Carcinosarcoma.
7. Unclassified tumours; these are malignant tumours where the cancerous nature is in doubt or pseudo-tumours.

This classification is generally accepted.

Prognosis

All mammary carcinomas can prove fatal and there are two principal factors involved in prognosis: 1. The behaviour of the tumour related to its histological type and, 2. Medical neglect of the pre-invasive malignancy. The fate of the subject with *invasive mammary carcinoma* is usually decided at the time of clinical presentation, for it is apparent that many, perhaps a majority, have occult bloodstream spread at that time. *Good prognostic factors are:*

1. A small tumour.
2. Absence of lymph node metastases.
3. Favourable histological patterns (modified after Hutter).
   (a) medullary carcinoma with lymphoid stroma.
   (b) colloid (or gelatinous) carcinoma.
   (c) papillary intracystic carcinoma with 10 years survival of around 70 per cent.
   (d) tubular (well-differentiated) carcinoma, a very low mortality indeed, tending to zero.
4. Absence of lymphatic invasion, vascular invasion and necrosis in the primary tumour and good cytological differentiation. Because of the irreproducibility of grading systems, only the extreme groups—well-differentiated and poorly-differentiated—have useful predictive characteristics.

The stage of the disease when the patient presents is the decisive factor. From a consideration of the pathology it can be seen that the larger the tumour, the more likely it is to prove fixed to the chest wall, to ulcerate, to be associated with lymphatic blockade of the skin (peau d'orange), regional node metastases and bloodstream spread.

That sutures placed in the specimen may reliably be used to accurately divide axillary lymph nodes into various groups is too hopeful. There are limitations on what may reasonably be achieved in the examination of pathological specimens. It must not be expected that the division of mammary carcinoma into several types based on histogenesis is absolute, since in the same microscopic section three different *in situ* phenomena may be exhibited, e.g. cribriform intraduct, *in situ* lobular and tubular patterns. Carcinoma of the breast in children of either sex does not differ pathologically from that of an adult. Heteroptic mammary gland, e.g. in the vulva or axilla, is subject to the same disease as the orthotopic organ.

Hormone Receptors: their value and application A receptor protein which mediates the intracellular action of circulating oestrogen is present in all normal cells which require oestrogen for growth and function. This is also true for hormone-sensitive breast tumours. Assays have been developed and are available to measure this protein. The number of specific binding sites within the tumour freely available to oestradiol are measured. The specimen for this test is taken at once at operation from the breast tumour or metastasis if available, and put in a dry container and frozen. At no time must it be in contact with any medium or fixative, e.g. saline or formalin; it is transported in a cold container to the assay laboratory.

This test has the following uses and values:

1. *In initial prognosis* it has been shown that women with oestrogen receptor positive mammary tumour have a less chance of early recurrence and survive longer than the negative group.
2. *In metastatic disease* when the receptor status has been determined at the stage of

primary treatment or from available secondary material. Those who are receptor positive will respond to hormone therapy by addition or deprivation, while the receptor negative group will not and can therefore be saved unnecessary treatment. Initial treatment by cytotoxic agents for this last group would be appropriate.

3. *In reinforcing adequate primary treatment*, a view which has some support, the patient's tumour receptor status will help to choose the most appropriate treatment. The receptor positive group could be influenced by adjuvant hormone therapy and Tamoxifen therapy could be used. The hormone insensitive, i.e. the receptor negative group, could be influenced by cytotoxic therapy.

The crucial role of histological diagnosis

A full histological examination is the final arbiter in the diagnosis of any breast lesion. Treatment can not be logically or ethically planned in its absence, nor should it be undertaken until this information is available. The microscopic differential diagnoses are also inevitably concerned with malignancy and its differential diagnosis. Granular cell myoblastoma, an unencapsulated proliferation of polyhedral cells with voluminous, eosinophilic granular cytoplasm and rather small nuclei, simulates a diffuse carcinomatous infiltration and the appearance of burst ducts with epithelial clumps in an inflammatory response in which foam cells are present, may resemble a polygonal cell carcinoma with an inflammatory stroma. Papillary carcinoma and innocent papilloma, epitheliosis and cribriform carcinoma, sclerosing adenosis and tubular adenocarcinoma of the breast are other pairs of lesions to be carefully differentiated. Lesions simulating mammary carcinoma grossly and microscopically also include: 1. neural invasion in association with sclerosing adenosis, a totally benign condition and, 2. periductal or plasma cell mastitis. This lesion simulates late carcinoma clinically and shows no tendency to resolve spontaneously. Histologically, it consists of ducts filled with purulent-like material and dense periductal inflammation rich in plasma cells and with scattered giant cells. The duct lining is hyperplastic, simulating comedo carcinoma. 3. Indurative mastopathy in which a sclerotic stellate lesion with distorted ducts has a constantly found prominent elasticity; the clinical, radiological, gross and microscopic appearances simulate carcinoma.

Fibrocytic disease, fibroadenoma and carcinoma in women receiving oral contraceptive hormones exhibit no specific changes; the histological picture is the same.

Lymphosarcoma and the inflammatory variant of malignant fibrous histiocytoma have to be distinguished from simple reactive changes in the mammary gland and an infiltrating fibromatosis must not be overdiagnosed as a fibrosarcoma.

The problems of clinico-pathological correlation

In the primary lesion it is quite usual for multiple pathology to be present in the breast and within one biopsy. There are the commonly found benign proliferations: adenosis, sclerosing adenosis, epitheliosis, cyst formation with a variable amount of apocrine gland metaplasia, papillomatosis, which may be solitary or widespread. The malignant changes are nearly always the carcinomas which have been described grossly. It is the experience of all pathologists that there is a continuum of epithelial appearances from innocence through atypia of cellularity and architecture to debatable and unequivocal malignancy. This is true for other sites but nowhere is this illustrated better, with all the inherent accompanying clinical problems, than in the breast. Therefore, there are limitations to the certainty of light microscopy in diagnosis. It must be stressed that *in situ* carcinoma is a form of malignancy and should have appropriate management.

The correlation of physical signs, pathological findings and other examinations which show evidence of local or metastatic spread of the disease is collected from the spectrum of evidence which is available to the clinician when assessing the patient. Some of this may not be absolute, in others it may be erroneous.

The classical physical signs of breast cancer are mainly those of late disease, often of disseminated disease, where local treatment is only part, may not be a major one, or is even applicable in the patients' management. Local spread is evidenced clinically, but attachment to the skin progressing to ulceration, attachment to underlying muscles and other structures and infiltration of the breast substance. Inflammation, acute or chronic, will also produce skin attachment.

Lymphatic involvement of the breast substance is shown first by skin oedema over the tumour.

This can be demonstrated and measured by mammography and correlates significantly with clinical stage and size of the tumour, and the status of the lymph nodes. It is available before operation. Its later progress is shown by *peau d'orange* and *cancer en curasse*. Each are signs of advanced disease and indicate a poor prognosis.

Peau d'orange is composed of two parts. Firstly, tethering of the oedematous skin by Coopers ligaments which are attached to its undersurface, ramify throughout the breast substance and are attached to the deep fascia. They therefore limit oedema and form skin pitting over the oedematous area. Secondly, by bulging of the intervening untethered oedematous skin between the pits, again this change can be caused by both underlying neoplasia or inflammation.

Lymph nodes. There is unfortunately no good agreement between the clinical assessment of the status of axillary lymph nodes in a case of mammary tumour, and their histological appearances. Enlarged nodes may be swollen from simple reactive changes, and very large nodes, one or two centimetres across may result from age change, fatty infiltration of the node (see later under T M and N). Undoubtedly, the demonstration of secondary cancer in the draining nodes generally signifies a worsening of prognosis. The final arbiter of nodes spread is meticulous and complete histological examination.

Is there a premalignant mammary lesion of significance, one which on diagnosis demands action from the Clinician? In the neighbourhood of excised carcinoma is found a higher frequency of the more advanced grades of mammary dysplasias from which it is inferred that these changes are precursors of carcinoma. Further, investigators from the Memorial Hospital in New York distinguished a group of "atypical hyperplasia", another way of expressing non-invasive epithelial findings similar to non-invasive carcinoma. In other words, where the spectrum of non-invasive epithelial proliferation approaches *in situ* carcinoma, a proportion of them are unrecognizable precancer, a proportion of them will, by virtue ot the diagnostic procedure, have undergone prophylactic surgery, and a proportion are either not precancer, or do not manifest their potential.

Cystosarcoma phylloides is a large enucleable fleshy cystic tumour and in its grossest form perhaps associated with ischaemic necrosis of the overlying skin. The name of the tumour was given by Muller in 1838 and refers to a fibroadenoma with a periductal hypercellular stroma and is a clinico-pathological spectrum, the benign nonrecurring forms having a stroma lacking significant numbers of mitoses (per high power field) and a sharply defined periphery; the malignant ones by contrast having a sarcomatous stroma, an infiltrating edge, a tendency to recur locally and metastases by the bloodstream. The malignant tumour is a stromal fibrosarcoma which does not metastasize to lymph nodes in more than 10 per cent of the cases. The sarcomatous forms have no specific naked eye appearances and may not be detectable on a random frozen section, therefore all fibroadenomas with a hypercellular stroma should be examined via several (10) large tissue blocks, since evidence of malignancy may have a restricted distribution.

Carcinoma arising in a fibroadenoma is an unrelated entity, and a chance finding; Hutter calls it an "early carcinoma".

Fat necrosis. Early on there may be a bruised appearance in the neighbourhood of the hard ill-defined lump, bisection of which reveals a flat yellow matt surface with small oil-containing cysts. Histologically, some phase of fat necrosis is present, but always glassy change in the cytoplasm of the fat cells, foamy macrophages and inflammatory cells are visible. The final stage is a scar in the breast.

Multiple pathology in the breast. In the past, breast pathology has been focused on the lump and the rest of the breast largely ignored. Recent studies on the whole mastectomy specimen have yielded much information on the multicentricity of breast cancer and the nature and incidence of associated benign diseases in the same breast.

In a series described by Hughes and Forbes, they state that all their specimens had some degree of ductal epitheliosis. Three quarters showed intraduct carcinoma or marked atypia. A further frank invasive focus of cancer of 0.5 cm or less in diameter was found in 50 per cent of those breasts examined. Duct ectasia, whose age incidence is similar to breast cancer, is commonly seen as are papillary lesions of the major and minor ducts. Benign breast tumours are often demonstrated as a coincidental finding.

The following facts about pre-invasive malignancy are essential in relation to management:

1. Large section and multiple block histological techniques and mammographic studies have revealed the frequency of multicentric, *in*

situ carcinoma, which is commoner than finding invasive tumours.

2. In the case of *in situ* lobular but no intraductal carcinoma bilaterality is frequent.
3. Consequently, there is a dilemma in the management of the second breast in the case of finding *in situ* lobular carcinoma. Thoughtful studies on this contraversial topic are those of Rosen *et al*. *In situ carcinoma of the breast is carcinoma at its most curable phase and is the presenting lesion of multicentric disease*.

There is no universally agreed answer to the question "how do you treat an equivocal breast lesion?" The choice lies finally between lumpectomy and regular surveillance through sector mastectomy preserving the breast to local mastectomy. No general rules can be made and each case should be managed after consultation between the surgeon and pathologist.

This problem has been discussed elsewhere in this chapter under Papillary Breast Lesions and Equivocal Breast Lumps. Our policy is that unless a diagnosis of malignancy can be given, local surgery with follow-up is advised. The pathogenesis and treatment of Paget's disease is well-summarized by Paone and Baker. Survival rates of patients with Paget's disease *and a palpable breast mass* are similar to those of patients with infiltrating duct carcinoma, but none of the patients with Paget's disease with no evidence of a breast mass developed recurrent carcinoma.

Mastectomy—late effects The best known, and hitherto the most dreaded sequela is the lymphangiosarcoma of the lymphoedematous upper extremity. Biopsy of the visible nodules reveals the quite unspectacular appearances of the lymphangiosarcoma which may be confused by those unfamiliar with the entity with chronic inflammation and some angiectasia.

Irradiation There is nearly always tumour regression, frequently total disappearance leaving a stellate scirrhous focus lacking tumour cells. More or less tumour regression is seen in the axillary metastases. The nodes are fewer in number than in a conventional radical mastectomy specimen and difficult to dissect from the fibrotic axillary tissues. Many years, perhaps decades later a variety of sarcomas are reported in the irradiated fields whether the breast is removed or not. Soft-tissue sarcomas include fibrosarcoma and malignant fibrous histocytoma, in the bones (scapula, clavicle and ribs) osteosarcoma, chondroma and fibrosarcoma, and in the skin, squamous cell carcinoma.

The impalpable tumour As a consequence of breast-screening projects the impalpable tumour is now a clinical entity. Only about 20 per cent of these lesions are proven cancers on histological examination. The pathology is either that of an established small carcinoma or a focus of pre-invasive carcinoma and does not differ from that found in palpable lesions. There is an appreciable risk of axillary nodal metastasis with an incidence of 20–30 per cent. The greatest benefit of mammography could be the discovery of the pre-invasive carcinoma. For the pathologist to identify the suspicious area markers of dyes and radio-opaque materials under X-ray control or X-rays of the specimen on a metal grid will define the area of the tumour for examination.

Breast lumps that can be mistaken for cancer These can be listed and discussed as follows:

(a) *An antibioma*. This is a consequence of incorrect treatment of a breast abscess (see later under the tender red breast) giving a chronic, hard, tender swelling with redness of the overlying skin. Treatment is directed to stopping antibiotic therapy and draining abscesses. The histological picture shows mature granulation tissue.

(b) *Fat necrosis*. Characteristically, this presents as a solitary hard lump in the breast with a history of trauma. However, the trauma history may be indefinite or replaced by evidence of injection into the breast.

(c) *Confluent periductal mastitis*. See under tender red breast and nipple discharges from duct ectasia.

(d) *Sclerosing adenosis*. This condition mimics many of the signs of carcinoma and only histological examination will differentiate it.

(e) *Huge benign tumours*. In this group it is often the patient's self-diagnosis of cancer, but malignancy may be present in the cystosarcoma phylloides group (see before, also see under fibroadenoma).

(f) The pathologist may be alerted to the possibility of *metastatic carcinoma* or other malignancy by the clinical summary on the pathology request form, e.g. in the case of a patient previously treated for ovarian carcinoma who presents with an adenocarcinoma *in* the breast.

(g) *Granular cell myoblastoma* (described elsewhere).

(h) *Diseases of the chest wall and intrathoracic lesions mimicking breast lumps*. In this connection one thinks of normal prominent ribs on self-examination and tuberculosis of the chest wall or of intrathoracic origin.

Breast lumps other than carcinoma

Breast cyst

There are many causes of this condition and the classification given here gives the clinical variations seen in a breast clinic, such as our own in the UK; variations clearly occur with geographic and pathological considerations. The cysts are diagnosed and treated by aspiration at first examination in the Clinic and unless complicated there will be no histopathology.

(a) *A simple cyst.* A single cyst in a granular, nodular, or clinically normal breast. The age range is from 15 to 70 with the majority occurring at 40 years. These occur with equal frequency with either breast, but are more common in the upper and outer quadrant. They are often cured by aspiration. The average aspirate is between 3–10 ml of watery greenish fluid. In a patient treated and cured by aspiration there is a 40 per cent chance of a further cyst occurring in that or the opposite breast during the following 15 years. Exfoliative cytology on the cyst contents is occasionally helpful. Some small cysts like the small multiple blue domed cysts regress spontaneously. All are alleged by the patient to change in size with menstruation. Local excision is advised when the cyst recurs on follow-up after six weeks following aspiration, when the aspiration is blood-stained suggesting an associated tumour, when a lump persists after aspiration as in co-incident disease or when there is a dry tap when a solid tumour is suspected.

(b) *Cystic carcinoma.* The fluid from the cyst is often, but not inevitably, blood-stained. Cytological examination of the aspirate may be positive and a lump thickening remains in the breast after aspiration.

(c) *Carcinoma in a breast in which there is also a cyst.* The clinical and pathological picture here is of two separate diseases.

(d) *Multiple, small, blue-domed cysts in a nodular breast.* These are often very small and tend to regress spontaneously.

(e) *Cysts associated with major duct systems of the breast.* These are usually retention cysts and must be differentiated from breast tumours, papillary tumours of the major ducts and periductal mastitis affecting a single or group of major ducts.

Histologically, breast cysts are spherical, fluid containing and of varied pathology. The commonest, single or multiple, are part of the cystic mastopathy group of mammary lumps and are thought to result from imperfect involutionary changes following the cyclical monthly proliferation of the terminal duct system. The lining varies but is a single layer of epithelium, perhaps backed by myoepithelium. Apocrine metaplasia (pink cell change) is common. A mixture of cysts varying in sizes and types of lining cells, lobular hyperplasia, intraductal distention by innocent proliferations of solid, cribriform or papillary type; all may be suggested by the naked eye appearances and their pleomorphic character readily confirmed by cryostat section. True carcinomatous change occurring in the wall of a breast cyst has the same histological appearances of any other breast cancer.

Fibroadenoma

Characteristically, a single mobile large or small lump in an otherwise normal breast which is non-malignant and treated by local removal. Pathologically they are described as: Pericanalicular, intracanalicular and papillary—the least common of the three. Giant fibroadenoma is a clinical description of size and will be discussed with cystosarcoma phylloides under the large breast.

Some fibroadenomas can be shelled out "breast mice" while others merge gently into the surrounding breast substance. The distinction of the two common patterns is not absolute, mixtures are frequent and all are benign. Breast cancer in fibroadenoma connotes two entirely distinct entities: first, carcinoma *in situ*, infiltrating with or without involvement of the contiguous breast and, secondly, a fibrosarcoma which, in this context is always called cystosarcoma phylloides. The first is not a clinical entity because of its total lack of features to distinguish it from a fibroadenoma, and is diagnosed only microscopically. The second is described earlier in this chapter.

Mesenchymal tumours, benign or malignant

The "mesenchymal" tumours form a miscellaneous group, which except for lipoma are not diagnosable clinically. Among them are seen liposarcoma, stromal sarcoma, lymphosarcoma, myelocytoma (chloroma), chondro- and osteosarcoma, and malignant fibrous histiocytoma, the differential diagnosis of the last being inflammatory conditions, acute or chronic, or inflammatory stroma associated with carcinoma. Critical assessment or paraffin sections of ostensibly inflammatory masses is always necessary. Angiosarcoma is a diagnosis which may be missed at biopsy for there is often preservation of lobular architecture and the well differentiated vascular neoplasia is unremarkable. Fibrosarcoma has a special relationship to cystosarcoma phylloides.

Papillary lesions of the breast

These may originate in the major duct system when they present as a para-areolar lump associated with a nipple discharge. Lesions originating from the minor ducts present as a palpable or radiologically demonstrable lump in the breast substance. Occasionally they are found by chance on examination of large breast substance. An associated nipple discharge is not common. The age range for each disease is as follows:

1. Single duct papillomata from 35 to 69 years.
2. Major duct hyperplasia from 20 to 40 years.
3. Papillomatosis of the breast substance from 17 to 45 years.

Duct papilloma

These occur in a single major duct; they are unifocal, said to possess no malignant potential but occasionally malignant and benign appearances can be seen in the same papilloma. They may present with a blood-stained or other type of nipple discharge with or without para-areolar swelling.

Papillary, cribriform and other intraductal or intracystic epithelial proliferations in the breast provide the most difficult region of differential diagnosis for the surgical pathologist. There is no single feature diagnostic of malignancy, rather a number of parameters to be considered.

Similarly, the sclerosing proliferations, papillary or simple glandular are distinguishable from papillary and tubular adenocarcinoma. Diagnosis is always easier when generous biopsy material, preferably the whole lesion, is obtainable. The following are the histological points taken into consideration:

1. The double layer characteristic of normal ductal epithelium is perpetuated in the fronds of benign papilloma.
2. Papillary carcinoma is frequently stratified with hyperchromatic monotonous nuclei. A double layer picture is absent.
3. Vascular cores to the stalks and a stroma are an important feature of innocence.

Papillomatosis of the ducts in the breast substance

A multifocal bilateral asymmetrical disease which may have no clinical presentation and is a chance finding on whole breast histological examination. Clinically, it presents as solitary, multiple and often recurrent lumps in one or both breasts in young men. Exogenous hormonal influences are suspected as the disease can disappear when these are removed. An initial tissue diagnosis with careful long follow-up including needle biopsy of other lumps is obligatory.

Some consider these to be unstable breasts and that it is a possible precancerous condition.

Two varieties of *in situ* carcinoma of the breast are recognized, intraduct or comedo, or cribriform pattern with or without involvement of lobules and *in situ* lobular carcinoma, and mixtures of the two are quite common. Interestingly, the intraduct carcinoma presents clinically or at screening, the *in situ* lobular is for all practical purposes a chance finding in association with some other diffuse mastopathy. Intraduct carcinoma treated by excisional biopsy alone is inevitably followed by local recurrence, in contrast with *in situ* lobular carcinoma.

Intraductal carcinoma is associated with the following:

(a) Discharge from the nipple in which carcinoma cells may be detectable.
(b) Paget's disease.
(c) Calcification, intraductal haemorrhage, periductal fibrosis and lymphocytic infiltration, multicentricity. When paraffin sections exclude infiltration, nodal metastasis is a great rarity.

The differential diagnoses in the gross do not correspond with those which present at microscopic level as a general rule. Whereas carcinoma may show some resemblance to fat necrosis grossly, there is no resemblance microscopically. A fibroadenoma with a very mucoid stroma may resemble a mucoid carcinoma grossly but not microscopically, and the same is true of the relationship of medullary carcinoma with lymphoid stroma and an inflammatory lymph node. However, a scirrhous carcinoma and sclerosing adenosis may be difficult to distinguish naked eye and microscopically, when the former has a well developed acinar pattern (see below).

The lumpy breast

Multiple breast lumps

This group has two clinical variations, the lumpy breast with large indefinite lumps and the granular breast. Both of these have a common pathology in cyclical changes, adenosis and fibrosis and drug- or-hormone induced changes. Granularity may be present on palpating normal breast tissue when breast tissue gets more prominent with age and when there is a loss of breast fat or when drug or hormone induced changes occur.

Biopsy may be helpful and normal breast tissue is rightly reported. An appreciation of the range in variations in the normal breast tissue at different ages needs to be appreciated both grossly and microscopically. Papillomatosis of the ducts in the breast substance described before also comes in this group. Occasionally the disease is asymmetrical or presents as a unilateral lumpy breast. The pathology of this lesion is the same as the above description.

Cystic mastopathy and other polymorphs, ill-defined mammary lesions

The synonyms for this group are legion. Forty years ago chronic mastitis was in vogue, now mammary dysplasia is favoured by some. From the surgeon's viewpoint the naked eye appearances embrace adenomatosis—brownish-pink nodular projections from the cut surface of the breast and an exaggeration of normal lobular architecture, papillomatosis, microcystic in character (epithelial hyperplasia perhaps cribriform or festooning in character with bland-looking small nuclei, apocrine gland "pink cell" metaplasia) and cyst formation.

Certainly allied to these changes are sclerosing mastopathies (sclerosing adenosis, sclerosing papillary proliferation) which have an entirely different significance because their naked eye and microscopic appearances simulate scirrhous carcinoma. The gross lesion is indurated, perhaps microcystic, and has a puckered appearance corresponding to a stellate centrally fibrotic appearance microscopically. The radiating fibrous bands merge peripherally with some or all of the varieties of cystic mastopathy. It is the central area which is problematic with its entrapped, perhaps distorted, epithelial structures. Two guides to the innocent nature of this radiating, scirrhous nodule with irregularly disposed tubules in it, are firstly the detection of the double-layered (epithelial and myoepithelial) nature of the tubules and secondly, the absence of such cords and tubules in the surrounding relatively normal areas away from the lesion. This entrapment of benign, double-layered epithelium is also seen in the sclerosing intraduct or intracystic papilloma.

Many clinicians regard a patient with a lumpy breast and a positive family history of breast cancer as a potential cancer risk and would follow them up carefully. Biopsy in these people shows benign disease or variations in age changes in the breast described elsewhere in this chapter.

The painful or inflamed breast

The tender red lump or the tender red breast

The conditions which need to be considered under this heading with their underlying pathology are as follows: *Acute and chronic abscess, mammary disorders of pregnancy including acute mastitis, confluent periductal mastitis*, a consequence of the coalescence of the primary lesion of the duct ectasia in several adjoining ducts, and finally *inflammatory cancer*, which has been described in the section on breast cancer. A clinical diagnosis of acute mastitis without pathological confirmation can be dangerous and amount to calling inflammatory cancer acute mastitis.

Breast abscess

The pyogenic type is most commonly caused by *Staphylococcus aureus*. Early treatment with antibiotics may cure without abscess formation. Late treatment, or use of an antibiotic to which the organism is insensitive, may result in an antibioma, a hard indurated mass in the breast made up of fibrous tissue in which there are abscesses of varying sizes.

Tuberculosis of the breast only occurs where tuberculosis is still common. The gross clinical lesions may be the only evidence of the disease or it may by one of several foci of tuberculosis in the patient. Presentation is either as a fluctuant abscess central in the breast or a poorly defined lump in the skin attachment and axillary lymphadenopathy. There may be fistulae through the skin. The pathology is the same as tuberculosis elsewhere. The condition should not be confused with para-areolar abscess.

The large breast

This may arise from a variety of causes. If bilateral it may be a normal variant of development. Unilaterally it may be due to large tumours such as fibroadenoma, cystosarcoma phylloides and large cysts. Occasionally normal breast growth in girls is asymmetrical. There is no known cause for this and, as in the bilateral cases, the histological picture is of normal breast tissue.

Breast augmentation

The various methods used by surgeons to augment the breast has brought with them a number of pathologies and clinical pitfalls especially when the patient omits to tell the surgeon of this treatment. Oil injections into the breast substance finally produce small hard painful breasts. The cut surface shows oil containing cysts of various sizes contained in fibrous tissue. Little, if any, of the breast substance remains and there are often associated palpable axillary glands. Silicone injections produce hard tender craggy breasts with sinuses which often become secondarily infected.

Pain in the breast

This fairly common symptom in breast disease is most commonly primary when there is an inflammatory, traumatic or allied lesion (see under the *Tender Red Breast*). In other instances it is part of the symptom complex and occurs in breast cancer as a presenting symptom with a lump or pricking pain preceding a lump. The aetiology is not explained in either case. Cyclical changes in the breast are often accompanied by pain. Pain in a clinically normal breast may defy diagnosis even when possible refered pain has been considered.

The causes of pain in the breast may be summarized as follows:

1. Association with a single breast lump as a first or later symptom.
2. Preceding a breast lump, e.g. preceding cancer.
3. Part of the symptom of inflammation.
4. Following trauma to the breast.
5. Associated with medicines and hormone preparations taken for other reasons but which may act on the breast substance.
6. Associated with a lumpy or granular breast.
7. Pain in a clinically normal breast.
8. Referred pain from elsewhere.

The surgical pathology of diseases of the nipple

These may be conveniently discussed under three clinical headings which are the patient's presenting symptoms.

The ulcerated nipple

The clinical lesions here include eczema which may be associated with poor hygiene or a contact dermatitis from detergents. Of the malignant causes, Paget's disease and an ulcerating cancer at the nipple are the most common. Generally a clinical diagnosis can be made on clinical examination but a biopsy is necessary to confirm the diagnosis.

The most popular explanation of the nature of Paget's disease of the nipple, that it is secondary intra-epidermal carcinoma associated with an underlying mammary carcinoma, may be true in some cases but does not account for (a) those cases in which the carcinoma is remote from the nipple; (b) those extragenital cases in which no underlying primary tumour is ever discovered; and (c) the ultrastructural demonstration of connections—desmosomes—between Paget cells and adjacent cells.

The hard nipple

Here the presentation is unilateral and may be the consequence of either infiltration from an underlying cancer, or from the benign condition of adenoma of the nipple, or from Paget's disease; histopathological study of such cases is essential. Adenoma of the nipple, a lesion presenting with a sore, ulcer discharge and crusting, is a tubular double-layered adenomatous structure, probably a hamartomatous lesion of the surface epithelium, an inverted adenoma by analogy with an inverted papilloma. It is a benign lesion and can be treated by local surgery. Most disease of the male breast are described by the patient as a hard swollen nipple.

Gynaecomastia

While the majority of these patients have an enlargement of the breast disc which is often idiopathic, bilateral and asymmetrical, the possibility of endocrine disease or causation from taking hormone preparations or other medicines should not be overlooked. The patient usually presents with a "hard nipple".

The male breast

Infantile and pubertal mastitis cases do not, or rather should not, provide biopsy material. Gynaecomastia, usually idiopathic, is associated with a wide range if clinical conditions: normal puberty, certain testicular tumours, spinal cord lesions, the dysthyroid state, liver disorders, Hodgkins disease, bronchial carcinoma and dialysis treatment of chronic renal failure. Diffuse or circumscribed grossly, it consists histologically of increase in duct numbers and proliferation of duct epithelium with multilayering papillary formation, some nuclear irregularity and mitoses in the most florid forms and the development of a fibroblastic stroma. The differential diagnosis of florid gynaecomastia is *in situ* carcinoma. There is a spectrum of appearances to a quite fibrotic form with a little increase in duct activity.

A proportion of cases of mammary carcinoma (10–20 per cent) occur in association with gynaecomastia. All types of mammary carcinoma of the breast seen in women occur in the male, including associated Paget's disease.

Nipple discharges

These are clinically divisible into those occurring through the nipple and those occurring from a para-areolar sinus or fistula. The cases in the first group are: duct ectasia, papilloma of the major and occasionally minor duct systems, multicentric hyerplasia of the major or minor ducts which is often a hormone stimulated condition associated with cystic disease of the breast, drug induced from hormone preparations and antidepressants and occasionally associated with endocrine tumours, i.e. from the pituitary. Where a nipple discharge is associated with a breast lump, attention should first be directed to the latter.

Mamillary fistula

Is characterized by a discharge near the nipple which may be uni- or bilateral and is either due to:

1. A single normal squamous lined duct of the major duct system connecting with the skin surface by a fistulous opening in the para-areolar region or through a Montgomery's tubercle in the areolar. It is often associated with an indrawn nipple and may be unilateral or bilateral and often occurs as a recurrent para-areolar swelling. It is not tuberculous althought it must be differentiated from tuberculosis if the breast in which multiple sinuses opening over the breast surface occur. There is no definite bacterial cause and any bacteria found are secondary invaders. There is no response to antibiotic treatment. Treatment consists of either laying open the fistula or excising the major duct system with the fistula en-bloc.

2. A similar picture is found in confluent periductal mastitis, a generalized disease of the major duct system requiring ablative surgery of the major ducts with fistula, en-bloc, to remove the disease.

Duct ectasia

This presents as a nipple discharge of various types including blood-stained, often occurring bilaterally but asymmetrically from more than one duct orifice. The age incidence stretches from 25 to 70 but usually the maximum incidence is between 40 to 55 years when clinical symptoms are prominent. The histological picture is made of two parts, duct dilatation and periductal mastitis. The major ducts become dilated, the lining epithelium is atrophic and the lumen is full of viscid secretion made of lipoid containing macrophages and their decomposition products. The change is reflected throughout the major duct system and of cellular infiltration of the substance of the breast starting in the periductal region and called periductal mastitis. The periductal cuffing is cellular in the acute stage but progresses to a healing stage with periductal fibrosis and thickening of the duct wall. The prominent cell in periductal mastitis is the plasma cell and for this reason the condition was known as plasma cell mastitis formerly. This is now thought to be a feature of duct ectasia and not a separate condition and the description periductal mastitis is preferred to plasma cell mastitis. The suggested mechanism of its production is that the dilated ducts whose epithelium may be atrophic or deficient allow a leak of the lipoid-containing secretion into the tissues. A non-suppurative cellular hypersensitivity reaction, characterized by plasma cells, giant cells and areas of fat necrosis, occurs. It varies from discrete periductal cuffing to confluence of these areas giving rise to the formation of an area of acute and sub-acute non-suppurative mastitis which may be mistaken for a carcinoma or an acute abscess. (See under the *Tender Red Breast*).

Duct papilloma

The true papilloma is usually single affecting one major duct. In the early stages it is a pedunculated tumour made of branching fronds and covered by a single layer of columnar epithelium. As the papilloma grows it becomes compressed and the tumour and the fronds adhere to each other, the villous appearance is lost and the tumour mass appears solid and velvety with secondary spaces in its substance. The delicate branching blood supply gives rise to recurrent haemorrhage from the nipple. The detailed histopathology has been previously described in this chapter.

Nipple discharge as a symptom of breast cancer

It is likely that some breast cancers can have a nipple discharge as part of their symptom complex. Study of published series gives a wide range of incidence from 15–30 per cent. Prospective studies with examination of the whole breast specimen post-operatively demonstrates lesions of the duct system such as duct ectasia and papilloma which could be the most likely cause of the discharge. However, 3–5 per cent of patients have no demonstrable associated pathology and the discharge must be ascribed to the cancer. In this instance a discharge of any sort may be present. It need not be, and often is not, blood-stained, but may contain blood and malignant cells. Papilloma and duct ectasia remain the most common causes of blood-stained discharge through the nipple.

The skin of the breast

Apart from the presence of blemishes and tumours which may occur on the body skin, e.g. the melanocytic naevi, low grade carcinoma of Bowen or basal cell type, there are conditions of special cancer to the clinician. Paget's disease is dealt with elsewhere. Peau d'orange, the chronic lymphoedema of the skin associated with the presence of a large carcinoma, is a bad prognostic sign. Dimpling of the skin is due to tethering by a carcinoma which may be quite small, and the physical sign may only be produced as a result of applying an appropriate clinical manoeuvre. Lymphoedema with reddening should always suggest inflammatory carcinoma before any lesser diagnosis.

Long after mastectomy, perhaps decades, one or more metastatic nodules may appear *near* the scar, rather than in it. To refer to these as scar recurrences is misleading, and suggestive of wound contamination, an unlikely explanation for a phenomenon which at present is not understood. Melanoma of mammary skin is a rarity and requires no special comment with regard to pathology and behaviour.

Further reading

Journals

Azzopardi JG, Chepick OF, Hartmann WH *et al.* The World Health Organisation histological typing of breast tumours—Second edition. *Am J Clin Pathol* 1982; **78**:806–16.

Carlson HB. Gynaecomastia. *N Engl J Med* 1980; **303**:795–9.

Gullino PM. Considerations on the preneoplastic lesions of the mammary gland. *Am J Path* 1977: **89**:413–30.

Hughes LE, Forbes JF. Early breast cancer: Part I: Surgical pathology and preoperative assessment. *Br J Surg* 1978; **65**:753–63.

Hutter RVP. The pathologist's role in minimal breast cancer. *Cancer* 1971; **28**:1527–36.

Love SM, Gelman RS, Silen W. Fibrocystic 'Disease' of the breast—a nondisease? *N Engl J Med* 1982; **307**:1010–14.

Paoni JF, Baker RR. Pathogenesis and treatment of Paget's disease. *Cancer* 1981; **48**:825–9.

Rosen PP, Senie R, Schottenfeld D, Ashikari R. Noninvasive breast carcinoma. *Ann Surg* 1979; **189**:377–82.

Rosen PP, Saigo PE, Braun DW, Weathers E, De Palo A. Predictors of recurrence in Stage I (TINOMO) breast carcinoma. *Ann Surg* 1981; **193**:15–25.

Stenkvist B, Bengtsson E, Eriksson O, Jarkrans T, Nordin B, Westman-Naeser S. Histopathological systems of breast cancer classification: reproducibility and clinical significance. *J Clin Pathol* 1983; **36**:392–8.

Books

Haagensen CD. *Diseases of the Breast*, Second edition. Philadelphia: W.B. Saunders, 1971.

Hadfield GJ. Benign Diseases of the Breast. In: Hadfield GJ, Hobsley M. eds. *Current Surgical Practice. Vol. I.* London: Arnold, 1976:250–261.

Hadfield GJ. Cancer of the Breast: Retrospect, Circumspect and Prospect. In: Hadfield GJ, Hobsley M. eds. *Current Surgical Practice. Vol. 3.* Arnold, 1981:292–307.

Harmer MH, ed. *TM and N Classification of Malignant Tumours*. 3rd edition rev. Geneva: I.U.C.C., 1982.

McDivitt RW, Stewart FW, Berg JW. *Tumors of the Breast*. Fascicole 2, Second series. Washington: Armed Forces Institute of Pathology, 1967.

Rosai J. *Ackerman's Surgical Pathology*, Sixth Edition. Two vols. St. Louis: Mosby, 1981.

2

Salivary Glands

M Hobsley and A C Thackray

Introduction

The surgeon meets problems concerned with the salivary glands in four main clinical situations:

1. A lump in the region of the parotid salivary gland;
2. Enlargement of one or both parotid salivary glands;
3. Disorders of salivation; and
4. Swellings in other salivary gland regions.

Lump in parotid salivary gland region

Fig. 2.1 shows the outline of the parotid salivary gland: it fills in the hollow between the ear and the posterior border of the jaw, extending upwards to the zygoma; it extends forwards onto the posterior third of the masseter muscle with an extension, the *accessory lobule*, along the parotid duct; it plunges deep into the neck to lie immediately posterior to the posterior pole of the submandibular salivary gland; and it extends backwards to overlie the mastoid process.

If one excludes any lump clinically attached to skin or to bone, most lumps in the parotid region turn out to be neoplasms of the parotid salivary gland itself.

In a personal series, no less than 250 of 299 con-

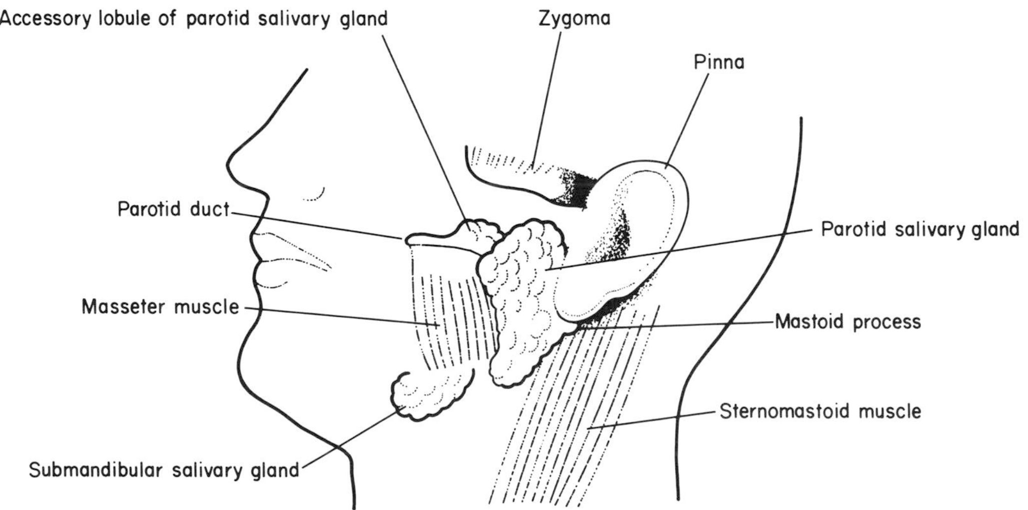

Fig. 2.1 Site and shape of the parotid salivary gland. See description in text.

secutive patients presenting with a lump in the parotid salivary region proved to have an epithelial tumour of the parotid gland, and only 49 other conditions such as connective tissue tumours or enlarged lymph nodes.

What was thought to be a tumour at the lower limit of the parotid gland may prove on subsequent microscopy to be a cervical lymph node enlarged by, for example, toxoplasmosis; conversely, what was provisionally diagnosed as an enlarged upper cervical lymph node occasionally proves to be a lower pole parotid tumour.

There are, however, actually within the substance of the parotid a few small lymph nodes which are liable to nearly all the possible causes of lymph node enlargement, and which then present clinically as parotid lumps, as also do tumours of the facial nerve in its course through the gland.

Clinical features such as symptoms, signs and simple radiological and haemotological investigations only rarely help to distinguish the various causes of a lump in the parotid region (see p. 26). It follows that for the unremarkable parotid lump the surgeon must proceed on the assumption, statistically based, that he is dealing with a parotid neoplasm and the form of treatment he adopts must aim at giving a good result with the common forms of parotid neoplasm. The scheme of nomenclature and classification adopted by the WHO is shown in the Table 2.1.

Table 2.1 Epithelial tumours of the parotid salivary glands.

Adenomas
Pleomorphic adenoma (mixed parotid tumour)
Monomorphic adenomas
Adenolymphoma
Oxyphilic adenoma (oncocytoma)
Other types
Mucoepidermoid tumour
Acinic cell tumour
Carcinomas
Adenoid cystic carcinoma
Adenocarcinoma
Epidermoid carcinoma
Undifferentiated carcinoma
Carcinoma in pleomorphic adenoma (malignant mixed tumour)

Incidence, classification and histopathology of parotid neoplasms

Salivary gland tumours are uncommon: their incidence has been assessed as between 0.25 and 2.5 tumours per 100 000 of the population. Among European races, salivary gland tumours account for less than 3 per cent of all neoplasms.

Nearly all parotid tumours are epithelial in origin, adenomas or carcinomas, derived from the ducts and acini of the gland. The majority are benign tumours, made up of the epithelial cells of the parotid ducts, but with the outermost layer of cells, the myoepithelium, often far more prominent than in the normal glandular tissue. In the commonest tumour of the parotid these myoepithelial cells take on a variety of appearances, resembling cartilage, myxoid tissue or smooth muscle in different parts of the same growth, and this led to these tumours for long being known as "mixed parotid tumours". The current term, "pleomorphic adenoma", stresses their essential benignity and their very variegated appearance (Fig. 2.2). Over 70 per cent of parotid tumours are pleomorphic adenomas. To contrast with this term, other much less common benign epithelial tumours are grouped together in the table as "monomorphic adenomas". Two of these, the oxyphilic adenoma or oncocytoma and the adenolymphoma, are made up of large eosinophilic cells having the characteristics of oncocytes. The oxyphilic adenoma is compact, whereas the adenolymphoma has a predominantly papillary-cystic arrangement and a lymphoid stroma.

Between 5 and 10 per cent of parotid tumours are adenolymphomas or "Warthin's tumours", and these are most often seen in men between the ages of 55 and 65. In about 5 per cent of cases further primary tumours subsequently develop in the same gland or in the opposite parotid. They grow slowly, and may remain stationary for a while. Adenolymphomas have a smooth outline, and their consistence varies with the tenseness of the cystic spaces within. The cystic spaces contain brownish viscid fluid which is quite characteristic if aspirated, though it is occasionally mistaken for pus. Adenolymphomas do very rarely become infected, with overlying redness, tenderness and increased swelling, and with real pus in the cavities and often with necrosis of much of the tumour. Biopsy of the lining of what was thought to be a simple parotid abscess may show adenolymphomatous tissue on microscopy.

The "other types" of monomorphic adenoma in Table 2.1 include a number of adenomas in which the ductal epithelium and myoepithelium, in varying proportions, present a much more uniform pattern throughout each tumour, without myxochondroid areas. Many names, based on the arrangement or cell type of these adenomas, have

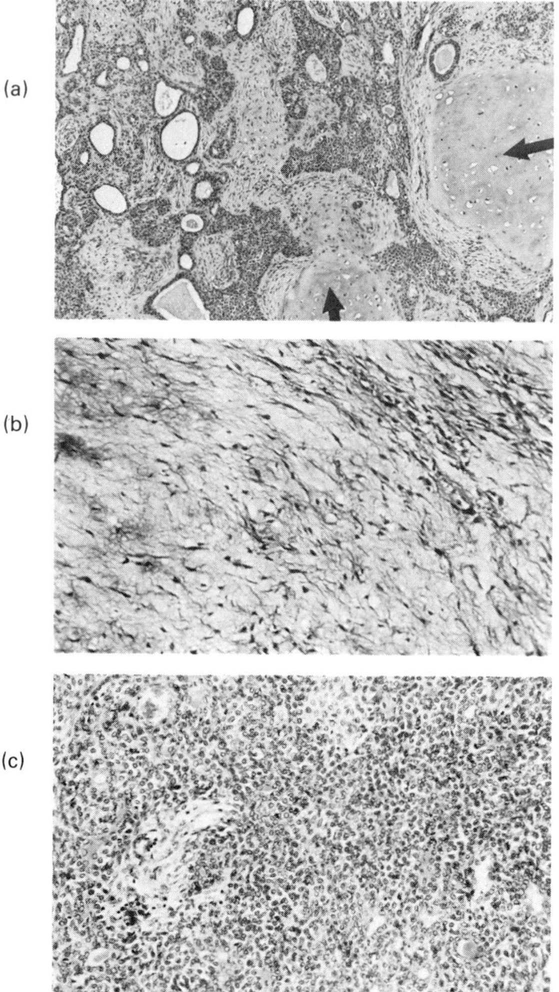

Fig. 2.2 (a) A characteristic field from a pleomorphic adenoma at a low magnification, showing chondroid areas (arrowed) as well as epithelial lined spaces; (b) Myxoid areas such as shown here are often a feature of pleomorphic adenomas, and this type of tissue may make up almost the whole tumour; (c) Considerable areas of pleomorphic adenomas may consist of solid sheets of polygonal or spindle shaped cells such as shown here.

been coined but further subdivision is of little practical value and they are usually just reported as "monomorphic adenoma". Some of them are cystic, and what appears at first to be a simple parotid cyst may prove to have tumour tissue in some part of its wall.

Three of the types of carcinoma listed in Table 2.1, adenocarcinoma, epidermoid or squamous cell carcinoma and undifferentiated carcinoma require no special mention here, as their behaviour is that of similar tumours elsewhere. Epidermoid carcinomas arise in ducts which have previously undergone squamous metaplasia. As these carcinomas have no histological features to indicate that they are of parotid origin it is important to keep in mind the possibility that the parotid lump may be a metastasis or extension from elsewhere.

The adenoid cystic carcinoma or cylindromatous carcinoma, although accounting for only about 3 per cent of parotid tumours, is important in that it combines a deceptively well-differentiated microscopic appearance with a habit of relentless, slow but widespread infiltration, often along nerve sheaths, far from the more or less circumscribed main body of the tumour (Fig. 2.3). This compactness of the main part of the growth is such that the surgeon may think he is dealing with an adenoma, but there is almost always local recurrence. By the time it is apparent that the tumour has recurred there is little chance of eradicating it. Lymph nodes are rarely if ever invaded, but after a number of years of persistent local extension, although checked by radiotherapy, distant metastases are found. Occasionally, at some time in its progress, the tumour undergoes a sudden access of malignancy and takes on the character of an undifferentiated carcinoma.

The term "carcinoma in pleomorphic adenoma" is a reminder of the danger that a neglected pleomorphic adenoma or unremoved local recurrences may, after many years, quite suddenly become malignant (Fig. 2.4). At one time the possibility of malignant change was denied, the tumour was said to have really been a carcinoma *ab initio*, but the long history of a slowly growing or even static lump, with the abrupt development of features of malignancy, and especially the fact that malignancy might develop in only one of a group of otherwise typical nodules of recurrent pleomorphic adenoma justify the concept of malignant change, and emphasize the importance of getting rid of parotid tumours at the first attempt. Almost any of the foregoing histological types of carcinoma may develop in a pleomorphic adenoma, even epidermoid carcinoma from the foci of squamous epithelium not infrequently present in pleomorphic adenomas.

The two tumours in an intermediate position in Table 2.1, the mucoepidermoid and acinic cell tumours, are both designated carcinomas by some writers. But many acinic cell tumours are well-differentiated and encapsulated and are cured by a sufficiently wide local removal; incomplete

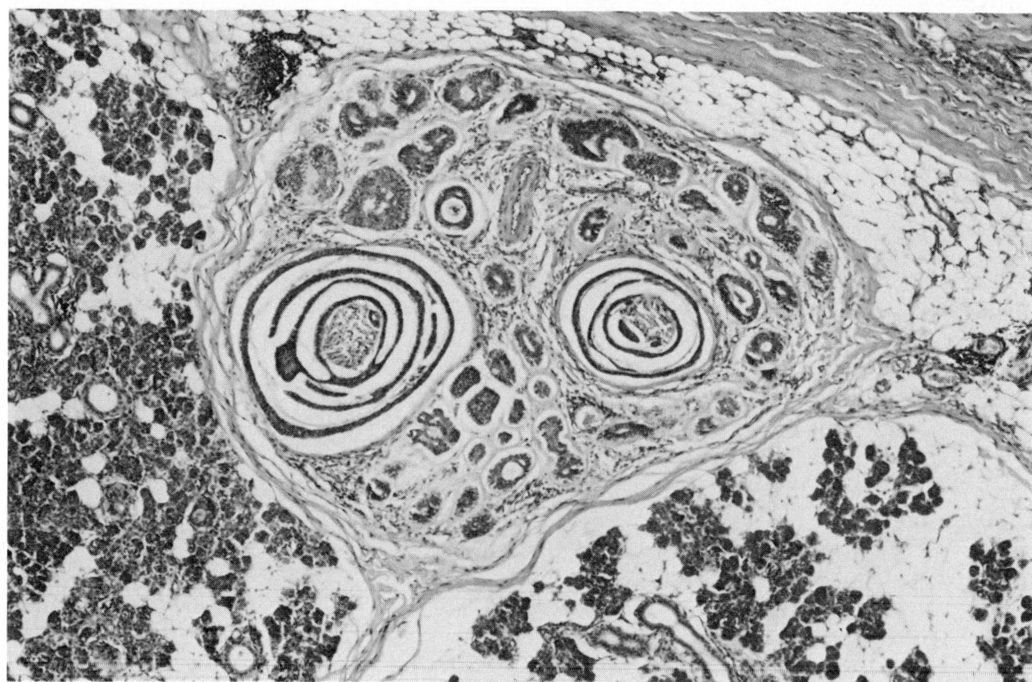

Fig. 2.3 An adenoid cystic carcinoma of the parotid has spread along perineural spaces (appearing as concentric rings) and is now invading the neurovascular bundle. The section is taken a centimetre away from the apparent edge of the tumour.

removal is of course followed by recurrence, but this may be controlled by further surgery. There is a possibility of glandular or even distant metastasis, but this is not great and the ultimate outlook is good.

Mucoepidermoid tumours arise from metaplastic duct epithelium and contain varying proportions of epidermoid and mucous cells. They are often well-differentiated, and though locally invasive and sometimes spreading to local lymph nodes, the prognosis is quite good.

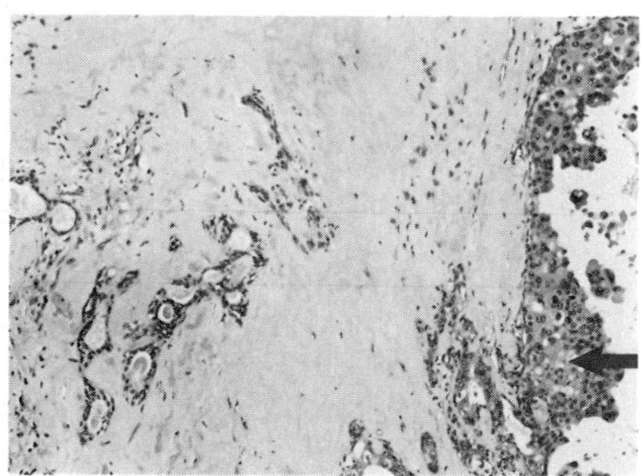

Fig. 2.4 Carcinoma in a PA. The greater part of the field shows a hyalinised, degenerate, but still recognisable, pleomorphic adenoma. At one end there is the edge of a carcinoma which developed in it (arrowed).

Connective tissue tumours are a rarity in the parotid. Malignant lymphomas may develop from the intra-parotid lymph nodes or exceptionally from lymphoepithelial lesions, (p. 32) and neurofibromas from the facial nerve. Lipomas occasionally develop in the parotid of adults, forming a rather soft lump which may be mistaken for a cyst, whilst in young children tumour-like angiomatous malformations present as rather diffuse bluish swellings.

The role of biopsy

It is commonplace for the surgeon, faced with a lump of unknown nature, to obtain a small piece of material from the lump for histological examination. Based on the histopathologist's report of the nature of the lump, and therefore its probable behaviour, a definite excision can then be planned. Indeed some surgeons do subscribe to the view that this procedure of preliminary biopsy should be applied to a lump in the parotid region. There are, however, two reasons for advising against this policy: the difficulties of parotid histopathology especially when the tissue sample is small, and the biological properties of the common parotid neoplasms with special reference to implantation recurrence.

Difficulties of salivary histopathology

Table 2.1 lists a series of apparently clear-cut entities. In practice, however, difficulties arise, mainly on the borderlines of malignancy. Quite a small biopsy may suffice for the diagnosis of a frank carcinoma, but the distinction between a well-differentiated adenocarcinoma and an adenoma with a degree of mitotic activity and other features suggestive of possible malignancy can be very difficult. If the whole tumour is available examination of the periphery for evidence of invasion is important, but with a small biopsy this is not possible. Another source of confusion is the occasional presence in adenomas of areas with an adenoid cystic pattern, but which are not necessarily of ominous significance, whilst adenoid cystic carcinomas are occasionally mistaken for benign tumours in small biopsies. Small biopsies of pleomorphic adenomas can resemble connective tissue tumours.

Malignant lymphomas may involve the intraparotid lymph nodes, but can also develop in the salivary glandular tissue; one of the most difficult histological distinctions to make can be between malignant lymphoma and the exuberant lymphoid hyperplasia of Sjogren's disease (p. 32) or a chronic inflammatory condition. This particular problem may be unresolved even if the entire lump is available for examination.

Salivary gland tumours and implantation recurrence

Pleomorphic adenomas have long been recognized to have a tendency to recur after local removal, and this may seem strange in what is essentially a benign tumour. There was at one time a suggestion that recurrences were fresh primary tumours elsewhere in the gland, but the recurrent nodules are so often outside the anatomical limits of the parotid—though always in the field of the original operation—that the explanation is surely that tumour tissue is left behind after what purports to be a complete removal. There may be only a few cells left in the wound, and as the tumour often grows slowly it may be 20 or more years before a noticeable swelling develops. Two characteristics of pleomorphic adenomas underlie this liability to recurrence. Firstly, areas of myxoid consistency in the tumour, sometimes sufficiently extensive to lead to a preoperative diagnosis of cyst, may account for the tumour rupturing during removal and spilling cells into the wound. Secondly, the tumours grow unevenly. Localized surface sprouts extend out through the fibrous surrounds (Fig. 2.5), and though they are soon walled off by fresh fibrosis, at one stage in their evolution they are liable to get separated and left behind if the plane of surgical removal is too close to the apparent surface of the growth. This uneven growth also results in pleomorphic adenomas becoming lobulated, and macroscopic lobules may similarly become detached and left behind if they have a narrow neck.

Local recurrences of infiltrative tumours require no explanation, for microscopic strands of tumour may extend far beyond the macroscopic limits of the tumour.

The only salivary gland tumour that is at all commonly truly multiple is the adenolymphoma, and recurrences of this are likely to be fresh primaries.

Implantation recurrences are particularly likely to be found in the scar of the previous operation, and this should be entirely excised. In planning an operation for recurrent pleomorphic adenoma it should be remembered that although only a single tumour nodule may be palpable, multiple scattered foci of tumour are nearly always found in the operative specimen.

A scheme of management

Of the 299 patients with a lump in the parotid gland in the series previously mentioned, the majority had no clinical features to enable the surgeon to make a diagnosis any more accurate than "lump in the parotid". However, the lump was attached to the overlying skin in four patients, to the underlying bone in one, and in five an exact clinical diagnosis could be made, e.g. a stone in the parotid duct. In 30 patients there were signs suggestive of malignancy, in 43 patients the lump was recurrent or persistent after previous surgery, and some histological material was therefore available, but in the remaining 213 patients there was no clinical clue to the nature of the lump.

Skin attachment

Attachment to skin means either that the lump arises in the skin or else it arises in deeper layers (probably in the parotid) but has gained secondary

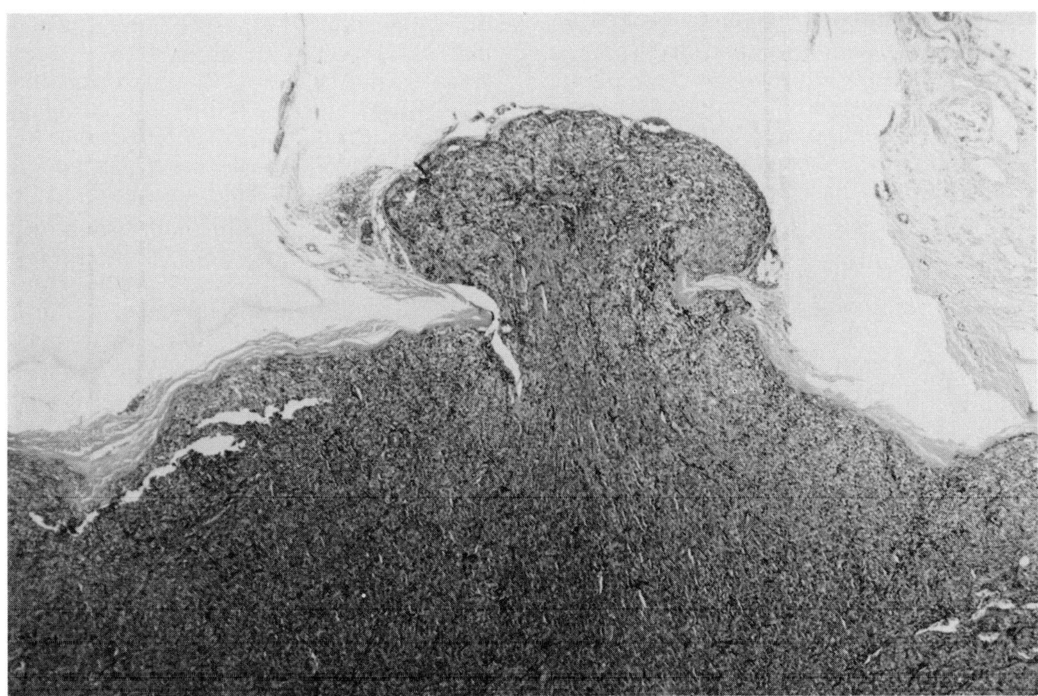

Fig. 2.5 The type of localized protuberance from the margin of a pleomorphic adenoma which is liable to become detached if the tumour is not removed with an adequate clearance. X55.

attachment to the skin. The common primary skin lesion is the epidermoid (sebaceous) cyst, and if the lesion has a characteristic punctum it is readily diagnosable. An epidermoid cyst is not invasive and therefore does not penetrate into the parotid so it can be safely excised without fear of damage to the facial nerve.

A lump in the parotid which has become secondarily attached to the skin is inflammatory or malignant (or both).

Attachment to bone

The bone involved may be mandible, zygoma or temporal. Like attachment to skin, attachment to bone means that the lump is inflammatory or malignant (or both) so that a diagnosis of pleomorphic or monomorphic adenoma is not feasible. Moreover any attempt to remove such a lump with a margin of normal tissue would result in severe deformity. Biopsy is therefore not only permissible but mandatory.

Actinomycosis is an example of a lesion that may be attached to bone but requires medical rather than surgical treatment.

Evidence suggesting malignancy

Clinical features suggestive of malignancy are either very rapid growth or facial nerve weakness, or both features combined.

The presence of rapid growth, often with an overlay of inflammatory features such as warmth, redness, oedema and pain make it quite clear that the patient is not suitable for an attempt at complete excision. Just as in the case of the so-called inflammatory carcinoma of the breast, an attempt to cut out such a lesion serves merely to spread the malignant cells even further afield.

The management should therefore be a preliminary biopsy. If the only evidence suggesting malignancy is a facial nerve weakness, the situation requires judgement and will be discussed later.

Previous histological evidence available

Always review any previous histological evidence with your own histopathologist. Histology of salivary glands is difficult, even for the expert, and a second scrutiny—particularly in the light of evidence that the lump has recurred—may result in a re-interpretation of the original histology.

Another very important point to remember is that parotid neoplasms show a tendency to become more malignant as time passes. It does not necessarily follow that the histology of a recurrent tumour is the same as that of the original tumour.

The unremarkable lump

For reasons already given, the management advised is to excise the lump with a wide margin of normal tissue and with preservation of the facial nerve provided the circumstances encountered at operation permit this. The principles are an early identification of the trunk of the facial nerve, followed by dissection forwards keeping as close to the plane of the nerve and its branches as possible.

If the lump is superficial to the nerve (85 per cent of cases) and does not invade the nerve, then this procedure removes the lump as a superficial conservative (i.e. with conservation of the facial nerve) parotidectomy. In 15 per cent of cases the lump is deep to the nerve. After the superficial parotid has been removed the deep part of the gland with its contained tumour is excised after mobilization of the facial nerve and its branches and division of the external carotid artery at the lower pole, and of the same artery or its two terminal branches, the superficial temporal and the maxillary, at the upper pole. Such an operation is a total conservative parotidectomy.

While the principles can thus be simply stated, the practice is not always so easy!

The lesion may approach very close to the nerve or one of its branches: if it appears that the lump is pushing the nerve aside it is reasonable to proceed with the dissection, always using sharp rather than blunt dissection and keeping the points of scissors directed towards the nerve rather than towards the tumour. It is when the nerve seems to be growing straight into the lump that one must accept that the lesion is invading the nerve in a malignant fashion. The difficult decision then has to be made whether the nerve (or in the involved branch) must be sacrificed to maintain the margin of normal tissue, or whether some other possibility should be explored. The decision in an individual case depends on a number of factors such as the age and sex of the patient and the area of facial territory that appears to be denervated by sacrificing nervous tissue. It might be considered acceptable to destroy the whole nerve in an elderly, retired man who lives alone, but to think twice about destroying a single branch in a beautiful young actress.

Fortunately the surgeon only rarely has to face this dilemma. Provided that he is sure that infiltration is occurring, it may be reasonable to cut into the lump to obtain material for immediate histological examination. The lesion could be a lymphoma, and local removal of as much as possible of the lesion plus radiotherapy later might give an excellent result with preservation of the function of the facial nerve. However, if any chance remains that the lesion is an expanding rather than an infiltrating one, our opinion is that the dissection should be proceeded with because expanding tumours like the pleomorphic adenoma are so much more common than infiltrative ones. As a final point on this subject, the surgeon may gain some comfort from the reflection that, with the solitary exception of the lymphomatous lesion, a parotid tumour that is infiltrating the facial nerve will destroy the function of the facial nerve even if he, the surgeon, chooses not to sacrifice the nerve.

Assessment of adequacy of removal The surgeon's own assessment of whether he has succeeded in removing the lump with a margin of normal tissue is usually accurate, especially if he is experienced in this branch of surgery. The pathologist can only make an assessment if the operation specimen reaches him intact. By inspection and palpation he will then identify any suspicious areas where tumour may be present on the surface of the specimen and take blocks for sectioning from such sites, possibly applying Indian ink to the free surface to identify it in the microscopic section. However, the infiltrative extensions of adenoid cystic carcinoma, for example, can neither be seen nor felt, and random sections may not show them. Such tumours may well recur, even though in the sections studied there appeared to be a margin of normal tissue outside the tumour.

Lump presenting with facial nerve weakness

This is a difficult problem because although our experience is that most such lumps prove to be malignant, there is no reason why a benign parotid tumour should not co-exist with a self-limiting Bell's Palsy. In the circumstances here visualized, the facial nerve weakness is the *only* evidence of malignancy: there is no question of rapid growth of the lump.

In other words, apart from the involvement of the facial nerve there appears to be no contraindication to attempting to remove the lump with a wide margin of normal tissue and preservation of the facial nerve provided that the findings at operation permit. Naturally if the nerve is involved it is much less likely that it will be possible to remove the lump with a margin and yet preserve the whole of the nerve. Nevertheless it might be possible to do so, or more probably it might be possible to sacrifice only one or two branches of the nerve and save the others. Whilst there cannot be any "correct" answer to this situation, our feeling is on the whole to ignore the facial nerve involvement and attempt to remove the lump with preservation of as much of the nerve as possible.

Management subsequent to histological report

The decision about further management depends upon whether the histopathology report specifies a diagnosis of pleomorphic adenoma, or of a lesion equally benign or a lesion more malignant.

Pleomorphic adenoma

If the surgeon's and the pathologist's assessment agree that the lesion was completely excised, we have never seen a recurrence of the lesion. The evidence for this statement is derived from two personal series totalling 178 patients in whom no recurrence has been noted in a follow-up lasting between four and 29 years. We therefore feel that no further treatment is necessary, but in order to maintain records we see these patients for a yearly follow-up.

Those who recommend lesser procedures should remember that a pre-operative provisional diagnosis of pleomorphic adenoma is by no means always confirmed by the pathological report, and although a certain line of treatment may be effective for subsequently confirmed pleomorphic adenoma, it is obviously desirable that the treatment should also be appropriate for unexpected well-differentiated malignant tumour.

Doubts about the completeness of excision may arise either because of the surgeon's findings at operation or because on one or more of the sections the tumour appears to reach very near the margin of the excision. In these circumstances we recommended the adoption of a "wait-and-see" policy.

There remains the problem of the pleomorphic adenoma that is known not to be completely excised, perhaps because the tumour burst during the operation with obvious spillage or because it was technically difficult to remove and the surgeon elected to leave the difficult part *in situ*.

Opinions differ as to the correct management if obvious spillage has occurred. Some clinicians advise radiotherapy, but the pleomorphic salivary adenoma does not respond well to radiotherapy and there is some evidence in the literature that radiotherapy encourages malignant change in a pleomorphic adenoma. We therefore rely on vigorous mechanical cleansing of the wound by irrigation with isotonic saline at the end of the operation and an expectant policy. Careful follow-up, at first at three month and later at six month intervals, should go on for ever and any nodules appearing are locally excised with the facial nerve having to take its chance.

For patients in whom tumour has been known to be left *in situ*, we have no doubt that a further operation should be performed by a surgeon experienced in this type of surgery in order to remove the residual mass with as wide a margin of normal tissue as possible, the wound being closed after vigorous irrigation in an attempt to remove seedling deposits.

Diagnosis as benign, or more benign than pleomorphic adenoma, or non-neoplastic

No further management of the parotid itself is needed except insofar as the histological diagnosis is of some disease that in its own right requires further treatment.

Diagnosis more malignant than pleomorphic adenoma

One cannot be dogmatic about the management of patients in whom the report has come back as a lesion that is more malignant than pleomorphic adenoma. Should one wait and see, or operate again and perform a radical parotidectomy, perhaps with cervical block dissection of lump nodes, or advise radiotherapy? Factors influencing the decision include the assessment of whether the excision was complete, the exact histology of the tumour, and other factors with respect to the health and general problems of the patient.

While it is impossible to deal with all the possible combinations of these factors, we can say that we tend towards an expectant policy for acinic cell tumour and muco-epidermoid tumour, but towards radiotherapy for adenoid cystic carcinoma and the frank carcinomas.

Multiple or bilateral parotid lumps

The only parotid tumour that is at all likely to be bilateral is the adenolymphoma. Despite its bilaterality or multiplicity, the adenolymphoma is entirely benign. Although a patient with a lump in both parotid regions is more likely to have an adenolymphoma than any other tumour, there is no reason why the histology might not be something else, for example pleomorphic adenoma. There is therefore no logical reason to treat the patient in any way differently and we would advise the usual management for a lump in the parotid region, first on one side and at a subsequent operation on the other.

The same logic applies to multiple lumps in the same parotid salivary gland. A formal parotidectomy should be performed in this situation as well. A careful search should however be made in such cases for lumps elsewhere, particularly in the neck, because the possibility that multiple nodules are due to a generalized disease of lymph nodes is high. If such nodules are found, it is a good idea to biopsy one of them rather than attacking the parotid in the first instance. For example if the diagnosis turns out to be a lymphoma, then the combination of radiotherapy and chemotherapy might be the correct management without the necessity for any parotidectomy.

Swelling of the whole parotid salivary gland

Enlargement of the whole parotid salivary gland may be acute, or chronic or recurrent, and may affect one or both glands. The swelling is usually inflammatory (either viral, bacterial or possibly auto-immune), but there are a few non-inflammatory causes of parotid enlargement for consideration later.

Acute swelling

Viral

Quite the commonest cause of acute parotid swelling, usually bilateral but sometimes unilateral, is mumps. In a child or young adult with a history of contact with other cases in the preceding few weeks, the diagnosis is obvious. Sporadic cases at any age may be confused with other causes of swelling of the gland, and in cases of doubt laboratory confirmation may be sought. The virus is present in the saliva and can be identified, or the serum can be tested for the presence of the V and S antibodies, though in doubtful cases the examination may need to be repeated a week later for a change in titre.

In recent years it has become apparent that a number of other viruses may cause parotitis, though they usually also affect other systems in the body, giving a clue to their identity.

Bacterial

Parotitis very rarely results from organisms reaching the gland by way of the blood stream. The usual route is by way of Stensen's duct from the mouth. There must therefore be suitable pathogenic organisms in the mouth and such sluggish or absent salivation that they are able to reach the gland without being washed out.

Acute parotitis

This was once a not uncommon post-operative complication when fluids were severely restricted and mouth hygiene neglected. Nowadays it is only seen in the debilitated, particularly when drugs with a side effect of reducing salivation are being given. The organisms responsible are most often penicillin-resistant staphylococci, but viridans streptococci or pneumococci may be found. It is desirable to identify the organism and its sensitivities and material from the mouth of the affected duct should be sent to the laboratory before treatment is started; should the antibacterial agent chosen prove ineffective, a change can be made when the sensitivities are reported.

Provided that pus is seen to be oozing from the affected duct orifice, the condition can confidently be expected to resolve with antibiotics and pain-relief together with the cleansing of the mouth.

In patients whose ducts are not draining pus, should local pain and tenderness and generalized constitutional symptoms such as fever and rigors not respond to antibiotics within a few hours a parotid abscess must be diagnosed and drained via an incision in the cheek. It is important not to wait for the appearance of fluctuance because the tough investing parotid fascia masks this sign.

Chronic or recurrent parotid swelling

Each episode of recurrent parotitis may be extremely acute, and the first such episode has usually mistakenly been diagnosed as mumps. It is only when the parotitis recurs that the original diagnosis becomes doubted.

Chronic parotitis means that the gland or glands are enlarged and painful or tender all the time, and there may or may not be acute exacerbations at intervals. Any condition which gives rise to recurrent acute parotitis is likely to result in chronic pain and swelling because each attack of acute inflammation increases the liability to chronic infection. The question whether recurrent or chronic parotitis is unilateral or bilateral is crucial to management, because bilaterality virtually excludes a common cause of unilateral disease, namely a stone in the parotid duct.

Unilateral recurrent or chronic parotitis

In a recent series of 109 patients with recurrent unilateral parotid swelling, the cause was proved to be a calculus in the parotid duct in 36 patients, and the same diagnosis was probable in another 59. Parotid duct calculus is therefore overwhelmingly the most important cause of recurrent unilateral parotitis. Only in 14 of these 109 patients did it appear unlikely that a stone was responsible. Note that the pain and swelling, especially when occurring in close association with eating, may merely be the result of the gland trying to function against the obstruction, and not always entirely due to concomitant inflammation.

Parotid duct calculi There are several clinical features suggestive of this diagnosis. These include a close relationship of the onset of the pain to eating, a sudden onset, a sensation of dryness in the ipsilateral half of the mouth during the attack, a duration of painful swelling of the salivary gland of less than one week and often of less than 48 hours, and a sudden termination of the attack, often with a gush of saliva into the mouth.

With regard to physical signs, the stone may be palpable—usually at the orifice in the mouth but occasionally in the cheek—and the orifice may look abnormal compared with its fellow on the opposite side, either pouting or oedematous or actually with a visible stone impacted within it.

The internal diameter of the main parotid duct is about a millimetre or less and therefore easily obstructed by a fairly small calculus. For this reason, and because not all parotid calculi are heavily calcified, plain radiology may fail to demonstrate the stone. The views most likely to be successful are the intrabuccal and the antero-posterior. Sialography should be deferred until the acute stage has passed: apart from the rather rare filling defect, appearances suggesting a stone include a sudden cut-off on the main duct at a point of fairly complete obstruction and an apparent 'stricture' with a proximal dilatation.

Treatment depends very largely on the position of the stone. If it is at or very near the parotid duct orifice, widening of the orifice by a plastic operation may permit the stone to be extracted immediately or it may pass spontaneously the next time it reaches the enlarged area. If the stone is further back, it may be reasonable to cut down on it from the cheek if it is clearly palpable. A 'blind' search for it through the cheek is a difficult procedure and hazardous because of the proximity of the buccal branches of the facial nerve. If the symptoms warrant a major operation, the best approach is to perform a superficial parotidectomy excising the duct with its contained stone.

Other causes of unilateral recurrent or chronic parotitis Clinical features suggesting that recurrent or chronic parotitis is not due to a calculus in the parotid duct include a lack of clear-cut relationship of the swelling to meals, gradual onset and gradual remission, duration of attacks in excess of one week and sometimes for as much as a month and chronicity itself—a chronic enlargement persisting between attacks is not very common in patients with calculus disease.

Most of the conditions producing non-calculous, unilateral parotitis can also produce bilateral chronic parotitis and so are considered below. Even when the disease appears to be restricted to one parotid, abnormalities of structure and function may also be demonstrable on the other side.

Bilateral chronic or recurrent parotid swelling

It is obviously possible for a patient to have a stone simultaneously in each parotid duct and so suffer from bilateral recurrent parotitis. We have seen two such patients. Nevertheless they constitute a rare and remarkable coincidence and the overwhelming majority of patients with bilateral symptoms and signs will be found not to be suffering from calculous disease.

There are certain clinical features which may help to distinguish some of the causes of the parotid swelling in this small group of patients. For discussion they can conveniently be subdivided into those that show punctate sialectasis on sialography, and those without sialectasis.

Sialectasis, or dilatation of the ducts of the salivary gland as shown by radiography after the injection of contrast medium, takes various forms. The fusiform dilatations and apparent strictures of the main ducts in calculous disease have already been mentioned. In another type a series of rounded opacities are seen along the course of the smaller ducts, looking rather like currants on their stalks; depending on the size of the berries this type is called punctate or globular sialectasis.

These globules in fact represent not pre-existing cystic dilations, but extravasations of contrast medium at points of rupture of the weak duct walls from the pressure of the injection. Although an artefact this type of sialectasis is a sure sign of inflammation, histological examination showing the extravasations to occur where the supporting tissue of the duct wall is weakened or destroyed by a dense inflammatory cell infiltrate.

Punctate sialectasis About 70 per cent patients with bilateral chronic or recurrent parotid swelling show punctate sialectasis on sialography.

There is a well recognized group of cases occurring in childhood, more often boys than girls. The acute attacks of inflammation, nearly always at first suspected to be mumps, last for a few days after which the swelling usually completely subsides until the next episode. The acute attacks rarely proceed to abscess formation. There is a strong tendency for the attacks to become less frequent as time passes so that the disease burns itself out before the patient is 25 years old. This being so, surgical interference is best avoided. On the rare occasions when a parotidectomy has been performed between attacks histological examination shows non-specific chronic inflammatory changes only, with cuffs of lymphoid tissue surrounding the ducts.

The organisms responsible are those normally found in the mouth, and for them to get along the duct to the gland there must be a reduced flow of saliva, but whether this is due to a congenital abnormality, to previous viral or bacterial inflammation or to some other cause is not clear.

When symptoms in association with punctate sialectasis first commence in adulthood, the prognosis is less certain and probably not so good. It is in adults that recurrent parotitis is often combined with the other clinical manifestations that were first described as a syndrome by Sjogren—swelling of other salivary and of the lacrimal glands, a dry mouth, dry eyes, and various manifestations of autoimmune disease such as rheumatoid arthritis. Eighty per cent of patients with the full syndrome have abnormal antibodies including antibodies to salivary gland tissue, and such antibodies are only present in about 20 per cent of patients without the syndrome.

In the early stages of Sjogren's disease the patient, more often a woman than a man, and middle-aged, may only complain of dryness of the mouth, the 'sicca syndrome', though even at this stage the sialogram may be abnormal, with areas of punctate sialectasis. Later, chronic or recurrent swelling develops, possibly at first a localized lump, but usually later involving the whole of both parotids and perhaps the submandibulars also. There are also characteristic chronic inflammatory changes in the minor salivary glands and biopsy of a labial gland has been suggested as a diagnostic procedure.

The changes in the parotid consist of a progressively dense infiltration with lymphoid tissue, often with germinal centres, around the inter- and intra-lobular ducts. The duct lining cells degenerate but the outer layers of epithelial cells proliferate to form solid masses which appear on cross section as the characteristic epimyoepithelial islands. Most ducts lose their lumen, but a few become cystic. With the blockage of the ducts and the increasingly heavy lymphocytic infiltrate the acini atrophy and disappear. As the acini atrophy and the ducts block, salivation is greatly reduced and there is liability to ascending infection superimposed on the autoimmune inflammatory process.

Parotid lesions of this histological type are sometimes seen in the absence of other components of Sjogren's disease, the changes then being designated the Benign Lymphoepithelial Lesion. Although almost always benign, there is a possibility of malignancy developing in either the lymphoid or epithelial component of Sjogren's disease or the lymphoepithelial lesion.

In some cases of recurrent or chronic parotitis in adults there is no evidence of autoimmunity, nor does the gland, if removed or biopsied, show the characteristic epimyoepithelial islands and other histological features of the lymphoepothelial lesion. Instead there is only non-specific chronic inflammatory cell infiltration and fibrosis around the ducts, not infrequently with microcalculi, and gradual fibrous replacement of the lobules. There may be quite marked dilatation of the larger ducts, and the duct linings may show squamous or mucous metaplasia increasing the viscosity of the saliva and still further slowing the flow. These cases are comparable with those seen in children, though with much less chance of spontaneous improvement.

In the absence of any clear understanding of the aetiology of these conditions, treatment is unsatisfactory. Apart from symptomatic measures to keep the mouth moist, steroids have been used in some patients with severe symptoms, but the results are variable. If recurrent attacks of the ascending infection with pain and swelling become a burden to the patient, the appropriate salivary gland can be removed surgically by conservative (usually total) parotidectomy.

Sialectasis absent Various conditions in which there is persistent or recurrent generalized enlargement of the salivary glands which is neither inflammatory nor neoplastic have been brought together by some writers under the heading Sialosis. The parotid glands are most affected; not only does sialography show no dilatation of the duct system in these conditions, there may even be narrowing, with scanty branching.

The conditions underlying this salivary gland enlargement may be either hormonal, nutritional or drug-induced. The hormonal disturbances involved are most often ovarian, so that the condition is more common in women, but bilateral parotid enlargement has been reported in diabetes and in thyroid dysfunction. The enlargement sometimes noted in acromegaly is probably only part of the general splanchnomegaly. Although the normal parotid is more easily seen and felt in emaciated patients, definite enlargement has been repeatedly noted in severe malnutrition, particularly where there is qualitative and quantitative lack of protein. This may also be the basis of the asymptomatic parotid enlargement which may be seen in alcoholic cirrhosis.

A number of drugs cause swelling of the salivary glands as an occasional side effect, sometimes with sufficient pain and tenderness to suggest mumps. This effect of iodides has long been recognized, with the label "iodide mumps" sometimes applied, Phenylbutazone therapy has also been recorded as a possible cause of parotid swelling, and there are several others listed.

Histologically, in most types of sialosis, the enlarged gland shows marked swelling of the individual cells of the serous acini, with compression and partial atrophy of the striated ducts. The hypertrophied acini eventually atrophy, with extensive infiltration of the gland by adipose tissue, leaving it still enlarged.

Sarcoidosis

The parotids are occasionally involved in cases of sarcoidosis, with gradual enlargement of the glands which become firm and finely nodular. The typical non-caseating tuberculoid granulomas are scattered throughout the gland and may compress and narrow the ducts, with appreciable dryness of the mouth. The lesions in due course fibrose. There is no sialectasis; there may be narrowing and reduction in numbers of the smaller ducts. Other lesions of sarcoidosis are usually present elsewhere in the body.

Hypertrophy of the masseter muscles

The alert clinician will not be tempted to misdiagnose a hypertrophied masseter muscle on one or both sides as a chronic enlargement of the parotid if he remembers the rhomboidal structure of the muscle and its exact position relative to the bones of the jaw and cheek.

Disorders of salivation

The complaint of making too much or making too little saliva is quite common. When it is accompanied by an anatomical abnormality such as a lump or swelling of the whole gland, the anatomical abnormality takes precedence in management. If there is no anatomical abnormality, then objective testing usually shows that the salivary secretion rate is within normal limits. The standard test is to collect parotid saliva under maximal stimulation with an intravenous injection of 10 mg pilocarpine nitrate and the normal limits are 3–13 ml of saliva from each parotid.

Hypersecretion

True hypersecretion is a very rare phenomenon, occurring with true hypertrophy of the parotid salivary glands.

Hyposecretion

Hyposecretion may occur in Sjogren's syndrome and in patients with the sicca syndrome (p. 32). Hyposecretion of saliva leads to dryness of the mouth or xerostomia. It is customarily divided into primary xerostomia, where a pathological condition of the salivary glands is present, and symptomatic or secondary xerostomia where no abnormality of the glands can be found. Primary xerostomia may be due to inflammation of the glands as in mumps or duct obstruction, to loss of glandular tissue following surgery or irradiation, or to involvement of the glands in Sjogren's syndrome or the sicca syndrome. In these latter dryness of the mouth may be the primary complaint before swelling of the glands or other manifestations of the disease develop. A reduced flow of saliva from any cause predisposes to infection from the mouth ascending the duct and causing inflammation, so that a vicious circle may develop.

Symptomatic or secondary xerostomia may be due to changes in the fluid or electrolyte balance of the body, as in dehydration, following severe haemorrhage or in diabetes insipidus, whilst many drugs, including drugs with an atropine-like action such as phenothiazine derivatives, tranquillizers and ganglion blocking agents also have this effect.

Swellings of other salivary gland regions

Submandibular salivary gland

There are two main clinical situations, one in which there is clinical and radiological evidence of calculous disease and the other in which there is no such evidence.

Calculous disease

A history of recurrent swelling of one submandibular salivary gland during meals is almost pathognomonic of a stone blocking the submandibular duct. The stone may be palpable in the duct in the floor of the mouth, and even if it is not, then plain X-rays and sialography clinch the diagnosis.

A stone in the submandibular duct will impede the flow of saliva, partly mechanically and partly in another way. The submandibular saliva contains a good deal of mucus and the duct is normally lined by ciliated epithelium to assist movement of the mucoid saliva. At the site of lodgement of the stone there is often squamous metaplasia of the epithelium, further impeding the flow. If the duct of a serous gland is blocked, the glandular acini atrophy, but mucous acini continue for a time to secrete against pressure so that the intralobular ducts are distended by the mucus and may rupture, with extravasation of mucus and fibrous reaction. Behind the obstruction there may be chronic inflammatory changes also. Whether the stone alone, or the whole gland is to be removed depends partly on anatomical considerations (the precise site of the calculus), partly on an assessment of the possibility of recovery of function of the gland. If it is hard and fibrous it is unlikely to recover.

No evidence of calculous disease

The part of the submandibular salivary gland palpable via the neck is roughly ovoid in shape, i.e. lacking the very characteristic shape of the parotid salivary gland. Therefore, an ovoid swelling in the submandibular gland region is often misdiagnosed as a swelling of the whole submandibular salivary gland when it is really a submandibular salivary gland tumour. In the absence of evidence of calculous disease, it should be assumed that a swelling of the submandibular salivary gland is a neoplasm.

If the swelling is ill-defined and rapidly growing there is some indication for a preliminary biopsy, possibly followed by radiotherapy if an undifferentiated carcinoma is diagnosed. If surgical removal of the gland and lump is decided on, the operation specimen will nearly always reveal an epithelial tumour of the submandibular gland. There are no lymph nodes within the substance of the submandibular gland, but occasionally the operation specimen will prove to be an otherwise normal salivary gland indented by an immediately adjacent lymph node enlarged by, for example, secondary carcinoma or tuberculosis. The other non-neoplastic condition that may be encountered is a curious chronic sclerosing inflammatory condition of the gland which leads to such induration that a tumour is suspected, the so-called Küttners tumour.

With these few exceptions the lump nearly always proves to be an epithelial tumour of the gland. Submandibular tumours are much less common than parotid neoplasms in an approximate ratio of 1:10. Pleomorphic adenomas are still the commonest submandibular tumour, but up to a third of all submandibular tumours are malignant, as against only about 15 per cent of parotid growths. Adenoid cystic carcinoma accounts for 17 per cent of submandibular neoplasms; most of the other submandibular malignancies are adenocarcinomas or undifferentiated carcinomas, though occasional epidermoid carcinomas occur, possibly following squamous metaplasia of the duct lining in the neighbourhood of a calculus. All these carcinomas are liable to get fixed to the mandible and invade it.

Sublingual and unnamed salivary glands

See Chapter 3

Further reading

Hobsley M. Surgery of the Salivary Glands. In: Hadfield J, Hobsley M (eds) *Current Surgical Practice*. Vol. 3 London: Edward Arnold, 1981.

Mason DK, Chisholm DM. *Salivary Glands in Health and Disease*. London, Philadelphia, Toronto: WB Saunders, 1975.

Rice DH, *Surgery of the Salivary Glands*. London: Mosby, 1983.

Thackray AC, Lucas RB. *Tumors of the Major Salivary Glands*. Washington: Armed Forces Institute of Pathology, 1974.

3

Mouth and Jaws

Sir Paul Bramley and C J Smith

Introduction

Although the mouth and jaws are the site of special pathology related to the presence of teeth, or the remnants of tooth-forming tissues, they also share many of the pathological processes of the rest of the body.

A brief review of the clinical and pathological aspects of the more important conditions likely to come the way of general surgeons is presented under the following headings:

1. The patient presenting with a swollen face.
2. White and red lesions of the oral mucosa.
3. Ulcers and bullae.
4. Conditions peculiar to the tongue and floor of mouth.
5. Localized intra-oral swellings.
6. The patient with inability to open the mouth.

The patient presenting with a swollen face

In most instances a perceptive history will give a strong lead to accurate diagnosis of the causative lesions. Whether the swelling is in soft tissues, in underlying bone, or in both, must be established, even though for acutely tender swellings this can be difficult.

Soft-tissue swellings

Most *acute inflammatory swellings* of the face originate from *acute pulpitis* or *acute pericoronitis* and their pathology is that of acute inflammation elsewhere, modified by local anatomy. They are usually preceded by localized toothache, which may become less intense just prior to appearance of the swelling; this coincides with release of pressure in a *periapical abscess* as it bursts through restraining cortical bone into overlying soft tissues. However, there may be no recent history of toothache and in these instances it is likely that an acute exacerbation has occurred within a chronic periapical granuloma or cyst associated with a long-dead tooth.

Although there will often be a readily identifiable grossly carious tooth near the swelling, vari-

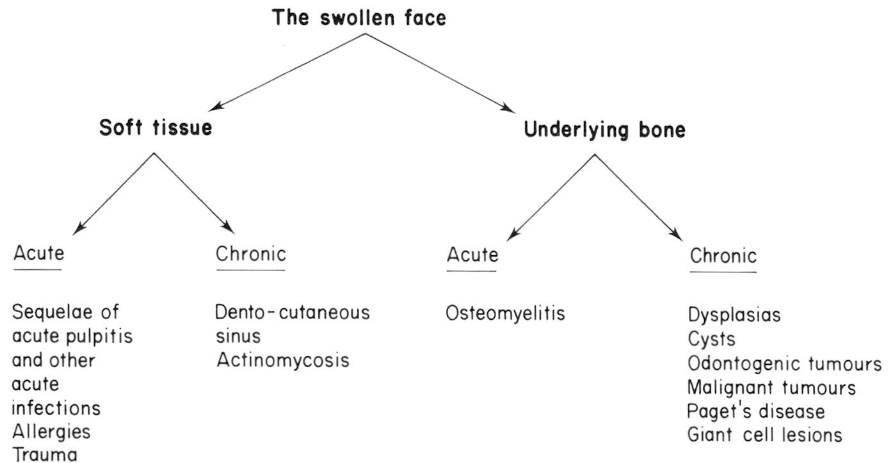

Fig. 3.1 A swollen face presentation.

ous restorative dental procedures or a blow to the tooth can also cause pulp death.

Early removal or drainage of the causative tooth is almost always the most humane, safe and effective treatment. If pus is localized in the soft tissues, tooth extraction or pulp extirpation alone is usually insufficient to establish full drainage.

The presence of pyrexia, cellulitis, enlarged regional lymph nodes and pus indicate vigorous antibiotic therapy, which is usually instituted before bacteriological identification and sensitivity testing. Both aerobic and anaerobic organisms are likely to be involved and the combined use of penicillin and metronidazole is a reasonable first step. When a specimen of pus can be obtained, more accurate antibiotic prescription and monitoring can follow.

Contamination with saliva should be avoided and the specimen sent at once to the laboratory, accompanied by a full history particularly mentioning the patient's recent antibiotic experience.

Amongst the less common causes of acute inflammatory facial swellings are acute suppurative sialoadenitis, mumps, acute maxillary sinusitis, acute dacryocystitis, boils, carbuncles and erysipelas.

Localized allergic reactions in soft tissues may present with a recent short history of relatively painless recurrent facial swelling. Cosmetic preparations, foodstuffs, local anaesthetic solutions, medicaments and dental restorative materials are occasionally identified as causative agents.

Facial swellings following *physical trauma* are often a combination of oedema and haematoma formation with or without underlying facial bone fracture. Similar swellings occur after difficult extractions, particularly of wisdom teeth, and local anaesthetic needles can damage small vessels with a resultant haematoma. Oedematous swellings are soft, and uninfected haematomas more solid and, if infected, tender to touch.

Chronic inflammatory conditions associated with non-vital teeth are sometimes difficult to diagnose. The patient presents with a mildly tender localized, reddened swelling on the skin of the face, with occasional episodes of discharge. It is often mistreated as a boil or an infected sebaceous cyst, until the true diagnosis of a *dento-cutaneous sinus* is made.

Early *cervico-facial actinomycosis* may present similarly, often at the anterior insertion of the masseter muscle. The history may show that some six weeks or more beforehand the oral mucosa was breached, perhaps by tooth extraction or mandibular fracture. Healing has taken place normally, but gradually a painless reddish-blue fluctuant lump has appeared. If previous discharges of pus have occurred, scarring may be followed by further abscess formation and discharge.

Bacteriological identification is important as energetic antibiotic treatment alone will effect a permanent cure. Characteristic so-called 'sulphur granules' may be found in the first outpouring of pus following incision. Such pus should be collected and sent immediately to the laboratory. Actinomyces colonies may sometimes be seen in tissue curetted from sites of infection but the diagnosis of actinomycosis depends both on the demonstration of colonies in pus or tissues and on culture of the organism.

Swellings within underlying bone

Almost all the mandible is accessible to bimanual palpation, but only the outer surfaces of the midfacial bones. Radiographs are essential for confirming clinical findings and also to begin the process of definitive diagnosis. The most useful general views are the rotational tomograph of the mandible and the standard occipitomental view for facial bones and anterior nasal sinuses.

Apart from acute osteomyelitis, most swellings originating in bone begin and may continue as silent, slow-growing expansions; many give rise to symptoms only if they become infected or, in the case of malignant neoplasms, ulcerated.

Dysplastic conditions of bone such as monostotic or polyostotic fibrous dysplasia and cherubism usually present in early life and may grow until the late teens. They can cause considerable deformity, usually as fusiform expansions of bone, displacing teeth and disturbing the normal sequence of eruption.

Fibrous dysplasia of mandible or maxilla is more frequently monostotic rather than polyostotic; if the latter, there may be accompanying skin pigmentation or endocrine dysfunction. The usual radiographic appearance is of the "orange-peel" or "ground glass" pattern, explained by the lesional tissue comprising numerous irregularly shaped trabeculae of metaplastic woven bone enmeshed in a stroma of vascular, fibroblastic fibrous tissue. Sometimes there is a more radiolucent, often multicystic, pattern on the radiograph, especially in the more aggressive form. In most instances growth ceases in early adult life.

There are no consistently abnormal serum chemical findings and biopsy is required for diagnosis, for which it is important to include adjacent normal bone; however, overlying expanded cortical plate is not particularly helpful. In fibrous dysplasia, lesional tissue merges with adjacent normal bone, whereas in ossifying fibroma, a benign neoplasm of continuous rather than restricted growth characteristics, tissue closely resembling that of fibrous dysplasia has a more distinct margin.

Cherubism is a hereditary condition and tends to arise at a younger age than fibrous dysplasia; multilocular radiolucencies are present usually in more than one quadrant of the jaws and are occupied by vascular fibroblastic tissue in which there are scattered foci of multinucleated giant cells.

By the time *cysts of the jaws* cause facial swelling, intraoral examination will usually reveal a large, painless, bluish fluctuant buccal expansion. The diagnosis of cysts is covered on p. 44.

Odontogenic tumours such as the ameloblastoma and the myxoma similarly are usually large before they become evident extraorally. Unlike cysts, they generally expand the bone at both cortices and remain solid to palpation. Although radiography is important, showing a typical multiloculated (though occasionally unilocular) radiolucency, a definitive diagnosis can be achieved only by examination of a biopsy. Treatment based on clinical and radiographic diagnosis alone has led to some unfortunate disasters.

The choice of biopsy site must be made with subsequent surgery in mind. It is preferable to use a mucoperiosteal flap whose repair line will be at a distance from the bone biopsy. Secondary infection of the tumour through a biopsy site causes unnecessary complications.

Although there are several histological variants of the *ameloblastoma*, they behave in a similar, locally infiltrative manner. Islands of neoplastic epithelium are often found within inter-trabecular spaces beyond the apparent radiological limits of the tumour. Consequently, treatment must ensure that surgical resection margins are made in normal bone, which is generally estimated to be 2 cm beyond the radiological margins distally and mesially. At the cortical plates, however, there is usually a well-defined limit to the tumour and only rarely is this breached, with extension of neoplasm into adjacent soft tissue. Where there is doubt, extra-periosteal resection is indicated.

It is useful to remember that approximately 80 per cent of ameloblastomas arise in the mandible, mostly in the angle or molar region.

The clinical and radiological features of the *odontogenic myxoma* are similar to the ameloblastoma, except for a more even distribution between mandible and maxilla. It has similar locally infiltrative behaviour and may be extremely difficult to remove from the interstices of adjacent bone, especially in the more gelatinous or mucoid forms. Unless wide resection is undertaken at the initial operation, local recurrence is to be expected.

Carcinomas may cause bony expansion. A squamous cell carcinoma or adenocarcinoma from the antrum may occasionally present as a swelling of the upper alveolar bone or palate. Either jaw may be the location for a secondary deposit from a carcinoma elsewhere, particularly the breast, bronchus or thyroid; primary carcinomas rarely arise from odontogenic epithelial remnants, or cyst lining epithelium. These possibilities should be particularly borne in mind when a swelling of the jaw bone is associated with the sinister sign of skin anaesthesia. Patients with *Burkitt's lymphoma* may show early jaw involvement in either single or multiple sites.

Paget's disease involving the mandible or facial bones occurs in middle and later life. In the mouth it often presents as a rather craggy expansion of bone covered with normal mucosa. If teeth are involved they may become loose or spaced; the edentulous patient may complain about dentures becoming ill-fitting, and there may be a history of dentures having to be made repeatedly over a period of years. Radiological changes show a variety of patterns, of which the commonest is a rather ill-defined mixture of radiolucent and radiodense areas. Teeth involved in affected bone often exhibit hypercementosis, which may lead to ankylosis. There may be accompanying neurological effects caused by compression of cranial nerves passing through foraminae. Selective skeletal radiography and serum chemistry should be undertaken, the latter to seek raised levels of alkaline phosphatase.

Histological changes in Paget's disease of bone appear to reflect a localized cyclical pattern. Some areas exhibit extensive osteoblastic deposition of new osteoid tissue and bone, whilst elsewhere there may be numerous osteoclasts undertaking removal of bone; hence the patchy radiographic appearances. Stromal fibrous tissue is often very vascular and within the bony trabeculae there is ample evidence of previous resorption and redeposition of bone such that the pattern of reversal lines produces a typical mosaic effect. Should teeth be extracted from within an area of bone affected by Paget's disease, these various microscopical features explain why in some instances excessive bleeding, in others subsequent infection and bone necrosis, and occasionally inadvertent removal of a considerable portion of accompanying ankylosed bone, may be associated undesirable complications.

Any surgical interference with Pagetoid bone, including biopsy, should be undertaken with a knowledge of the difficulties. If biopsy is essential to diagnosis, it is better to raise a mucoperiosteal flap and take a bone specimen at a distance from the soft-tissue repair line.

Central giant cell lesions within the jaws are most commonly granulomas but occasionally are associated with hyperparathyroidism. Presentation tends to be as a slowly expanding swelling that may eventually undermine the cortical plate to such an extent that a bluish hue is imparted to overlying mucosa and "egg-shell crackling" may be elicited. Radiologically, the features are those of a multiloculated (occasionally unilocular) radiolucency, and histologically lesional tissue comprises numerous multinucleated osteoclast-like giant cells supported by vascular, fibroblastic stroma of delicately fibrillar connective tissue. Bone or osteoid may divide lesional tissue into lobules and account for the delicate septae sometimes seen on radiographs. Central giant cell granulomas are commonest in childhood and early adult life, affect females more than males and the mandible more than the maxilla. Local removal and curettage is usually followed by normal healing.

When tissue typical of a giant cell granuloma is recovered from a jaw lesion, it is necessary to eliminate the possibility that the patient is suffering from hyperparathyroidism, in which the microscopical features can be identical. Raised serum calcium levels will usually point to hyperparathyroidism and lead to further appropriate investigation and treatment. Loss of the radiological lamina dura around teeth is not an absolutely reliable sign of hyperparathyroidism.

White and red lesions of the oral mucosa

Normal oral mucosa exhibits different hues of pink depending upon local site variations in keratinization, vascularity and elasticity. Disturbances to the normal pattern of colour largely arise because of changes in the keratinization properties of the stratified squamous epithelial lining or within the epithelium itself. Sebaceous glands, "Fordyce's spots", may occasionally become prominent enough to concern the patient. The accurate diagnosis of white and red lesions is important because they include some pre-cancerous states and very early invasive carcinomas.

The term "leukoplakia" still causes much confusion. Some use it clinically to describe any white patch on oral mucosa, others reserve it for white patches with malignant potential, whilst still others use strict histological criteria. The WHO definition confines its use to a clinical lesion and is one of exclusion—A white patch or plaque which cannot be removed by rubbing and which cannot be classified clinically or histologically as any other diagnosable disease. The approach adopted here is to avoid the use of the term and to describe the various causes of the more important white and red lesions of oral mucosa and to give guidance for their diagnosis and management. While many of the conditions described may sometimes present as purely white or purely red lesions, they are often mixed. The following subdivision is based on the predominating colour.

Biopsies of these lesions should include normal adjacent mucosa and be sufficiently deep to provide the pathologist with adequate and representative material. Appropriate fixation is essential. From the diversity of conditions that can produce similar clinical appearances, it will be obvious that a full history and description should accompany each specimen to the laboratory.

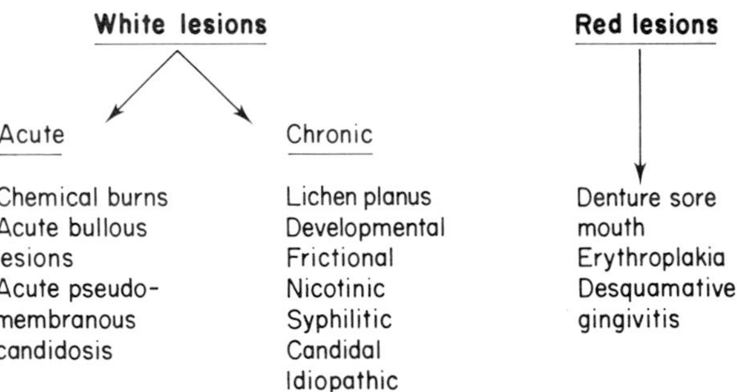

Fig. 3.2 White and red lesions of the oral mucosa.

White lesions

White patches with an *acute history* are usually the result of sloughing and waterlogging of surface epithelium. This may be caused by *chemical burns* (e.g. by aspirin, or misplaced dental medicaments and materials). Similar white patches follow *acute bullous lesions* as seen in the Stevens-Johnson syndrome (erythema multiforme exudativum). In addition any ulcerated oral surface rapidly becomes covered by a whitish-yellow infected film of fibrin.

Acute pseudo-membranous candidosis, or thrush, is more common at the extremes of age and in patients on antibiotic, steroid, irradiation, immunosuppressive or antimetabolite treatment, or suffering from diabetes mellitus or other debilitating disease, including AIDS. The patches can be scraped off to reveal an erythematous base. Blastospores and hyphae typical of *Candida albicans* can be demonstrated in smears made from the white slough and the organisms can also be cultured.

White patches of longer standing are of more importance.

The lesions of *lichen planus* may occur in the mouth with or without skin lesions. Although there are many variations in appearance, the commonest is a reticular pattern of interlacing white lines, sometimes against an erythematous background, that are often bilaterally placed on the buccal mucosa in the molar regions. Palliative treatment is all that can be offered to symptomatic lichen planus sufferers, but the possibility of a lichenoid drug reaction should be excluded as early resolution usually follows withdrawal of the causative drug.

Hyperkeratosis and epithelial hyperplasia presumably account for the white striated pattern, whereas atrophic areas of epithelium most probably are responsible for erythematous patches.

Oral lichen planus is usually regarded as a completely innocent condition, but carcinoma has been occasionally reported arising in the erosive form.

Developmental keratoses are uncommon, but need to be identified. As far as is known, they have no pre-malignant potential. The so-called "white sponge naevus" is usually first noticed in childhood. All areas of the oral mucosa may be affected. The lesion is white and furrowed, and sometimes the surface is flaky. Both clinically and histologically it has "spongy" characteristics, expressing saliva when compressed and showing pronounced intra-cellular oedema in the epithelial prickle cell layer.

The abnormal formation of keratin in non-keratinized areas of oral mucosa and its excessive formation in normally keratinized areas result in white adherent patches; at first these are thin and filmy but go on to thickened, fissured and sometimes nodular lesions.

Chronic friction may be caused by a denture clasp, an ill-fitting denture base, a rough dental restoration or cheek chewing. Malignant change is extremely rare and resolution usually follows removal of the cause.

Excessive exposure to tobacco, whether chewed, smoked or snuffed, is related to a raised incidence of keratosis and oral cancer. The problem is seen most commonly in the Indian subcontinent and in South-East Asia.

The condition in the United Kingdom is less frequent and less florid, *tobacco keratosis* being limited to a specific area of insult, the soft palate in heavy pipe smokers where the hard palate is protected by a denture, on the tongue related to the pipe stem, or in the buccal mucosa adjacent to the parking place of a tobacco quid.

Patients can often be alarmed by the sight of their palate exhibiting bright red spots surrounded by well-defined whitish-grey plaques. The explanation is usually the straight-forward one that increased keratinization has blocked minor salivary gland ducts and caused a localized swelling from the dammed back saliva. Subsequent trauma to the most prominent parts removes keratin and leaves red exposed areas.

Cessation of the tobacco habit often leads to considerable improvement in appearance of the mucosa.

A keratosis appearing on the tongue should always call for serological examination for syphilis. Syphilitic keratosis of the tongue, which is now a rare occurrence, has a relatively high malignant potential compared with other types.

Hyperkeratotic patches may be associated with long-standing infection by *Candida albicans*. *Chronic hyperplastic candidosis* is particularly prone to occur at the angles of the mouth, sometimes extending onto skin as angular cheilitis or along the occlusal line of buccal mucosa. Both hyperplastic and atrophic areas of epithelium are usually present; when the latter are prominent, the clinical appearance is of a red and white "speckled" lesion. Such a speckled appearance, and the presence of Candida organisms, is associated with a greater likelihood of subsequent malignancy. The extent of any increased risk is uncertain, however, as there are many examples of chronic hyperplastic candidosis that behave innocuously. Nevertheless, it would seem that the wisest course is to see how the lesions respond to antifungal treatment, and to remove any remaining white patch for further microscopical examination. Patients with this condition may be more likely to suffer from systemic diseases, such as anaemia and diabetes mellitus.

Most keratotic white patches have no demonstrable cause and few satisfactory generalizations can be made concerning their malignant potential. However, *keratotic areas on the floor of mouth and the ventral surface of the tongue* have a high incidence of carcinomatous change (in one series as high as 50 per cent) and must be managed with great care and thoroughness. Recently, so-called "hairy" leukoplakia has been associated with AIDS.

Management of keratotic patches

1. Confirm presumptive diagnosis by biopsy and, in the tongue, also by specific serology. No further action is necessary for developmental keratoses.

2. Search for possible causes and correct them. If the biopsy report indicates no evidence of epithelial dysplasia, keep the lesion under observation.

3. If there is no progressive resolution, remove the whole keratotic area with a surrounding margin of normal mucosa and keep the site under subsequent observation.

Where the biopsy has indicated dysplastic changes, laser or cryoprobe destruction render serial sectioning and examination of the whole excised lesion for evidence of invasive change impossible and may place the surgeon and patient in a temporary fool's paradise.

There is no place for putting a dysplastic lesion on probation and following it with repeated biopsies.

4. *Biopsy*—The selection of biopsy site should take into account those areas where epithelial dysplasia or early carcinomatous change is more likely to be found. The following clinical appearances may act as a guide—white speckling on an erythematous mucosa, loss of keratin in a particular area in an otherwise homogeneous white plaque, areas of superficial ulceration, areas of cracking and fissuring, and where there is nodular thickening or excrescence.

Biopsy in this part of the body is a relatively simple procedure and, in the face of ready access and visibility, half measures such as exfoliative cytology or intra vitam toluidine blue staining have little or no place. Both of these methods produce too many false results. It is worth re-emphasising the need to ensure that a biopsy is of sufficient depth to enable the pathologist to study uncompromised areas of the underlying connective tissue, where he may be in doubt as to whether micro-invasion has already occurred. It may be helpful in further management if the biopsy is marked in some way, perhaps by passing a suture through a relatively unimportant part; this assists the pathologist in orientating the specimen to determine the micro-anatomical location of any dysplasia.

Red lesions

Most red lesions of the oral mucosa are inflammatory in origin; the commonest is the so-called "*denture sore mouth*", which is usually precisely defined by the fitting area of an upper denture. The mucosa is dark red and boggy and sometimes is associated with papillary hyperplasia, which may exhibit pseudo-epitheliomatous hyperplasia and can be the cause of overdiagnosis if a superficial biopsy is sent to an unsuspecting pathologist. It is produced by the prolonged wearing of an ill-fitting and insanitary denture. Candidal infection can usually be demonstrated by culture from swabs of both the mucosal and denture surfaces, and is often associated with an angular cheilitis.

Defined, fiery red, velvety changes of the oral mucosa should be viewed with suspicion and submitted to biopsy. *Erythroplakia* is characterized by epithelial atrophy, epithelial dysplasia, carcinoma-in-situ or invasive carcinoma. It is a similar condition to Bowen's disease and must be submitted to early surgical excision and close follow-up.

"*Desquamative gingivitis*", in which the gums are bright red and sore, is usually due to lichen planus or benign mucous membrane pemphigoid.

Red and white lesions, more common on, or exclusive to, the tongue are covered on p. 42.

Ulcers and bullae

Any oral bullous or vesicular lesion is readily broken down by trauma to form a shallow erosion or ulcer. Bullae or vesicles are, therefore, more likely to be observed in protected parts of the mouth, such as the buccal sulci, and many ulcerated lesions may have a short-lived vesicular stage that is rarely observed.

Infections

Acute primary herpetic gingivostomatitis is mainly a disease of children. Prodromal irritability and

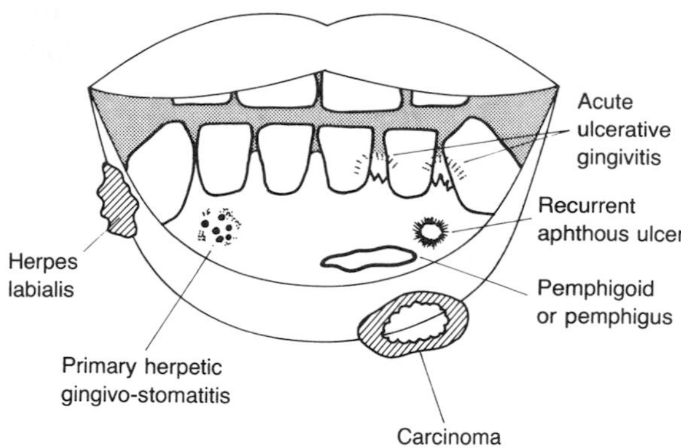

Fig. 3.3 Ulcers and bullae.

malaise is followed by intense erythema of the gums and oral mucosa on which scattered vesicles appear. There is high fever, salivation and enlargement of cervical lymph nodes; the condition is often mistakenly ascribed to "teething". Diagnosis is almost invariably achieved from the history and clinical examination, and only rarely is it necessary to resort to cytological examination or virological tests. The vesicles are caused by degeneration of epithelial cells which may be aggregated to form typical multinucleated forms and exhibit viral inclusion bodies.

A more familiar expression of the same virus is the secondary form, *herpes labialis* or a "cold sore", seen mainly in adults. The vesicles occur usually in localized sites at the junction of the vermilion border and the skin, only very rarely being found intra-orally. The vesicles usually rupture early to leave a crusted ulcer that heals in 7–10 days; recurrent crops occur from time to time, often being precipitated by fatigue, exposure to sunlight or fever. The virus probably lies dormant in local neural ganglion cells between such events.

Herpes zoster can also affect oral mucosa, where the vesicles are distributed over the area supplied by the affected nerve. Histopathological features of the vesicle are identical to those of the other herpetic infections.

A distinctive infection characterized by non-specific ulcers at the tips of the gingival interdental papillae is *acute ulcerative gingivitis* (Vincent's infection). The causative organisms are Borrelia vincenti and Bacillus fusiformis, which can be observed in smears from the affected gingiva. In addition to ulceration, the gingival tissue is swollen, inflamed and bleeds easily; there is a distinctive halitosis. Successful treatment is achieved by vigorous oral hygiene and metronidazole or penicillin. Malnourished children compromised by a recent acute infection may suffer spread of acute ulcerative gingivitis to other parts of the oral cavity, where tissue necrosis and destruction is known as "*cancrum oris*".

Tuberculosis and *syphilis*, in their various stages, may also be responsible for chronic ulceration of oral mucosa, the tongue being the commonest site affected.

Trauma

Mechanical, chemical or physical trauma can all be responsible for *non-specific ulceration* of the oral mucosa. A greyish-yellow slough covers a defect in the epithelium and is surrounded by reddened mucosa. If healing does not occur within a few days after the source of irritation has been removed, then the ulcer should be biopsied as a suspected carcinoma.

Autoimmune

The early diagnosis of *benign mucous membrane pemphigoid* and *pemphigus* is important; the former because early treatment can prevent conjunctival scarring, and the latter because of the high mortality in untreated cases. In both cases biopsy is essential and, in addition to the usual histopathological examination, immunological staining techniques are employed on frozen sections of fresh biopsy material.

Unknown aetiology

Many agents have been suggested as a cause of recurrent *aphthous ulcers* but there is no conclusive proof. These ulcers are common and occur at irregular intervals. They are shallow and painful, being classified as major, minor or herpetiform types in decreasing order of size. Healing occurs in 7–10 days but is sometimes delayed and accompanied by scarring in the major type. Failure to heal indicates that a biopsy should be taken to exclude malignancy. There are no distinctive microscopical diagnostic features of recurrent aphthae. An association with certain deficiencies or diseases has been established in some instances and appropriate replacement therapy can prevent further recurrences. The possibilities of coeliac disease, or deficiencies of oestrogen, vitamin B_{12}, folic acid or iron should all be considered. Local traumatic factors may act as precipitators and should be eliminated.

Ulceration may also be a component of *erythema multiforme* and oral *Crohn's disease*, though the latter is often more noted for the "cobblestone" features of the buccal mucosa.

Most serious of all is the *squamous cell carcinoma*, for which ulcerated mucosa is the commonest form of presentation. Any non-healing ulcer with induration and everted margins should be considered malignant until proved otherwise. Biopsy should include a portion of adjacent normal mucosa. No site in the mouth is exempt from this possibility, for which the most significant aetiological factor would appear to be combined abuse of tobacco and alcohol. If the mandible is involved, there may be rapid spread along the inferior dental canal, with consequent neural symptoms. Metastasis to regional lymph nodes is common in late stages but more widespread secondary deposits are relatively uncommon. Patients may exhibit "field change" of the oral mucosa and those who have already had one carcinoma of the upper digestive or respiratory tract are particularly susceptible to a second.

Conditions peculiar to the tongue and floor of mouth

Patients who put their tongues out far enough are often worried by what they see. The foliate papillae or the circumvallate papillae are occasionally presented to the surgeon as a focus for cancer phobia.

The so-called "*median rhomboid glossitis*" not only causes anxiety to patients but may well result in mismanagement. A midline, slightly raised and sometimes sunken rhomboid area devoid of papillae is occasionally seen at the junction of the posterior one-third and anterior two-thirds of the tongue. It is not a neoplastic condition; although some believe it to be an embryological remnant, there is increasing evidence implicating a candidal infection.

Histopathologically, there are grounds for confusion between an early invasive carcinoma and median rhomboid glossitis because the surface epithelium frequently exhibits pseudo-epitheliomatous hyperplasia. It is important that surgeons and pathologists should be aware of this particular difficulty and should also take into account the fact that carcinoma in this site is very rare.

Geographic tongue, or erythema migrans, exhibits a curious and varying loss of filiform papillae on the dorsum of the tongue. The lesion is painless, very superficial, usually erythematous and has an irregular whitish outline which changes over a matter of days. Its cause is unknown and it has no sinister significance. The diagnosis is visual.

Black hairy tongue in contrast is caused by a massive overgrowth of the filiform papillae mixed with saprophytic micro-organisms and stained by tobacco smoke and foodstuffs. It has no sinister significance and the diagnosis is again visual.

The presence of a single, shallow, relatively painless ulcer at the tip of the tongue should raise suspicion of a *syphilitic chancre*.

Lichen planus on the dorsum of the tongue may produce a horseshoe-shaped loss of papillae so that smooth patches are seen on either side of the

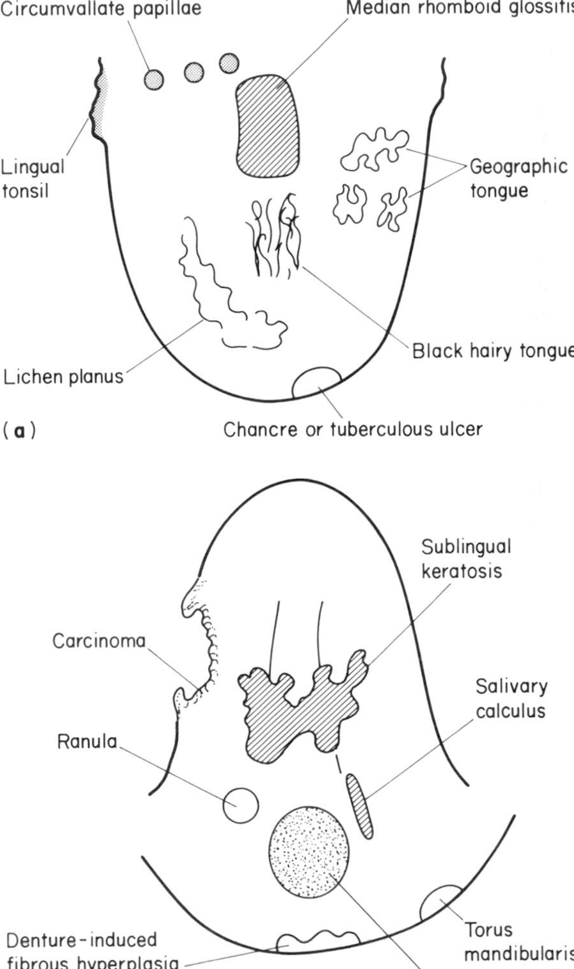

Fig. 3.4 Conditions peculiar to the tongue (a) and floor of the mouth (b).

mid-line with union just behind the tip. More pronounced effects include shallow ulceration over a similar distribution. White striae may be evident in the areas of smooth mucosa but in mild cases these can sometimes be revealed only by observing the dorsum of the tongue through a glass slide applied firmly to it.

White patches on the ventral surface of the tongue and adjacent floor of the mouth have been mentioned above (*see* p. 40).

The lateral aspect of the tongue and the paralingual gutter are common sites for *squamous cell carcinoma*. In examining these areas, the tip of the tongue should be grasped with dry gauze and the area effectively displayed to eye and finger. Normal lingual tonsillar tissue may be mistaken by both patient or surgeon for something more sinister.

Unilateral lesions in the floor of the mouth include *ranula* and *submandibular salivary calculus*. Both swellings lie superficially in the line of the submandibular duct. The calculus is hard and, when anteriorly placed, reveals its yellowish colour through the stretched mucosa. The ranula is usually a retention or extravasation cyst associated with the sublingual salivary gland. Its swelling is pinkish-blue and often covered by a greatly thinned mucosa. The excised ranula and associated sublingual gland should be submitted for histopathological examination, as a salivary gland neoplasm can sometimes present with a similar clinical picture.

A rounded, pudgy, soft tissue midline swelling may rightly be diagnosed as a *sublingual dermoid*. However, it could also be *ectopic thyroid tissue* and that tissue be the only functioning part of the gland. Incisional biopsy, or aspiration of contents for examination of a stained smear to detect squames, is therefore a necessary preliminary to more radical surgery.

A common place for hyperplastic reaction to the irritation of a denture is over the genial tubercles.

Localized intra-oral swellings

Most localized soft-tissue swellings in the mouth are due to reactive hyperplastic tissue responses. True neoplasms, benign or malignant, are relatively uncommon by comparison. In spite of this clinical generalisation, all excised tissue must be submitted for microscopical examination however innocent and obvious the diagnosis may appear to be.

Reactive hyperplasia

Although the *epulides* may be separately classified and described, it is generally recognized that they are all different stages of a hyperplastic reaction to irritation, possibly from a carious tooth cavity, an overhanging filling or sub-gingival calculus. The initial reaction is in the form of red, bleeding, ulcerated granulation tissue adjacent to an interdental papilla. This soon becomes epithelialized and replacement by fibrous tissue occurs. The epulis is now firm, pink and does not bleed. In a few cases, giant cells may be a feature and the lesion is more vascular, looks purplish instead of pink, and bleeds more easily. A *peripheral giant cell lesion* appears to be confined to the region of the former temporary dentition. The so-called *pregnancy granuloma* starts as an enlarged interdental papilla on the background of a generalized marginal gingivitis. The lesion gradually enlarges and usually recedes after the birth, leaving a fibrous remnant.

Just occasionally a *secondary deposit* from a distant site such as bronchus, breast, or thyroid can present as a rather friable epulis.

Ill-fitting dentures are a source of chronic irritation and particularly at their periphery may induce a cycle of superficial ulceration and repair by fibrous tissue. As the bone supporting the denture resorbs, so the denture sinks further and induces another round of ulceration and repair. The eventual result may be multiple, firm, raised, pink ridges and furrows parallel to the edge of the denture.

Where there is a substantial inflammatory element, an ulcerated and infiltrated area of reactive hyperplasia can resemble clinically a primary squamous cell carcinoma. Although carcinomatous change is rare within such lesions, one must be wary of the carcinoma that mimics *denture-induced hyperplasia*, particularly the *verrucous carcinoma*.

All denture-induced hyperplasias improve enormously once the denture is not worn for several days. The inflammatory element resolves, leaving only fibrous remnants to be dealt with.

A smooth, rounded, pink swelling which may be sessile or pedunculated and growing from the buccal mucosa is often incorrectly termed "fibroma". True fibromas are rare and this type of lesion is usually described clinically as a *fibro-epithelial polyp*; it probably represents the end stage of a reactive lesion.

Infective conditions

Acute or chronic *sequelae of pulpitis* may give rise to localized oral swellings. A periapical abscess usually points buccally into the mouth. Teeth with deeply placed apices and those towards the posterior part of the mouth, depending on their relationship to the buccinator attachment, are exceptions to this and may point onto the skin of the face.

The subperiosteal abscess rapidly becomes a fluctuant submucous swelling; it is often yellowish and is closely related to the causative tooth. Once the abscess has discharged, it leaves a leaking sinus; this is what most patients refer to when they complain of a "gum boil".

Lateral periodontal abscesses should be distinguished from periapical abscesses as management may be different. These abscesses are usually associated with pre-existing, chronic, destructive periodontal disease. They are situated part of the way down the root surface and not at the apex. The diagnosis can be confirmed by gentle probing down the associated periodontal pocket, as this usually releases pus.

Mucosal soft-tissue around partially erupted teeth, more frequently in the lower wisdom tooth area, is often subject to acute inflammatory episodes. The pocket under the flap of gum partially covering the tooth becomes infected, the overlying tissue swells and then is traumatized by an upper tooth. The gum around the involved tooth is swollen and oedematous, and pus is usually to be seen exuding from the pocket. Diagnosis and treatment of such *acute pericoronitis* are usually carried out without recourse to laboratory tests.

Lesions of minor salivary glands

Apart from the main aggregations in the parotid, submandibular and sublingual salivary glands, salivary tissue is present in most areas of the mouth and can give rise to localized swellings when it is involved in cystic or neoplastic changes.

A *mucocoele* or *mucous extravasation cyst* most commonly presents as a rounded, bluish, clearly cystic lesion between ½ cm and 1 cm in diameter. The history is usually one of several episodes of discharge and recurrence.

The commonest tumour of the salivary glands is the *pleomorphic adenoma* and its usual site is near the junction of the hard and soft palate and the tuberosity region of the maxilla.

The swelling is rounded, fixed to underlying structures and may have the elastic feel of a squash ball. As it enlarges, the overlying mucosa becomes bluish and finally ulcerates.

Occasionally, malignancy supervenes in long-standing pleomorphic adenomas, or they may be malignant from the outset. This takes the form of a carcinoma, and the presence of necrosis or haemorrhage within the tumour may alert the pathologist to it.

One of the characteristic microscopical features of the benign pleomorphic adenoma is the tendency to have satellite foci beyond the limits of the apparent edge of the neoplastic tissue. Their presence explains the high frequency of recurrence if simple enucleation is attempted rather than excision.

Of the other salivary gland neoplasms, the *adenoid cystic carcinoma* is most common in the palate (of intra-oral sites) and presents clinically as a fairly slowly growing swelling. The propensity for this malignant tumour to extend along perineural spaces makes it difficult to eradicate. Nonetheless, surgery remains the treatment of choice.

Both pleomorphic adenomas and adenoid cystic carcinomas, when in the palate, usually prove to extend more deeply into palatal bone than their surface features might suggest. The use of computerized axial tomography is particularly helpful in revealing their approximate limits.

Cysts of the jaws

The physical signs produced by most jaw cysts are very similar. They are slow-growing, symptomatically silent, and cause damage by displacement and not by invasion; consequently, adjacent teeth are tilted and displaced but rarely eroded and neurovascular bundles are pushed aside but function is not altered.

A hard, smooth buccal expansion is usually first noted. As the cyst enlarges, overlying bone is resorbed and the swelling becomes softer and in parts fluctuant; later still, overlying tissues become so thin that the swelling appears to be blue-black.

A midline fluctuant swelling in the incisive foramen region is likely to be a naso-palatine cyst. Sometimes this type of cyst is responsible for an otherwise inexplicable salty taste in the patient's mouth, a small communication being undetected.

Radiologically, a smooth, well-defined outline to a radiolucent area is suggestive of a cystic condition. Close relationship of the cyst to a non-vital tooth suggests an inflammatory origin, a *radicular cyst*, though it has to be remembered that an involved tooth may have been previously extracted. A tooth crown inside a cystic area is suggestive of a *dentigerous cyst*, but is not diagnostic; similar radiological appearances may occur in the ameloblastoma or the odontogenic keratocyst.

Both radicular and dentigerous cysts are usually lined by stratified squamous epithelium; the former more often shows a variable degree of inflammation and the latter is more likely to have cuboidal and mucous cells within the lining.

The pre-operative diagnosis of the *odontogenic keratocyst* is essential as its well-founded reputation for recurrence may demand a different approach to management.

Although the odontogenic keratocyst can occur anywhere in the jaws, it typically presents as a large cystic swelling at the angle of the mandible. Indeed it might be a useful aphorism to state that "all large cysts at the angle of the mandible are odontogenic keratocysts until proved otherwise".

There are certain radiological hints to diagnosis. The outline of the radiolucent area, although clear cut, may be lobulated or crenated, rather than a single smooth sweep. Multiloculation is a fairly common feature and the rare occurrence of more than one tooth apparently inside the cyst should raise suspicions. The odontogenic keratocyst, although having many clinical and radiological features of the ameloblastoma, rarely causes resorption of adjacent teeth.

The odontogenic keratocyst has the most distinctive lining of all the jaw cysts. As its name implies, it is keratinized and there is a regular layer of supporting stratified squamous epithelium that often exhibits basal cell palisading and a smooth junction with the underlying thin fibrous tissue wall. These features tend to be lost if the cyst becomes inflamed and the lining is then indistinguishable from other types of cyst. It is thought that the relatively flimsy nature of the keratocyst wall may lead to portions of it being retained when removal is attempted and that these contribute to the high recurrence rate. Of more significance in this regard, however, is the frequent presence of "daughter cysts" around the periphery of the main cyst.

Pre-operative confirmation of the diagnosis can sometimes be made by electrophoretic analysis of fluid aspirate and a film examination for keratin squames. Aspiration is best achieved by using a wide bore needle with a second one for an air inlet if necessary. Infection can prejudice the subsequent management and accurate microscopical diagnosis; aspiration should therefore be done under sterile conditions and antibiotic cover.

The presence of cholesterol crystals in aspirated fluid will almost certainly be indicative that a cyst is present, and that it is probably either a radicular or dentigerous cyst. Keratin squames point strongly to an odontogenic keratocyst, as does a finding of less than 4 g/100 ml protein in the cyst fluid. If the cyst is inflamed, however, neither of these tests will be helpful. When submitting tissue for microscopical examination, either the whole cyst or if marsupialisation is indicated the whole of the portion removed, should be sent; small snippets from the wall are likely to be at best unhelpful and at worst misleading. Needless to say, a clear account of the state and relationships of associated teeth should accompany the specimen.

There are less common types of jaw cyst that apparently arise from various odontogenic or other epithelial remnants as well as some uncommon, non-epitheliated cysts.

As will be apparent from other sections of this Chapter, several different conditions may present as a localized swelling of jaw bones with similar physical signs to those produced by cysts.

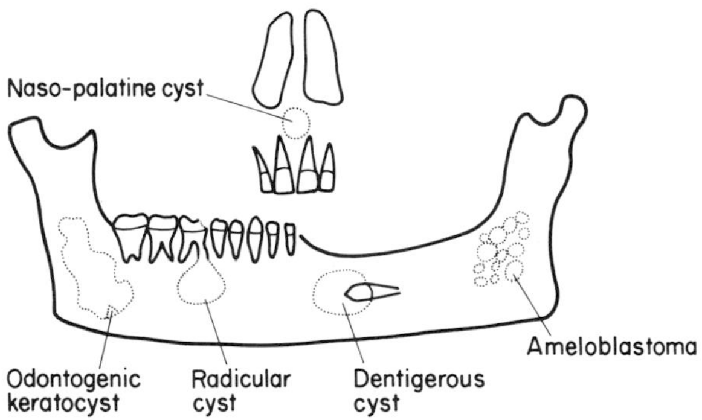

Fig. 3.5 Cystic lesions of the jaws presenting as intra-oral swellings.

Benign neoplasms and developmental anomalies

Benign neoplasms of bone, fat, connective tissue, epithelium, nerve and vessels all occur in the mouth from time to time and exhibit the same characteristics as elsewhere in the body. However, the haemangioma and the lymphangioma have probably greater significance in the mouth.

The *cavernous haemangioma* usually presents as

a purple, lobulated swelling which fills up when the head is lowered and which can be emptied on finger pressure. It can affect any part of the mouth, and even small cavernous haemangiomas may be protuberant and can cause embarrassing bleeding if damaged during chewing. Treatment is indicated if such a risk is present.

The *lymphangioma* usually presents as a thickening with a clear or pink, bubbly surface and is occasionally the site of haemorrhage, when it can swell alarmingly. Lymphangiomas affecting tongue and pharynx are potentially dangerous to the airway, particularly if they are of any size.

Squamous cell papillomas are small, benign, epithelial neoplasms with a white, cauliflower-like surface; they may be confused with warts on the oral mucosa. Microscopical examination is necessary to exclude verrucous carcinoma.

Torus palatinus is the name given to a symmetrical, rounded overgrowth of bone situated at the maxillary midline suture; it is covered with normal mucosa and usually noticed in middle life. A similar symmetrical condition known as *torus mandibularis* sometimes appears on the lingual aspect of the alveolus in the lower premolar region. Tori only have clinical significance if they interfere with the fitting of a denture.

Malignant neoplasms

Carcinomas or sarcomas arising from oral tissues may in their early stages present as localized swellings, as may secondary deposits to various oral sites or extensions from adjacent regions such as the maxillary antrum. Leukaemias can present as swelling of the gums.

The patient with inability to open the mouth

The term "trismus" is now loosely and almost universally used for the symptom of inability to open the mouth fully whatever the underlying cause.

Most trismus is temporary in nature, but it should not be forgotten that to some patients it carries overtones of "lockjaw" or disabling rheumatism.

Temporary conditions

Acute infective conditions in the tissues adjacent to the jaw joint are associated with pain on opening the mouth. Muscle guarding must be the principal cause of this type of trismus, although there may be some element of inflammatory infiltration of the muscles of mastication.

Acute pericoronitis associated with a partially erupted lower wisdom tooth, acute sore throat, quinsy or mumps are common causes.

Some degree of trismus almost inevitably follows the *removal of an impacted wisdom tooth* with its associated oedema and haematoma formation. If the symptom is not improving after two or three days, then infection should be considered as an additional cause.

Occasionally, an *inferior dental block* injection may be followed by trismus, either due to fortuitous minor vascular damage by the needle point with haematoma formation, the introduction of infection or a chemically-contaminated local anaesthetic solution, or merely by injecting an excessive quantity of local anaesthetic solution.

A blow to the jaw may cause haemarthrosis, an intracapsular fracture or an extracapsular fracture of the mandible, or a dislocation, all of which render the patient unwilling or unable to open the mouth.

Internal joint derangement need not necessarily be caused by sudden trauma. It can occur in the *mandibular pain-dysfunction syndrome* as a result of abnormal chewing habits, faulty mandibular posture or occlusal anomalies.

Amongst the *medical causes of trismus*, tetanus, tetany and the spasmodic trismus which sometimes follows the use of the phenothiazine group of drugs should be considered.

Conditions of longer standing

Extra-articular causes

Burns, major surgery, radiotherapy or oral submucous fibrosis can cause such *scarring of soft-tissue* as to limit severely the movement of the mandible. The diagnosis is usually clear, but the management can prove extremely difficult.

Intra-articular causes

Bony or fibrous ankylosis sometimes follows intracapsular fractures and pyogenic infections of the joint in early childhood.

Disorganization of the joint when involved in *osteoarthritic or rheumatoid change* often results in pain and limitation of movement but rarely in ankylosis.

Psychological disturbances are sometimes the cause of trismus. The symptom usually dates from some form of dental treatment or minor jaw injury. Apart from the inability to open the mouth, no other physical abnormality can be identified and the jaw opens fully and freely as soon as the patient is submitted to a general anaesthetic. On return to consciousness, trismus returns.

If the cause, be it intra- or extra-articular, is unilateral, the chin will deviate to the abnormal side when the patient is encouraged to thrust his jaw directly forward with the teeth together. The small amount of forward movement required to demonstrate this physical sign is present even in severe, unilateral ankylosis cases.

Tomographic radiography is often required to clinch the diagnosis in cases of longer standing. Laboratory investigations have little if any role to play.

Further reading

Pindborg JJ, Hjørting-Hansen E. *Atlas of Diseases of the Jaws*. Copenhagen: Munksgaard, 1974.

Kiley HC, Kay LW, Seward GR. *Benign Cystic Lesions of the Jaws*, 3rd edition. Edinburgh: Churchill Livingstone, 1977.

Wahi PN, Cohen B, Luthra Usha K, Torloni H. *et al. Histological Typing of Oral and Oropharyngeal Tumours*. International Histological Classification of Tumours No. 4, World Health Organization, 1971.

Pindborg JJ, Kramer IRH, Torloni H. *et al. Histological Typing of Odontogenic Tumours, Jaw Cysts and Allied Lesions*. International Histological Classification of Tumours No. 5, World Health Organization 1971.

Renson CE, ed. *Oral Diseases*. London: Update Books, 1978.

Lucas RB. *Pathology of Tumours of the Oral Tissues*, 4th edition. Edinburgh: Churchill Livingstone, 1984.

Shafer WG, Hine MK, Levy BV. *Textbook of Oral Pathology*, 4th edition. Philadelphia: W. B. Saunders, 1983.

4

Oesophagus

RM Kirk and JE McLaughlin

Introduction

The oesophagus is simply a conduit between the pharynx and stomach. Its function depends upon the existence of an adequate lumen and the correct sequence of neuromuscular peristaltic contractions to propel the contents. The direction is reversed in regurgitation and vomiting.

Apart from developmental abnormalities requiring urgent or early correction the four fundamental pathological processes affecting the oesophagus are:

1. Neuromuscular disorders including both involvement in systemic diseases of nerve and muscle and local mechanical disorders resulting in the development of a hiatal hernia or diverticulum.
2. Inflammation, often the result of reflux of gastric acid and leading to stricture formation.
3. Neoplasia, usually of the epithelium, but also including the connective tissue elements, and secondary involvement.
4. Bleeding associated with oesophageal varices and traumatic damage.

The outstanding symptoms are dysphagia, heartburn, regurgitation, pain on swallowing (odynophagia), and bleeding. Because the symptom is not an accurate indicator of the pathology, a knowledge of the latter is important and the help of the pathologist is often adjunct to clinical and radiological findings in the management of patients.

Appearances

Normal

The oesophagus is a thin-walled conduit 24 cm long with constrictions at the upper cricopharyngeal and lower cardiac sphincters and an indentation where it is crossed by the aortic arch. It is enormously distensible, stretching until its walls are translucent. It has no peritoneal covering except for the lower 2–3 cm which lies in the abdomen. The muscle coat is striated in the upper eighth, then mixed, becoming totally smooth in the lower half. The prominence of the longitudinal muscle coat is unique to the oesophagus. H. Daintree Johnson accounted for this by proposing that gastro-oesophageal reflux is normally prevented on straining because the lower, intra-abdominal segment of oesophagus is compressed like a flutter valve during straining, as intra-abdominal pressure rises. However when it is necessary to belch or vomit, the longitudinal muscle contracts: since it is attached through the pharyngeal constrictors to the base of the skull, the gastric cardia is drawn into the chest. Straining and increasing intra-abdominal pressure no longer compresses the lower oesophagus which lies in the chest, and gastric contraction now forces fluid past the weak intrinsic lower oesophageal sphincter up into the mouth. The oesophagus is lined with squamous epithelium.

During swallowing barium meal X-rays show that the bolus is projected posteriorly by compression of the tongue against the palate, over the epiglottis into the pharynx, where the cricopharyngeal sphincter is relaxed to permit the fluid to enter the upper oesophagus. Heavy barium drops rapidly by gravity. In supine subjects and in some people even when they are upside down, the barium still travels towards the stomach, driven by a wave of peristaltic contraction preceded by a wave of relaxation. The lower oesophagus behaves now like the remainder of the gullet, relaxing to allow the swallowed fluid to enter the stomach. The oesophagus appears smooth and flaccid, with a few longitudinal folds at the lower end which is normally collapsed.

At endoscopy the oesophagus presents a smooth

cylindrical tube, often with a few annular peristaltic constrictions moving distally. The epithelial lining is pale pink and opaque. At the lower end there is frequently a sudden crenated line of junction with the shiny red, florid, gastric mucosa.

Atresia

This is often not a solitary congenital defect but may be accompanied by other malformations. It is possible that vascular anomalies result in atresia. The upper segment ends blindly in most cases, while the lower end tapers proximally towards a fistulous connection with the lower trachea (Fig. 4.1). Less frequently both upper and lower ends are blind, or the upper end has a fistulous connection with the trachea. Another infrequent anomaly is the existence of a tracheo-oesophageal fistula with an intact oesophagus. In the presence of atresia the blind segment of oesophagus may be represented by a fibrous cord. Radiological examination is often not carried out but in the most usual type there is gas in the intestine, reaching it from the trachea. If radio-opaque material is instilled it shows the dilated blind upper pouch. Endoscopy is inappropriate and the diagnosis is made by detecting excessive pharyngeal mucus aspiration at birth.

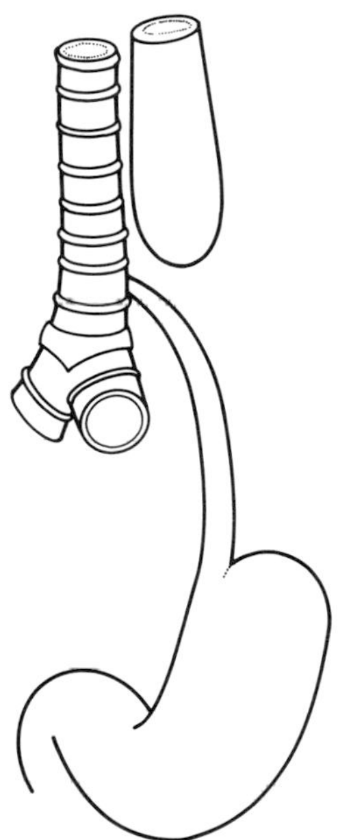

Fig. 4.1 Oesophageal atresia. This is the commonest type with a blind upper end and a fistulous track between the trachea and the lower end.

Dilatation

The oesophagus dilates slowly above an obstruction and does not usually develop hypertrophy. The obstruction may be intraluminal such as polypoid neoplasm, or be from benign or malignant stricture, or develop as a result of external compression such as mediastinal or bronchial neoplasm. In dysphagia lusoria (*L. lusorius* = deceitful) the oesophagus is compressed by an aberrent right subclavian artery passing behind or in front of it. At endoscopy the oesophagus above an obstruction may contain food debris producing inflammation and excoriation.

Gross dilatation is nearly always secondary to neuromuscular myenteric ganglion degeneration. This is frequently but not always accompanied by achalasia of the cardia, that is failure to relax when a food bolus descends. The thin-walled oesophagus often becomes serpentine as retained food or fluid distends it until sufficient head of pressure overcomes the achalasic lower oesophageal sphincter. The epithelium often becomes inflamed and excoriated. There is an increased risk of carcinoma developing in this condition.

A fluid level is sometimes seen on a plain X-ray of the chest. Barium swallow X-rays demonstrate the dilated oesophagus narrowing smoothly down to the cardia (Fig. 4.2). When sufficient head of pressure is built up the cardia opens and the barium runs freely into the stomach.

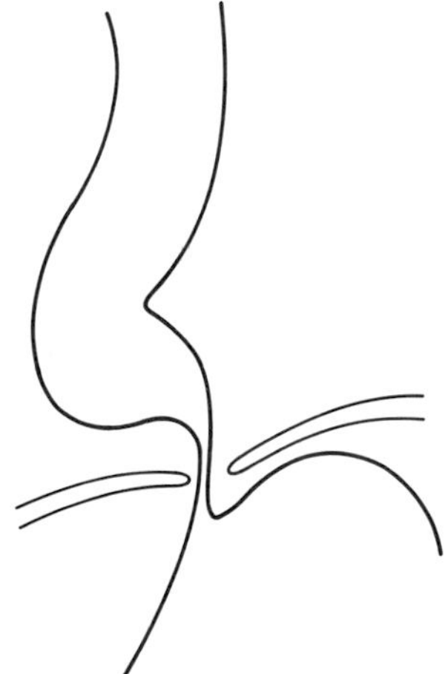

Fig. 4.2 Dilated serpentine oesophagus in achalasia of the cardia.

At endoscopy the dilated oesophagus may display inflammation and excoriation at its lower end, but there is no stricture and the endoscope passes smoothly into the stomach.

In South America Chagas' disease (infection with *Trypanosoma cruzi*) is rife. One manifestation is gross dilatation of the oesophagus. The myenteric plexus is probably destroyed as the result of an immune reaction to the Trypanosoma antigen.

Benign strictures

The level of an oesophageal stricture gives an important clue to its origin.

Postcricoid web

At the upper end is the stricture associated with the Plummer-Vinson or Paterson-Kelly syndrome of sideropaenic web. It may be genetically determined, associated with gastric atrophy or pernicious anaemia. It develops in middle-aged women as a web at the postcricoid level. Histologically there is a basal cell hyperplasia with nuclear hyperchromatism. The epithelial changes are sometimes premalignant. At endoscopy a concentric short stricture is visible which dilates easily.

Caustic

Strictures following ingestion of caustics typically appear at the site of temporary hold up of the injurious substance, where it remains longer in contact with the epithelium. These are the cricopharyngeal region, the level at which the aortic arch crosses and indents the oesophagus, and the cardia. They are typical sites of caustic excoriation and subsequent stricture formation. No specific features are found but the stricture is usually smooth, fibrous and dilatable at endoscopy. The smooth narrowing, of variable length, can be seen on barium swallow X-rays.

Peptic stricture

Peptic stricture of the oesophagus develops whereever squamous epithelium is in continuity with gastric epithelium, although the exact mechanism is unknown. Two types of peptic stricture are known. In one it is assumed that reflux of gastric acid provokes oesophagitis and the resulting scarring produces a stricture. This develops above a sliding hiatal hernia and is seen at all ages, including neonates. In a proportion of subjects a discrete peptic ulcer is seen and the pathology then resembles the stenosis from chronic peptic ulceration that is well described in the stomach and duodenum.

At endoscopy oesophagitis and peptic ulceration may be seen. In some patients a hiatal hernia is detected, and there is an upper loculus of stomach in the chest. As the patient inspires, the neck of the loculus where it joins the body of the stomach, is partially constricted as the diaphragmatic crus tightens around it.

If the patient swallows barium, the smooth short stricture is seen, sometimes with a projecting flake of barium in an ulcer crater, in the lower oesophagus. When the barium has entered the stomach it will often reflux into the gullet especially if the patient is place head down, and then asked to strain or swallow. In some, but not all, a sliding hiatal hernia can be demonstrated: an upper loculus of stomach lies above the diaphragm, (Fig. 4.3) lined with thick longitudinal gastric folds. The stricture lies at the oesophago-gastric junction.

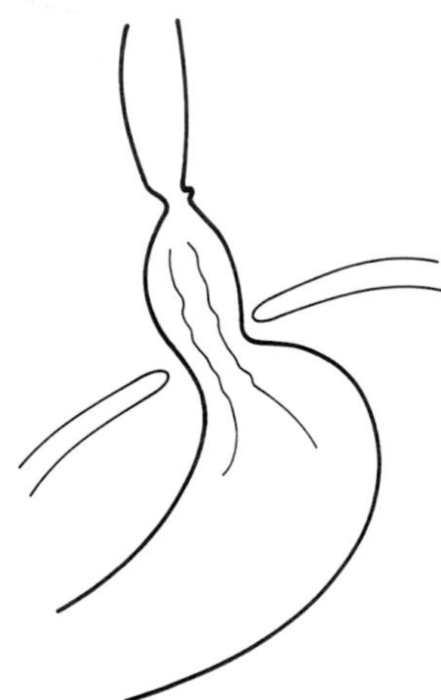

Fig. 4.3 Peptic ulcer with stricture at the gastro-oesophageal junction. There is a sliding hiatal hernia with gastric mucosal folds visible in the upper loculus of the stomach.

Congenitally short oesophagus

In this fascinating condition, often called Barrett's syndrome, the lower oesophagus is lined with columnar epithelium of the type found in the cardiac region of the stomach. During development the oesophagus is for a period lined with columnar epithelium but at 6 months the middle third is already lined with stratified squamous epithelium. It was formerly considered that the oesophagus was congenitally short and that the lower columnar-cell lined segment was stomach. The junction has been demonstrated to migrate upwards. Probably gastro-oesophageal acid reflux produces oesophagitis, ulceration of oesophageal mucosa, with replacement by cardiac gastric mucosa.

Ulceration causes stricture formation and this is often higher than is seen in sliding hiatal hernia. Barium swallow X-ray may show a short stricture in the mid-thoracic oesophagus with apparently normal oesophagus below it. At endoscopy the diagnosis can be made with certainty only by obtaining mucosa from below the stricture to demonstrate that it is cardiac gastric mucosa. A peptic ulcer is sometimes demonstrable radiologically and endoscopically at the level of the stricture.

This condition should not be confused with the fixed shortening of the oesophagus that may occur as a result of hiatal hernia. Sliding hiatal hernia implies that the oesophagus is capable of lengthening so that the hernia can be reduced. Sometimes, probably as a result of fibrosis the hernia is fixed and cannot be reduced under radiological control and the surgeon cannot restore the cardia into the abdomen at operation because the oesophagus is permanently shortened.

Schatzki's ring

This is a diaphenous mucosal diaphragm which is sometimes seen on barium swallow X-ray about 2–3 cm above the cardia. At endoscopy the ring is easily dilated. The reason why it forms is unknown.

Malignant stricture

The factors which cause oesophageal carcinoma are unknown. Oesophageal obstruction from postcricoid web, peptic or caustic stricture and achalasia may be important, although no convincing link with hiatal hernia has been found. Ingested substances such as alcohol, nitrosamines and smoking may be important.

Epidemiological studies display marked differences in the incidence of oesophageal cancer throughout the world varying from 5 cases per 100 000 of the population in England and Wales, through 6 in US whites, 20 in US blacks and in Japan, 23 in Hong Kong, 25 in France, to 28 in black South Africans. It is estimated that there are 109 deaths per 100 000 south of the Taihang mountains of Northern China and no less than 262 deaths per 100 000 in the Caspian littoral of Iran.

Although many factors are indicted in the associations and epidemiological studies, no single aetiological factor has been identified.

Cancer may develop at any level of the oesophagus but is most frequent either in the postcricoid region or in the middle and lower thirds of the thoracic oesophagus. Narrowing results from two factors—the first is infiltration and thickening of the wall which narrows the lumen and secondly from tumour expanding into the lumen to block it (Fig. 4.4). Oesophageal growths are usually squamous cell carcinomas but may be adenocarcinomas in less than 10 per cent. Adenocarcinoma of the cardiac region of the stomach often invades the oesophagus from below.

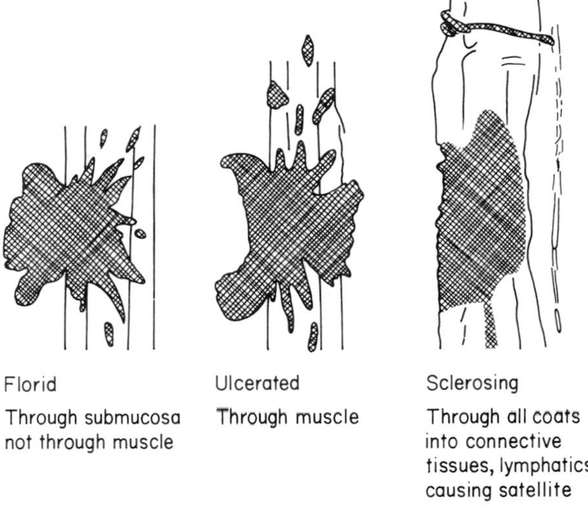

Fig. 4.4 Oesophageal cancer: different types and degrees of penetration. In each drawing the mucosa is on the left, then submucosa with the muscularis on the right.

In some cases there is a minor degree of irregularity of the mucosa, or ulceration, classically with rather everted edges to the ulcer. In proliferative lesions, the growth bulges into the lumen (Fig. 4.4). As a rule by the time the carcinoma is detected a large proportion of the oesophageal circumference is involved and some tumours produce an annular thickening with the proximal and distal ends of the annulus protruding into the lumen.

It is well known that the macroscopic limits of the tumour do not represent its full extent and lymphatic submucosal and peri-oesophageal spread may extend for up to 12 cm on either side, beyond the limits of macroscopic growth, and also produce "skip" lesions at a distance from the primary (Fig. 4.4). In addition it may directly invade the trachea, pleura, lung, pericardium, dia-

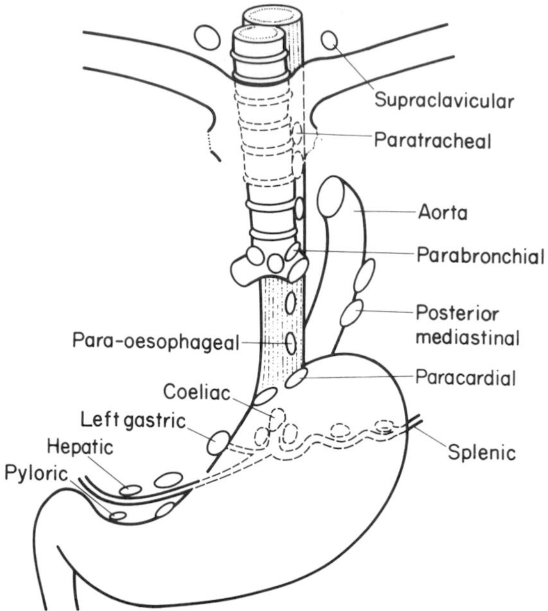

Fig. 4.5 Glandular spread of oesophageal carcinoma.

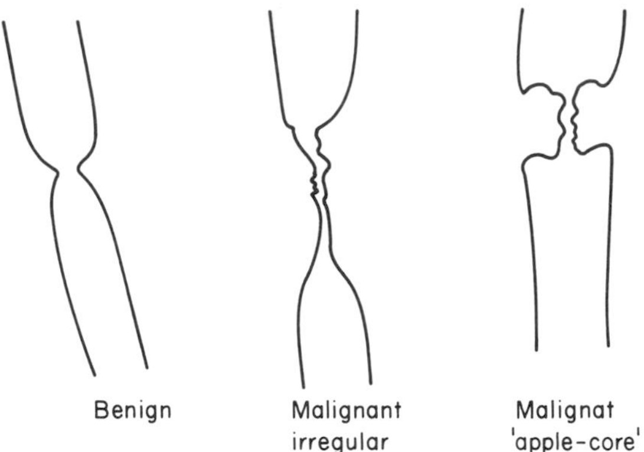

Fig. 4.6 Benign and malignant strictures.

phragm, recurrent laryngeal or phrenic nerves, and aorta or other blood vessels.

Oesophageal carcinoma does not spread segmentally although a high proportion, usually more than 60 per cent, have mediastinal glandular involvement and almost as many have involvement of the upper gastric glands. However the supraclavicular, perigastric, coeliac, hepatic and splenic glands may be involved in the absence of mediastinal nodal invasion. Thus the finding of uninvaded glands at tumour level is no guarantee against distant glandular spread (Fig. 4.5). Blood stream spread to the liver, lungs and adrenal glands and bones does occur, but the patients are usually dead before such metastases become clinically important.

Radiological studies classically display a longer stricture than is seen in benign strictures, and it is often irregular (Fig. 4.6). Projection of the tumour may produce "shouldering" and sometimes the classical "applecore" effect is seen. It is rare except when radiological screening is carried out, to make the diagnosis of early carcinoma by observing a superficial filling defect, converging, tortuous or interrupted mucosal folds, and spasm and stiffness representing early or carcinoma in situ.

At endoscopy the tumour, which may be ulcerated, can sometimes be seen bulging into and filling the lumen. There may be merely irregularity or roughening of the mucosa, or an ulcer which appears benign. Cytological brushings or biopsies are required to prove the diagnosis. The neoplasm may infiltrate upwards under normal mucosa so that at endoscopy a smooth stricture is seen and superficial biopsies reveal no abnormality. Cellular diagnosis is made only when deeper bites are made, or biopsies and cytological brushings are obtained from within the stricture.

Primary adenocarcinoma of the oesophagus accounts for 6–10 per cent and is assumed to arise in the oesophageal mucus-secreting glands, glands resembling those of the gastric cardia, or from islands of ectopic gastric mucosa that can be found especially in the upper third of the oesophagus.

Other tumours

Benign neoplasms infrequently develop in the oesophagus and include lipoma, leiomyoma, lymphangioma and papilloma. These and pseudotumour, fibrovascular polyp, and epithelial oesophageal cyst, are mainly important because they may be confused with malignant tumours.

Malignant leiomyosarcoma, rhabdomyosarcoma, fibrosarcoma, lymphoma, carcinosarcoma, pseudosarcoma, and melanoma are rare. Carcinomatous invasion occurs directly not only from the stomach but also from the bronchus. Lymphatic and blood-borne spread infrequently affects the oesophagus from breast, thyroid, pancreas, and larynx.

Inflammation

The oesophageal mucosa is inflamed in a number of conditions.

Peptic oesophagitis

The inflammation is from contact with gastric acid or bile because of functional or organic incompetence of the antireflux mechanism. Reflux may accompany sliding hiatal hernia, surgical damage to, or excision of the gastro-oesophageal junction, or develop in the absence of anatomical factors. The lower oesophageal mucosa may be reddened, thickened and thrown into longitudinal folds often with whitish deposition. There may be erosions or ulceration. However it may appear macroscopically normal and can be detected only by observing increased vascularity in biopsy specimens. The upper oesophagus usually appears normal.

Barium swallow radiological studies show only a slight irregularity of the mucosa but may demonstrate gastro-oesophageal reflux when the patient lies with head down, especially on straining or swallowing. If there is a hiatal hernia, the upper loculus of stomach is demonstrated above the diaphragm.

At endoscopy the mucosa varies so much that the diagnosis cannot always be confidently made visually since it appears normal. Very often refluxed contents can be seen. In the presence of a hiatal hernia the endoscope passes through the cardia into an upper loculus of stomach. Oesophagitis may be seen in the unusual condition of Barrett's oesophagus above the junction of oesophageal and gastric mucosa.

Acute oesophagitis

This develops after severe irritation of the oesophagus by ingestion of caustics, hot liquids or other irritants. The mucosa is inflamed and oedematous. It may be excoriated, especially at the sites of hold up where contact is increased with the irritant at the cricopharyngeus, the crossing of the aortic arch, and the cardia. It is usually unwise to carry out radiological or endoscopic examination during the acute phase.

Candida albicans

This may flourish in the oesophagus in patients treated with antibiotics, immunosuppressive drugs, and steroids. It usually starts in the mouth and spreads secondarily to the oesophagus, producing whitish plaques with underlying inflammation and excoriation.

Crohn's disease

Crohn's disease affecting other parts of the gastrointestinal tract may produce similar lesions in the oesophagus.

Rigid oesophagus

The oesophagus may become rigid because of involvement with systemic sclerosis (scleroderma). Collagenous sclerosis develops in the submucosa and muscularis mucosa. The lack of contractility results in a flaccid and sometimes dilated oesophagus but the mucosa is quite normal. Barium swallow X-rays confirm the reduction in motility but no abnormality is seen at endoscopy.

Malignant infiltration occurs early, extending in the submucosa and spreading through all coats. Peristalsis does not pass through the invaded segment so that food and fluid fall through by gravity. The extent of invasion is much greater than is visible to the naked eye. Loss of suppleness is an early radiological sign and especially when the rigid endoscope is used, the induration can be felt.

Ulcerated oesophagus

Peptic ulceration

This develops just above the junction of gastric and oesophageal mucosa in the presence of gastric acid reflux. It forms in the absence of any anatomical abnormality, or above a sliding hiatal hernia. In patients with the lower oesophagus lined with gastric mucosa the ulcer appears at about the middle of the thoracic oesophagus and is called a Barrett's ulcer. This is a typical peptic ulcer with shelving and oedematous margins, a slough in the crater, and a fibrous base.

Barium swallow X-rays show a projection seen tangentially or as a concentration of barium seen *en face*. Endoscopically the ulcer should demonstrably be at the junction of the two different mucosae.

Erosions are frequently seen in oesophagitis, whether this results from gastro-oesophageal reflux or from retention of food and debris. The mucosal irregularity is visible both radiologically and at endoscopy.

Malignant ulceration

This classically develops in a tumour so that the edges are everted. The tumour often extends far beyond the base of the ulcer. Radiologically the tumour is seen as a filling defect in the lumen and the ulcer base should lie within the oesophagus. At endoscopy the crater is sometimes invisible and all that can be seen is the raised everted edge proximal to it. The tumour base may invade the trachea, and necrosis in the malignant ulcer base then can form a tracheo-oesophageal fistula. Oesophageal contents now spill over into the trachea causing pulmonary collapse and infection.

Early carcinoma

The oesophageal mucosa is a little irregular, nodular, raised, sunken or ulcerated (Fig. 4.7).

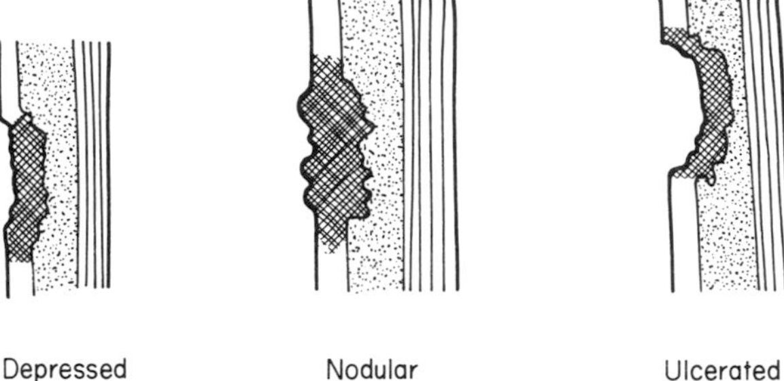

Fig. 4.7 Early cancer of the oesophagus. The mucosa is on the left, the muscularis is on the right with the submucosa between them.

The carcinoma may be very early, still confined to the mucosa. This is in-situ carcinoma. It is not known how long it is before the carcinoma becomes invasive, successively penetrating the submucosa, and the muscular coats.

At the stage of early carcinoma there are no symptoms. Barium swallow X-ray using double contrast techniques may show slight mucosal irregularity, thickening, tortuosity, interruption, destruction or convergence of the mucosal folds, or spasm and stiffness of that segment of the oesophagus.

The diagnosis is confirmed at endoscopy by biopsy of suspicious areas and brush cytology. In China the diagnosis is made by screening asymptomatic patients using a balloon covered in a net: the patient swallows the balloon, it is inflated and drawn up, scraping off epithelial cells. The net is wiped onto slides, fixed and stained to display the presence of malignant cells.

Diverticula

These occur most frequently at the upper end, or in the middle and lower thirds of the oesophagus. The most frequent surgically important diverticulum is not truly oesophageal. Zenker's diverticulum or pharyngeal pouch arises between the circular and oblique fibres of the cricopharyngeus muscle. It is assumed that as a food bolus arrives the muscle fails to relax and the posterior pharyngeal wall bulges between the two parts of the cricopharyngeus muscle. As it bulges more and more the diverticulum often extends to the left and comes to lie vertically beneath the pharynx with the oesophagus opening high on its anterior wall. Thus food does not spill over until the pouch is filled or until the patient bends or lies down.

Lateral views of barium swallow X-rays reveal the pouch lying behind the cervical oesophagus sometimes containing food debris. When endoscopy is attempted the tip of the endoscope always enters the blind pouch unless it is carefully directed forwards into the oesophageal opening at the upper anterior lip. A long-standing pharyngeal pouch occasionally develops carcinomatous changes in the mucosa.

Diverticula in the mid-oesophagus are usually small and have been attributed to traction from tuberculous lymph nodes in the region of the tracheal carina but tuberculosis can often not be demonstrated in such patients. Thus they may be pulsion diverticula as are those seen in the lower thoracic oesophagus.

Varices

Venous drainage of the oesophageal mucosa is from subepithelial veins which drain into submucosal veins lying deeper. These in turn drain into extrinsic veins. Blood from the thoracic oesophagus normally passes into the azygos and hemiazygos systemic veins while the lower 2 or 3 cm lying normally within the abdomen drains into the left gastric vein. Portal venous hypertension can develop because of extrinsic obstruction of the main vein, or thrombosis before it enters the liver. Most frequently obstruction occurs in the liver as a result of cirrhosis, but obstruction rarely develops beyond the liver when thrombosis develops in the hepatic veins draining into the inferior vena cava—the Budd-Chiari syndrome.

In the presence of portal venous hypertension, blood finds its way into the systemic venous system through portal-systemic anastomoses. These are present in the haemorrhoidal veins, the retroperitoneal veins and the periumbilical veins but the effect is most notable in the anastomoses around the lower oesophagus. Dilated, tortuous, subepithelial veins form irregular longitudinal columns, bulging into the lower oesophageal lumen. Varices may extend into the cardiac end of the stomach. Infrequently gastric varices occur in the absence of visible oesophageal veins. The varices are easily seen as irregular filling defects on barium swallow X-rays, and at endoscopy where they are thinly covered with mucosa. Abrasion or ulceration produces copious venous bleeding.

Traumatized

External injury to the cervical oesophagus is usually accompanied by severe and often fatal injuries to the vital vessels and trachea. The thoracic and abdominal oesophagus are both deeply placed and protected from external injury by the rib cage and spinal column. Trauma of sufficient force to injure the oesophagus almost always damages the heart, great vessels, lungs or spine and this is usually fatal.

Oesophageal trauma is mostly iatrogenic from instrumentation. During the passage of, especially rigid, instruments the cervical oesophagus may be crushed between the instrument and the bodies of the cervical spine, usually when osteoarthritic osteophytes project forwards from the vertebral bodies. The mucosa alone may be bruised or broken, or the whole wall may be disrupted. Swallowing action now forces air through the break and into the cervical connective tissues producing air emphysema. If fluid is extruded into the neck an abscess may form. The site of existing disease makes it fragile and susceptible to injury. Thus strictures, ulcers, inflammation and neoplasms are a risk. Particularly dangerous is the dilatation and pulsion intubation of malignant strictures. Perforation occurs into the posterior mediastinum. If the lower third is damaged the left pleural cavity is often breached. Near the cardia the breach may communicate with the abdominal cavity. Oesophageal contents including air and mucus leak into the surrounding tissues. Infection rapidly causes mediastinal cellulitis or abscess. The oesophagus may be accidentally traumatized during operations such as vagotomy or it may leak following operations upon it especially if an anastomosis is formed. If the wound was drained, leakage sometimes produces an external fistula through the track.

Straining during vomiting or retching may tear the mucosa at the cardia and cause bleeding in the Mallory Weiss syndrome. Much rarer is Boerhaave's syndrome of spontaneous rupture of the oesophagus. The tear is usually longitudinal and follows a strain such as retching or vomiting. The rupture is nearly always on the left side.

Clinical presentation

Dysphagia

This can be defined as difficulty in swallowing or inability to swallow. It can develop in the absence of oesophageal disease as in pharyngitis but usually results from obstruction or failure of propulsion in the oesophagus. Dysphagia may be merely the sensation of momentary hold up of solid food, ranging through difficulty with soft foods, to difficulty or even total inability to swallow liquids, including saliva. The degree of dysphagia has no diagnostic significance, however, since a slight hold-up may result in impaction of a lump of food, causing total obstruction. A frequent presentation is progressively increasing dysphagia in an elderly person who has lost a little weight. Usually there are no abnormal physical signs except in those patients with the features of aspiration of oesophageal contents into the respiratory system.

In all such patients carcinoma must be excluded. Carcinoma of the middle and lower thirds is more frequent in men, usually 57–67 years old. It affects women at 54–62 years although postcricoid carcinoma affects women at 40–50 years. The diagnosis may be fairly certainly made using contrast radiology with barium—a short smooth stricture being typical of a benign cause and a longer, irregular stricture in keeping with malignancy. However, debris within the obstructed oesophagus may mislead, and the final diagnosis can be made only by pathological examination.

Endoscopic biopsy specimens should be obtained either through the flexible fibre-optic oesophagoscope or through the rigid instruments. The biopsy forceps used with flexible instruments are small and cannot bite deeply: side-biting forceps that can be passed through rigid instruments will obtain specimens from within a stricture, which may first need dilating. This is important since a tumour can infiltrate under the normal mucosa and if the upper end of the narrowed segment is biopsied no abnormality will be revealed. Specimens should also be taken at the edges of lesions where possible, as well as at places showing severe change. Make sure that the biopsy forceps cut cleanly, and always take specimens from each quadrant around the circumference.

Specimens are usually placed into formol saline, keeping separate biopsies taken from different regions so that the level of origin can be recognised later. It is usual to measure the distance of the

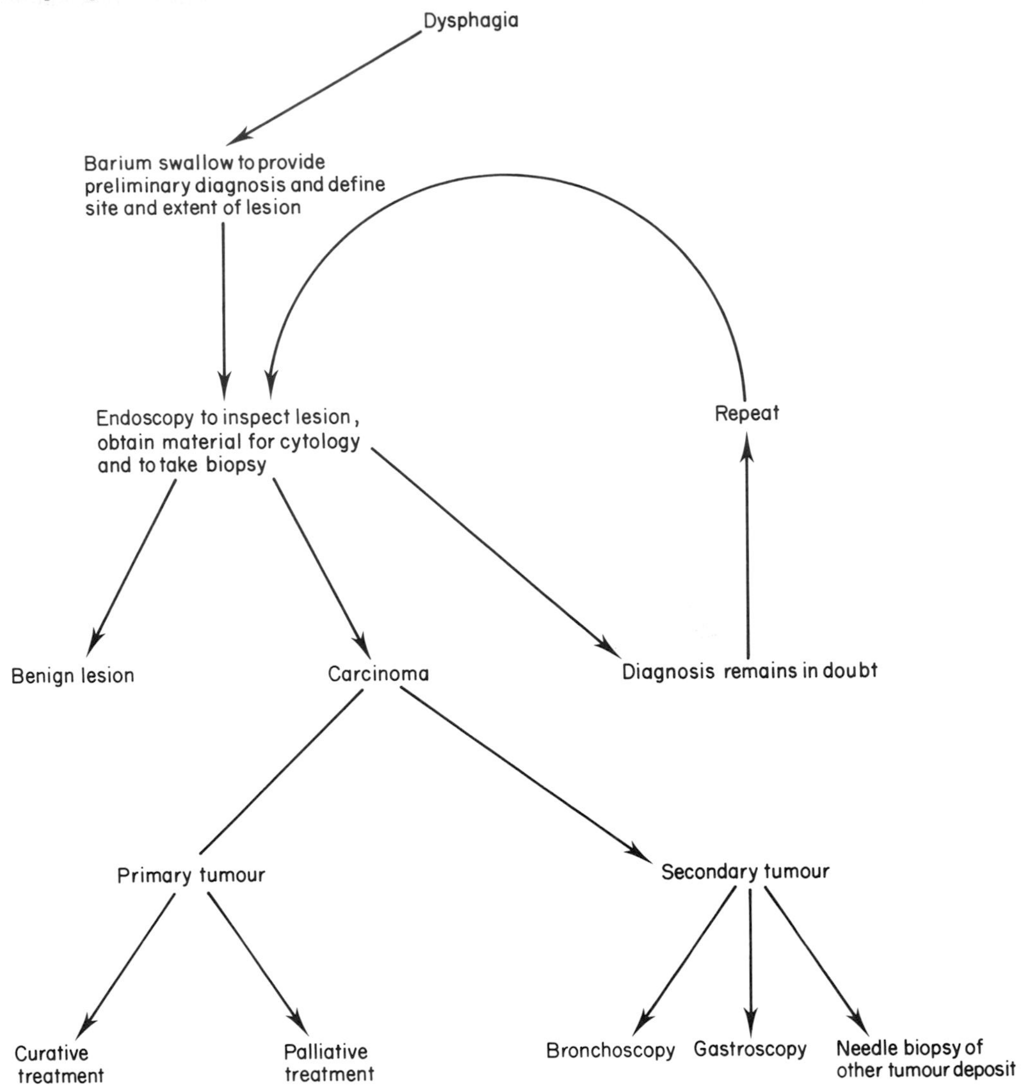

Chart 4.1 The major stages involved in the investigation of acquired dysphagia.

tumour from the incisor teeth, and both flexible and rigid endoscopes have distance marks to enable the length of insertion to be determined.

If tumour is seen the histologist will be able to give information about the cell type of the neoplasm—whether it is a squamous carcinoma, which is usual in the oesophagus, or an adenocarcinoma which may develop in the oesophagus but more frequently results from invasion of the lower oesophagus by a gastric carcinoma. If the latter is suspected, a flexible gastroscope should be passed through the stricture if possible, and the interior of the stomach examined and biopsies taken. The oesophagus may be secondarily invaded from mediastinal and bronchial tumours. In case of doubt, and routinely if the stricture is in the mid oesophagus, a bronchoscope should be passed to examine and if necessary biopsy the bronchial tree. This may reveal a primary bronchial neoplasm, or secondary invasion of the bronchus from oesophageal or mediastinal tumour. The upper oesophagus may also be invaded by head and neck carcinomas by perineural spread, causing dysphagia.

The ability to make a diagnosis depends much upon the skill and experience of the endoscopist in recognising what is seen and obtaining good specimens. If the diagnosis is suggestive of neoplasia and the biopsies do not confirm this, repeat the endoscopy and take further biopsies.

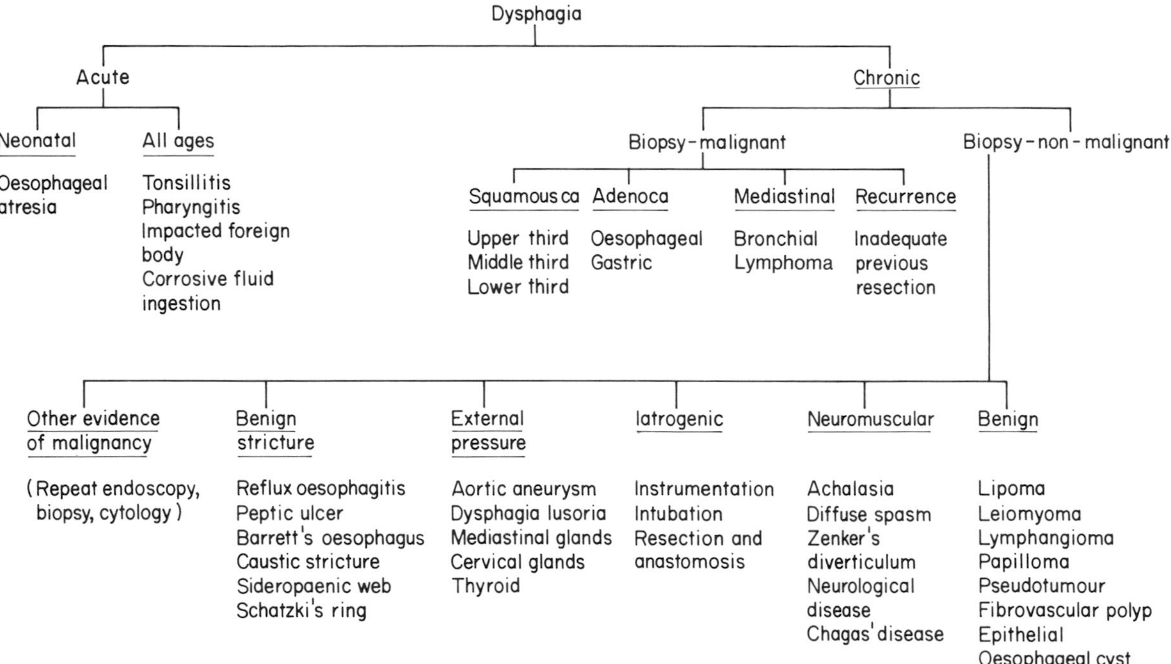

Chart 4.2 Classification of dysphagia (Adapted with permission from *Pathways in Surgical Management* Edited by Michael Hobsley, Edward Arnold, London, 1979).

Diagnostic accuracy has been enhanced in the last few years by the application of cytological diagnosis. A cylindrical brush that can be passed through the biopsy channel of a flexible endoscope is rotated against the suspect area, withdrawn and wiped immediately onto clean microscope slides. The slides are placed in fixative which will be subsequently centrifuged and the deposit stained together with the slides for expert examination. In countries where carcinoma of the oesophagus is frequent, screening for cancer may be done simply by asking the patient to swallow a balloon which is wrapped in a fabric net. The balloon is inflated and withdrawn and the net wiped onto microscope slides to obtain cells for cytology. Sometimes cytology reveals neoplastic cells but the cell type cannot be determined, and endoscopy and biopsy should then be carried out.

Some elderly patients with progressive dysphagia present with lymphadenopathy involving either supraclavicular fossa. In these cases a gland should be removed for histological section to assess the nature and extent of the disease. The high incidence of involvement may make it advisable to biopsy these glands before embarking on radical surgery. A CAT scan may reveal clinically undetectable glands here. In others an epigastric mass, or hepatomegaly in the presence of dysphagia suggests either gastric adenocarcinoma or advanced oesophageal carcinoma. Abnormal liver function tests may suggest liver metastases but imaging techniques such as ultrasound, computerized tomography or radio-isotope scans are more reliable in defining suspected secondary deposits. Histological confirmation can follow guided needle biopsy or cytological aspiration.

It is important to remember that dysphagia in elderly people is not always from malignant disease, although if it arises de novo with no preceding history of gastro-oesophageal reflux, there is a high chance that this is a malignant stricture and not a stricture from peptic oesophagitis. Peptic oesophagitis usually starts in middle life. In our experience more than half the strictures that arise above a hiatal hernia demonstrated on barium meal X-rays are malignant. In all cases confirmation of malignancy by histological or cytological methods is essential because surgical treatment is hazardous. If there is any doubt about the histology, repeat the examination using a rigid endoscope with side-biting forceps and obtain a number of specimens from each quadrant at different levels along the stricture, in addition to obtaining cytological brushings.

Biopsy or cytology shows malignancy

Carcinoma of the oesophagus is squamous in 80–90 per cent of patients and is radiosensitive. If it arises in the upper third many surgeons opt for radiotherapy treatment as an alternative to excision by pharyngo-laryngectomy. Of course if there is any metastatic disease, surgical excision is valueless. Middle third growths that appear to be localized with no bronchoscopic evidence of invasion are amenable to resection with mobilization of the stomach and anastomosis to the upper cut end of the oesophagus. If there is any evidence of spread then bypass, intubation and radiotherapy should be selected, and some surgeons would offer this as a first choice because the results of surgical excision, at least in Western countries, is so poor. In contrast in Japan and parts of China early carcinoma detected by screening asymptomatic high risk populations responds well to excision. Lower third growths are more frequently resected, provided there are no obvious metastases but again radiation treatment, intubation and bypass are used when the growth is unresectable or resection is not indicated because of spread of the growth or if the patient is unfit for the major opera-

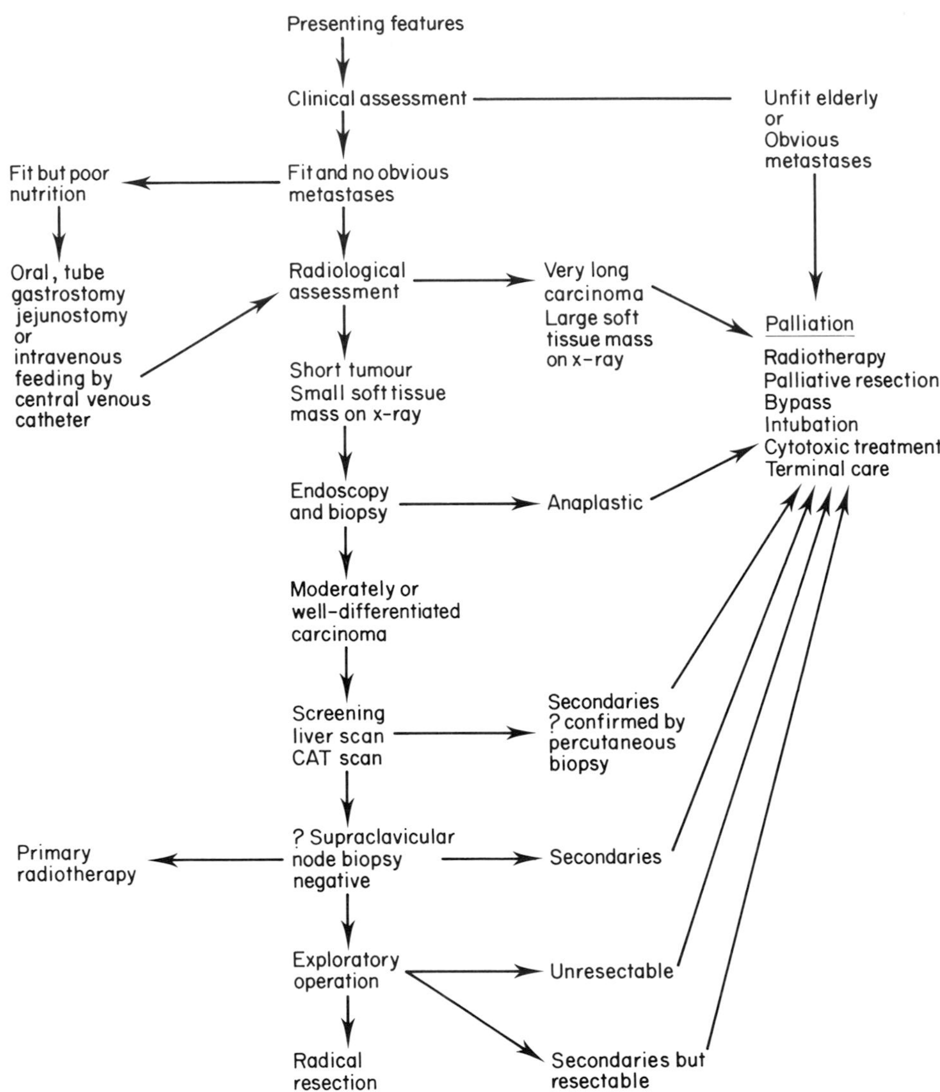

Chart 4.3 Treatment of oesophageal carcinoma.

tion of resection. Irradiation has been claimed to give results at least as good as surgery, as first choice treatment.

Adenocarcinoma occasionally develops in the middle and upper thirds of the oesophagus, presumably from glands in its wall. More frequently it is found in the lower third and represents extension from adenocarcinoma of the gastric cardia. This tumour is relatively radio-resistant and resection provides the only hope of cure for the patient. If the growth cannot be resected, or has produced metastases, then bypass or intubation is necessary to relieve dysphagia. The operation to bypass the growth carries risk and can only be contemplated if the patient is expected to live several months.

Spread Both oesophageal squamous carcinoma and adenocarcinoma of the gastric cardia spread extensively deep to the epithelium in both directions and may produce skip lesions at a distance from the primary growth. It is estimated that following resection, approximately one quarter of cases of oesophageal carcinoma have residual growth in the cut ends. Frozen section histology of the cut ends is not a certain guarantee that they are free, and at least 12 cm should be resected on both sides beyond visible growth when dealing with squamous carcinoma of the oesophagus or adenocarcinoma at or near the cardia of the stomach invading the oesophagus. A palliative resection that leaves growth in the cut ends or in the skip lesions not only carries a high operative risk but also leaves the surviving patient at risk from recurrent malignant dysphagia. On the other hand in early carcinoma wide excision does not appear to be necessary, but this is infrequently seen in Western countries.

It is also necessary to be aware of the extensive lymph node spread that occurs both with squamous carcinoma and adenocarcinoma within the posterior mediastinum and along the gastric lesser curve, around the coeliac axis and along the upper border of the pancreas. Residual tumour will extend from these sites and invade the oesophageal replacement conduit causing recurrent malignant obstruction. In patients submitted to operation the pathologist may help by examining, by frozen section histology, any suspicious enlarged nodes. If these are widely infiltrated with carcinoma then resection is often fruitless and a palliative procedure is more appropriate. In such cases, metal clips may be placed at the tumour margins to delineate the growth for planning subsequent radiotherapy.

Specimen Following resection the specimen should be pinned out and submitted together with a drawing, or at least an accurate verbal description of what is included for histological examination. The pathologist then reports the size and cell type of the growth, its degree of differentiation, its penetration through the visceral wall or extension to peri-oesophageal tissues and lymphatics, and its extension longitudinally. He will also be able to demonstrate any skip lesions and report whether the ends of the specimen are free of growth. Finally he will demonstrate the extent of lymph node involvement.

Prognosis This information allows the prognosis to be estimated. If the growth and any extension appears to be totally encompassed, the patient has a good chance of being cured. If there is an extension to the limit of the specimen, either longitudinally or into the peri-oesophageal tissues and lymph nodes, then eventual recurrence is highly likely. In such cases a patient with squamous carcinoma may be offered adjunctive radiotherapy after recovery from surgery.

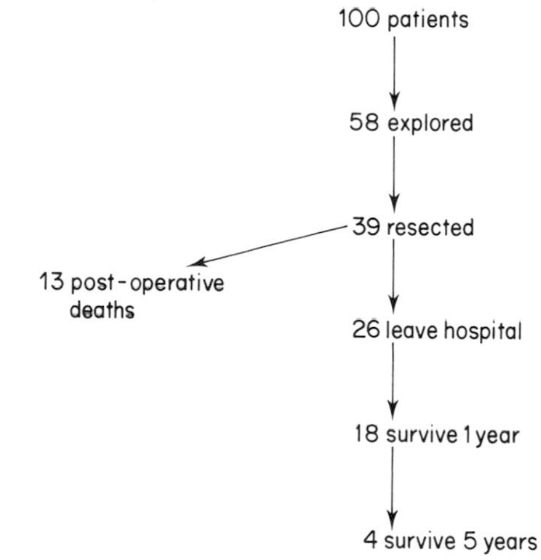

Chart 4.4 Survival rates for surgery of oesophageal carcinoma (Adapted with permission from Earlam R, Cunha-Melo JR. Oesophageal squamous cell carcinoma. In: A critical review of surgery. *Br J Surg* 1980; **67**:381–90)

Some early successes have been claimed using cytotoxic drugs and it is hoped that these may offer valuable palliation in the future. For the present it seems to be worth trying their effect in patients with adenocarcinoma who were unsuitable for resection or in whom resection has shown pathologically to be incomplete. They may also be used in patients with squamous carcinoma if the tumour has been shown to have spread beyond the field suitable for local irradiation, such as to the liver.

Biopsy and cytology are both negative

Do not accept failure to demonstrate malignancy as exclusion of malignancy. If there is any doubt, repeat the examination using a rigid endoscope and side-biting forceps, taking cytological specimens with small gauze swabs on rigid swab holders. Take four quadrant biopsies at all levels of the stricture. Be willing to repeat the examination again at all levels of the stricture, and yet again if the results are still inconclusive.

Peptic stricture If dysphagia does not result from malignant disease it may be from benign stricture associated with reflux oesophagitis. This is usually but by no means invariably associated with sliding hiatal hernia, where the stomach and lower oesophagus slide through the diaphragmatic hiatus into the mediastinum. The condition is usually acquired in late adult life, possibly related to increased intra-abdominal pressure from obesity or to spasm and shortening of the longitudinal muscle of the oesophagus from irritation, drawing the upper stomach into the chest. The stricture develops following inflammatory changes in the lower oesophagus. A peptic stricture may also develop following damage to the cardiac antireflux mechanism by trauma or surgery, including resection of the lower oesophagus with anastomosis of the stomach to the thoracic oesophagus. The endoscopic appearances vary but biopsy specimens show inflammation, vascular malformation, erosions and hyperplasia of the basal layer of the epithelium.

Severe peptic stricture sometimes develops in infancy and must be recognized early and treated effectively.

Barrett's oesophagus Occasionally as a result of reflux the lower oesophageal epithelium undergoes metaplastic change to a columnar epithelium, sometimes including more distally goblet cells and specialized gastric cells. This is Barrett's oesophagus and ulceration and stricture may develop higher than would be expected, in the mucosa proximal to the junction between normal and metaplastic oesophageal mucosa. The diagnosis can be made only by obtaining biopsy specimens from the oesophagus below the level of the stricture after dilating it, and demonstrating metaplastic columnar epithelium.

Medical treatment The management of benign peptic stricture is initially conservative with dilatation, and a regime to reduce gastro-oesophageal reflux. This includes weight loss, avoiding stooping and bending, sleeping propped up, avoiding tight abdominal clothing, and in reducing the acidity of any refluxed fluid. For many years patients have been asked to suck or chew antacid tablets or drink liquid preparations of antacids and these have often been successful. Some antacids contain alginates to form a protective coat to the oesophageal mucosa, or dimethicone which is intended to prevent reflux. An H2 receptor-blocking drug such as cimetidine or ranitidine is effective in profoundly reducing the acidity of the refluxed fluid. Carbenoxolone is also claimed to improve healing of the inflamed mucosa. Dilatation of the stricture alone merely allows free reflux and consequent restenosis.

Peptic stricture in infancy is best treated by keeping the baby vertical and never allowing it to lie flat. This can be achieved by placing it in a specially designed chair. Provided this regime is assiduously maintained the condition usually resolves.

Surgery If the stricture recurs frequently then surgical treatment is indicated to prevent gastric acid reaching the damaged oesophageal mucosa. In some cases this is achieved by the operative repair of the sliding hiatal hernia. If gastric acid secretion is high, especially when there is a duodenal ulcer and associated delay in gastric emptying, a peptic ulcer operation may be added, usually vagotomy and an adjunctive procedure to improve gastric emptying, such as gastroenterostomy, pyloroplasty or gastrectomy. In recent years the antireflux operations associated with Nissen and Belsey have gained favour either on their own or in conjunction with the other procedures. They rely on reformation of the area of the gastric cardia to produce a valve-like action, preventing reflux.

Caustic If a benign stricture is not associated with gastro-oesophageal reflux it may be the result of scarring following mucosal damage from previously ingested caustics. This occurs typically in sites where there is mechanical hold-up of swallowed fluids – the cricopharyngeal sphincter, the aortic crossing and the cardia. There are no specific pathological features. The condition usually responds to intermittent dilatation, but as carcinoma may be a late complication, biopsies should be taken.

Plummer-Vinson A post-cricoid web-like

mucosal stricture developing usually in a woman classically suffering from hypochromic anaemia, but probably genetically determined, constitutes the Plummer-Vinson syndrome. The web is easily dilated, but a biopsy specimen should be removed because change to carcinoma occurs in some patients.

Schatski's ring Infrequently a mucosal diaphragm develops in the lower oesophagus causing dysphagia. This is Schatski's ring which easily responds to dilatation and biopsy confirms its benign nature.

Iatrogenic strictures These are quite frequent, but fortunately, not usually severe. The irritation from a nasogastric tube may cause inflammation resulting in scarring and a stricture at the cardia. Where an anastomosis has been formed a benign stricture may develop. If the anastomosis was carried out as part of an operation for malignant disease, biopsy specimens should be taken to exclude recurrent malignant stricture. Sometimes following a hiatal hernia repair or vagotomy, the patient develops dysphagia. This nearly always improves rapidly. If not, pass a mercury-filled Hurst's bougie.

External compression This produces dysphagia but usually no mucosal abnormality is seen at oesophagoscopy. In the neck, thyroid and lymph node enlargement may compress the pharynx and oesophagus and perineural spread may occur from head and neck squamous carcinoma. In the chest the oesophagus may be invaded and compressed by bronchial carcinoma or lymph nodes secondary to the lung disease or from lymphoma and other conditions. Neck nodes are amenable to excision biopsy. Bronchoscopy and biopsy may confirm bronchial carcinoma when the presence of oesophageal involvement precludes treatment by radical surgery. Aneurysm of the aortic arch may compress the oesophagus as may an anomalous right subclavian artery in dysphagia lusoria. Iatrogenic compression of the lower oesophagus often follows surgical repair of a hiatal hernia – indeed many surgeons welcome a temporary mild hold-up indicating a satisfactory tightening of the hiatal margins.

Diverticula of the oesophagus These do not cause dysphagia although diffuse oesophageal spasm may be associated both with dysphagia and the development of pulsion diverticula. Zenker's diverticulum or pharyngeal pouch is not strictly speaking an oesophageal lesion. It is a pulsion diverticulum developing above the lower fibres of the cricopharyngeal sphincter. Incoordination of this sphincter causes dysphagia and pouch formation above it. Rarely a squamous carcinoma develops in the pouch but diagnosis of the presence of the pouch does not require pathological assistance. The treatment is excision of the pouch with myotomy of the lower cricopharyngeal sphincter muscle.

Benign tumours Dysphagia rarely results from ledge formation associated with benign lesions such as lipoma, leiomyoma, lymphangioma, squamous papilloma, inflammatory pseudotumour, fibro-vascular polyp and epithelial oesophageal cyst. Biopsy through the endoscope confirms that the lump is benign and it may be removed locally.

Neuromuscular Dysphagia may result from oesophageal involvement in systemic neuromuscular disease such as syringobulbia, muscular dystrophy and myasthenia gravis, where oesophageal biopsy is usually not indicated.

Achalasia It is postulated that the primary lesion is in the ganglion cells of the oesophageal plexus. These cells appear reduced in number and there is failure of the cardiac sphincter to relax with uncoordinated peristalsis in the oesophagus proximally. The diagnosis is not made by muscle biopsy but oesophagitis is often present in the lower oesophagus with leukoplakia which may be premalignant, so remove biopsy specimens from suspicious areas before proceeding to cardiomyotomy or forcible dilatation of the cardia using a Plummer-type hydrostatic bag.

Chagas' disease Degeneration of the ganglion cells of the oesophagus is also seen in Chagas' disease due to infection by Trypanosoma cruzi, resulting in a dilated, flaccid oesophagus.

Scleroderma The smooth muscle of the oesophagus may degenerate and be replaced by fibrous tissue but the mucosa remains quite normal.

Heartburn

This is a substernal burning sensation which often spreads up into the neck and to the jaw, caused by contact of the sensitive oesophageal mucosa with gastric acid or with alkaline duodenal juice, and consequent inflammation. The irritating fluid reaches the oesophagus because of weakness of the cardiac sphincter mechanism, usually, but by no means always, associated with sliding hiatal hernia. It can be iatrogenic following cardiomyotomy or excision of the oesophagogastric junction and re-anastomosis.

Diagnosis

It is often difficult to confirm oesophageal inflammation by endoscopy. Hyperaemia with contact bleeding and mucosal exudate may not always be evident, although there are sometimes erosions and ulceration. The vascularity is said to be very variable over even a short period. Biopsy gives more positive diagnosis in case of doubt. There is distortion of the vascular pattern, and the increased rate of cell turnover is evident from the thinning of the mucosa, increased height of the papillae and hyperplasia of the basal cell layer. Where the inflammation has progressed to ulceration or scarring and stricture, biopsies must be taken to ensure that there is no malignant change since this will influence the management of the patient.

Medical treatment

Provided malignant change is excluded, uncomplicated gastro-oesophageal reflux and oesophagitis are treated conservatively. Overweight patients are adjured to lose weight, avoid tight clothing, avoid stooping and bending, sleep propped up, and take an antacid to neutralize refluxed acid. Alginates may protect the mucosa, dimethicone may reduce reflux, and cimetidine lowers the acid content of gastric fluid, usually resulting in the healing of a peptic ulcer. Carbenoxolone slows the rate of cell turnover and so improves the mucosal resistance to acid or alkaline attack.

Surgical treatment

This is rarely required for uncomplicated gastro-oesophageal reflux. Occasionally when all methods of conservative management have been assiduously followed but the patient remains incapacitated, surgery is employed. To prevent gastro-oesophageal reflux, ideally the lower oesophageal segment is restored to the abdomen and the diaphragmatic crus is repaired in front or behind it, from below through the abdomen, or from above through the left chest. Sometimes the oesophagus is shortened and fibrotic. In this circumstance the gastric fundus is wrapped around the lower oesophagus in the Nissen fundoplication or the fundus is sutured up on to the oesophagus to form an inkwell type of plication in the Belsey Mark IV operation. Both techniques prevent reflux and are in vogue even when hiatal hernia is fully reduceable.

Barrett's oesophagus

Heartburn may be the presenting symptom of Barrett's oesophagus. The diagnosis can only be made if biopsy specimens can be taken of the mucosa below the junction between normal and metaplastic mucosa. This condition is treated with cimetidine as a rule but there is no doubt that this can be pre-malignant, so endoscopic assessment and biopsy should be performed at intervals.

Odynophagia

This is pain on swallowing related to spasm of oesophageal muscle and is similar in character to the pain of cardiac ischaemia, being predominantly substernal, often radiating through to the back. Acute odynophagia results from oesophageal obstruction with consequent over-distension of the upper oesophagus, or from spasm which may be spontaneous. It may follow trauma to the mucosa by swallowed objects, instrumentation, or mucosal tears from straining, as in the Mallory-Weiss syndrome. Oesophageal perforation from swallowed objects or surgical instruments produces odynophagia which, if ignored, results in mediastinitis with pyrexia, toxicity, leucocytosis and cardiac irregularities. The pathological cause must be sought.

Minor tears of the cervical oesophagus following instrumentation, often accompanied by air emphysema of the neck, can usually be treated conservatively but intrathoracic rupture is usually best explored, repaired, and drained. Severe damage may demand temporary defunctioning of the oesophagus by producing a proximal cervical oesophagostomy and a distal feeding stoma such as a gastrostomy.

Correction of spasm from neuromuscular incoordination is not usually possible, but an impacted foreign body must be removed and a stricture causing the obstruction must be assessed, biopsied and dilated if necessary. Mucosal tears are usually treated conservatively.

Bleeding

Haematemesis or melaena from the oesophagus are usually associated with only 4 conditions.

Mallory-Weiss syndrome

This is the condition in which straining to retch or vomit causes mucosal tears of the lower oesophagus and gastric cardia. Operative suture repair is occasionally necessary, but usually the tears are not severe, and can be treated expectantly.

Peptic ulcers

Oesophageal peptic ulcers that bleed must be confirmed pathologically at a later stage when they have stopped bleeding. They rarely bleed sufficiently severely to demand urgent surgical control.

Oesophagitis

This is an infrequent cause of severe bleeding but chronic blood loss may produce hypochromic anaemia; it demands vigorous medical management and if this fails, surgery to prevent reflux, after correcting the anaemia.

Oesophageal varices

The most dramatic oesophageal bleeding is usually from portal venous hypertension with oesophageal varices. The pathologist has no part in assessment during acute bleeding phases but may have helped in the diagnosis of an underlying cirrhosis from needle biopsy of the liver. Moderate bleeding may be controlled by lowering the portal venous pressure with intravenous infusion of pitressin. In severe bleeding, the patient is transfused, a Sengstaken tube is passed into the stomach where the balloon is inflated and traction is then exerted on the balloon to obstruct the flow of portal venous blood into the varices.

Three second line treatments are at present on trial. The varices may be injected through an endoscope in a similar manner to varicose vein injections, in the hope of producing thrombosis. Percutaneous transhepatic cannulation of the left gastric vein allows the varices to be visualized with radio-opaque media, then injected to embolize them. The rather difficult operation of porto-systemic disconnection has been simplified by using the circular stapling device.

Portocaval, splenorenal and mesenteric-caval anastomoses for diverting portal venous blood directly into the systemic circulation are infrequently used in Britain for the emergency control of severe bleeding. Portal vein decompression may however be used as an elective procedure to prevent future bleeding.

Trauma

External trauma is obvious but when other structures are damaged oesophageal trauma may be missed. Radiology and endoscopy or careful surgical exploration may reveal the damage. The oesophagus must be repaired and drained.

Trauma resulting from instrumentation or intubation is recognised because the patient develops pain, may collapse and display air emphysema in the neck and chest. Radiology and endoscopy confirm the diagnosis. Small tears of the cervical oesophagus are often treated conservatively but more severe injuries and all intrathoracic injuries should be explored, repaired and drained.

Mallory Weiss mucosal tears reveal themselves by bleeding. The diagnosis should be confirmed by endoscopy but the condition nearly always responds to conservative management. Boerhasve's syndrome of spontaneous oesophageal rupture produces collapse and air emphysema in the neck and chest. The diagnosis is confirmed by endoscopy and radiology. Surgical exploration is urgently required with repair and drainage.

Atresia

The only hope for survival is early operation. The fistulous track is disconnected from the trachea. The two ends of the oesophagus are united. Provided the baby does not have other congenital defects, and the operation is carried out before the neonate has developed pneumonia from spillover of oesophageal contents into the trachea and bronchi, the outlook is usually good.

Further reading

Akiyama H, Tsurumaru M, Kawamura T, Ono Y. Principles of surgical treatment for carcinoma of the esophagus. *Ann Surg* 1981; **194**: 438–46.

Barrett NR. Chronic peptic ulcer of the oesophagus and 'oesophagitis'. *Br J Surg* 1950; **38**: 175–82.

Burrell RJW, Roach WA, Shadwell A. Esophageal cancer in the Bantu of the Transkei associated with mineral deficiency in garden plants. *J Cancer Institute* 1966; **36**: 201–14.

Cook P. Cancer of the oesophagus in Africa. A summary and evaluation of the evidence for the frequency of occurrence, and a preliminary indication of the possible association with the consumption of alcoholic drinks made from maize. *Br J Cancer* 1971; **25**: 853–80.

Doll R. Cancer in five continents. *Proceedings Royal Society of Medicine* 1972; **65**: 49–55.

Jacobs A, Kilpatrick GS. The Paterson-Kelly Syndrome. *Br Med J* 1964; **11**: 79–82.

Kirk RM. Double indemnity in oesophageal carcinoma? *Br Med J* 1982; **286;** 582–83.

Kirk RM. Oesophagoscopy. In: *Rob and Smith's Operative Surgery*, 4th Edition. Edited by Dudley H and Pories W: Upper Gastrointestinal Surgery. London: Butterworths, 1983.

Miller C. Carcinoma of thoracic oesophagus and cardia. A review of 405 cases. *Br J Surg* 1962; **49**: 507–22.

Morson B. The spread of carcinoma of the oesophagus in Tumours of the Oesophagus (Eds) Tanner NC and Smithers DW, Vol IV in *Neoplastic Disease at Various Sites* (Ed Smithers DW). Edinburgh: Churchill Livingstone, 1961; 136–145.

Morson BC, Dawson IMP. *Gastrointestinal Pathology*. 2nd Edition. Oxford, Blackwell: 1979; p 33–57.

Pearson JG. The present status and future potential of radiotherapy in the management of oesophageal cancer. *Cancer* 1977; **39**: 882–90.

Sannohe Y, Hiratsuka R, Doki K. Lymph node metastases in cancer of the thoracic esophagus. *Amer J Surg* 1981; **141**: 216–18.

Smith EI. The early development of the trachea and esophagus in relation to atresia of the esophagus and tracheo-esophageal fistula. In: *Contribution to Embryology*. Vol 36. Washington, D.C.: Carnegie Institute, 1957.

Tuyns AJ. Cancer of the oesophagus: further evidence of the relation to drinking habits in France. *Int J Cancer* 1970; **5**: 152–156.

5

Dyspepsia, Haematemesis and Melaena

J B McFarland and D W Day

Introduction

Dyspepsia has no precise meaning but is a commonly employed term for a collection of symptoms—dysphagia, heartburn, waterbrash, nausea, vomiting, food related pain, abdominal distension/bloatedness and anorexia—arising from disease of the stomach and duodenum and the small intestine (the topics in this chapter) and also the oesophagus, appendix, colo-rectum and associated alimentary canal adnexa (which are described elsewhere).

Haematemesis is the vomiting of blood, and melaena is the passage of changed blood per rectum. Both require that there is haemorrhage into the alimentary canal, usually the upper part. Such haemorrhage may be a complication of one of the conditions which can give rise to the symptom complex listed above. Not only is it by far the most dramatic, but special problems are posed and for this reason it will be dealt with separately in this chapter.

Dyspepsia

Symptoms

It is not always possible to explain the abdominal symptoms outlined above on the basis of pathology, and confusion may well arise when extra-abdominal disease leads to a close simulation of alimentary canal symptoms, particularly pain (e.g. myocardial ischaemia, tabetic crises, porphryia, etc.).

There are other problems. The numbers affected by dyspepsia are unknown, response is variable, and significance (possibly leading to a consultation request) may be attributed differently according to personal, social, ethnic circumstances and, of course, the age of the patient. Furthermore, the development or association of symptoms may place them in a different light. For example, the extension of nausea to frank vomiting (with whatever characteristics) may cause increased alarm, as may loss of weight (when this cannot be given an apparently rational explanation) in association with any of the above symptoms.

At the other extreme, every clinician is aware that gross pathological change may develop in any of the organs most commonly associated with such complaints without the subject admitting to any suffering; in other words serious illness may be present with no awareness of disease. Examples range from the carrier of silent gallstones to the subject whose impending demise from extensive peritoneal metastatic cancer is signalled only by, at most, an increase in abdominal girth noted by her dressmaker.

Neither is it easy to be entirely logical when a ubiquitous dyspeptic symptom (e.g. food-induced nausea) may lead to the diagnosis of disease of the oesophagus, the liver, the pancreato-biliary system, the small or large bowel or develop into an acute abdominal problem.

However, the policy in this book is for such organ-related problems to be dealt with in the appropriate sections. The concern of this chapter is with conditions of interest to the surgeon and pathologist who deal with diseases of the stomach, duodenum and small intestine. This would include disordered bowel habit and inflammatory bowel disease, but these are given detailed consideration elsewhere (Chapter 8).

Pathology

The lesions of the upper gastrointestinal tract most commonly associated with dyspeptic symptoms are, firstly, chronic peptic ulcer of the stomach and duodenum and, secondly, gastric cancer.

Inflammation of the stomach and duodenum, that is gastritis and duodenitis, have a less clearly defined association with dyspepsia. Rare causes are hamartomas (e.g. Peutz-Jeghers polyps, Brunner's gland "adenoma") and benign and other malignant tumours of the stomach and small intestine.

Gastric ulcer

The majority of patients with gastric ulcers have a stimulated acid output which is within or beneath the normal range. Invariably gastric ulcers are associated with local or regional inflammation, usually most marked in the antrum and extending for a variable distance proximally. Histological examination shows that many ulcers arise at the junction of antral and body mucosa, a site which tends to be higher on the lesser curve in women than in men. Reflux of duodenal content, which is demonstrable in the majority of gastric ulcer patients, may be an important factor leading to gastritis, disruption of the gastric mucosal barrier, and ulceration. Several studies have shown an association of chronic gastric ulcers with aspirin abuse. In such cases the ulcers may be multiple and more often involve the greater curve of the antrum; the adjacent mucosa shows little or no gastritis.

The majority of chronic gastric ulcers occur on the lesser curve, with a minority on the anterior and posterior walls, and approximately 5 per cent on the greater curve. They are mostly single and approximately three-quarters of them are less than 3 cm in diameter. However about 10 per cent of benign ulcers are greater than 4 cm in diameter so that size alone does not differentiate a benign from a malignant lesion. In appearance the typical peptic ulcer is round or oval with a punched-out appearance and relatively straight walls perpendicular to the base or a slightly overhanging mucosal margin particularly at its proximal end. At endoscopy an active ulcer may show a slightly raised and injected margin but it is smooth and well demarcated. During healing the ulcer becomes progressively linear. The depth of the ulcer can vary considerably but by definition has penetrated the mucosa and involves the submucosa and muscle coats to a variable degree. Penetration of the entire stomach wall may occur and occasionally pancreas, liver or omental fat may form its base.

Microscopically four zones are recognized in the base of an active peptic ulcer. The luminal aspect consists of a thin layer of fibrino-purulent exudate beneath which is a layer of eosinophilic necrotic tissue. Then a zone of granulation tissue containing fibroblasts, mononuclear cells and variable numbers of capillaries is present which blends with the deepest layer of collagenous scar tissue in which lymphoid aggregates may be a prominent feature. Vessels in the fibrous tissue are often thickened and occasionally thrombosed. Regenerative changes are present in the mucosa at the ulcer margins. Healing takes place by the growth of a single layer of epithelium over the defect, and in time simple mucus glands may develop, but a completely normal mucous membrane is not regenerated.

Duodenal ulcer

It has been estimated, from an extensive autopsy study, that, over the age of 35 years, at least 13 per cent of men and 5 per cent of women have a duodenal ulcer, and 3.9 per cent of males a gastric ulcer. Gastric ulcers found in the pre-pyloric area, often in association with duodenal ulcer, have more in common with duodenal ulcers than with ulceration elsewhere in the stomach. Taken as a group these ulcers are associated with high basal and stimulated acid secretion levels and occur in a younger age group, with a greater preponderance of males, than gastric antral and lesser curve ulcers. However, the finding of a wide range of secretory responses in duodenal ulcer patients suggests that duodenal ulcer disease is not an entity but rather a heterogeneous group of disorders. Factors which contribute to duodenal ulceration include excessive and inappropriate secretion of acid, and excessively rapid emptying of the stomach contents, with defective buffering of acid within the duodenum.

Chronic ulcers are sited usually in the first part (duodenal bulb) just distal to the junction of pyloric and duodenal mucosa but can occasionally be post-bulbar. In 10–15 per cent of cases they are multiple. There is usually some degree of surrounding duodenitis. Ulcers of the distal duodenum and jejunum are characteristic of the Zollinger-Ellison syndrome although recent experience suggests that such patients may present with an uncomplicated, proximally sited duodenal ulcer, or even with erosive duodenitis.

Acute superficial, early duodenal ulceration may fully resolve but chronic, deep, prolonged or recurring ulceration leads to distortion of this relatively narrow tube from which it is unlikely to recover fully. The ultimate degree of the resulting deformity is constriction of the duodenum to a point where the passage of contents is held up. This is misleadingly called "pyloric stenosis". If labelled "benign" it may be distinguished from obstruction of the pyloric canal by carcinoma ("malignant pyloric stenosis") but the stenosis is, in fact, almost always in the first part of the duodenum *beyond* the pylorus. Exceptions to this are the relatively uncommon situation where an ulcer is situated precisely at the pylorus and fibrous contraction has dragged the mucosa together to leave only a tiny opening, and also the entirely separate condition of infantile pyloric stenosis due to pathological hypertrophy of the circular muscle layer of the stomach at this point. In each condition there is a work hypertrophy of the stomach proximal to the *incomplete* obstruction. This varies according to the rate of development of the obstruction. Thus, the stenosis of chronic duodenal ulceration will give rise to the largest stomachs whilst distal gastric carcinoma may be associated with little or not gastric distension.

Of course, considerable structural damage may also derive from benign ulceration of the stomach (e.g. an "hour-glass" deformity caused by a fibrous stricture at its mid-point) but this much larger organ is so much better able to accommodate the deformity that symptoms may be negligible.

The other complications of ulceration are also common to viscera lined with acid/pepsin secreting mucosa. They are the haemorrhage that arises from the erosion of a vessel in the ulcer's base (see later) and perforation of the base of the ulcer, either into a contiguous organ or freely, allowing the gastric or duodenal contents to flood into the peritoneal cavity. These may be sterile and, thus, it could be argued that the peritonitis resulting from this catastrophe is a chemical one. In practice the coverings of the intestinal viscera are damaged so extensively that there is no longer any major barrier to the transmural passage of faecal bacteria and thus a pyogenic peritonitis will develop within hours. The incidence of ulcer-cancer, that is carcinoma developing in a pre-existing chronic peptic ulcer, has long been a matter of controversy. The two essential criteria for the diagnosis are firstly that there must be definite evidence of a pre-existing ulcer on histological examination and secondly that there is definite evidence of malignant change at the ulcer edge quite distinct from any attempt at epithelial regeneration. Current opinion is that malignant change occurs in approximately one per cent of chronic peptic ulcers of the stomach.

Gastric carcinoma

Although its incidence is decreasing, gastric cancer is the third commonest fatal malignancy in the United Kingdom, lying only behind cancer of the lung and colorectum. In 1973, in England and Wales, there were 12 191 deaths from malignant neoplasms of the stomach, the vast majority of which were adenocarcinomas. A common presenting symptom is of epigastric pain often relieved by food and antacids, i.e. similar to the pain of peptic ulcer disease, but as the disease progresses the patient almost invariably becomes anorexic and there is associated weight loss. The tumours occur predominantly in the prepyloric region, the pyloric antrum and on the lesser curve and are less common at the cardia and in the body of the stomach. About 10 per cent are diffuse lesions. Grossly, they may be nodular, ulcerating, fungating or infiltrative in type. Ulcerated gastric cancers are commonest and usually occur in the antrum or in the region of the lesser curve. They differ from benign peptic ulcers in a number of ways. They have an irregular margin with raised edges, and surrounding tissue is firm and appears thickened, uneven and infiltrated. The ulcer has a necrotic, shaggy, often nodular, base. Mucosal folds radiating from the ulcer crater do not have a regular appearance as with benign ulcers and frequently show club-like thickening and fusion. Malignant ulcers tend to be larger than their benign counterparts. Fungating and nodular tumours typically consist of friable masses which project from a broad base into the cavity of the stomach. They tend to occur in the body of the stomach, in the region of the greater curve, posterior wall or fundus and at the time of diagnosis are usually large, when surface ulceration and bleeding may be prominent features. Infiltrative cancers may spread superficially in the mucosa and submucosa giving rise to plaque-like lesions with flattening of the rugal folds and an opaque appearance of the mucosa. Superficial ulceration may supervene. More frequently infiltration involves the entire thickness of the stomach wall usually over a limited area in the region of the pylorus, but rarely extensively, to produce the so-called linitis plastica or 'leather-bottle' stomach. In these cases the wall is markedly thickened and assumes a cartilaginous consistency due to an extensive fibrotic response to tumour cells in the submucosa, muscle coats and subserosa. Some gastric cancers which produce large amounts of mucin giving their cut surface a gelatinous appearance are referred to as colloid carcinomas.

The histological appearances show marked variability not only between tumours but not infrequently within the same tumour. One classification of gastric adenocarcinoma divides them into two main groups, intestinal type and diffuse type. The former have a glandular pattern in which component cells are columnar and have a brush border, and the tumours tend to have a well-defined margin of growth with an associated stromal inflammatory reaction. Atrophic gastritis with intestinal metaplasia is usually marked in the surrounding mucosa. Diffuse cancers consist of scattered solitary cells or loose aggregates of cells which often contain secretory products and are separated by fibrous tissue. Signet ring cells contain large amounts of mucus which compresses the nucleus to the cell border. The margin of diffuse cancers is poorly defined and intestinal metaplasia is absent or inconspicuous.

Intestinal type cancers, which are the predominant variety in areas where the incidence of gastric cancer is high, have a better prognosis than diffuse cancers when the same stage of disease is considered. Although this classification is of considerable interest from the point of view of epidemiology and pathogenesis, the most important factor which determines the prognosis of gastric cancer is the degree of spread through the gastric wall and the involvement of regional lymph nodes by metastases.

Gastric carcinomas are highly infiltrative tumours and in resection specimens the majority have extended into the subserosa. Penetration of the gastric serosa may result in direct extension to the greater and lesser omentum, liver, pancreas, spleen, large bowel, diaphragm and abdominal wall. Involvement of the peritoneum can give rise to transcoelomic spread and when deposits affect the pelvic peritoneum may be felt as hard masses on rectal examination in cases of inoperable disease. Bilateral ovarian metastases (Krukenberg tumours) may occur which can lead to endocrine dysfunction. Tumours at the cardiac end of the stomach infiltrate freely into the oesophagus both along the mucosal surface and within the wall, and at the distal end extension into the duodenum, observed microscopically, is not uncommon, particularly with carcinomas located less than 1 cm from the pyloric ring. Macroscopical observation and palpation cannot be relied upon to define the margins of either early or advanced gastric cancer at operation and frozen section examinations of resected margins, particularly where the margin of excision is less then 4 cm, are desirable to ensure that recurrence does not occur in the gastric remnant.

Metastasis to lymph nodes is frequent in surgically resected stomachs and is in part related to the size and degree of penetration of the primary tumour. However, it is not uncommon for a large tumour, particularly of the polypoid type, to be accompanied by few or no nodal metastases, whereas a small ulcerating carcinoma may be associated with widespread lymph node involvement. The distribution of metastases varies according to the location of the tumour. Involvement of nodes along the lesser and greater curves is common and extension to the next zone, namely the para-aortic nodes and those of the coeliac axis is often seen. Tumours of the mid-portion of the stomach may give rise to metastasis in pancreatic and splenic nodes and lesions high in the stomach can metastasise to mediastinal lymph nodes. Spread by way of the thoracic duct to the left supraclavicular nodes (Virchow's gland) can occur and may be the presenting sign of gastric carcinoma and occasionally growth takes place along the ligamentum teres with presentation of tumour at the umbilicus.

Spread via the blood stream particularly to the liver results from invasion of tributaries of the portal venous system and may occur even in the absence of lymph node metastases.

The dismal overall prognosis of gastric carcinoma, with five year survival rates of between 20–30 per cent for advanced cancer after gastrectomy, has led to much endeavour towards earlier diagnosis. The experience of the Japanese has shown that diagnosis and surgery of early gastric cancer, that is cancer which has spread no further than the submucosa and whether or not local lymph node metastases, are present, results in five year survival rates of the order of 80–90 per cent.

Gastritis

Chronic gastritis is a frequent finding in biopsies from the stomach, even in asymptomatic individuals, and epidemiological investigations have shown that, where the incidence of gastric cancer is high, it increases in prevalence and severity with age to affect a majority of the older population. The antrum is the site most commonly affected and spread of gastritis, which is often a patchy process, occurs proximally, preferentially along and adjacent to the lesser curve. The obvious exception to this is in individuals with pernicious anaemia where it is body mucosa which is primarily involved with eventual glandular atrophy causing achlorhydria and loss of secretion of intrinsic factor. Antibodies to parietal cells are commonly demonstrable in the serum and intrinsic factor antibodies may also be present. Serum gastrin levels are usually increased.

The pathologist describes chronic gastritis, on the basis of histology, as a superficial type involving the supraglandular mucosa, and an atrophic type in which there is variable destruction of glands often associated with metaplasia to an intestinal type of epithelium. Areas of intestinal metaplasia usually consist of mucosa with characteristics resembling that of the small intestine namely the presence of goblet cells secreting non-sulphated acid mucins, absorptive cells with a microvillous brush border and Paneth cells at the base of the glands. Less commonly the metaplasia involves a transformation to goblet cells resembling those present in the large bowel which secrete sulphomucins. In a number of studies this variety of metaplasia has been particularly associated with intestinal type cancers and the finding of this change in biopsy material may indicate an increased risk of developing stomach cancer.

A proposed aetiopathogenetic classification of gastritis, based on differing clinical features and topographical distribution of the inflammation, recognizes autoimmune, hypersecretory, and environmental types.

Duodenitis

Non-specific duodenitis, like chronic gastritis, shows a poor correlation with dyspeptic symptoms. Its relationship to ulcer disease is still controversial although follow-up studies have shown that a significant proportion of people with duodenitis develop duodenal ulcers.

Gastric polyps

Polyps in the stomach derived from the epithelium may be conveniently considered under three headings, namely those of hyperplastic or regenerative type, neoplastic and harmartomatous (e.g. Peutz-Jeghers, juvenile) polyps.

Hyperplastic or regenerative polyps are those most frequently seen in the stomach and constitute from 50 to 90 per cent of the total. They are smooth-surfaced, oval or hemispherical, rarely larger than 1.5 cm in diameter and may show a central erosion. They can be single or multiple and can occur anywhere in the stomach although the antrum is the commonest site. They may occur at the site of, or bordering, ulcers and erosions and at gastroenterostomy stomas. Histologically they consist of markedly hyperplastic and elongated foveolae, and cyst formation may be conspicuous. Although the malignant potential of this type of polyp is low they may be associated with an independent carcinoma elsewhere in the stomach.

Neoplastic polyps consist of adenomas and of polypoid carcinomas. Endocrine cell tumours may also be polypoid. Adenomas are rare in the stomach and are sessile or broad-based, mostly single, and predominate in the antrum. They may reach very large sizes. Microscopically they are composed of dysplastic epithelium often with a tubulo-villous or villous architecture. Unlike hyperplastic polyps, adenomas have a significant potential for malignant change which in reported series has averaged 40 per cent.

Hamartomatous polyps are uncommon and usually associated with similar polyps elsewhere in the gastro-intestinal tract.

Other tumours of the stomach

Primary lymphomas make up about 2 per cent of malignant tumours of the stomach, being the commonest non-epithelial malignancy. They may arise at any site although more common on the posterior wall and along the lesser curvature of the body and antrum. Grossly many of the tumours are ulcerated with rolled elevated margins. Others may be polypoid or infiltrating giving rise to marked thickening of the gastric wall and sometimes resulting in the formation of rigid, giant rugal folds. In about twenty-five per cent of patients multiple tumours may be present. None of the macroscopic appearances is pathognomonic and distinction from carcinoma is only possible after biopsy and histological examination. The vast majority of gastric lymphomas are non-Hodgkin's in type, and comprise approximately equal numbers of high and low grade tumours. The prognosis is better overall than for gastric adenocarcinoma and relates to the stage of disease rather than the histological type. In one series, after surgical resection for cure, the overall 5 year disease free survival was 47 per cent, with 78 per cent of patients without spread to perigastric lymph nodes surviving this interval, decreasing to 29 per cent where local nodal involvement was present. Although there is an increasing tendency to incorporate chemotherapy and radiation in the management of gastric lymphoma, surgical exploration is considered by many an essential step in establishing the extent of disease to plan therapy. Surgical resection is the most effective treatment of localised gastric lymphoma and may also be employed in more extensive disease to avoid the complications of haemorrhage and perforation associated with chemotherapy and irradiation.

Smooth muscle tumours are very common in the stomach at autopsy but only the larger ones give rise to symptoms during life. The majority are benign but malignant smooth muscle tumours make up about one per cent of all malignant tumours of the stomach. The tumours are apparent at endoscopy as submucosal circumscribed masses which as they grow project into the lumen and may become pedunculated. Ulceration of the mucosa overlying the tumour may occur and be the cause of haematemesis or iron-deficiency anaemia. Endoscopic biopsies may fail to provide diagnostic material because of the submucosal location of the tumour. It is often difficult to predict the behaviour of smooth muscle tumours from their histological appearances. Malignant tumours tend to be larger, have a high mitotic index and show infiltration of surrounding tissues. They arise more commonly in the body and fundus of the stomach than in the antrum. Perforation of the tumour into the lesser sac may occur. Provided surgical excision is complete the prognosis is good, but local spread to liver, pancreas or retroperitoneal tissues may be present at operation. Blood stream metastasis to the lungs may occur but lymph node metastasis is rare.

A variety of other benign and malignant tumours are uncommonly encountered in the stomach. They include neurogenic tumours, lipomas, and vascular tumours. Aberrant or heterotopic pancreatic tissue presents clinically as a submucosal tumour within 3 cm of the pylorus and characteristically shows a central dimple corresponding to a ductal opening.

Towards a diagnosis

History and physical signs

The importance of the most careful taking of the patient's history can never be over-emphasized, for, in alimentary canal disease, direct physical signs are commonly absent. Objective signs of disease must be carefully sought, both locally (e.g. abdominal masses, a stomach splash, an area of tenderness, any unusual feature of rectal examination, etc.) and generally (e.g. loss of weight, anorexia, skin lesions, etc.).

Investigations

These may conveniently be considered as "direct", that is the study of the effects of the disease on the organ; or "indirect", the study of how such disease has affected the rest of the body.

1. *Direct Study*

First order tests	Radiology—straight and contrast, e.g. Barium meal Endoscopy
More complex tests	Other imaging techniques—arteriography, ultrasound scan, computerized axial tomography, isotope scintigraphy Secretion studies, e.g. for gastric acid secretion Pressure studies

2. *Indirect Study*

First order tests	Standard haematology Standard biochemistry Standard faeces tests
More complex tests	Haematology involving bone marrow sampling, dynamic studies, etc. Biochemistry involving specialized assays, absorption studies, etc. Immunology

The relative merits of radiology and endoscopy in the investigation of dyspepsia are a matter of debate. Using double-contrast barium examinations it is possible to demonstrate mucosal lesions down to a diameter of 2–3 mm. In some situations (e.g. detection of oesophageal reflux) radiology is paramount; but endoscopy, in most cases, provides the most direct view of the problem and also the possibility of removing material for microscopic examination. External inspection of much of the upper abdominal viscera may be obtained at laparoscopy (peritoneoscopy) when a rigid laparoscope is introduced into the inflated peritoneal cavity. Biopsies may be obtained under direct vision from the liver and from peritoneal metastases, by introducing an appropriate cannula (e.g. Tru-cut) through the abdominal wall opposite the lesion. At laparotomy there is the opportunity for the more detailed inspection and handling of diseased and normal organs.

It is at these points of the most critical importance to the patient, namely the endoscopy session and the operation, that the closest liaison between surgeon and pathologist is essential. The techniques of obtaining, labelling and processing material should be mutually approved and the lines of communication foolproof. To this end the presence, from time to time, of the pathologist in the endoscopy room and theatre, and of the surgeon in the laboratory is invaluable. Regular clinico–pathological meetings, where the histology of material removed at endoscopy or operation is demonstrated, are valuable for pathologist and surgeon.

At endoscopy, tissue is obtained with biopsy forceps and in the case of polyps, by a polypectomy snare, and cytological material by brushing or directed washing of lesions. At operation, it may be gained by much more generous biopsy or by resection of the whole or part of an organ.

Cytology

The frequency with which specimens for cytology are taken during endoscopic examination where malignancy is suspected, or a possibility, is usually related to the availability of local expertise to evaluate the samples produced. In particular situations, such as with strictures of the oesophagus and in pyloric stenosis, it may be difficult or impossible to biopsy under direct vision and, although samples may be taken blindly if the forceps can be advanced through the narrowing, they are not always contributory. In these circumstances brush cytology is particularly valuable. Cytology may also be helpful in diffusely infiltrating carcinoma of the linitis plastica type and in the diagnosis of lymphomas, situations where biopsies may not provide a tissue diagnosis. Where cytology is carried out it is preferable if it is done prior to biopsy so that excessive contamination with blood is avoided. Histology of biopsies is unaffected by prior brushing cytology. Touch smears from forceps biopsies have been reported to add to the sensitivity of biopsy alone in the diagnosis of malignancy.

The handling and preparation of specimens for cytological examination may be carried out by staff from the cytology laboratory or by a trained endoscopy nurse. Ideally the interpretation of the cytology and of the biopsy specimens should be carried out by the same pathologist but where different people are involved, the assessment benefits from a collaborative approach.

Biopsy

It is essential for proper patient management, and particularly before major surgery is embarked upon, that the clinician is aware of the lesion with which he is dealing. Endoscopy has provided the facility for this by allowing targeted biopsies to be taken under direct vision. Several studies have demonstrated the importance of taking multiple biopsies in the diagnosis of malignancy of the upper gastrointestinal tract and the accuracy of diagnosis is directly related to the number of biopsies taken. Ulcerated lesions should be biopsied from their margins or their base. It is important that a tissue diagnosis is made, since a number of lesions, particularly ulcers, which appear benign endoscopically, prove to be malignant on histological examination and vice versa. In the latter situation (that is where the endoscopist considers he is dealing with a malignant lesion but the biopsies fail to confirm this), repeat endoscopy and careful follow-up are necessary. Where endoscopy is repeated, biopsies should always be taken even if the ulcer appears to be healing, since it is known that this may occur in malignant ulcers following drug treatment to lower the amount and concentration of gastric acid.

Apart from enabling a pre-operative diagnosis to be made in the case of advanced gastric tumours, the advent of endoscopy has resulted in detection of an increasing proportion of gastric cancers at an early stage (carcinoma limited to the mucosa or submucosa of the stomach, irrespective of lymph node metastases). These early gastric cancers can be polypoid, slightly elevated, flat, slightly depressed or ulcerated lesions and not infrequently require meticulous examination of the stomach for their discovery. In fact, the efficiency of gastric diagnosis in an institution can be measured as the percentage of cancers that are diagnosed at an early stage. In the best centres in the USA and Europe the figure is currently around 10 per cent. The importance of always biopsying these lesions was demonstrated in a recent series where only 50 per cent of the early gastric cancers diagnosed were suspected of being malignant at endoscopy.

There are other situations where it is important to biopsy the gastric mucosa. People with pernicious anaemia are known to be at increased risk of developing adenomas and carcinomas of the stomach which have a tendency to occur in the body or fundus of the stomach rather than in the pyloric antrum. Patients who have had a partial gastrectomy for benign peptic ulcer may develop a carcinoma in the gastric stump many years later. These usually arise close to the stoma on the gastric side and at endoscopy only marked inflammatory changes, not infrequently with polyp formation, may be noted. Multiple biopsies should be taken particularly from the region of the stoma to detect epithelial precancerous change (referred to as epithelial dysplasia) and early malignant change. The exact risk of malignancy in these high-risk groups is unknown and is a subject of current research.

Whenever possible gastric polyps seen at endoscopy should be removed *in toto* for histological diagnosis since small biopsies may not give representative samples.

Biopsies should be sectioned at different levels and our practice with standard-sized material is to examine three levels. With biopsies obtained with instruments having a large biopsy channel, extra levels can be cut. Whether or not biopsies from the upper gastrointestinal tract should be orientated is a matter of debate, and our own view is that in general there is no advantage. The reasons for this are several.

1. The biopsies are small and attempts to handle them may result in traumatic artefact.
2. The biopsies tend to curl up with their luminal aspect outwards and an experienced technician can embed them in such a way that problems of orientation are obviated.
3. Although a well-orientated biopsy is preferable to a poorly-orientated one, the pathologist is usually not concerned, in the same way as he is with neoplastic lesions of the large bowel, in assessing whether or not neoplastic tissue is present beneath the mucosa.
4. The number of biopsies taken in a single case (which may be from 10 to 20 with a suspicious-looking ulcer) makes it impracticable to orientate them individually.

The one obvious exception to these opinions regarding orientation occurs with biopsies taken from the second part of the duodenum from patients with dyspeptic symptoms in whom the diagnosis of coeliac disease may be suggested. In this situation, or when a small intestinal biopsy is taken using a suction capsule technique (such as the Crosby capsule), the tissue samples should be placed submucosal surface downwards on a suitable surface such as a ground-glass slide or nylon mesh before being placed in formalin. This can be facilitated by the use of a dissecting microscope, thus ensuring that in the laboratory the biopsies after processing can be embedded in such a way that sections may be cut perpendicularly through the mucosa. In this way the pathologist can optimally assess the architecture of the intestinal villi.

Operative specimens

At operation in patients with malignancy of the upper gastrointestinal tract, frozen section diagnosis may be employed to confirm the impression of widespread disease and to assess whether resection margins are free from tumour. Immediate cytology of lymph nodes removed during operations for cancer of the stomach has been used to decide whether or not radical surgery should be carried out.

It is important that resection specimens should reach the pathologist fresh and unfixed. In practice this is readily achieved by a member of the theatre staff contacting the laboratory as soon as the specimen is ready. Copies of operation lists should be available to the pathologist so that he is aware, in advance, of proposed surgery. On receipt of the specimen it should be carefully opened. In the case of a stomach this is usually along the greater curve or in such a way as to avoid cutting across any tumour present. The specimen is then pinned out flat on a cork board which is placed in buffered formaldehyde. In certain instances tissue may be taken from the fresh specimen for further study, such as hormone assay or electron microscopy, e.g. when pre-operative biopsy material suggests an endocrine tumour, or when there is doubt as to whether a particular tumour is a carcinoma or malignant lymphoma. After fixation the specimen should be photographed, a rough outline drawing made recording the site of the tumour, any blocks removed, and the lymph nodes and major blood vessels. Blocks should be taken of the whole diameter of the tumour (or representative blocks in very large tumours or in extensive diffusely infiltrating growths) and of the area of deepest spread of the tumour through the gastric wall as well as the resection margins. A meticulous search for lymph nodes is essential and all should be sectioned.

Handling of the specimens in this way enables the pathologist to impart the maximum amount of information to the surgeon particularly regarding histological typing and, on the basis of spread through the stomach wall and involvement of lymph nodes, staging of the tumour, so that an assessment of prognosis can be made in the individual patient. In some cases of early gastric cancer the changes on macroscopic examination may be very subtle, and only apparent when the specimen is handled properly. It is often very informative for the endoscopist/surgeon to see the specimen in these cases before blocks are taken, particularly when malignancy was not suspected at the endoscopic examination.

Comment

If, as seems probable, gastritis/gastric ulcer and duodenitis/duodenal ulcer are diseases of mucosa with spectra of severity, the pathologist's knowledge of these, and particularly of possible initiating factors (steroid therapy, uraemia, burns, other high stress situations etc.) may be of inestimable clinical value.

Possible problems in the post-operative situations (immediate, mid-term, long-term) may also be mentioned here. For duodenal ulceration, the recent tendency has been (very rightly) towards a decreasing rate of treatment by surgery and, when this *is* undertaken, for the operation to be of a less radical nature than heretofore. Yet there is still a very considerable number of operated patients and a wide range of clinical problems left as a consequence of the more radical surgery of past times. Furthermore, gastrectomy is probably still the form of surgery most widely used for non-healing gastric ulcer, and it is the only option in extirpative treatment of gastric carcinoma.

Much of the assessment is by indirect studies (haematology, biochemistry) but there are also direct effects (e.g. of bile reflux on gastric or oesophageal mucosa) to be looked for and studied. Great vigilance is necessary if the rare case of carcinoma developing in the operated, previously benign, stomach is to be found early enough for any help to be offered.

There are, of course, techniques of therapy other than surgery that may be considered in gastric carcinoma. Although radiotherapy and chemotherapy may, as yet, have no more than a trial place in this condition, the pathologist has a responsibility for tissue and organ assessment with this in mind, even if for no other reason than the extremely dismal outlook with present therapeutic measures, singly or in combination.

The small intestine

Apart from the acute abdominal conditions discussed in Chapters 6 and 7 and the spectrum of inflammatory bowel disease, Chapter 9, jejuno-ileal disease is more usually of concern to the gastro-enterologist than to the surgeon. Excluding congenital anomalies, which will almost invariably present in the neonatal period, primary conditions of the small intestine usually come to light following (sometimes very extensive) alimentary canal studies. Only in particular circumstances (*) will there be a high risk of direct clinical suspicion for such lesions which include:

1. *Hamartomatous conditions*
   (a) Peutz-Jeghers syndrome*
   (b) Hereditary haemorrhagic telangiectasia (Rendu-Osler-Weber disease)
   (c) Arteriovenous malformations (Angiodysplasias; vascular ectasias)
2. *Benign tumours*
   (a) Epithelial (adenomas)
   (b) Connective tissue (leiomyoma, lipoma, angioma, neurofibroma).
3. *Malignant tumours*
   (a) Adenocarcinoma
   (b) Lymphoma*
   (c) Leiomyosarcoma
4. *Endocrine cell (APUD) tumours**
5. *Diverticula*
   (a) Duodenal diverticula may arise as a consequence of healing of duodenal ulceration. Otherwise they are congenital, as are

* The Peutz-Jeghers syndrome will be suspected when the characteristic mucocutaneous pigmentation is observed.
* There is an increased incidence of malignant lymphomas of the small bowel in subjects with coeliac disease and in immuno-suppressed patients.
* The lead to an endocrine cell tumour may be given by its systemic effects (e.g. the carcinoid syndrome).

(b) Jejunal diverticula—usually symptomless.
(c) Meckel's diverticulum. The major significance of this solitary congenital diverticulum, arising from the antimesenteric border of the terminal ileum (within 90 cm from the ileo-caecal valve), is that it may become inflamed, or be the site of haemorrhage arising in association with ectopic gastric mucosa.

If surgical treatment is indicated, this is by excision, with appropriate restoration of intestinal continuity.

Haematemesis and Melaena

Presentation

Vomited blood may be fresh, clotted, or having the appearance of "coffee grounds" (the haemoglobin converted to haematin by gastric acid). Blood which has been degraded during its passage through the gut will be passed per rectum as melaena, black and tarry with a characteristic odour. Only when intestinal transit time is exceptionally rapid, which may occur with very profuse proximal haemorrhage, is such blood passed relatively less changed, in which situation the patient is nearly always shocked. Similar bleeding occurs from lesions of the large bowel (Chapter 8) when shock may or may not be present, depending on the severity of the haemorrhage. Bleeding from mucosal ulceration in a Meckel's diverticulum will more usually present in the manner of colonic haemorrhage, and shock is unlikely.

Unless there is total alimentary canal occlusion below the point of haemorrhage, bleeding giving rise to haematemesis will always lead to the passage of some changed blood per rectum, although constipation may obscure this to a relative degree. The reverse is not the case. Bleeding from the uppermost reaches of the alimentary canal does not necessarily lead to the vomiting of blood. Whichever presentation is paramount it is common for there to be a single bleeding point, even in the presence of two lesions.

Assessment

Clinically, assessment of the amount of haemorrhage is notoriously difficult. Acute major haemorrhage will usually be associated with hypotension and tachycardia, although this may be absent even when significant blood loss has occurred. Severe anaemia is not usually manifest within twenty four hours of an acute haemorrhage, as the haemoglobin concentration and haematocrit do not give an accurate indication of the amount of blood lost because of the time required for haemodilution. A raised blood urea occurs following breakdown of blood in the gut and there can be a transient rise in bilirubin concentration. A blood urea greater than 8.5 mmol/litre with a normal serum creatinine indicates a blood loss of at least one litre into the gastrointestinal tract.

It is from the assessment of these indirect features that the measures for the resuscitation of the patient are decided. Such action may be urgently necessary and thus take precedence over the establishment of a precise diagnosis. Furthermore, any degree of haemorrhage from the upper alimentary canal, although initially minor, may presage catastrophic bleeding. This is not usually self-limiting, as is the case when the site is more distal (e.g. from diverticulitis coli, etc.), probably because the acid/pepsin milieu is itself one of the initiating and perpetuating factors. This has important diagnostic and therapeutic implications. For example, gastric carcinoma does not usually give rise to major persisting haemorrhage because of the associated hypo- or achlorhydria; and effective gastric acid suppression or neutralization can be of considerable benefit in situations such as erosive gastritis.

Causes

In approximately 95 per cent of patients presenting with haematemesis or melaena the site of bleeding is in the oesophagus, stomach or duodenum. The sources of haemorrhage which account for the vast majority of these cases are relatively few, namely:

1. Oesophagitis and oesophageal ulcer
2. Mallory-Weiss tear
3. Oesophageal (and gastric) varices
4. Erosive gastritis and gastric ulcer
5. Erosive duodenitis and duodenal ulcer

Bleeding from oesophageal lesions has been discussed in Chapter 4 and will not be considered here except to re-affirm that in this area, as elsewhere, the demonstration of a lesion should not automatically lead to the conclusion that it is the site of haemorrhage. In this respect, oesophageal varices are noteworthy; on a barium meal X-ray their presence may be very evident and distract attention from a haemorrhagic erosive gastritis. Conversely, repeated retching in association with a gastric ulcer may lead to a Mallory-Weiss tear, with alarming haemorrhage from this radiologically obscure lesion. In both instances endoscopy should allow the correct diagnosis to be made.

Acute gastric and duodenal ulcers and erosions

These lesions constitute an important source of upper gastrointestinal bleeding. An erosion consists of a superficial defect of the mucosa which does not penetrate the muscularis mucosae. It may heal or, if it extends through the muscularis mucosae, progress to an acute ulcer, when major bleeding is more likely because of the rich vascular network in the submucosa.

Acute gastro-duodenal erosions and ulcers, which are often multiple, can arise in a number of clinical settings. In some cases there is a history of ingestion of drugs such as salicylates, steroids or nonsteroidal anti-inflammatory agents such as indomethacin and phenylbutazone. The debate about the role of many of these drugs as a cause of peptic ulcers and bleeding in the upper gastrointestinal tract can be related to the disparate conclusions drawn by different authors from the same body of evidence.

Other clinical situations where erosions and acute ulcers can arise are after trauma, sepsis and post-operative complications, after major burns (Curling's ulcer) and following intra-cranial trauma or operation (Cushing's ulcer). These are usually referred to as stress ulcers and are associated with a high mortality. Damage to the gastric mucosal barrier resulting in excessive back diffusion of acid may result from a number of factors including mucosal ischaemia secondary to shock, reflux of upper gastrointestinal content and, in the case of Cushing's ulcer, hypersecretion of acid.

A serial endoscopic study has demonstrated differences in the distribution and progression of stress ulcers and erosions related to trauma and sepsis compared to those following aspirin ingestion. Thus stress ulcers and erosions are first observed on the greater curve of the fundus close to the gastro-oesophageal junction and progress distally, with time, to reach the junction of body and antrum. Erosions following aspirin ingestion involve all segments of the stomach from the outset.

Chronic gastritis and duodenal ulcers

Haemorrhage is the commonest complication of chronic peptic ulcers and occurred in 16 per cent of patients in a 15 year study in general practice. Postbulbar duodenal ulcers and stomal ulcers are particularly prone to bleed. Peptic ulcers in females, although less frequent than in males, may be more likely to undergo haemorrhage. Recurrent bleeding from peptic ulcers is common, occurring in approximately half of duodenal ulcer patients within 10 years of an initial bleed. The mortality rate for this complication has been of the order of 5–10 per cent in different series, being higher with gastric ulcers than duodenal ulcers.

The endoscopist, surgeon and pathologist may each have good reason to appreciate why the haemorrhage from such lesions may be catastrophic and persistent. A deeply penetrating chronic ulcer may erode a major artery (e.g. the gastroduodenal artery or left gastric artery) lying outside the gastric or duodenal wall. Although large vessels incorporated in an ulcer base usually show endarteritis obliterans this may not be present if the ulcer is rapidly progressive. Even when present, although the lumen of the vessel is narrowed, surrounding fibrosis prevents contraction of the vessel wall and only occlusive thrombus will stop the bleeding in the absence of surgical intervention.

Other causes

Less commonly, tumours, either benign or malignant, can cause acute gastrointestinal haemorrhage but they rarely account for more than 2-4 per cent of the total, and the majority are gastric cancers. Bleeding can arise from vascular abnormalities such as rupture of an aortic aneurysm into the gut or from angiomatous lesions. Gastrointestinal bleeding may be a feature of certain inherited disorders such as hereditary haemorrhagic telangiectasia (Rendu-Osler-Weber disease, mentioned above), pseudoxanthoma elasticum, the Ehlers-Danlos syndrome, haemophilia and von Willebrand's disease. Rarely, bleeding into the biliary tree (haemobilia), or secondary to pancreatitis, may result in haematemesis and/or melaena. Bleeding into the upper alimentary tract can be an occasional complication of a variety of disorders such as Crohn's disease, polyarteritis nodosa, systemic lupus erythematosus and systemic sclerosis. However, even when haematemesis or melaena occurs in association with one or other of these diseases, the site of haemorrhage is as likely as not to be from one of the common sources (e.g. a chronic peptic ulcer or erosive gastritis).

Endoscopic examination of the upper gastrointestinal tract soon after an episode of bleeding will identify the site in most cases and has shown that even where a potential source of haemorrhage is present the bleeding is not uncommonly occurring from other sites, e.g. patients with portal hypertension and oesophageal varices may bleed from acute gastric erosions or peptic ulcers. Endoscopic series of acute upper gastrointestinal haemorrhage differ markedly from those of the pre-endoscopic era when the diagnosis was made on clinical, radiological or operative grounds.

There is, as well, considerable variation between different series on a regional and national basis, reflecting not only differences in collation and interpretation of material but also related to such factors as the drinking habits, analgesic consumption and social status of the patients studied.

Management

Such debate may matter little to the clinician dealing with the individual problem, at least initially. His brief may be considered in three stages:

1. Attainment and continuation of a proper haemodynamic balance
2. Control of the haemorrhage at its source
3. Long-term management so as to minimise the possibility of further haemorrhage or any other complications.

The principles of general management of haemorrhage from the upper alimentary tract are well established. They are:

1. Accurate system monitoring—especially haemodynamic, but also respiratory, urinary, etc.
2. Appropriate fluid, cystalloid, colloid and blood replacement.
3. Adequate oxygenation, protection against infection, etc.

The details and the technology are quite complex and are discussed elsewhere (see Chapter 35 on 'Shock'). As an ideal, the management of patients requiring such support should be in an 'Intensive Care' environment with joint consultative supervision by appropriate clinicians. It is in such a unit that the indication for, and timing of, surgical intervention may best be gauged. Such a decision may be extremely difficult and general guidelines are almost impossible to formulate precisely. When specific direct action does become necessary, precision in diagnosis must be the basis for the best management. Although reference has already been made to the debate about the relative merits in such diagnosis of emergency radiology and emergency endoscopy, commonsense tells us that there can be no substitute for actually seeing active, or very recent haemorrhage, and the best diagnosis rate overall is in series employing both radiology and endoscopy.

Furthermore, a view of the matter may be of greater importance in immediate prognosis for it has been shown that the endoscopic findings of bleeding, fresh clot, or a visible vessel ('stigma of recent haemorrhage') in gastric or duodenal ulcers is associated with a high rate of re-bleeding.

While such knowledge means that, increasingly, the surgeon can make his decisions from a position of strength, it is disappointing that, so far, no real improvement in the overall mortality rate from acute gastrointestinal haemorrhage has been achieved. To some extent, this may be because death is not from exsanguination, but its likelihood is heightened by associated cardiac, respiratory, or liver disease and the odds are loaded unfavourably for, and in direct relationship to, the decades over the age of sixty. If these statistics seem somewhat dismal, it is also difficult to see much improvement in mortality figures looked at separately for operated patients, whether for gastric ulcer (15 per cent and 12 per cent) or duodenal ulcer (9.9 per cent and 9.8 per cent). These figures represent a mean from over ten collected series for each condition. In each instance the former percentage refers to the results of vagotomy and a drainage procedure and the latter to gastrectomy, with or without vagotomy. They suggest that the choice of operation in the individual case should be that which the surgeon would carry out in the elective situation, gastrectomy being favoured for gastric ulceration, and vagotomy with a drainage procedure and ulcer oversewing, for duodenal ulceration. The same author's collected figures for post-operative mortality for erosive gastritis are far worse (34 per cent and 43 per cent) and indicate that surgery is inappropriate in this condition.

Comment

It has been suggested that, as the average age of the population rises, this static mortality rate may conceal real improvements in the management of alimentary tract bleeding resulting from modern techniques of investigation and treatment. However, the lack of agreement in the management of patients, once the diagnosis has been established endoscopically, has been brought out in a recent investigation analysing the practice of United Kingdom gastroenterologists in cases of acute upper gastrointestinal haemorrhage. This particularly concerns indications for surgical intervention and management of the elderly patient.

Perhaps the surgeon may gain some comfort from the knowledge of the therapeutic ground gained by the physician; less aggressive—gastric acid depression by H2 receptor antagonism (Cimetidine, Ranitidine); or more aggressive direct approach to the bleeding vessel by electrocoagulation, thermal coagulation, laser photocoagulation, or clips, glue, etc. The latter is still a new area of study and reports are eagerly awaited but, as with the direct approach to bleeding oesophageal varices, (i.e. endoscopic injection) such methods would seem to offer the best chance of controlling the haemorrhage with the least constitutional disturbance to the patient.

Such less-extensive (though not less skilled) manoeuvres may convert the clinical situation into the stage 3 situation (see above), which is the subject of the first part of this chapter. In other words, the problem of long-term management remains but has been heightened by the event of serious haemorrhage. It could be considered that a more radical approach initially would have obviated this, but such an argument becomes circular; the best timing for operative treatment is when other circumstances are as normal as possible; the best decision to do so must be based on a very sound knowledge of both surgery and pathology.

Acknowledgement

The authors wish to thank Mr C. J. Stoddard, FRCS, Senior Lecturer in Surgery, University of Liverpool, for his constructive comments relating to this chapter.

Further reading

Allan R, Dykes P. A study of the factors influencing mortality rates from gastrointestinal haemorrhage. *Quart J Med* 1976; **45**:533–50.

Bennett JR, Dykes PW. Ulcerative disease of the stomach and duodenum. In: *Gastrointestinal Haemorrhage* pp 34–48. Ed. by P. W. Dykes and M. R. B. Keighley. Bristol: John Wright, 1981.

Browse N. *Symtoms and Signs of Surgical Disease.* London: Edward Arnold, 1978.

Classen M. Endoscopy in benign peptic ulcer. *Clinics in Gastroenterology* 1973; **2**:315–27.

Correa P. The epidemiology and pathogenesis of chronic gastritis: three etiologic entities. In: *Frontiers of Gastrointestinal Research—The Stomach*, pp 98–109. Ed. by L. van der Reis. Basel: Karger, 1980.

Cotton PB. Upper gastrointestinal endoscopy. *B J Hosp Med* 1976; **15**:7–15.

Green PHR, O'Toole KM, Weinberg LM, Goldfab JP. Early gastric cancer. *Gastroenterol* 1981; **81**:247–456.

McFarland J. The impact of gastrointestinal endoscopy on surgical practice. In: *Current Surgical Practice—Vol. 3*, pp 32–47. Ed. by J. Hadfield and M. Hobsley. London: Edward Arnold, 1981.

Morson BC, Dawson IMP. *Gastrointestinal Pathology.* Oxford: Blackwell Scientific Publications, 1979.

Sakita T, Oguro Y, Takasu S, Fukutomi H, Miwa T, Yoshimori T. Observations on the healing of ulcerations in early gastric cancer. The life cycle of the malignant ulcer. *Gastroenterol* 1971; **60**:835–44.

Schrompf E, Serck-Hanssen A, Stadaas J, Aune S, Myren J, Osnes M. Mucosal changes in the gastric stump 20–25 years after partial gastrectomy. *Lancet* 1977; II:467–69.

Thomas GE, Cotton PB, Clark CG, Boulos PB. Survey of management in acute upper gastrointestinal haemorrhage. *J Royal Soc Med* 1980; **73**:90–95.

Venables CW. Gastroduodenal surgery. In: *Gastrointestinal Haemorrhage*, pp 337–56. Ed. by P. W. Dykes and M. R. B. Keighley, Bristol: John Wright, 1981.

Watkinson G. The incidence of chronic peptic ulcer found at necropsy. A study of 20,000 examinations performed in Leeds in 1930–49 and in England 1960; and Scotland in 1956. *Gut* **1**:14–30.

6

Acute Abdomen: Section I

N V Addison and G I Horsfield

Introduction

The term "acute abdomen" is generally used to imply abdominal pain caused by peritonitis which may be local or generalized. The cardinal clinical features of peritonitis are pain, rigidity, and distension of the abdomen. These symptoms and signs are present when the peritoneum is inflamed or irritated by blood, bile, urine or pancreatic enzymes. Simple mechanical obstruction of the intestine is also considered to be an acute abdomen but the classical signs of peritonitis may not be seen until the late stages of obstruction.

Abdominal pain and tenderness do not necessarily mean that a patient has a peritonitis but following irritation of the parietal peritoneum by an inflammatory process, rebound tenderness and rigidity develop. These two physical signs are generally regarded as minimum criteria for the diagnosis of true peritonitis.

Diagnosis

The abdominal muscles over the inflamed peritoneum are tightly contracted, and if this rigidity is localized to one area it usually indicates the site of the causative lesion. For example, in acute appendicitis there may be rigidity only in the right iliac fossa. However, in diffuse or generalized peritonitis when the whole abdominal wall is rigid and motionless and does not move on deep inspiration, the cause of the peritonitis may not always be immediately obvious. The surgeon must, therefore, look for further evidence, such as in the age and history of the patient, which will assist him in making an accurate diagnosis. For instance, a history of previous indigestion and the sudden onset of upper abdominal pain followed by the signs of diffuse peritonitis, are classical features of a perforated peptic ulcer. Pain in the right shoulder tip occurs when the peritoneum of the right diaphragm is irritated and this may be present both in acute cholecystitis and in perforated peptic ulcer. In abdominal trauma pain in either shoulder tip suggests the possibility of a ruptured liver or spleen. If the peritonitis localizes, the rigidity passes gradually away and an abscess may become palpable through the relaxed abdominal wall or, in the case of a pelvic abscess, palpable by rectal examination. Where the peritonitis remains diffuse, peristent rigidity is ultimately followed by abdominal distension with the signs of paralytic ileus and profuse vomiting. This late stage in peritonitis is almost inevitably fatal unless the cause of the infection is removed.

Causes of peritonitis

Infection reaches the peritoneal cavity:

(a) from a perforation of the gastrointestinal tract;
(b) from an inflammatory process in one of the intraperitoneal viscera;
(c) after operation on a hollow abdominal viscus;
(d) directly from an abdominal wound;
(e) by direct spread from the outside via the female genital tract;
(f) from trauma causing rupture of a viscus;
(g) from blood infection.

The changing face of the acute abdomen

During the last 25 years the general surgeon has witnessed an interesting change in the relative incidence of the common abdominal emergencies (Table 6.1). Whereas acute appendicitis was formerly at the top of the list of causes, it has now been replaced by acute cholecystitis in the United Kingdom. The incidence of perforated peptic ulcer has also decreased, and we have seen in an ageing population the emergence of ruptured abdominal aortic aneurysm, which is now a fairly common abdominal emergency. Trauma is an increasingly frequent cause of acute abdominal pain and therefore must be considered in this context.

Table 6.1 Relative incidence of common acute abdominal emergencies undergoing emergency operation.*

	No. of cases	*% of total*
Acute cholecystitis	923	34.8
Acute appendicitis	914	34.6
Peritonitis secondary to diverticulitis	255	9.6
Small intestinal obstruction	168	6.4
Large intestinal obstruction	130	4.9
Perforated peptic ulcer	108	4.0
Acute pancreatitis	76	2.9
Abdominal trauma	47	1.8
Ruptured abdominal aortic aneurysm	27	1.0
	2648	

The majority of patients with cholecystitis and gallstone pancreatitis underwent operation during the same emergency admission.
* These patients were under the care of one of us (NVA) during the period 1971–1980.

Geographical variations in incidence

In general there is a striking contrast between patterns of disease in the tropics and the rest of the world, and this applies also to the acute abdomen. Acute appendicitis is rare in African negroes who consume a high roughage diet and have frequent bowel actions. Its incidence in the USA in negroes is similar to that in the Caucasian population. The incidence of acute appendicitis is increasing in Ghana in the upper social class who have adopted Western eating habits. Diverticulitis of the colon is considered to be uncommon in developing countries and is regarded as virtually absent from the black population of Africa. Contrary to these facts, diverticular disease of the colon is now appearing in Ghana and Uganda. Environmental factors are probably important in the incidence of peptic ulceration. Although the incidence of perforated duodenal and gastric ulcer in the United Kingdom has fallen during the last decade, the frequency of perforation of duodenal ulcer in the Madras region of India is rising. In Africa the same trends have been observed in districts such as South Nigeria, North Tanzania and North Ethiopia.

In the USA the type of hospital and the locality in which the hospital is situated affect the frequency of causes of an acute abdomen. In the Ben Taub General Hospital in Houston, Texas, the most frequent lesion is trauma which accounts for more than 50 per cent of all patients undergoing emergency operations for acute abdominal conditions.

Investigations

If there are definite clinical signs of peritonitis in the abdomen, then rapid decision making and operative intervention are mandatory for reduction of morbidity and mortality. It is important to realize that diagnosis is based on careful history taking and the recognition of certain pathognomonic signs, and the absence of certain clinical features can be just as important as the presence of others. It is only by taking a careful history that one can exclude extra-abdominal diseases and rare general causes of abdominal pain, such as porphyria, sickle cell disease, lead and other poisons producing abdominal symptoms. Modern investigatory techniques which have been introduced into all branches of surgery cannot replace clinical observation, particularly in the acute abdomen.

Once a clinical diagnosis of generalized peritonitis has been made, the following investigations may be helpful to the surgeon in confirming the diagnosis.

1. Plain abdominal X-rays
2. Grey scale ultrasound
3. Peritoneal tap
4. Haematological and biochemical tests

Plain films of the abdomen, supine and erect, are diagnostic in acute intestinal obstruction. In a perforated peptic ulcer there may be free gas under the diaphragm and this may be seen occasionally in perforation of colonic diverticular disease. Radio-opaque gallstones (10–15 per cent) are diagnostic in acute cholecystitis and gallstone pancreatitis in the United Kingdom, and in intestinal obstruction if gas is seen in the biliary tract this is conclusive evidence of gallstone ileus.

Other helpful findings on a plain X-ray include the loss of the psoas shadow in a leaking abdominal aortic aneurysm and the presence of stones in the renal tract. A plain X-ray of the abdomen is mandatory for abdominal injury, both blunt and perforating in type.

During the last few years non-invasive grey scale ultrasound has proved to be of great value in the diagnosis of acute cholecystitis and pancreatitis. In the early stages of rupture of an abdominal aortic aneurysm, by demonstrating the increase in the transverse diameter of the aorta, ultrasound may be the most rapid and accurate method of making an early diagnosis. More recently, computerized axial tomography has been used in the early diagnosis of an expanding aneurysm.

Aspiration of fluid from the abdominal cavity to aid the diagnosis of intra-abdominal disease is an invasive test which has been practised for years, but its role in the acute abdomen is very limited except in trauma and acute pancreatitis. When aspirated fluid is bloodstained, a decision has to be made whether the amount of blood is sufficient to require operative intervention following a blunt injury. A count of between 20 000 and 100 000 red cells per cubic millimetre is now regarded as a positive tap. The examination of peritoneal fluid for white cells is not helpful in the early stages of the acute abdomen as it takes several hours for the development of a leucocytosis. In our opinion the main indication for a peritoneal tap is in the detection of haemorrhage in abdominal trauma, especially in the unconscious patient. It can, however, be very helpful in diagnosis of a distended abdomen in the late stages of peritonitis.

Other tests which have been employed include a white blood count, but again in the early stages of a generalized peritonitis there is no appreciable leucocytosis and therefore this test is not reliable. On the other hand, in patients with acute cholecystitis and peritonitis from colonic diverticulitis, there may be an associated pyrexia and a neutrophil leucocytosis. A raised white cell count in a patient who has subacute intestinal obstruction may indicate probable strangulation of the bowel. Routine blood tests are not justifiable in a patient who is suffering from peritonitis due to acute appendicitis or a perforated peptic ulcer except in the late stages. Laparoscopy or peritoneoscopy has a limited value in the diagnosis of an acute abdomen except in tuberculous peritonitis and gynaecological conditions.

Acute upper abdominal pain

One of the commonest causes of acute upper abdominal pain seen today in a general surgical ward is acute cholecystitis, and the incidence has been rising steadily during the last few years in the United Kingdom. It affects men and women of all ages, occurring in the very young, and seen in increasing numbers in the older age group. In 90 per cent of patients with acute cholecystitis the cause is gallstones, but acute acalculous cholecystitis is not uncommon. In the young patient with acute cholecystitis, the possibility of associated haemolytic disease must be borne in mind.

The pathological process in acute cholecystitis is identical to that of an acute obstructive appendicitis, when the base of the appendix is obstructed by a faecolith. In the case of the gall bladder, obstruction is usually due to a stone in the cystic duct. The natural sequence of events to obstruction is perforation, but this does not occur so often in acute cholecystitis and unlike appendicitis it is uncommon in less than 3 to 4 days after the onset of symptoms. The wall of the gall bladder may already be thickened due to repeated attacks of cholecystitis and therefore is less likely to perforate. Because of this fact, many surgeons still adopt conservative measures in the management of acute cholecystitis. If there is an acute inflammatory reaction in the gall bladder wall, this may lead to a small gangrenous patch at the fundus and a local perforation may occur. This does not usually lead to generalized peritonitis as the upper surface of the gall bladder is in contact with the liver bed and the lower surface is almost always protected by very adherent greater omentum and transverse colon. The end result of a local perforation is a small abscess, which may eventually burst into the peritoneal cavity leading to a generalized peritonitis. The response by the peritoneum to bile irritation depends on whether or not the bile is infected, being more marked when the biliary peritonitis is secondary to acute cholecystitis although this is uncommon. Occasionally, in acute cholecystitis there may be a biliary peritonitis without evidence of perforation of the gall bladder. This is a rare occurrence and may be due to distension of the gall bladder by inflammatory exudate producing ischaemia of the gall bladder wall which becomes permeable to bile.

The diagnosis of acute cholecystitis can usually be made on clinical grounds alone. Pain is usually severe and may be colicky, often with radiation into the back between the shoulder blades, and occasionally pain is experienced in the right shoulder tip. If there is a tender palpable mass under the right costal margin, and there are radio-opaque gallstones on a plain X-ray film, then no further investigations are deemed necessary. Abnormal liver function tests, particularly a raised serum alkaline phosphatase, are valuable confirmatory laboratory investigations. The white cell count is often raised, but may be normal and quite often the serum amylase is high. On clinical examination a tinge of jaundice in the conjunctiva and a trace of bile in the urine also help to confirm the diagnosis. Conventional methods of X-ray investigation of the gall bladder and biliary tract are dependent on the excretion of the contrast medium by the liver. If there is abnormal liver function, which occurs in acute cholecystitis and pancreatitis, then oral cholecystography or intravenous cholangiography either fails or is of limited value. On rare occasions there can be a normal functioning gall bladder and yet at operation there is an acute cholecystitis with a stone impacted in Hartmann's pouch, so one should not be misled by this radiological finding. Infusion tomography with contrast medium has been advocated in the diagnosis of acute cholecystitis in the early stages of the disease, and TcHIDA scanning. There is no doubt that the greatest advance in diagnosis is the use of grey scale ultrasonography. An overall accuracy of 82 per cent can be achieved by this non-invasive technique which can be carried out shortly after admission. Ultrasound may demonstrate a thickened inflamed gall bladder wall and therefore is of value in a diagnosis of acalculous cholecystitis.

Acute perforation of a peptic ulcer remains a common cause of acute upper abdominal pain, although in the second half of this century the incidence has undoubtedly declined. The proportion of patients with a perforated chronic duodenal ulcer is falling and the majority now seen, between 60 and 70 per cent, are acute ulcers with little or no history of ulcer symptoms prior to perforation. This trend may be due to a change in environmental factors, more efficient treatment with specific drugs such as cimetidine, and finally to earlier surgery in the case of chronic duodenal ulcers. However, 10 per cent of all peptic ulcers do perforate and several studies have shown that analgesic ingestion is associated with the perforation of gastric ulcer. Stress induced ulcers of the stomach and duodenum have become more common, occurring in those patients who have had several major operations, including transplantation procedures, or are being treated for multiple trauma, or extensive burns. The aetiology of these ulcers is probably related to mucosal ischaemia, aggravated by hypotension, sepsis and hypoxia. The majority of these ulcers are complicated by active bleeding but acute perforation can occur (10 per cent). These complications are usually preceded by a marked increase in the volume and acidity of gastric contents which contain bile. Other acute gastric mucosal lesions which may perforate are said to be caused by injurious agents such as corticosteroids and anti-inflammatory drugs which are now commonly used. As far as corticosteroids are concerned, this topic has been dealt with in major reviews and it may be concluded that acute ulcers in patients on steroids are not more common than expected by chance and no association of steroids with haemorrhage or perforation has been documented.

In an ageing population it is not uncommon to find a perforation of an anterior wall duodenal ulcer concomitant with bleeding from a posterior wall ulcer. These ulcers tend to be of the chronic variety and the onset of perforation may be insidious. Those who die of perforation, and that is one third of ulcer deaths, are often undiagnosed before death.

The differential diagnosis of acute upper abdominal pain includes acute cholecystitis, acute pancreatitis, perforation of a peptic ulcer or of a pericolic abscess secondary to diverticulitis and acute appendicitis.

Upper abdominal pain with tenderness and guarding mainly on the left side may be due to splenic infarcts in sickle cell disease occurring in those patients of Central African origin who carry the gene.

Serum amylase remains the most accurate laboratory test for confirming the diagnosis of acute pancreatitis in the first 24 hours and any level above 1000 iu is significant. It should be remembered that many other conditions including perforated peptic ulcer, intestinal strangulation, myocardial infarction and acute cholecystitis can be responsible for a raised serum amylase. In a blunt injury to the abdomen a raised serum amylase indicates damage to the pancreas.

On a plain X-ray of the abdomen free gas under the diaphragm is seen in about 80 per cent of patients with a perforated peptic ulcer, so that its absence is not always diagnostic. When there is board-like rigidity of the whole of the abdominal wall and peritoneal tenderness on rectal examination, the most likely diagnosis is a perforated peptic ulcer rather than cholecystitis or pancreatitis, unless the gall bladder has actually perforated and infected bile has caused a generalized peritonitis. In the early stages of acute pancreatitis there may be generalized tenderness and rigidity but not as marked as in a perforated ulcer. Profuse vomiting associated with signs of peritonitis is common in acute pancreatitis and there is back pain in about 50 per cent of cases.

The white cell count is usually normal in a perforated peptic ulcer but raised in acute cholecystitis and diverticulitis, especially when the patient is seen several hours after the onset of symptoms. The medical condition which may mimic an upper abdominal emergency is a diaphragmatic pleurisy secondary to an infected condition in the lung. In this situation, abdominal pain and rigidity may be very marked affecting the upper half of the abdomen. The physical signs in the chest, positive X-ray findings, or a raised white cell count may favour the diagnosis of a thoracic cause of the rigidity. Just as acute appendicitis can mimic a perforated duodenal ulcer, the reverse situation may occur. The ulcer perforates and a little fluid escapes and, tracking down the right paracolic gutter, produces tenderness and rigidity in the right iliac fossa, and the remainder of the peritoneal cavity is free from contamination.

Injuries to liver and spleen

The lower ribs protect the liver and spleen from injury, but lacerations in both organs may be caused by blunt trauma. In adults there is usually evidence of rib injury or fracture, but in children this is not always the case as the rib cage is very pliable and so trauma to upper abdominal viscera must always be considered if there is tenderness and guarding in the upper abdomen. The spleen is more liable to damage by trauma if it is pathologically enlarged and occasionally ruptures spontaneously as in infectious mononucleosis and chronic malaria. Shoulder tip pain is an important symptom indicating free blood in the peritoneal cavity, and if this symptom is induced by raising the foot of the bed this is a diagnostic index of blood in the peritoneal cavity following a history of abdominal injury. A peritoneal tap using a catheter to irrigate the peritoneal cavity may be employed to help establish the diagnosis.

Surgical management of generalized peritonitis

The dangers of generalized peritonitis depend on two potentially lethal factors. Firstly, infection, due to the absorption of toxic products in a septicaemia and the failure of localization, and secondly, hypovolaemia, due to plasma and electrolyte loss. A knowledge of the pathological response of the peritoneum to infection helps the surgeon to understand the natural history of peritonitis and in consequence aids the planning of surgical management.

The peritoneum, which consists of flat mesothelial cells, basement membrane and vascular connective tissue, acts as a semipermeable membrane. In the initial stage of acute peritoneal inflammation there is swelling and desquamation of the mesothelial cells with replacement of the cells by a thin layer of fibrin enclosing neutrophils and cellular debris. The vascular response induced by chemical mediators, such as bacterial toxins together with histamine and vasoactive substances from mast cells, is characterized by dilatation and a rapid outflow of fluid rich in protein. Additional potent mediators of acute inflammation are the prostaglandins with some prostaglandins such as PGE_1 and PGE_2 producing vasodilatation directly and others potentiating the actions of histamine and kinin. One source of prostaglandins is the platelet which contains prostaglandin forming enzymes, and the inhibition of prostaglandins and serotonin release from platelets by corticosteroids probably explains why corticosteroids may mask symptoms and signs of inflammation especially in the acute abdomen. In peritonitis the large plasma exudate passes into the peritoneal cavity where it tends to collect in the dependent parts of the abdominal cavity, such as the rectovesical pouch, the paracolic gutters and the subphrenic region. The fluid increase helps to dilute the bacterial toxins and is rich in antibodies and fibrinogen which is converted later to solid fibrin by local thromboplastin. The resulting fibrin may serve to trap bacteria and seal local perforations. However, infection may spread rapidly in subserosal lymphatics and in severe cases septic thrombosis of mesenteric veins may lead to portal pyaemia and liver abscess formation. Clinically the peritoneum becomes pink and injected, losing its sheen due to the thin layer of fibrin which forms on its surface. These changes lead to the affected part becoming sticky, and coils of intestine adhere together. The amount of fibrin deposit depends on the causative organism, being greatest with an *E. coli* infection where there is a thick matting of fibrin around a perforation of the bowel. The fibrin deposit forms a protective adherent covering and limits the spread of the disease, leaving a raw surface if it is removed. Following treatment, the fibrin can either reabsorb completely leaving a clear peritoneal cavity, or become organized by the ingrowth of fibroblasts to form established adhesions which can be an important cause of postoperative morbidity such as small intestinal obstruction. If the peritoneum and other tissues are subjected to vascular damage caused by crushing, suturing, or ligation, then indeed adhesions develop due to vascular ingrowths of newly formed vessels into the ischaemic tissue. There is clinical evidence that some patients are particularly prone to develop peritoneal adhesions even after simple exploration of the abdomen. In general, however, the nature of the infective agent and the degree of chronicity of the peritonitis are important factors in the formation of temporary or permanent, localized or generalized, adhesions.

A second immediate peritoneal defence mechanism is the removal of bacteria and small particulate matter by lymphatics of the diaphragm helped by the natural upward circulation of peritoneal fluid and increased intraperitoneal pressure. The stimulation by bacterial products and other foreign material causes a marked influx of neutrophils which reaches a peak at 24 hours. This is due to chemotaxis and the most likely agents are the activated components of Complement. The influx of neutrophils is later followed by mononuclear cells which remove cellular debris.

The greater omentum plays a major role in the body's defences in peritonitis. Its mobility helps to localize infection and even sometimes it can seal off a perforation. It can wrap itself around an acutely inflamed appendix, preventing further contamination of the peritoneal cavity. At operation the position of the omentum is usually a guide to the cause of the peritonitis. However, in children the omentum is thin and flimsy and does not contribute to localization of infection to the same extent as in the adult. This difference is clearly seen in the case of an appendix abscess where in a child the infection is contained by loops of small intestine rather than the omentum as in the adult. Because of this fact, an abscess in a child should always be treated by operation. A more severe infection may spread directly over the surface of the peritoneum by the movement of the bowel and a diffuse peritonitis results. The peritoneal exudate is firstly a thin watery fluid (serous) but soon becomes cloudy due to the presence of leucocytes and bacteria. It may be purulent at the site of origin of the infection but still serous some distance away.

Pathological investigations, haematological and biochemical, may help in the diagnosis of the primary cause in generalized peritonitis, for example—acute pancreatitis. They are essential in the pre- and post-operative assessment of the degree of metabolic derangements of patients with severe generalized infective peritonitis, where early operation is essential. If the body's defence mechanism is unable to rapidly control intraperitoneal infection there is a depression of the level of plasminogen locally and thus of the fibrinolytic system in the peritoneum. Fibrin deposits remain for days and fibroblasts grow into the strands producing dense adhesions. Foreign material such as glove powder or barium also reduce the level of plasminogen as does intestinal trauma. Continuing infection with reflex small bowel ileus commonly gives rise to bacteraemia with a consequent reduction of the opsonic alpha-2-globulin responsible for the removal of particulate matter from the blood by the reticuloendothelial system. The failure to remove split products of fibrin digestion results in multiple organ failure in prolonged sepsis. Saba has shown that replacement of the opsonic protein reversed the organ dysfunction in some of his patients.

When the defence mechanisms of the body fail to overcome bacterial infection, abscess cavity formation occurs. Due to the natural upwards movement of peritoneal fluid such a cavity is commonly found in a subdiaphragmatic position. Alternatively as a result of gravity the infection tends to localize in the pelvis. A failure to localize by abscess formation under these circumstances can occur in patients receiving steroids, cytotoxic drugs, immunosuppressive drugs and with antibiotic lowered resistance or following previous radiotherapy. Under these conditions opportunistic pathogens may appear and cause septic complications. Debridement of the peritoneal space alone is highly desirable since the procedure removes foreign material, bacteria, fluid and dead and dying leucocytes. Floating bacteria are difficult to engulf by leucocytes and large volumes of fluid occurring naturally or introduced at operation by the surgeon also result in lowered oxygen potential and so inhibit the leucocytes since they require oxygen and prefer bacteria on a surface such as fibrin. There is a possibility that some abscesses may be the result of a self-perpetuating process of continued neutrophil influx resulting in tissue digestion and further neutrophil influx and abscess formation without bacterial infection.

Peritonitis can be either primary or secondary although the former is rare and usually occurs in children, accounting for about 2 per cent of abdominal emergencies in childhood. Spontaneous bacterial peritonitis also occurs in patients with ascites due to hepatic or renal disease. In cirrhotics, from being a rare unrecognized syndrome, primary peritonitis has quickly come to be considered a common manifestation of this disease. Any organism may be involved; classically pneumococcal peritonitis occurs in young girls and streptococcal peritonitis in boys. However, the occurrence of primary anaerobic peritonitis in young adults without ascites illustrates the need for expert bacteriological examination in these cases and it cannot be emphasized too strongly that this must include anaerobic culture. An immediate Gram stain on the pus in purulent peritonitis obtained from the lowest point possible in the abdomen, may yield vital information and direct rational antibiotic therapy. Gram negative bacteria appear to be occurring more frequently and their presence raises the possibility of an anaerobic infection. In patients with ascites the presence in the ascitic fluid of leucocyte counts greater than 1000 cells/mm^3 with more than 85 per cent granulocytes suggest a high likelihood of infection. In these patients the gram stain may not be so rewarding and centrifugation of the fluid to concentrate the bacteria is important. The predominance of organisms usually considered part of the normal bowel flora, particularly *E. coli*, has been demonstrated in several series. Whereas primary peritonitis is characterized by the presence of a single organism there is usually a mixture of bacteria in secondary peritonitis since in general it follows perforation of an organ. The site of perforation may be helpful in deciding primary antibiotic therapy. Gastric perforations release lactobacilli, candida and anaerobic gram positive oral organisms. Duodenal perforations are generally sterile due to the high acid content. The jejunum contains lactobacilli and streptococci in the upper part with replacement by colonic bacteria including enterobacteriaceae, enterococci and gram positive non-sporing anaerobes. In the large intestine water is reabsorbed and high concentrations of bacteria chiefly anaerobes are found. It is evident from experiments that despite the mixture of bacteria initially many survive for only a short time. In practice *E. coli* is the most commonly isolated aerobe and *B. fragilis* the most commonly isolated anaerobe. Coliforms lower the oxygen potential and allow the growth of obligate anaerobes such as bacteroides. It is evident that a combination of bacteria may be more virulent than a single species and it has been shown that any combination of an aerobe and an anaerobe results in marked abscess formation at least in experimental animals.

Effects of plasma and electrolyte loss

If a generalized peritonitis is not treated the exudation of plasma remains unchecked. As a result of this, the intestines become paralysed and dilated and the patient vomits profusely losing extracellular fluid in the form of saline. The loss of plasma by exudation into the peritoneal cavity and extracellular fluid from vomiting and small bowel dilation, ultimately lead to hypovolaemic shock and death unless treated.

In the early stages there is only loss of plasma, and the plasma protein concentration does not alter since the fluid loss is the plasma itself. At this point the plasma protein concentration is normal and the haematocrit reading is high. This situation also arises in acute pancreatitis in the early stages and the logical method of treatment in both peritonitis and acute pancreatitis is the intravenous infusion of plasma to restore plasma loss and improve the general condition of the patient. When a paralytic ileus develops in peritonitis there is a superadded loss of water and electrolytes in the extracellular fluid. At this stage the haematocrit reading is still high but the plasma protein concentration is also high due to fluid loss. The treatment then should be replacement intravenously of the lost fluid and electrolytes. The simultaneous measurement of haematocrit and plasma protein concentration enables the surgeon to distinguish between a pure plasma or extracellular fluid loss, or both, and thus treat the patient accordingly.

Treatment of generalized peritonitis

When the surgeon opens the peritoneal cavity, identification of the type of exudate is imperative for diagnosis and management. Escape of gas usually indicates perforation of a peptic ulcer, less commonly perforation of the small or large intestine, and only occasionally perforation of a pericolic abscess secondary to colonic diverticulitis. If the gas is under pressure this indicates a tension pneumoperitoneum but this condition should be diagnosed by physical and radiological signs preoperatively when gas is seen both inside and outside the wall of the intestine. Very rarely, gas may be caused by a gas forming organism such as anaerobes, in peritonitis. The presence of clear or turbid peritoneal fluid usually indicates a perforation of a peptic ulcer, appendicitis, of pericolic abscess from diverticulitis. Frank pus may be seen if the peritonitis is advanced. The nature and quantity of the free fluid in the peritoneal cavity is not always related to the physical signs in the acute abdomen. There may be extreme boardlike rigidity yet at operation there is only a little serous exudate present. On occasions, a rigid abdomen may be due to a localized acute appendicitis without perforation and no free fluid is found in the abdomen. In these circumstances, it is difficult to explain this variable response to peritoneal irritation but one should be aware that this situation occurs. In a primary pneumococcal peritonitis the exudate is profuse and typically sticky, greenish and odourless, and in primary streptococcal peritonitis the exudate is thin and cloudy. It is obviously of vital importance to identify the organism in primary peritonitis as quickly and accurately as possible. To do this it is essential to take a sample of peritoneal fluid from the lowest point possible in the abdomen, but if insufficient fluid is present, a swab will be adequate. Under ideal conditions the specimen should be sent immediately to the laboratory so that the chances of growing the organism are increased. The age of the patient must be stated on the request form. At night it is usually sufficient to place the swab in Stuart's transport medium. However, it is not unreasonable in a case of primary peritonitis for the surgeon to ask the laboratory to examine the sample at any time. Early identification of the organisms in primary peritonitis will lead to the rapid institution of specific therapy. In these patients it is often advantageous to give metronidazole routinely especially if an anaerobic infection is suspected. In acute tuberculous peritonitis, which usually simulates acute appendicitis in children and young adults, there is a thin straw-coloured exudate, and both visceral and parietal peritoneum are studded with fine white tubercles. In this type of peritonitis ascitic fluid should always be sent for microscopy and culture for acid fast bacilli, and a tubercle should be sent to the pathologist for histological examination.

Table 6.2 Causes of haemoperitoneum.

1. External trauma
2. Other conditions
   (a) Ruptured ectopic gestation
   (b) Rupture of aortic or other abdominal aneurysm
   (c) Internal strangulation of intestine and mesenteric thrombosis
   (d) Acute haemorrhagic pancreatitis
   (e) Rupture or torsion of ovarian cyst or intestinal tumour
   (f) Torsion of great omentum
   (g) Rare causes such as ulceration of a leiomyoma of the intestine or spontaneous rupture of the spleen

The presence of blood in the peritoneal cavity is either due to trauma or many other conditions which may occur spontaneously. (Table 6.2.)

Bile can be present in the peritoneal cavity following upper abdominal trauma, perforation of a duodenal ulcer, following surgery, and cholecystitis (Table 6.3). The presence of bile salts causes peritoneal irritation and a great outpouring of fluid into the abdominal cavity.

Table 6.3 Causes of bile in the peritoneal cavity.

1. External trauma
   (a) biliary tract
   (b) duodenum and jejunum
2. Perforation of a duodenal ulcer
3. Postoperative
   (a) biliary surgery
   (b) gastric surgery
4. Acute cholecystitis
5. Rarely in common bile duct obstruction

Management of upper abdominal pain

The timing of surgery in acute cholecystitis remains controversial, but there is no doubt that early cholecystectomy in the first few days after the onset of symptoms gives excellent results, especially in the elderly where perforation of the gall bladder is more common. Removal of the gall bladder is technically easier in the first few days than if carried out 3 months after the acute attack has settled down. There is a well-defined plane of cleavage between the gall bladder wall and the liver bed which consists of soft, oedematous inflamed connective tissue. This is well-illustrated in the case of an acute empyema or mucocele when it is very easy to remove the gall bladder if dissection commences at the fundus and is carried down to the cystic duct before this is divided. Finally, it is essential to send bile for culture in all patients undergoing cholecystectomy, especially when the gall bladder is acutely inflamed.

In a perforated peptic ulcer the abdominal cavity usually contains serous exudate which may be bile-stained in 10 to 15 per cent of patients who have perforation of a duodenal ulcer. It is essential for the surgeon to recognize the distinguishing features between an acute and chronic duodenal ulcer.

In the acute ulcer there is usually only a small perforation with little surrounding induration, and it may already be sealed off with a small fibrin plug. Minimal surgery is indicated in an acute ulcer and a single suture covering the perforation with an omental patch is adequate. In a chronic ulcer the perforation is usually larger and there is more induration and fibrous tissue surrounding it. Definitive surgery such as vagotomy and drainage should be carried out for chronic ulceration especially if this is associated with some stenosis or haemorrhage. Provided the patient is reasonably fit to undergo this surgical procedure the results are excellent.

Peritoneal lavage with saline and the instillation of antibiotics into the peritoneal cavity has been advocated, but simple removal of free peritoneal fluid by suction is usually adequate in most cases, especially when operated on in the early stages of the condition.

The majority of gastric ulcers which perforate are usually chronic and are situated along the lesser curvature of the stomach from the pylorus to the cardia. Simple closure is not always practicable owing to the chronicity of the ulcer, and if minimal surgery is to be carried out, then biopsy is mandatory. Ideally an immediate Bilroth I or Polya type partial gastrectomy is the treatment of choice for a chronic gastric ulcer as healing may not always occur after simple closure or the perforation may be in a carcinomatous ulcer. An ulcer situated on the greater curvature of the stomach is almost always malignant, and so a Polya type partial gastrectomy should be carried out.

Further reading

Addison NV. The clinical value of ultrasound in biliary tract and pancreatic disease. *Ann Roy Coll Surg Engl.* 1979; **61**:448–51.

Archampong EQ, Christian F, Badoe EA. Diverticular disease in an indigenous African community. *Ann Roy Coll Surg Engl* 1978; **60**:464–70.

Bartlett JG, Onderdonk AB, Thomas L, Kasper DL, Gorbach SL. A review. Intra-abdominal sepsis. *Arch Surg* 1978; **113**:853–7.

Bouchier IAD. *Recent Advances in Gastroenterology No. 4* pp. 27. Edinburgh: Churchill Livingstone, 1980.

Conn HO. Bacterial peritonitis: spontaneous or paracentetic? *Gastroenterol* 1979; **77**:1145–6.

Ellis H. The causes and prevention of intestinal adhesions. *Br J Surg* 1982; **69**:241–3.

Jordan GL. *Advances in Surgery Volume 14* pp. 260. Chicago: Year Book Medical Publishers, 1980.

Keddie NC, Gough AL, Galland RB. Acalculous gall bladder disease: a prospective study. *Br J Surg* 1976; **63**:797–8.

Kent SJS, Menzies-Gow N. Biliary peritonitis without perforation of the gall bladder in acute cholecystitis. *Br J Surg* 1974; **61**:960–62.

Matthews P. Primary anaerobic peritonitis. *Br med J* 1979; **2**:903–4.

McCartney JE, Fraser J. Pneumococcal peritonitis. *Br J Surg* 1922; **9**:479–89.

McDougal WS, Izart RJ jun., Zollinger RM jun. Primary peritonitis in infancy and childhood. *Ann Surg* 1975; **181**:310–13.

Morson BC. The Peritoneum. In: *Systemic Pathology*, Vol. 3 2nd Edition. 1182–1183. Ed. by W St C Symmers. Edinburgh: Churchill Livingstone, 1978.

O'Callaghan JD, Verow PW, Hopton D, Craven JL. The diagnosis of acute gall bladder disease by technetium-99m-labelled HIDA hepatobiliary scanning. *Br J Surg* 1980; **67**:805–8.

Onderdonk AB, Bartlett JG, Louie T, Sullivan-Seigler N, Gorbach SL. Microbial synergy in experimental intra-abdominal abscess. *Infection and Immunity* 1976; **13**:22–6.

Piper DW. *Peptic Ulcer*. pp. 37–39. Sydney: Aldis Health Science Press, 1982.

Robarts WM, Parkin JV, Hobsley M. A simple clinical approach to quantifying losses from the extracellular and plasma compartments. *Ann Roy Coll Surg Engl* 1979; **61**:142–5.

Saba TM. Prevention of liver reticuloendothelial systemic host defence failure after surgery by intravenous opsonic glycoprotein therapy. *Ann Surg* 1978; **188**:142–52.

Simmons RL, Ahrenholz DH. Pathobiology of peritonitis: a review. *J antimicrob Chem* 1981; **7**:Supplement A, 29–36.

Stephen M, Loewenthal J. Generalised infective peritonitis. *Surg Gyn Obst* 1978; **147**:231–4.

Stone HH, Kolb LD, Geheber CE. Incidence and significance of intraperitoneal anaerobic bacteria. *Ann Surg* 1975; **181**:705–15.

Targan SR, Chow AW, Guze LB. Role of anaerobic bacteria in spontaneous peritonitis of cirrhosis. *Am J Med* 1977; **62**:397–403.

Totten J. Primary anaerobic peritonitis. *Br med J* 1979; **2**:1225.

Weinstein MP, Iannini PB, Stratton CW, Eickhoff TC. Spontaneous bacterial peritonitis. *Am J Med* 1978; **64**:592–8.

7

Acute Abdomen: Section II

D A Macfarlane and J N Harcourt-Webster

Introduction

In the management of the acute abdomen the most important aspect is the judgement of the clinician. A knowledge of the common causes and to a lesser extent rarer ones is imperative. These mainly lie in the gastro-intestinal tract but reference must be made to trauma, genital lesions, vascular and metabolic causes as well as extra-abdominal pathology. The role of the pathologist is to assist in confirming the diagnosis and hence influence the surgeon in his decision to operate, or at times to deflect his intention and to encourage a more conservative approach. To obtain the best results teamwork between the surgeon and the pathologist must be close and full clinical information must be conveyed to the latter if a correct diagnosis is to be reached. The acute abdomen has to be regarded as an emergency and the decision facing the surgeon is whether a laparotomy is immediately necessary. A pre-operative report of urinary porphyrins is an example of what would be a contra-indication. It is the responsibility of the surgeon, aided by the anaesthetist, to assess the patient's general condition and overall suitability to withstand surgery. To this end the pathologist should be requested to provide a base line of tests, albeit in the majority of instances simple ones which support clinical acumen, but in addition which will aid resuscitation when necessary and assist future management. The acute upper abdomen has been discussed in the previous chapter and the features of the acute lower abdomen will be dealt with here.

Table 7.1 Acute lower abdomen presentations.

Inflammation:	Appendicitis Diverticulitis Crohn's disease Salpingitis Primary peritonitis Actinomycosis Amoebiasis
Perforation:	Colon and rectum Duodenum Obstructed bowel Infarcted bowel
Colic:	Ureteric Large bowel Appendix Ovarian
Obstruction:	Mechanical – Carcinoma of large bowel Diverticulitis Volvulus Intussusception Adynamic
Genital:	Testicular torsion Epididymo-orchitis Gynaecological
Vascular:	Infarction Ischaemic colitis Rectus muscle haematoma Rarer – polyarteritis nodosa, scleroderma
Metabolic:	Diabetes Porphyria Sickle cell anaemia Rare – lead, syphilis
Extra-abdominal:	Herpes zoster Spinal – vertebra – OA collapse – cord – tumour, compression Hip joint disease Bornholm disease

Presentation

The mode of onset of pain can be related to the underlying pathology. Visceral, parietal and referred pain should all be considered. Typical of visceral pain is the dull central abdominal discomfort associated with the early stages of acute appendicitis and produced by inflammation, distension or ischaemia of an autonomically innervated intra-abdominal organ. At a later stage, when the inflammation becomes more pronounced, the overlying parietal peritoneum also becomes inflamed and the pain can be felt in the right iliac fossa due to a nerve supply from the intercostals. Referred pain due to extra-abdominal causes has to be considered, although it is less frequent. Spinal lesions, such as osteoarthritis, spinal cord tumours or herpes zoster may simulate an acute abdomen, as well as may diseases of the hip joint or testicular torsion.

The rate of onset of the pain is affected by the underlying pathology. A gradual onset usually denotes an inflammatory cause, in the right lower quadrant, commonly due to appendicitis, although acute diverticular disease in an elongated sigmoid colon or salpingitis may be responsible. Leakage of gastric juice or contents down the paracolic gutter from a perforated peptic ulcer should be considered. It is unlikely that acute Meckel's diverticulitis will be diagnosed other than at operation. A sudden onset of severe pain is usually caused by rupture of a hollow viscus such as the appendix, the caecum due to distal obstruction or intrinsic carcinoma, or a vascular accident such as massive intestinal infarction or a ruptured aortic aneurysm. In intestinal infarction pain and guarding are generally more widespread than in the right lower quadrant alone, whilst bloody diarrhoea often occurs. There is sometimes a history of recent cardiac infarction or of atrial fibrillation and, in any event, where this diagnosis is likely, cardiac studies are essential. Biliary colic is unlikely to cause right lower quadrant pain, except in low lying gall bladders, but renal colic requires exclusion.

The age of the patient can also affect the diagnosis. The lack of an accurate history in infants and young children or a non-appreciation of pain in the elderly can account for many late presentations of perforated appendicitis, particularly when an epidemic of gastroenteritis is in existence. Mesenteric adenitis is common in children and difficult to differentiate from acute appendicitis, but a history of recent upper respiratory tract infection may be helpful. In addition the relatively few symptoms experienced by the post-partum patient in perforated appendicitis enjoins the necessity of accurate history-taking.

Additional symptoms other than pain may be important in obtaining the correct diagnosis in acute abdominal conditions. Anorexia, nausea and vomiting may occur in acute appendicitis, but are seldom dominant and generally occur after the onset of pain. If anorexia, nausea and vomiting are present before the pain and particularly if associated with diarrhoea, gastro-enteritis should be suspected, although pelvic appendicitis requires exclusion. If associated with blood, ulcerative colitis, Crohn's disease and the dysenteries must be considered, as should ischaemic colitis. Although the symptoms of diverticulitis resemble left-sided appendicitis, nausea and vomiting are usual. If the underlying pathology is more marked with severe pericolic inflammation, attachment to the bladder with urinary symptoms and even pneumaturia may be present. Severe and sharp lower abdominal colic, particularly in the elderly, and accompanied by sudden gross distension, can be due to sigmoid volvulus. The missed or scanty period may suggest ruptured ectopic pregnancy. Inflammatory pelvic disease often presents at the end of a menstrual period and the acute colicky pain of a twisted ovarian cyst is characteristic. The absence of anorexia and nausea and the occurrence midway between two periods can differentiate 'mittelschmerz' from acute appendicitis.

Previous administration of antibiotics may mask many symptoms and in turn such information should be made available to the pathologist for a correct interpretation of bacterial growth and culture. Other drugs such as steroids or even analgesics may complicate the clinical picture and communication between general practitioner, surgeon and pathologist is essential. Finally, in the history-taking it is important to remember that abdominal pain may occur in the ketotic state of diabetics and in those races susceptible to sickle cell anaemia.

Examination

Careful examination may elicit a number of important features. Where peritonitis is present the patient lies still, as unnecessary movement exacerbates the parietal pain, thus differentiating it from the writhing associated with ureteric or other colic. Abdominal retraction may be apparent in cases of perforation, or a mass noted in an appendix abscess or diverticular disease. In earlier stages of appendicitis, the mass may be composed of an inflamed appendix surrounded by oedematous omentum. Therefore in the first few days it is unlikely that an abscess has formed, and despite the presence of a mass it is wiser to explore the region and perform an appendicectomy. After 5–6 days the mass felt may enclose an abscess and the tissue response has sealed off the area. It is then wiser to await conservative resolution. At times pain, tenderness and a soft mass in the right iliac fossa are caused by caecal distension due to distal obstruction.

Obvious pallor and lower abdominal pain in a female are suggestive of a ruptured ectopic pregnancy, particularly if associated with a missed or scanty period. These symptoms may also be noted following trauma which has produced a severe rectus muscle haematoma. A severe haemoperitoneum requiring laparotomy may occasionally follow rupture of a luteal cyst midway between periods. Mesenteric occlusion with infarction and bowel strangulation are other known causes, as well as intra-peritoneal trauma from blunt or incised wounds.

Pre-operative investigations

These are of limited value to the surgeon confronted with an acute abdomen due to inflammation or haemorrhage. They are more helpful in acute intestinal obstruction, described later. They may be discussed under two headings: (a) radiological and (b) laboratory.

Radiological investigations

A plain radiograph of the abdomen may demonstrate a radio-opaque stone in the line of the ureter, or the presence of free gas in the peritoneal cavity in erect and supine films may be noted. The psoas shadow may be absent in the presence of a large intra-abdominal abscess or retro-peritoneal haematoma. Chest radiography may show metastatic disease, helpful in differentiating benign from malignant obstruction. Localized intra-peritoneal or pelvic abscesses may be recognised and defined by ultrasound or CAT scans. Angiography is the best method of diagnosing mesenteric occlusion or vascular bleeding.

Laboratory investigations

Haemoglobin estimation can be of value in all cases of suspected or actual blood loss, but especially in chronic bleeding, for example neoplasia or diverticular disease of the colon. It is an essential pre-requisite to assessment for anaesthesia in the elderly and in all cases involving haemorrhage or metabolic insufficiency. Race or country of origin may suggest the possibility of sickle cell disease or trait, requiring a search for HbS by electrophoresis. In the acute abdomen the surgeon prefers a simple sickle cell test as a matter of urgency. The PCV can be helpful in assessing the degree of hydration or blood loss.

An elevated or rising white cell count indicates well established inflammation or lymphoma, but a normal or low count does not eliminate such changes in their early stages, particularly in the very young or elderly. A differential count may help in rare cases such as eosinophilia or punctate basophilia. The blood sugar level may be diagnostic in diabetes and the urea and electrolytes should be measured, not only as a base line for future management, but to exclude uraemia, at times simulating the acute abdomen.

Normal or ectopic pregnancy is quickly and reliably excluded by confirming the absence of chorionic gonadotropin in urine using an agglutination-inhibition reaction based on latex particles as in the Roche Pregnancy Slide Test.

Cardiac enzymes and electro-cardiography may be required in the investigation of severe abdominal pain accompanied by gross shock; whilst this combination may well suggest a catastrophe such as torsion of an internal organ or rupture of a blood vessel or viscus, the possibility of referred pain from ischaemic heart disease such as a myocardial infarct must not be ignored. Microscopy for faecal organisms in peritonitis and biochemical estimation of serum amylase in suspected pancreatitis may be helpful. However, high levels of amylase, often above those usually found in pancreatitis, may accompany duodenal ulceration, volvulus, gangrenous cholecystitis, ruptured aortic aneurysm and mesenteric thrombosis; further, most patients with a raised amylase, from whatever cause, also have gall stones. Enteropathogenic bacteria, such as *Campylobacter jejuni*, *Yersinia enterocolitica* and *Clostridium difficile*, may cause abdominal pain and mimic acute appendicitis. If surgery is undertaken the appendix is usually normal but acute mesenteric lymphadenitis or terminal ileitis may be noted. If suspected, stool cultures should be undertaken and a search made for the responsible organism.

Operative management

On opening the peritoneal cavity by an adequate incision, careful attention must be paid to the escape of gas, indicating a perforated viscus, and the nature of any intra-peritoneal fluid observed. Clear fluid from a gastric or duodenal perforation may have tracked down into the pelvis and turbid fluid usually indicates an inflammatory process. Frank pus may be seen; bile is uncommon. Blood stained fluid denotes infarction or strangulation of the bowel, a twisted ovarian cyst or pancreatitis, the latter being accompanied by yellow-white flecks of fat necrosis around the pancreas and in the omentum and elsewhere. Actual blood is due to trauma, a gynaecological condition such as ruptured ectopic gestation or occasionally a ruptured aneurysm.

With suspected or proven infection microbiology is important, only culture determining the flora and its sensitivity to antibiotics. Whilst a plain swab may suffice, sampling into Stuart's transport medium is to be preferred. Where the organism may be the gonococcus, then Amies variant of Stuart's media, with its incorporated charcoal, is essential and, if possible, there should be direct inoculation on to a Thayer Martin culture plate. The value of an immediate Gram stain on pus obtained should be remembered and then initial antibiotic therapy can be commenced.

Table 7.2 Common pathological states encountered at laparotomy.

Inflammation
Perforation
Obstruction
Trauma
Vascular

Inflammation and perforation

The type of surgery performed in inflammatory conditions is governed by the pathological stage of the disease and by the age and general condition of the patient. In inflammation the changes develop to a varied time scale so that in the appendix or any other viscus, the external appearance does not always reflect the rate at which they are developing. The earliest visible change in both the appendix and its neighbour, the Fallopian tube, is dilatation and congestion of the small vessels of the serosa, going on to local or general hyperaemia. Swelling, especially of the distal appendix, may occur, and a patchy, purulent exudate dull the surface. The tip, sometimes the whole organ, becomes soft, purple and haemorrhagic as necrosis develops, and these changes indicate imminent rupture in any hollow organ. Local and general peritonitis may ensue following, as before, perforation, particularly in the young; if the patient survives, pus may accumulate in the pelvis or sub-phrenic spaces.

With less acute changes, or when the organ is retrocaecal or retrocolic, the disruption may be walled off by adhesions and a local abscess form; the adhesions may well involve omentum or loops of small intestine. Abscesses at these sites may 'point' and communicate with rectum or vagina and fistulae into bladder or gastro-intestinal tract can develop.

Such changes may suggest actinomycosis and this should be suspected if sinuses or fistulae follow appendicectomy; microbiological examination of any discharge and the inflammatory tissue is essential.

Appendicectomy is usually feasible in appendicitis but with the finding of a large abscess, particularly in an elderly and poor risk patient, drainage is usually wiser. In children, where localization is less effective, the appendix should be removed. In all instances histological examination must not be omitted, as occasionally underlying carcinoid disease or even carcinoma may be found, requiring further surgery, except where the carcinoid is found in the distal appendix.

When correctly diagnosed, Crohn's disease and acute diverticulitis will have been treated conservatively, but failure of response or the development of complications may necessitate exploration.

Acute Crohn's disease may mimic appendicitis, but is recognisable at laparotomy by thickening of the terminal ileum, by the presence of skip lesions and by mesenteric lymphadenitis. The classical picture is that of strictures with short or long, single or multiple segments of narrowing such as the "hose pipe" appearance seen in the terminal ileum. The bowel wall is considerably thickened, often with spread of the inflammation to peri-intestinal fat and neighbouring serosa, followed by fibrosis and adhesions with later sinuses or fistulae. Regional lymph nodes may be normal, but more often they are enlarged though soft and discrete.

The appearance of the disease at surgery is fundamentally the same at all levels of the gastro-intestinal tract, any variations being due to differences in anatomy and physiology as well as the different stages of the disease. Many patients and especially those where the disease affects the colon have anal lesions at some time during the illness; the peri-anal area ranges from dusky blue, oedematous skin, to one with chronic fissures and anal fistula. Sometimes the anal changes may be the presenting sign of clinically latent Crohn's disease higher up the gastro-intestinal tract.

As the full extent of the disease cannot be assessed in the acute phase, resection should not be performed, but if not involved, the appendix can be removed. If the disease has progressed to perforation or obstruction, resection may become necessary and in the large bowel this may mean extensive or total colectomy. Frozen section histology may prove useful at the edges of resection as more conservative removal is being performed at present. By-pass procedures may be the only alternative in fixed and irremoveable masses, but carry an increased risk of closed loop obstruction and carcinoma in the excluded segment.

The development of peritonitis or perforation in acute diverticular disease may require laparotomy, when it may be difficult or impossible to locate the exact perforation site. Diverticula may be restricted to the bowel wall or penetrate to extramural tissue; inflammation tends to begin at the apex so that initially it is the pericolic and mesenteric fat which swells, becomes dusky and inflamed. A small abscess may form around a sac and within the fat, but later local peritonitis occurs followed by fibrosis and adhesions to neighbouring structures with distortion; ultimately a mass develops. During this stage fistulae may form and there may be chronic obstruction because of the narrowed lumen. In such findings the possibility of carcinoma, even a small one tucked between the muscular folds, must not be overlooked.

Diverticular disease is most common in the sigmoid colon and may only involve a small segment, but spread with diverticulosis of the whole colon does occur quite often; it is not found in the rectum where the problem is one of duplication with complete or partial formation of a second tube.

If the general condition is reasonably good and the surgeon experienced, immediate resection has the advantage of removing all the affected tissue in one stage. An alternative is to remove the affected area, close the bowel distally and perform a proximal colostomy—Hartman's operation. It is probably a safer procedure and continuity can usually be restored at a later date. In some instances the diseased bowel may be exteriorized and opened to act as a colostomy. When the general condition does not allow these major procedures, a transverse colostomy can be undertaken and the abscess or perforation site drained. Carcinoma of the colon, if perforated, may be similarly treated. Biopsy of any residual mass will indicate whether resection has been complete and it is often helpful to delineate any questionable area with a circle of metal clips for later radiotherapy should neoplasia be diagnosed.

Primary peritonitis, occasionally due to pneumococci and occurring in children, is now an uncommon entity. Diffuse in nature, it can be confirmed by swab and culture, but is more often found today in cirrhotics with ascites. Peritonitis due to starch powder from surgical gloves can be encountered. The risk of it occurring can be diminished by thoroughly rinsing the gloves in water prior to opening the peritoneal cavity; the small white granulomatous masses may be seen on the peritoneal surface resembling tuberculosis or carcinoma. The pathologist should be warned of the possibility of the condition when a biopsy is taken so that it can be examined by polarized light, and it must not be confused with the fat necrosis accompanying pancreatitis.

Trauma

Injury to the lower abdomen, whether blunt or by penetrating wound, has increased markedly in the last decade as the result of a greater number of road traffic accidents and of mounting national and international civilian violence. Penetrating wounds are of two types: those due to high velocity missiles travelling at over 1200 feet per second, and fired by rifles, and smaller calibre missiles of lower velocity reaching about 850 feet per second and discharged by a hand gun. The latter type of wound is more commonly seen in civilian practice, but the amount of local destruction is greater following high velocity wounds when the bullet usually traverses the abdomen, leaving a gaping exit hole. Stab wounds are daily seen in our larger cities and can penetrate the peritoneal cavity, causing localized but severe damage.

Difficulties in diagnosis may arise in closed abdominal injuries, particularly in the unconscious patient with an associated head injury. In the presence of obvious shock and haemorrhage which is not responding to active resuscitation, little time should be wasted in getting the patient to the operating theatre. Plain radiography may denote the site of a low velocity missile, but laboratory help is of limited value except in the provision of adequate supplies of blood for transfusion. It is valuable to administer systemic antibiotics. In less obvious cases of intraperitoneal injury, peritoneal lavage may establish the presence of blood and is more reliable than a four quadrant tap. A haematocrit of 1 per cent or more in the returned lavage solution indicates significant bleeding. Previous abdominal surgery producing adhesions renders the procedure more difficult. Occasionally laparoscopy can be undertaken in a doubtful case where the general condition is stable. Despite positive peritoneal lavage it may show that surgery is not required for minimal injuries, thereby saving a laparotomy, particularly if there is drug intoxication or head injury.

At operation, full and adequate debridement of devitalized tissue is essential in the avoidance of infection. In civilian practice wounds are seen at an earlier stage than in war, and being more often due to low velocity missiles, there is less extensive soft tissue damage. Small intestinal injuries can be sutured or, where extensive, resected. Unlike military casualties the incised less contaminated wound in civilian injuries often permits primary colonic closure, unless associated with liver or pancreatic damage. A proximal colostomy or caecostomy may be an advantage or the wound can be exteriorised. An increasing number of foreign bodies are being encountered in the rectum. Some have perforated the upper part of the sigmoid colon and similar principles apply. Retroperitoneal haematomas resulting from gun-shot wounds should be explored as they may cover penetration of the large vessels or retroperitoneal organs.

Vascular problems

There are two principal pathological problems of vascular origin which may be encountered in the surgery of the acute abdomen. The first of these is a ruptured aortic aneurysm and the second is superior, less commonly inferior, mesenteric occlusion. The latter is usually arterial, either from an embolus or thrombosis due to atherosclerosis, but may at times be venous, which is known to be associated with the taking of the contraceptive pill. These pathological states are discussed fully elsewhere, but mention is made at this juncture as urgent operative management is essential for survival. Often, being asymptomatic, aortic aneurysms may be undetected until, at laparotomy for severe abdominal pain and gross shock, a large pulsatile and diffuse retroperitoneal mass is encountered. Rapid control of the aorta proximal to the aneurysm is mandatory and an aortic graft prosthesis is inserted. In delayed recognition the operative mortality is high.

With mesenteric or any vascular occlusion there is necrosis of the mucosa, with ulceration, haemorrhage and later progression to infarction. The affected intestine is oedematous and deep plum coloured, the outer surface developing a mottled, purple or greenish hue, as the wall becomes thin and friable and free blood leaks into the peritoneal cavity. Infection follows and toxaemia hastens death. Operation is often undertaken for suspected intestinal obstruction or perforation, but the blood stained fluid and necrotic bowel establish the diagnosis. In arterial obstruction the limits of infarcted bowel follow the distribution of the blood supply, whilst an oedematous mesentery and the finding of thrombi in the veins, suggests venous occlusion. In non-occlusive ischaemia the less sensitive muscle and outer tissues may remain relatively unaffected, whilst the mucosa and submucosa become haemorrhagic and ulcerate; typically, this is seen in acute ischaemic enterocolitis. In all cases resection should be undertaken if possible, unless incompatible with life, but out-patient parenteral nutrition may be necessary for prolonged survival.

When the changes associated with infarction are seen in an acutely dilated colon, usually the transverse segment, with some inflammatory exudate on the surface, the diagnosis is fulminating colitis (toxic megacolon); as with perforated ulcerative colitis at any site, treatment is partial or total colectomy.

Intestinal obstruction

Classification into the two main types; mechanical and adynamic ileus, is essential to the surgeon for the diagnosis and management of this condition. Mechanical obstruction may be partial or complete and due to causes within the lumen, in the wall or from external compression. In most instances it is found to be uncomplicated and called simple obstruction, but the blood supply may be curtailed or completely occluded, causing the more serious form known as strangulation, when the affected tissue has the appearances described above, as for infarction. If simple obstruction occurs at more than one point, the condition of closed loop obstruction results which, like strangulation, has serious effects. Adynamic ileus is the result of ineffective peristalsis. It is a usual occurence after intra-abdominal surgery due to intestinal handling, and believed to be a reflex response to injury. It is often secondary to sepsis, intestinal ischaemia or metabolic disorder such as hypokalaemia; or it may be due to extra-abdominal causes such as spinal trauma or burns.

The two types of obstruction must be differentiated from pseudo-obstruction occasionally found in the elderly due to faecal impaction, or in some instances associated with collagen disease or myxoedema.

Most cases of simple obstruction are due to intestinal adhesions affecting the small intestine, but the presence of a femoral hernia in an obese patient can be easily overlooked. All obvious external hernial sites must be carefully examined, but the possibility of a rare obturator hernia causing referred pain in the knee should be remembered. Diagnostic difficulties also arise in a closed loop obstruction. Localized tenderness is an important sign of strangulation. Intussusception in children can be overlooked if the patient is seen between attacks of colic, but blood and mucus in the stool and a palpable tumour provide the diagnosis. At times barium enema examination is both diagnostic and curative. The occasional gall stone ileus is easily misinterpreted as further biliary colic unless considered. At times the stone can be seen and air found in the bile ducts on plain radiography. Rarely small intestine ulceration follows drug therapy causing stenosis. Sigmoid volvulus is the main cause of sudden progressive abdominal distension and like caecal volvulus can be confirmed by abdominal radiography. The latter can show large bowel obstruction due to the commoner causes of carcinoma and diverticular disease or localized narrowing in ischaemic colitis or chronic inflammatory bowel disease.

At laparotomy the principles to be followed are to relieve any mechanical obstruction in the form of bands or adhesions when initial conservative treatment has failed or when strangulation or perforation has supervened. Over-sewing or resection of small intestine may be required. In large bowel obstruction where the lesion involves the right half of the colon and is resectable, right hemicolectomy should be undertaken, unless the general condition only permits a by-pass procedure. In left colon lesions in fit patients, resection with an end colostomy is preferable, otherwise a proximal colostomy or caecostomy may be advisable. A caecal volvulus should be untwisted and anchored. If a sigmoid volvulus cannot be decompressed rectally, resection is required without immediate anastomosis.

Genital disorders

In the male these will tend to be straightforward in their localization, although referred pain may be misleading in the initial assessment. Exquisite pain and tenderness, with or without swelling and discolouration, will concentrate attention on the scrotum and testis; the possibility of incomplete or mal-descent of that organ must always be considered in considering inguinal and low pelvic disease.

The cysts and neoplasms of both the ovary, uterus and related structures are often quiescent or almost so symptomatically, but they may present as an acute abdomen for a variety of causes. Examples are corpus luteum haemorrhage with haemoperitoneum; ovarian torsion with infarction and a dull, deeply congested, almost purple outer surface; and intestinal obstruction, with or without necrosis, when bowel has looped around the stalk of a cyst or neoplasm or become caught within a band due to previous inflammation.

Histopathology

The prime aim behind the histopathology examination of surgically excised material is to determine the final or, where that is not possible, the likely diagnosis; with that goes the extent of the pathology including the completeness of excision or the degree of spread and involvement of lymphatics and blood vessels from which an opinion on prognosis is formulated.

Small and shallow or crushed biopsies which cannot be orientated are valueless. The size and condition of material, and especially that from the edge of an ulcer or sinus, must be such that the various tissue layers can be clearly recognized, if necessary with a hand lens, so that after processing the sections are in the correct plane for microscopic interpretation. When neoplasia is suspected both the abnormal and adjacent normal tissue should be included, but as with all biopsies from hollow viscera care must be taken to avoid perforation. The tissue removed must be fixed straight away in 10–15 per cent formol saline, unless frozen section examination has been arranged. Similarly when infection is possible fixation must be avoided and fresh material including selected, or halved, lymph nodes submitted direct to the microbiologist, refrigerated until that is possible or treated as previously indicated. This is particularly important with chronic lesions and sinuses, such as in Crohn's disease, tuberculosis and actinomycosis.

With larger surgical specimens they should preferably be submitted to the laboratory fresh, unopened and unfixed; those taken out of normal laboratory hours can be placed in a plastic bag and safely refrigerated at +4°C until the next day. On opening the specimen the pathologist can thoroughly examine it, take any fresh material for special investigations such as histochemistry and electron microscopy, arrange for photography, complete a carefully detailed diagram-assisted description with an ultimate record of the site of tissue blocks and lymph nodes removed and pin it out to avoid distortion after fixing in formol saline. Colour photographs and lantern slides before fixation or, if unavoidable, after recolourizing and black and white at any time, make excellent adjuvants to the descriptive report and are invaluable for teaching. Surgeons and histopathologists routinely observing these procedures will be contributing greatly to the provision of high quality diagnosis and prognosis.

Where resection is the treatment it is essential that wherever possible the lesion, be it neoplasm, necrosis or inflammation as in ulcerative colitis or Crohn's disease, should be totally removed with viable non-involved cuffs of tissue on either side. All lines of excision must be examined microscopically to confirm completeness of removal, although in some instances the surgeon may not be able to achieve this for technical reasons. With inflammation the regional lymph nodes should be sampled and may materially assist diagnosis, as in Crohn's disease and tuberculosis, whereas with neoplasms all the nodes, their origin carefully recorded, should be removed and, however small, examined.

In many pathologies important information includes the degree of penetration into or through the tissue involved, the involvement of peritoneum, lymph node changes and vascular findings. This applies particularly to atherosclerosis with infarction, thrombosis accompanying inflammatory disorders and permeation by carcinoma. Furthermore, the surgeon must be aware of the possibility of mixed pathology such as appendicitis with carcinoid or carcinoma, ulcerative colitis with carcinoma and intussception with an adenomatous polyp.

Further reading

Bouterie RL. The assessment and diagnosis of the patient with abdominal trauma. *Int Surg* 1981; **66**:59–61.

Greenlee HB. Acute large bowel obstruction: an update. *Surg Ann* 1982; **14**:253–76.

Jones PF. Gynaecological disorders and the acute abdomen. In: *Emergency Abdominal Surgery*. Oxford: Blackwell Scientific Publications, 1974.

Morson BC. The large intestine. In: *Systemic Pathology, Vol 3* (Ed Symmers W St C). Edinburgh: Churchill Livingstone, 1978.

Powell DC, Bivins BA, Bell RM. Diagnostic peritoneal lavage. *Surg Gyn Obst* 1982; 257–64.

Price AB, Day DW. Pseudomembranous and infective colitis. In: *Recent Advances in Histopathology, Vol II* (Ed Anthony PP, MacSween RNM). Edinburgh: Churchill Livingstone, 1981.

8

Disturbances of Bowel Habit: Malignant Disease

R J Nicholls and B C Morson

Introduction

The first aim of the surgeon is to cure disease, and the second is to provide treatment in a way most satisfactory to the patient. With large bowel cancer the emphasis in the last 30 years has been very much on the latter, since survival rates have not improved during this time. The two greatest advances have been the introduction of endoscopic removal of polyps (saving many patients a laparotomy with the morbidity of colotomy) and the increasing use of sphincter-preserving operations for carcinoma of the rectum. The latter does not appear to have prejudiced cure rates and this is largely the result of appropriate selection of patients based on histopathological data. Pathology is fundamental to diagnosis, choice of treatment, prognosis and strategy of follow-up of patients with large bowel tumours, both benign and malignant.

The general pathology of large bowel tumours has been long established and forms the framework on which the specific attributes of a tumour in a particular patient are set. Whilst the clinician must be familiar with the framework, he also relies on the pathologist for guidance in the treatment of the individual case. In this chapter an account of the pathology of large bowel tumours is followed by an attempt to relate abnormalities to clinical features and management.

Pathology

Polyps

A polyp is a localized lesion forming an elevation on the mucosal surface. It is therefore a term which describes the morphology of the lesion and not its histological type. Polyps can be neoplastic or non-neoplastic (Table 8.1). Neoplastic polyps can be benign or malignant while non-neoplastic polyps are either metaplastic, inflammatory or hamartomatous. Some polyps may have stalks which can be short or long. Others are flat, although raised up above surrounding normal mucosa. They vary in size from tiny nodules to large pedunculated lesions or large sessile tumours.

Table 8.1 Classification of large bowel polyps.

Non-neoplastic:	Metaplastic
	Inflammatory
	Hamartomatous – Peutz-Jeghers
	– Juvenile
Neoplastic:	Benign adenoma
	Malignant carcinoma

Non-neoplastic

Metaplastic polyps are common, always very small and occur in 5–10 per cent of patients examined by sigmoidoscopy. This lesion can be considered to be a deformity of the normal epithelium in which there is cystic dilation and elongation of the crypts. The cells themselves are indistinguishable from normal large bowel epithelial cells. Metaplastic polyps have no malignant potential and have therefore no pathological significance, their importance being that they may be confused by the clinician with other types.

Inflammatory polyps occur in "colitis" and develop where ulceration has occurred. Neighbouring intact mucosa becomes undermined and relatively raised up, giving rise to a mucosal tag which can sometimes mimic the morphology of an adenoma.

Hamartomatous polyps are rare and occur in two forms—as juvenile polyps and in the Peutz-Jeghers syndrome. Although different histologically they share the common features of hamartomas which include the presence of morphologically normal epithelial cells arranged within an excessive stroma of connective tissue elements. Juvenile polyps may occur sporadically when they are solitary or few in number or as Juvenile polyposis, which is a rare genetically predetermined syndrome. Juvenile polyposis has a low malignant potential for colorectal cancer. The latter is an exceedingly rare complication of the Peutz-Jeghers syndrome; most cancers complicating this genetically predetermined type of gastrointestinal polyposis occur in the stomach and small intestine. Both types of hamartomatous polyps are pedunculated. Juvenile polyps have a particularly slender pedicle owing to the absence of connective tissue elements.

Neoplastic

A benign neoplastic polyp is called an adenoma and a malignant polyp is the result of carcinomatous change in an adenoma. The former is confined to the mucosa and lies superficial to the muscularis mucosae. In malignant polyps neoplastic cells have spread across the muscularis mucosae into the submucosa or stalk of the polyp. A neoplastic polyp is characterized by two basic abnormalities; first a change in morphology of individual epithelial cells and secondly in the normal arrangement of crypt glands. Thus there are both cytological and architectural abnormalities.

Neoplasms are often multiple, the term *synchronous* being used to describe simultaneous lesions. The term *metachronous* is used to describe a lesion separated in time from the occurrence of the first.

Adenoma

An adenoma is a process of cellular proliferation called epithelial dysplasia. The cells show enlargement of nuclei which demonstrate varying degrees of pleomorphism and mitotic activity. In normal crypts the nuclei lie consistently at the base of the cell adjacent to the basement membrane but this regular arrangement is lost, the nuclei being found at variable points between the base and apex of the cells. This feature is known as loss of polarity of the nuclei.

There are two basic types of altered architecture, tubular and villous. A tubular adenoma consists of compactly-arranged tubules resulting from excessive branching. In a villous adenoma epithelial proliferation occurs outwards into the lumen as frond-like processes covered by dysplastic cells with the stroma lying as a core within the epithelial elements. In a tubulo-villous adenoma the morphological pattern is intermediate between these two types.

Tubular and villous adenomas differ in their macroscopic appearance. The former are more usually pedunculated and the latter sessile. Villous adenomas are on the whole more extensive, i.e. involve a greater surface area of mucosa, than tubular adenomas. Tubulo-villous adenomas present as either pedunculated or sessile tumours. Malignant change is more likely to occur in adenomas with a villous component in their histology. The term adenomatous polyp and villous papilloma should no longer be used.

It is uncommon for there to be more than five or so synchronous adenomas in any given individual. In the rare condition of familial adenomatosis however, hundreds or even thousands may be present.

When one adenoma has formed, there is a tendency for metachronous adenomas to develop in the future. The likelihood appears to be greater if more than one adenoma was present at initial presentation.

Carcinoma

Adenoma-carcinoma (dysplasia-carcinoma) sequence Adenomas are premalignant lesions and it is probable that most carcinomas arise within a preexisting adenoma. Invasion through the muscularis mucosae by an adenoma is a common finding and the cytological appearances of adenoma and well differentiated carcinoma may be indistinguishable. Except for the uncommon instance of malignant change developing in ulcerative colitis, small carcinomas arising *de novo* without surrounding adenoma tissue have not been observed. In fact, many carcinomas contain areas of adenoma especially if they are not locally advanced. About 20 per cent of patients presenting with large bowel cancer have synchronous adenomas and the distribution of adenomas and carcinomas within the large bowel is similar, the majority of lesions occurring in the sigmoid colon and rectum.

A patient with an adenoma is liable to develop a metachronous carcinoma and vice versa. Those with multiple adenomas are at increased risk of developing carcinoma which rises to 100 per cent in familial adenomatosis. There is a well-documented epidemiological association of carcinoma and large adenomas and some (although not conclusive) evidence that destruction of rectal adenomas may reduce the incidence of colorectal cancer.

Evolution of carcinoma The essential step in the development of a carcinoma from an adenoma is the invasion of adenomatous tissue through the muscularis mucosae into the submucosa. Since this is the sole criterion used by the pathologist to diagnose carcinoma, the emotive term carcinoma-*in situ* is confusing and should be avoided; the neoplasm is either a carcinoma or an adenoma.

The carcinoma may spread from the submucosa by direct local extension, lymphatic spread, venous invasion and transcoelomic spread.

Direct local extension

Direct local extension can take place in three directions; usually outward through the bowel wall into the extramural tissues, occasionally around the bowel wall in a circumferential manner and, rarely, longitudinally within the bowel wall.

There is a general tendency for colorectal carcinoma to spread along lines of least resistance, e.g. via tissue planes or along the course of vessels or nerves. As it grows, parts become ischaemic resulting in ulceration as well as necrosis of the original adenoma. There is usually a surrounding fibrotic or desmoplastic reaction. Local spread outward through the bowel wall and beyond results in vascular invasion and penetration of other surrounding structures. The degree of local spread, therefore, has a most important influence on prognosis.

Venous and lymphatic invasion

Carcinoma in the submucosa comes into close contact with venous channels. When veins are invaded tumour permeates along the lumen and metastasises by embolization. Except for the lower rectum and anal canal, the venous drainage of the large bowel is via the portal system. The liver is therefore the commonest site for metastasis. In the lower rectum drainage along the middle rectal veins to the iliac veins may result in systemic venous spread. Invasion of veins outside the bowel wall is much more likely to result in metastasis than when intramural veins only are involved. There is some evidence that manipulation of a tumour may release tumour cells into the circulation but it is doubtful whether these implant and produce metastases.

Lymphatic invasion leads to metastases in regional lymph nodes from which spread to more central nodes may occur. In the colon and upper rectum drainage is to mesenteric and preaortic nodes while in the lower rectum spread along lymphatics in the lateral ligaments may lead to involvement of nodes in the lateral pelvic wall draining to the iliac and para-aortic nodes. In the lower anal canal drainage occurs to the inguinal nodes.

Lymph nodes in a lymphatic chain are usually involved in a serial manner, starting from the node nearest to the carcinoma.

Transcoelomic spread

Tumour cells can spread within the peritoneal cavity and implant on peritoneal surfaces. Initially small seedlings are formed but they may grow into large nodules. This form of spread takes place where the primary tumour has invaded through the serosa and does not therefore occur where the bowel lacks a serosal covering, e.g. in the lower rectum. Transcoelomic spread may be responsible for metastasis to the ovary.

Relationship of pathology to clinical features

Polyps

Non-neoplastic

Metaplastic Metaplastic polyps do not appear to produce symptoms.

Hamartomatous polyps Juvenile polyps produce mucus which has a yellowish hue. Owing to the slender pedicle there is a tendency for torsion to occur leading to sloughing (autoamputation). The shed polyps may be seen in the stool by the patient or parents. Patients with Peutz-Jeghers polyps usually present with intermittent small bowel obstruction and large bowel symptoms are rare; obstruction is caused by intussusception due to the polyp being propelled by peristalsis.

Inflammatory polyps There are no special symptoms due to inflammatory polyps.

Neoplastic

Adenoma Many adenomas less than 10 mm in diameter are asymptomatic, being found incidentally on investigation. The commonest symptom is bleeding due to ulceration. It is usually intermittent and small in amount. As with carcinoma (*see below*) screening studies using faecal occult blood testing have shown that bleeding is often unnoticed by the patient.

Adenomas may produce mucus and villous adenomas of the rectum in particular often secrete large amounts. Diarrhoea which occurs in some patients is probably due to the admixture of mucus and faeces resulting in a fluid stool.

Carcinoma As with adenoma, bleeding and mucus production result from the presence of the lesion within the lumen but other features of carcinoma are due to invasion into the bowel wall and beyond. Stenosis is both due to the carcinoma *per se* and to constriction by the surrounding desmoplastic reaction. Initially it is likely to cause a change in bowel habit with diarrhoea and constipation, resulting ultimately in obstruction. There is a tendency for left-sided colonic lesions to be more likely to constrict the bowel than right-sided or rectal carcinomas. A low lying rectal carcinoma may cause tenesmus, which is probably caused by the tumour or impacted stool above it stimulating the defaecation reflex.

Penetration through the bowel wall may result in the involvement of neighbouring structures. Nerve invasion (e.g. of the lumbosacral plexus by a rectal or rectosigmoid carcinoma) may cause sensory or motor disturbances of a peripheral or segmental distribution. The external iliac veins and lower limb lymphatics may become obstructed (especially on the left side), leading to swelling of the leg. Obstruction of the ureter leads to hydro- or pyo-nephrosis and occasionally to bilateral obstructive uropathy. Involvement of the bladder may cause an entero-vesical fistula producing pneumaturia and recurrent urinary infection. In the female a tumour may erode into the uterus or vagina and if fistula formation occurs, faeces and flatus are passed per vaginam. Involvement of a loop of small bowel may present with the features of small bowel obstruction.

Besides obstruction, abdominal distension may be caused by ascites formation. In large bowel cancer this is usually due to peritoneal metastases. General dissemination leads to systemic symptoms such as anorexia and weight loss.

The influence of pathology on management

Benign polyps

Treatment is influenced by two main pathological factors. First the histological type of polyp and second the number of polyps present. Based on these premises the clinical steps in management can be divided into five phases: first the identification of the presence of a polyp; secondly the identification of synchronous polyps; thirdly their removal for histological diagnosis; fourthly the follow-up of the patient (depending on histological type); and fifthly the construction of a family tree if there is a genetic factor causing the disease.

Identification

A polyp is usually seen either on the initial sigmoidoscopy or on a barium enema examination. Up to a few years ago, rigid sigmoidoscopy was the only means of inspecting the bowel at the initial presentation of the patient, but recently flexible sigmoidoscopy has been introduced for outpatient use. This enables the sigmoid colon to be examined in about 80 per cent of cases and the colon to the splenic flexure in about 40 per cent. As a result more polyps are being identified on the first consultation, the ratio of polyps diagnosed on flexible compared with rigid sigmoidoscopy being about 4:1.

Synchronous polyps

Having identified a polyp the next stage is to determine the number present. If not already carried out, the more effective way of doing so is by double contrast barium enema examination. Colonoscopy should be reserved for those patients in whom contrast radiology is unsatisfactory or negative despite reasonable clinical evidence that further lesions exist.

Occasionally hundreds of polyps may be demonstrated, indicating a polyposis syndrome and a few other patients may be found to have a carcinoma.

Removal technique

The method of removal depends on the site of the polyp and on whether it is pedunculated or sessile.

Over 90 per cent of polyps can be removed by colonoscopic snare polypectomy. These include all pedunculated lesions and sessile polyps up to about 2.5 cm in diameter. The latter can be raised from the muscularis propria by traction to create a false pedicle. Larger sessile polyps and those in which malignant change is suspected should be removed by formal surgical resection. In the mid and lower rectum it is usually possible to do so by local submucosal excision via an endoanal approach; in the rectosigmoid region and colon a segmental resection of bowel is necessary.

The technique of submucosal excision relies on the pathological anatomy of a benign polyp. Since the lesion is entirely confined to the mucosa, it is possible to separate it from the muscularis propria by scissor dissection in the submucosal plane. This is facilitated by expanding the submucosa with saline introduced by simple injection to raise the mucosa bearing the polyp off the rectal wall.

Histological examination

The pathologist has two tasks: first to make a histological diagnosis and secondly to determine in the case of adenomas whether malignant invasion has taken place. As a general principle, therefore, a polyp should be removed by complete excision biopsy so that surrounding normal tissue containing muscularis mucosae is present. With a pedunculated polyp it is therefore necessary to remove some of the stalk along with the head. With a sessile polyp the specimen should be removed intact and have a surrounding margin of normal mucosa.

An excised sessile polyp should be fixed to resemble its configuration *in vivo*. The surgeon can assist the pathologist by pinning the specimen out onto a cork board directly after removal to minimize contraction and distortion before fixation. This allows well-orientated sections to be cut, enabling the pathologist to determine the microscopic relationship of the adenoma to the muscularis mucosae.

Formalin pots should be big enough to accommodate these specimens. All polyps must be numbered and sent to the pathologist in separate labelled pots and their corresponding sites recorded on a diagram in the hospital notes. The location of any that have undergone malignant change will thus be known.

Features suggesting malignant change in adenomas

In some cases it is only possible to diagnose malignant change by microscopic examination of an excised adenoma. There are however, certain pathological features which may suggest invasion before removal. There is a clear relationship between size and the likelihood of malignant invasion into the submucosa and as can be seen in Table 8.2 an adenoma greater than 25 mm has a high chance of already being a carcinoma. The morphology of an adenoma, whether tubular or villous, sessile or pedunculated, is also related to the presence of malignant change. Ulceration of an adenoma suggests malignancy and an adenoma which has areas of hardness or induration on digital palpation should be regarded as a carcinoma. The desmoplastic reaction which to a large extent accounts for this induration may also be responsible for the important radiological sign of indrawing of the base seen on barium enema. Here the normal smooth contour of the barium representing the profile of the mucosal surface is drawn towards the lumen at the base of the lesion (Fig. 8.1).

Table 8.2 The relationship between type and size of adenoma and the presence of malignant change.

Histological Type	*Percentage with carcinoma*			*Total*
	<1 cm	1–2 cm	>2 cm	
Tubular	1	10	35	5
Tubulo-villous	4	7	46	23
Villous	10	10	53	41

Follow-up

The need for further action depends on the histological type. A metaplastic polyp is of no pathological significance but patients with hamartomatous polyps may develop metachronous lesions and have an increased risk of malignancy (*see below*).

Adenomas excluding those occurring in multiple familial adenomatosis are common and follow-up by regular surveillance of the large bowel may strain medical and diagnostic services. It is, however, apparent that these patients are at increased risk of developing metachronous adenomas and carcinoma. The risk is cumulative over the years and probably amounts to about 40 per cent for adenoma and 10 per cent for carcinoma over a 20 year period. The risk appears to be greater if synchronous adenomas were originally present and if the patient was over 60 years at initial diagnosis. There is a suggestion that a family history of large bowel cancer also increases the risk.

The optimal frequency of follow-up has not been established and it is not yet known whether an adenoma follow-up system is effective in cancer prevention. At the present time a full examination of the large bowel, preferably by colonoscopy at 1–3 years depending on risk factors, is being used in some centres. Villous tumours of the rectum

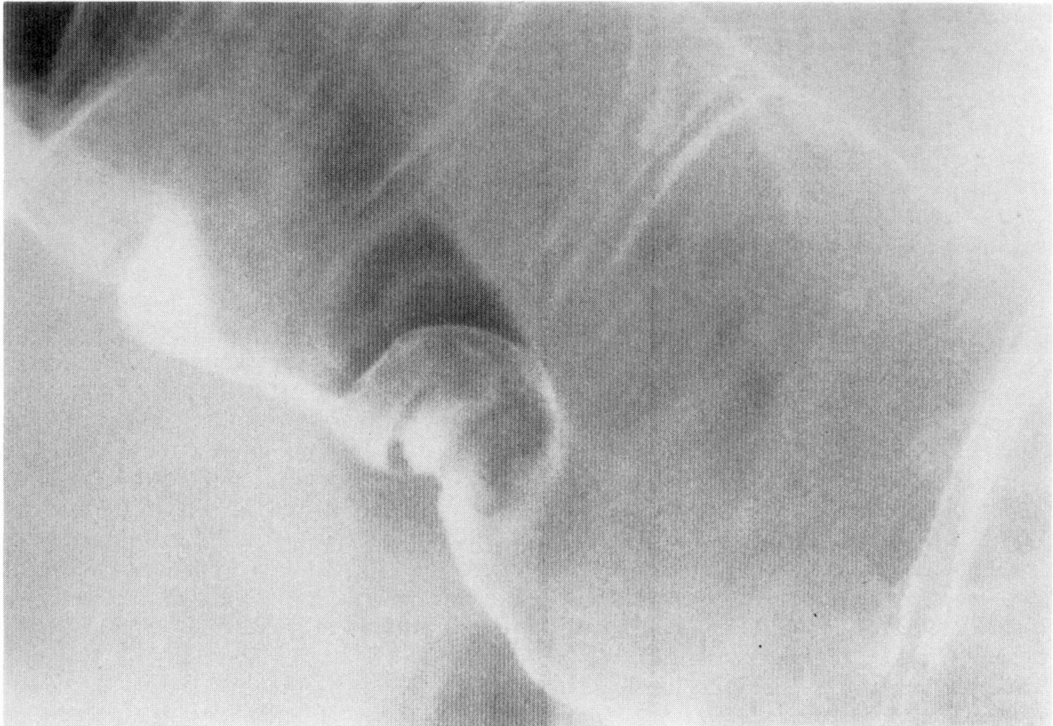

Fig. 8.1 X-ray showing indrawing of the base of an adenoma seen on barium enema.

treated by local excision recur locally in about 30 per cent of cases and regular digital examination and sigmoidoscopy are essential.

Family history

A family history must be taken from patients with hamartomatous polyps and adenomas owing to their high familial incidence. Even in the case of sporadic adenomas there may be an increased risk of large bowel cancer among close relatives.

Polyposis syndromes

Polyposis syndromes (Table 8.3) are rare and with the exception of metaplastic polyposis, they are genetic diseases inherited as a Mendelian dominant.

Table 8.3 Classification of polyposis syndromes.

Non-neoplastic:	
Metaplastic	
Hamartomatous	– Juvenile
	– Peutz Jeghers
Neoplastic:	
Familial adenomatosis	

Metaplastic polyposis

The occasional case with numerous metaplastic polyps may be mistakenly treated as for familial adenomatosis. This can only be avoided by establishing the diagnosis by microscopic examination of a polyp obtained by biopsy. No treatment for metaplastic polyposis is required.

Juvenile polyposis

The colon is primarily affected and there is a small but increased risk of large bowel cancer. There is no need for major surgery since the polyps are easy to remove by colonoscopic snare polypectomy owing to the long slender stalk. A colonoscopy at 1–2 yearly intervals thereafter should be carried out.

Peutz-Jeghers polyposis

The diagnosis is made on the demonstration of small bowel polyps by a small bowel barium meal examination accompanied by the presence of circumoral and perianal skin pigmentation. Surgical removal of the polyps through multiple small bowel enterotomies is necessary if symptoms due to intussusception are present. Large bowel polyps are uncommon and should be removed by snare polypectomy.

Familial adenomatosis

It is now realized that the entire gastrointestinal tract is affected in this condition, although the large bowel is chiefly involved. Adenomas begin to form in adolescence and rapidly increase in number. If untreated the development of cancer appears to be certain. Symptoms usually occur after the age of thirty. By this time cancer will be present in about two-thirds of patients. Adenomas may occur in the duodenum, and carcinoma of the duodenum, the biliary tree or peri-ampullary region may develop. Gastric polyps are often present but are almost always hamartomatous. Some patients also have tumours of connective tissues, e.g. fibromas, osteomas, intra-abdominal desmoids and epidermoid and odontal cysts. The association of these lesions with gastrointestinal adenomatosis is known as Gardner's syndrome.

Identification There are always over 100 adenomas in the colon when the disease is fully developed and this is the essential feature which distinguishes patients with familial adenomatosis from those with sporadic adenomas, where synchronous lesions seldom exceed five in number. The diagnosis will therefore be suspected after full examination of the colon by endoscopy and barium enema has revealed such numbers. Gastroduodenoscopy to look for upper intestinal neoplasms should also be carried out.

Removal Since there is no practical way of controlling all polyps by endoscopic means it is necessary to remove the colonic disease by surgical resection. Before doing so, histological examination of a biopsy of a polyp is essential to confirm adenoma. Failure to do so may result in unnecessary operations on patients with metaplastic or juvenile polyposis. A colectomy with ileorectal anastomosis achieves the aim of removing the bulk of large bowel at risk while avoiding a stoma. The rectum can readily be kept under surveillance by regular sigmoidoscopic examination and polyps destroyed by diathermy fulguration. During follow-up any area of induration or ulceration suggesting the development of carcinoma should be biopsied. A three-monthly sigmoidoscopy, and gastroduodenoscopy every 2–3 years are advisable.

Patients who are likely to be unable to attend for follow-up and those who develop cancer should not be treated by colectomy with ileorectal anastomosis owing to the risk of malignancy developing in the rectal stump. For these a proctocolectomy is indicated. It is now possible to avoid an ileostomy when this operation is necessary, by constructing an ileo-anal anastomosis with an ileal reservoir, provided adequate clearance of any established cancer is assured.

Family history

The dominant gene is likely to be widely distributed among members of the family, unless it has arisen as a mutation in the individual presenting. A typical distribution is shown in Fig. 8.2, from

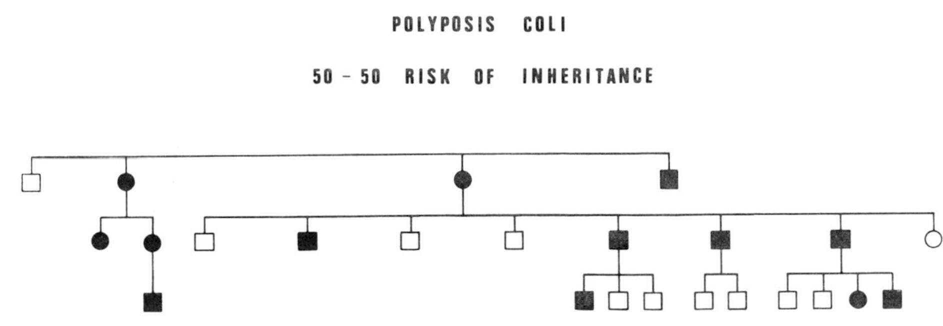

Fig. 8.2 Pedigree from a family affected by familial adenomatous polyposis.

which it can be seen that offspring from a heterozygous gene carrier have about a 50 per cent chance of being affected. The gene is rare, occurring in about one in 20 000 of the population.

Since the aim is to identify those at risk either at the present or in the future, a full family history involves the following: construction of a family tree; entering the family details on a register; identification of members at risk; and updating as children are born.

With this information, it will be possible for those at risk to be brought up for examination in the hope of identifying the disease before cancer has developed.

Carcinoma

Pathological stage

The pathological stage of a carcinoma is the most important factor which determines prognosis and consequently it has considerable influence on the choice of treatment. Survival is otherwise affected only by operative mortality and by inadequate treatment leading to avoidable recurrence.

The disease may be confined to the immediate location of the primary carcinoma and regional lymphatic and vascular drainage, or it may be disseminated beyond. Patients with disseminated carcinoma have little prospect of long-term survival in contrast to those with locally confined disease. In these, however, survival is related to the local extent which in part has been formalized in Dukes' classification, but is also influenced by the degree of local extra-mural spread in continuity with the primary tumour and by the presence or absence of venous invasion.

The stage is determined by clinical examination before or during operation, by imaging techniques and by histopathological examination of the resected specimen. The presence of dissemination is largely established by the first two methods, whilst the local stage is determined largely by the third. Ideally it would be preferable if the local stage were known pre-operatively so that the optimal choice of treatment might be made. In rectal cancer there has been some progress towards a clinical staging system which accords sufficiently with the pathological stage to be useful in practice.

Histopathological grading of biopsy material obtained pre-operatively may give valuable information on the histological grade which also is related to survival and local recurrence and may therefore be useful when selecting treatment.

Dukes' classification

The Dukes' classification is based on the degree of penetration of the bowel wall and the presence or absence of lymph node metastases. Carcinomas are divided into Stages A, B and C as shown in Fig. 8.3. Stage C is sub-divided into Stage C1 and Stage C2 according to whether or not the lymph node adjacent to the surgical ligature of the vascular pedicle is involved. There is no Dukes' stage to denote disseminated disease, although, as would be expected, locally advanced growths are more likely to have associated metastases.

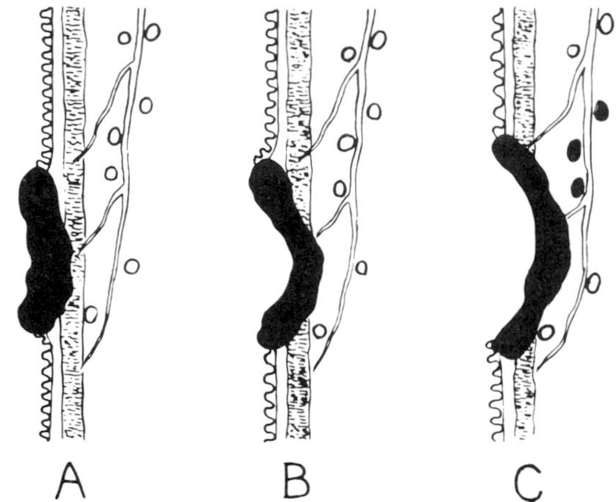

Fig. 8.3 Dukes' classification: carcinomas are divided into three stages A, B and C.

There have been several attempts to modify Dukes' classification, but most have tended to confuse definitions and have not usefully added to the accuracy of prognostic prediction. The relative proportions of Dukes' stages and corresponding survival rates are shown in Table 8.4.

Table 8.4 The prevalence of Dukes' stages and their relationship to survival.

Stage	*Proportion (%)*	*Age-corrected 5-year-survival (%)*
A	15	95–100
B	40	65–75
C_1	35	30–40
C_2	10	10–20

Extent of local spread

Extramural In his classification, Dukes distinguished only two degrees of local spread, namely confinement to the bowel wall and penetration into the extramural tissues. He recognized, however, that spread outside the bowel wall could vary considerably. It was clear that the outcome of treatment of a tumour that had just penetrated the bowel to invade the surrounding fat by a few millimetres was quite different from that of a tumour that had extensively invaded into surrounding structures. Accordingly local spread was divided into nil, slight, moderate and extensive as a complement to Dukes' classification. The criteria of these subdivisions are as follows: *nil*: confined to the bowel wall; *slight*: invasion of the outer margin of the bowel wall with commencement of invasion of the extra-mural tissues; *moderate*: well-established spread into the extramural tissues; *extensive*: deep invasion of the extramural tissues possibly involving other organs.

The importance of local spread as an indicator of prognosis is shown in Table 8.5. It can be seen that

Table 8.5 Rectal Cancer – The influence of direct local spread on survival and local pelvic recurrence.

	Extrarectal Spread			
	Nil	Slight	Moderate	Extensive
5-year-survival (%)	97.5	75	57	31*
Local recurrence (%)	NIL	0.9	5.9	16.8**

* Dukes & Bussey, 1958
** Morson *et al.*, 1963

besides its relationship to survival, local spread is also related to the development of local recurrence after surgery.

Intramural The microscopic spread of carcinoma within the bowel wall beyond the macroscopic limit is an important factor when considering the extent of surgical removal. Unlike carcinoma of the oesophagus or stomach where intramural microscopic spread may extend for several centimetres, large bowel carcinoma tends to remain confined to the macroscopic lesion. There are numerous pathological studies showing that microscopic spread beyond 1 cm distal to the macroscopic limit of the carcinoma occurs in only about 5 per cent of cases and where it does so, the carcinoma is usually poorly differentiated. If a sphincter preserving operation is proposed (e.g. anterior resection or local excision), local clearance must be adequate and it would seem that a margin of normal bowel greater than 3 cm is exceedingly likely to obtain clearance of any intramural spread provided the carcinoma is well or moderately differentiated.

Venous invasion

Invasion of veins in the vicinity worsens the prognosis as shown in Table 8.6. It is not surprising that

Table 8.6 The prognostic influence of venous invasion.

	Extramural venous invasion	
	Absent	Present
5-year-survival (%)	71.7	32.3
Distant metastases at presentation (%)	14.2	35.1

venous invasion is frequently associated with lymphatic invasion and with metastases to the liver. The prognosis is worse only when extramural rather than intramural veins have been invaded.

Lymphatic invasion

Involvement of lymph nodes tends to occur in a gradual manner from those in the vicinity of the tumour to those more central. It is uncommon for a node in the chain of drainage to be bypassed by invading tumour. The marked difference in survival of Dukes C1 and C2 cases indicates the prognostic importance of the extent of lymphatic involvement.

Histological grade

Based on certain morphological microscopic features it is possible to grade carcinomas into those that are well-differentiated, moderately well-differentiated and poorly-differentiated. It should be recognized that histological grading is a subjective assessment by the pathologist. There is consequently considerable observer variation in distinguishing well from moderately-well differentiated carcinomas, although agreement in identifying poorly differentiated lesions is much greater.

The relative proportions of grades in a large pathological series is shown in Table 8.7, and it can

Table 8.7 The prevalence of histological grades and their relationship to survival.

Grade	*Proportion (%)*	*Age-corrected 5-year-survival (%)*
Well-differentiated	20	80–90
Moderately-differentiated	60	60–70
Poorly-differentiated	20	25–30

be seen that each grade is related to different survival rates.

In grading a preoperative biopsy the pathologist can contribute to management particularly in identifying a poorly-differentiated carcinoma. It must be recognized however that a preoperative grade sometimes does not correspond to the grade determined from examination of the operative specimen. The surgeon can help the pathologist by supplying a large biopsy specimen taken from the edge of the carcinoma where the tumour is more viable and necrosis is minimal.

The influence of pathology on management

Resectability rate

The most important surgical factor which can be related to survival is the resectability rate, i.e. the proportion of patients in whom the primary tumour is removed. The inability to resect is usually due to extensive direct local spread from the primary into surrounding structures. Thus the chief factor determining resectability is pathological. There is, however, some evidence that resectability may also be surgeon-related. Table 8.8 shows the results obtained by two groups of surgeons working in the same hospital. The "aggressive" surgeons were characterized by a willingness to resect the primary wherever possible, in contrast to the 'conservative' surgeons who tended to leave the growth when other organs were involved. It can be seen that the different survival rates were largely accounted for by the different resectability rates. The surgeon should therefore do all he can to maintain as high a resectability rate as possible.

Table 8.8 Large Bowel Cancer: The influence of resectability on survival.

	Resectability rate (%)	*5-year-survival (%)*
Aggressive surgeons	92	47
Conservative surgeons	72	35

Peloquin, 1973

Disseminated disease

Nevertheless, about 30 per cent of patients already have disseminated disease at diagnosis and with few exceptions are incurable at the present time. Most present with obstruction or perforation and about 50 per cent of patients admitted with these emergencies have disseminated disease.

Dissemination may modify treatment, which should be limited to obtaining control of the local disease. In general, this involves removal of the primary with the most limited resection that will achieve this aim. Usually a major abdominal operation is necessary but occasionally a rectal carcinoma may be successfully controlled by local means including local excision, radiotherapy or diathermy fulguration. It is, of course, desirable for the patient if a colostomy can be avoided and with the various techniques available for preservation of the anal sphincter this is now possible for most rectal cancers. However, it should be appreciated that the return to acceptable bowel function after very low anterior resection may take many months, perhaps more than the patient's life expectancy. Under these circumstances the removal of a low-lying rectal carcinoma by total rectal excision may offer better palliation.

Survival of patients with liver metastases is related to their number and distribution, mean survival times of those with bilobar, unilobar multiple and unilobar solitary metastases being about 6, 12 and 24 months respectively. Patients with a solitary metastasis are important to identify since long-term survival (e.g. 30 per cent at 5 years) is possible following surgical resection.

Local disease

Synchronous neoplasms

As with managing an adenoma, a search preoperatively for synchronous neoplasms by barium enema of colonoscopy should be made. In about 2 per cent of cases a second cancer will be found and about 20 per cent of patients will have at least one synchronous adenoma.

Principles of surgical removal

The aim of surgery is to remove if possible all malignant tissue. In most cases, this is done by radical resection based on the direction of pathological spread. A radical resection includes removal of the primary tumour with an adequate surrounding of normal tissue and as complete a removal of the segmental mesenteric drainage as is anatomically possible. This is the standard operation for all colonic carcinomas.

The anatomical relationship of the anal sphincter makes the rectum a special case, however, and the alternative operations to total rectal excision have been devised solely to avoid a permanent colostomy. While anterior resection fulfills the criteria for a radical operation, local treatment does not. To some extent the choice of operation depends upon clinical factors, for example, the age, general fitness and build of the patient and the patient's wishes, but it is chiefly influenced by the local pathological features. The most important include the level of the tumour, the extent of direct local spread, the presence of local lymph node invasion and the histological grade. It is possible by clinical and histological examination to obtain much useful information when planning treatment pre-operatively. Sigmoidoscopy will give the level of the tumour and the microscopic examination of a biopsy the histological grade. Local extent and lymph node involvement can however only be determined by digital examination per rectum.

Clinical stating

Tumours up to 10–12 cm from the anal verge are palpable per rectum. Based on the physical signs of mobility and the presence of palpable extrarectal carcinoma (felt through neighbouring normal rectal wall) it is possible to identify four degrees of penetration of the rectum and extrarectal tissues correctly in about 75 per cent of cases. Stage 1 tumours are still confined to the rectal wall; stage 2 tumours are either confined or have penetrated beyond to a slight degree (approximately <1 cm); stage 3 tumours have penetrated the extrarectal tissues more extensively and stage 4 tumours have very extensive local spread whereby resectability is in doubt. It can be seen that each stage is related to markedly different survival and local recurrence rates following surgery (Table 8.9). Lymph node metastases can also be identified correctly in about two-thirds of patients.

The staging system is most useful in identifying tumours suitable for local excision but can also aid the decision on whether to perform an anterior resection or a total rectal excision or whether pre-operative radiotherapy should be carried out.

Radiotherapy is being used in combination with surgery in the primary treatment with the hope of reducing the rate of local recurrence. The clinical staging system may be useful in case selection for pre-operative radiotherapy by identifying those with locally extensive tumours who are at greatest risk. Postoperative radiotherapy can be based on the pathologist's examination of the resected specimen. Radiotherapy is not applicable to colonic cancer owing to the risk of small bowel irradiation damage.

Table 8.9 The relationship of the clinical stage of rectal cancer to survival and local recurrence rates.

Stage	*Extrarectal spread*	*5-year-survival (%)*	*Local recurrence (%)*
1	Nil	98	1
2	Nil + slight	86	4.5
3	Moderate + extensive	42	17
4	Extensive	<27	>17

Nicholls *et al.*, 1982

Major resections

There are many techniques for joining the colon to the rectum or anal canal and the indications for anterior resection are determined more by pathological considerations than by any shortcomings in the methods available. The amount of tissue removed by total rectal excision and anterior resection is similar proximally and laterally, the chief difference being the extent of distal clearance. Distal spread below the lower border of the tumour greater than 1 cm is exceedingly uncommon provided the growth is not poorly differentiated and a distal margin of normal rectum below the tumour of 3 cm long does not prejudice cure. Thus, carcinomas in the mid and upper rectum, i.e. above 8 cm from the anal verge, are suitable for anterior resection provided they are not poorly differentiated. Distal spread with these extends sometimes for several centimetres and total rectal excision would seem to offer the best prospect of cure. It should be appreciated, however, that the histological grade of a preoperative biopsy may not agree with the grade reported on examining the resected specimen. This is partly due to an error of sampling and partly to differences in interpretation by different pathologists.

The degree of extrarectal spread may also influence the decision, since it is inadvisable to carry out an anastomosis after removal of a growth (for example, stage 4), which is likely to recur locally, or where local clearance is known to be incomplete. Conversely stage 1 and some stage 2 lesions in the upper part of the lower third may be amenable to anterior resection without vitiating the patient's prospect of cure.

Local excision

Local excision is only appropriate where the alternative is total rectal excision with a permanent colostomy or when the patient is considered too unfit to withstand a major operation. It can cure carcinomas which have not metastasized to local lymph nodes and which are unlikely to recur. This depends chiefly on two pathological factors; first the absence of penetration of the bowel wall by the carcinoma and secondly a preoperative histological grading of well or moderate differentiation. With such growths the incidence of lymph node metastasis is less than 10 per cent compared with 50 per cent for those that have penetrated the rectal wall. Thus, adequate local excision should theoretically remove the tumour in about 90 per cent of cases.

Suitable growths are therefore those assessed as Stage 1 without palpable nodes and they should also be small enough for complete local excision to be technically feasible.

The pathological examination of the excised carcinoma is an integral part of the management. The pathologist will be able to determine whether the pre-operative clinical assessment and histological grade were correct. He will look particularly for penetration of the bowel wall and invasion of lymphatics and veins in the specimen. As with sessile adenomas, his task is made easier if the surgeon pins out the carcinoma on a cork board immediately after removal and before fixation. If the pàthological examination shows that the clinical assessment was wrong, removal of the rectum is indicated. With other methods of local treatment, e.g. radiotherapy and electrocoagulation, no specimen is available.

Follow-up

The purpose of follow-up is four-fold. First to identify treatment failure in the hope of being able to carry out some salvage procedure; secondly to discover any missed synchronous neoplasms; thirdly to identify a metachronous neoplasm; fourthly to establish the results of the primary treatment.

A purely clinical approach is inadequate in fulfilling all but the fourth aim. Clinical examination has therefore been combined with rigid sigmoidoscopy, examination of the large bowel by barium enema and fibre endoscopy and more recently by the monitoring of the serum CEA in an attempt to improve the first three.

Local recurrence

Local recurrence occurs in about 10 per cent of cases and is related to the local extent of the original tumour. It may, however, not be the chief cause of death in most patients dying of large bowel cancer. A detailed epidemiological study found that only 8 per cent of patients with local recurrence examined at post mortem were free of disseminated disease. It is however a most serious cause of suffering.

Attempts have been made to resect local recurrence. There is now considerable experience on the results of surgery used either where recurrence is clinically detected or when applied as a "second look" strategy. Only about 10–15 per cent of recurrences are apparently completely resectable and less than 5 per cent of patients have survived for five or more years, a salvage rate similar to the surgical mortality of these operations.

It is argued that the poor results of salvage surgery might be improved if recurrence were detected before clinical presentation. Monitoring of the serum level of CEA has been shown to achieve this, anticipating clinical recurrence sometimes by several months. There is some preliminary evidence suggesting that operations prompted by a raised CEA titre may have a greater prospect of resulting in the resection of all apparent tumour, but further reports are required before this can be confirmed. Often the CEA level is not raised when local recurrence predominates over disseminated disease.

Metachronous neoplasms

About 3 per cent of patients followed over a 15 year period will develop a second primary carcinoma. It has been shown that metachronous carcinomas among patients who have regularly attended for follow-up are of a less advanced pathological stage when compared with patients who have not done so. Adenomas which develop can be removed as previously described.

Further reading

Berge T, Ekelund G, Mellner C, Wenckert A. Carcinoma of the colon and rectum in a defined population. *Acta chir Scand* 1973; Supplement 438.

Bussey HJR. *Familial polyposis coli.* Baltimore and London: The Johns Hopkins University Press, 1975.

DeCosse JJ. *Large Bowel Cancer.* Edinburgh, London, Melbourne and New York: Churchill Livingstone, 1981.

Dukes CE. The classification of cancer of the rectum. *J Pathol Bacteriol* 1932: **35**:323–32.

Dukes CE, Bussey HJR. The spread of rectal cancer and its effect on prognosis. *Br J Cancer* 1958; **12**:309.

Enker WE. *Carcinoma of the Colon and Rectum.* Chicago and London: Year Book Medical Publishers Inc, 1978.

Goligher JC. *Surgery of the anus, rectum and colon.* Fourth Edition. London: Baillière Tindall, 1980.

Morson BC and Sobin LH. *Histological typing of intestinal tumours.* Geneva: World Health Organisation, 1976.

Morson BC, Dawson IMP. *Gastrointestinal Pathology*, 2nd edition. Oxford: Blackwell Scientific Publications, 1979.

Nicholls RJ, York Mason A, Morson BC, Fry IK, Dixon AK. The clinical staging of rectal cancer. *Br J Surg* 1982; **69**:404–9.

Thomson JPS, Nicholls RJ, Williams CB. *Colorectal Disease.* London: Heinemann, 1981.

9

Changes in Bowel Habit: Inflammatory Bowel Disease

J Alexander-Williams and H Thompson

Introduction

Diarrhoea is usually defined as three or more watery or urgent stools per day. Broadly, it can be steatorrhoea or malnutrition due to malabsorption. They can present as constipation or as distension. The first and last two manifestations often coincide but sometimes patients with malabsorption can be both constipated and malnourished. The pathologist is frequently able to provide the clinician with the appropriate diagnosis and guidance if adequate specimens are taken for histological examination.

Diarrhoea

Diarrhoea is usually defined as three or more watery or urgent stools per day. Broadly, it can be classified aetiologically as small or large bowel diarrhoea. Small bowel diarrhoea tends to be a loose, watery or frothy stool passed many times a day and at night. If it is associated with specific malabsorption of fat, the stool will tend to float, to be malodourous and the patient will usually be malnourished.

Large bowel diarrhoea often occurs particularly in the morning. The consistency of the stool varies from watery to hard solid pellets, sometimes with the two coexisting. Large bowel diarrhoea is frequently intermittent with alternating constipation and large bowel diarrhoea is more likely to be associated with pain than is small bowel diarrhoea.

When the clinician investigates the patient with disordered bowel habit, he will require the assistance of radiologist, bacteriologist and biochemist in his quest for a diagnosis, but he will rely heavily and often exclusively on the assistance of the histopathologist in achieving a final diagnosis. The clinician will want to know whether the disordered bowel habit is due to intestinal, microbiological or parasitic pathogens.

Although he will utilize and explore bacteriological services to assist him in the diagnosis he will also be providing the histopathologist with biopsy material obtained principally at endoscopy and relatively rarely at operation. He will look for confirmatory evidence of specific pathogenic disease such as Salmonellosis, Shigellosis or amoebiasis. Many of these specific enteric inflammatory diseases will be discussed in the next section. The clinician will need to know how best to procure, fix if necessary and to transport material for pathological examination. He should know specifically what question he is asking of the pathologist. He should also know how difficult is the task that he is setting the histopathologist when he sends a specimen to him with a specific request for diagnosis.

Infective diarrhoea

Although this is usually a self-limiting disease which responds to antibiotic and anti-diarrhoeal treatment, some cases go on longer than expected and mimic the picture of inflammatory bowel disease. Bacillary dysentery, salmonella infection and coliform diarrhoea are probably the commonest varieties but there is a long list which includes campylobacter diarrhoea, pseudomembranous colitis associated with *Clostridium difficile* infection, amoebic dysentery, staphylococcal enteritis, gonorrheal and chlamydial proctitis, infection with herpes virus, crytosporidiosis, leptospirosis, blastomycosis, infection with *plesiomonas shigelloides* or *aeromonas hydrophilia* and infestation with *balantidium coli*, etc.

The endoscopic appearances of these diseases are usually those of non-specific hyperaemia and friability. Some experts claim to be able to recognize such conditions as gonococcal proctitis on the sigmoidoscopic appearances of acute oedema and hyperaemia with thin mucopus in the lumen but such specific appearances will only raise suspicion. The diagnosis should rest on microbiological and histological criteria.

Acute infective diarrhoea produces oedema of the mucosa, neutrophils in the lamina propria and epithelium, inflammatory hyperaemia, erosion of surface epithelium, epithelial regenerative changes and a zone of oedema between the base of the crypts and the muscularis mucosae. Crypt abscesses and inflammatory erosions are usually scanty. Plasma cell infiltration is not a feature and lymphoid hyperplasia is usually absent. Rectal biopsy and bacteriological investigation indicate the correct diagnosis.

Chronic infective diarrhoea can occur in certain patients with amoebic or bacillary dysentery, cryptosporidiosis or chlamydial proctitis. In such cases plasma cell population is increased and there is a greater resemblance to inflammatory bowel disease.

A few patients with infective diarrhoea progress to true inflammatory bowel disease. In such circumstances the infection has acted as a trigger for ulcerative colitis or Crohn's disease. Certain patients with established proctocolitis develop superimposed infective diarrhoea which can only be detected on bacteriological investigation.

Pseudomembranous colitis due to *Clostridium difficile* infection

This represents a special variety of infective diarrhoea which follows the use of antibiotic therapy. Rare cases develop spontaneously in the absence of the administration of antibiotics. It is an important infection since it has a 40 per cent mortality rate in untreated postoperative patients. Furthermore, if it is not suspected it may be overlooked in clinical practice.

On sigmoidoscopy the mucosa of the colon and rectum is usually seen to be studded with multiple small yellowish plaques representing a pseudomembrane composed of fibrin, mucin and leucocytes. However in some areas the sigmoidoscopic appearances are normal. Histological assessment of rectal biopsy material is usually diagnostic. The faecal toxin test is positive in the majority of cases and *Clostridium difficile* may be isolated from the stools and swabs using special culture techniques.

The development of the final histological appearances can be divided into three main stages.

Summit lesion

Microscopic inflammatory erosions are visible consisting of fibrino-leucocytic exudate and mucin streaming upwards from the lamina propria on to the surface of the mucosa (Fig. 9.1).

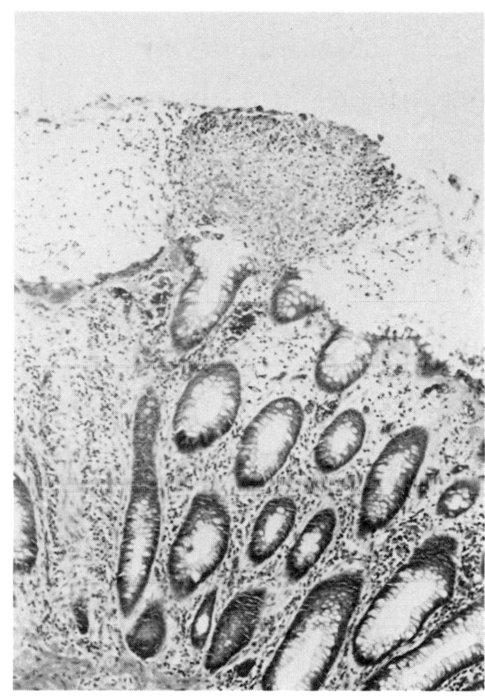

Fig. 9.1 Pseudomembranous colitis with summit lesion on surface of mucosa.

Pseudomembrane stage

A pseudomembrane formed by coalescence of a series of summit lesions corresponds to the yellowish plaques studded over the mucosa. Crypts in the vicinity of the pseudomembrane are frequently distended with mucin.

Necrotic stage

The mucous membrane shows necrosis probably due to toxaemia and ischaemia.

Non-specific acute inflammatory changes occur prior to the stage of the summit lesion during which neutrophils appear in the lamina propria and the surface epithelium shows regenerative syncytial changes with tufting. These appearances resemble those found in infective diarrhoea and the pathologist should warn the clinician of the possibility of pseudomembranous colitis if he discovers histological changes of this kind.

Pseudomembranous colitis responds to treatment with oral vancomycin or metronidazole. If the infection is not treated it can persist for more than one month. Occasionally, even after treatment, patients may suffer a relapse. Patients undergoing abdominal surgery for colerectal cancer are at particular risk and on such units the surgeon, physician and pathologist maintain constant vigilance so that pseudomembranous colitis can be detected and treated in its early stages.

Amoebic dystentery

This disease is most likely to occur in cities which are international ports. Accurate diagnosis helps to avoid the mortality associated with unnecessary colectomy in these cases since the disease can be treated medically. *Entamoebae histolytica* with or without ingested red cells may be identified by the pathologist in exudate covering a rectal biopsy. If doubt exists about identification of the amoebae then bacteriological examination of the fresh warm stool will resolve the diagnostic problem since the motility of the amoebae is highly characteristic.

Schistosomiasis

Ova or larval forms may be identified in the mucosa and this disease also can be corrected by medical treatment, so that unnecessary operations can be avoided by accurate diagnosis. Occasionally patients suffer from both schistosomiasis and inflammatory bowel disease.

Disaccharidase deficiency

When diarrhoea and distension are due to lactase deficiency specialized biochemical methods are required for diagnosis from material obtained by Crosby capsule or endoscopic biopsy.

Lactase deficiency leading to lactose intolerance is the commonest abnormality. Enzyme activity is assessed by preparing a homogenate from a jejunal biopsy and incubating it with the appropriate substrate and then measuring the yield of glucose. The biopsy should be taken from the first 30 cm of the jejunum where lactase is uniformly distributed in the brush border of the epithelium. Other tests for lactase deficiency include lactose tolerance tests and breath tests.

Primary lactase deficiency can be associated with abdominal discomfort, flatulence and looseness of bowel action but also it may be asymptomatic. Secondary lactase deficiency occurs in a variety of diseases including adult coeliac disease, tropical sprue, postgastrectomy diarrhoea, duodenal ulcer, ulcerative colitis and adult giardiasis. Secondary lactase deficiency can also occur in children with intestinal infection and Kwashiorkor.

Sucrose isomaltase deficiency represents another variety of disaccharidase deficiency which produces trehalase intolerance and discomfort after eating mushrooms.

Choleraic or bile salt diarrhoea

This does not produce any specific histopathological abnormalities but malabsorption due to a wide variety of disease entities can result in lipofuscin deposition due to vitamin E deficiency. Brownish pigmentation of the muscularis propria is due to excess accumulation of lipofuscin pigment in the muscle cells which can be corrected by giving alpha tocopherol. It is encountered in untreated adult coeliac disease, Crohn's disease, the postgastrectomy syndrome and Whipple's disease. In some cases the pigmentation is so striking that the name *brown bowel syndrome* is applied.

It is beyond the scope of this chapter to include important disease entities such as adult coeliac disease associated with subtotal villous atrophy, Whipple's disease characterized by PAS positive macrophages in the lamina propria, lymphangiectasia or alpha chain disease. These specific entities can be diagnosed by jejunal biopsy technique, by laparotomy or by serum electrophoresis.

The pathologist is occasionally required in the diagnosis or assessment of specific deficiency such as vitamin B_{12} deficiency when multiple gastric biopsies from the body of the stomach have to be assessed for absence of parietal cells.

Giardiasis

This is an important cause of travellers' diarrhoea. It can also occur in association with coeliac disease, hypogammaglobulinaemia, postgastrectomy syndrome etc. The endoscopic appearances are non-specific. Bacteriological examination of the stool or of jejunal mucus may reveal the parasite which can also be identified by jejunal biopsy technique where the giardia are found lying close to the surface of the mucosa. The condition responds readily to treatment with metronidazole.

Apudomas

These are islet cell tumours of the pancreas or carcinoid tumours of gastrointestinal tract, pancreas, etc. They represent slow growing tumours which secrete polypeptide hormones such as vasoactive intestinal peptide or amines such as hydroxytryptamine. These secretory products may be responsible for diarrhoea. It is rare for preoperative biopsy evidence to be *obtained* but the pathologist may be required to express an opinion on a frozen section during laparotomy.

Ischaemic colitis

Ischaemic colitis and ischaemic proctitis are particularly difficult to differentiate from inflammatory bowel disease. The history may give an indication of an ischaemic aetiology if there has been recent surgical treatment of an aortic aneurysm or any major operation, contraceptive pill therapy, cardiovascular disease, polyarteritis nodosa, autoimmune disease, strangulated hernia, major trauma, mesenteric vascular disease, carbon monoxide poisoning, renal transplantation, colorectal carcinoma, recent parturition or abortion, Behcet's syndrome, intussusception or volvulus.

Barium enema examination may show diagnostic thumb printing features. Endoscopic findings are occasionally misleading particularly if there is a pseudomembrane but usually there is ulceration which may be diffuse, patchy, irregular or linear. Ischaemic colitis normally resolves within 6 weeks, unless there is superimposed infection or recurrent ischaemia. Rectal biopsy may be diagnostic but at times the features are indistinguishable from those of proctitis.

The principal features of ischaemia vary from haemorrhagic infarction to ischaemic ulceration and intestinal necrosis with or without pseudomembrane. The depth of ulceration may extend through the muscle coat into the pericolic mesenteric tissues. The intervening mucosa can assume a cobblestone pattern and perforation and haemorrhage occur occasionally.

The histological features include ulceration, haemorrhagic infiltration, necrosis and leucocytic infiltration but the diagnostic feature is ischaemic necrosis of the muscle coat associated with leucocytic infiltration. Thrombosis of submucosal and subserosal veins is also prominent. In the later stages macrophages laden with haemosiderin granules can be identified; these give a positive Prussian blue reaction (Perl's test). A peculiar variety of fibrosis occurs in the submucosa which experienced observers can recognize as ischaemic. Thrombosed arteries are occasionally identified.

It has been established that almost all stercoral ulcers occurring in association with colorectal cancer or faecal impaction represent ischaemic lesions. The least common type of ischaemic lesion is a stricture which can be misinterpreted as inflammatory bowel disease.

Ischaemic lesions of the terminal ileum may present as surgical problems necessitating laparotomy. The aetiology is diverse and includes mesenteric vascular disease, thrombosis, embolism, reduction of strangulated hernia without resection and radiation therapy. The history and circumstances combined with the histological features enable a confident diagnosis of an ischaemic lesion to be made. The gross and histological appearances closely resemble Crohn's disease but necrosis of the muscle coat is characteristic and granulomas are usually absent. Ischaemic lesions can be misleading since they can be followed by recurrence after resection as in Crohn's disease.

Irradiation colitis

Following an irradiation dose of 3000–4000 cGY for the treatment of pelvic malignant disease, the sigmoid colon and rectum sustain mild reversible damage with oedema and hyperaemia leading to incomplete evacuation, diarrhoea and tenesmus. Radiation induced necrosis is a more serious complication that occurs 6–12 months after treatment or years later associated with ulceration, fibrosis and stricture; it is accompanied by diarrhoea, rectal bleeding, pain and constipation. These late complication are most likely to occur as a complication of treatment of Stage III carcinoma of the cervix with radiation dose exceeding 600 cGY in 6 weeks. Endoscopic appearances are those of a florid haemorrhagic mucosa with an undistensible rectal wall. Rectal or colonic biopsies may show ulceration, necrosis and vascular changes which include fibrinoid necrosis, endarteritis obliterans, thrombosis or telangiectasia associated with oedema and fibrosis. Epithelial dysplasia may be a confusing feature.

Diverticular disease

This condition may present as diarrhoea, altered bowel habit or as left-sided abdominal pain. Rectal bleeding may occur, but is uncommon and should always raise the suspicion of an associated carcinoma. The clinician should always remember that diverticular disease is extremely common and can be associated with other common disorders such as carcinoma, ischaemia and Crohn's disease. The role of histopathology in diagnosis is limited, nevertheless it is invaluable in differentiating it from ischaemic bowel disease and Crohn's disease. Therefore, as part of the evaluation of the supposed diverticular disease, endoscopic mucosal biopsies may play an important part.

The histological examination of resected material in diverticular disease is also important. On rare occasions, frozen section histological diagnosis is necessary at the time of the emergency operation to exclude carcinoma. When attempting to determine the source of such complications as haemorrhage or perforation, histopathological examination is also extremely important.

In diverticular disease a series of sacs project into the pericolic fat, principally of the sigmoid colon and in some cases these may be complicated by perforation, abscess or fibrosis. The diverticular sac may contain faecal material or purulent exudate. There is muscle thickening of the wall of the colon and sometimes there is a stricture with fibrous contracture causing concertina-like folds showing excess interdigitary bands of smooth muscle. Foci of ulceration may be present within the diverticula or on the mucosal surface. Foreign body giant cell reaction is frequently present in the pericolic tissues and granulomata are occasionally present in the muscle coat and other layers. It is important to remember that patients with Crohn's disease or ulcerative colitis may also have diverticular disease and that specimens of resected diverticular disease may show features of inflammatory bowel disease as well as diverticular disease. Muscle thickening alone may precede the development of diverticula and small diverticular bulges are seen in the prediverticular state.

Differentiation between diverticular disease and carcinoma can be difficult on gross examination in the resected specimen or at autopsy and therefore detailed histological examination is necessary. Ischaemic bowel disease is also occasionally superimposed on diverticular disease. Polyps within a deformed stricture segment may be difficult to demonstrate and may be missed.

Irritable bowel syndrome

This presents a common diagnostic problem. The diagnosis of the irritable bowel syndrome is one of exclusion and is helped by the findings of negative laboratory tests and normal histology in colorectal biopsies.

Colonic disorders of uncertain significance

Intestinal spirochaetosis has been found in 9 per cent of rectal biopsies by Harland and Lee. A blue haze is identifiable at the surface of the epithelial cells and under electron microscopy the spirochaetes measure 3 μm in length and 0.15 μm in diameter. The condition is probably of no clinical significance but it has been cited as a rare cause of diarrhoea and as an association with homosexuality.

Collagenous colitis is a rare condition characterized by a narrow zone of subepithelial collagen. It has been described as being responsible for watery diarrhoea and can clear up without treatment.

Malakoplakia can also occur in the rectum and colon.

Self-inflicted disease

Purgative abuse is a well known pitfall in diagnosis of diarrhoea, which has to be borne in mind; the characteristic sigmoidoscopic appearance of melanosis coli will give the diagnostic clue in most cases.

It is also useful to consider the possibilities of Munchausen's syndrome, ingestion of foreign bodies or introduction of instruments or foreign bodies into the rectum in subnormal or mentally disturbed patients. Some drugs, particularly antibiotics, are frequently associated with diarrhoea. Mefenamic acid (Ponstan) has recently been reported as precipitating colitis with recurrence on re-exposure. Diarrhoea associated with poisoning by arsenic or other poisons is fortunately rare.

Other causes of diarrhoea

There are many other causes of diarrhoea or altered bowel habit including amyloid infiltration of intestinal mucosa, vagotomy diarrhoea, etc.

Constipation

Constipation can be due to faulty diet or faulty habits such as inadequate bulk intake, ignoring the call to stool, lack of exercise, change of drinking water or, paradoxically, to laxative abuse.

Disorders of motility such as idiopathic slow transit and the irritable bowel syndrome, idiopathic megacolon or megarectum have no specific histological abnormality to aid in diagnosis or to guide in the treatment. However, such diagnoses are made only after specific disorders such as Hirschsprung's disease have been excluded on histological grounds.

Melanosis coli

Melanosis coli may be appreciated on endoscopy and can be confirmed on examination of biopsies.

Black pigmentation of the mucosa is due to accumulation of lipofuscin pigment (pseudomelanin) granules in macrophages within the lamina propria. The discolouration of the mucosa is associated with purgative abuse particularly with the anthracene group (cascara, senna, aloes, etc.) and the mucosa may also show the features of the cathartic colon, which has a characteristic snake skin appearance of the mucosal surface.

Endocrinal and metabolic causes of constipation

These include hypothyroidism, diabetes mellitus, hypopituitarism, phaechromocytoma, hypokalaemia, hypercalcaemia, uraemia and porphyria. Histopathological information is only of indirect value in the assessment of these conditions.

Chronic recurrent obstruction

When the cause of disordered bowel function is due to a mechanical obstruction the diagnosis is more likely to be made radiologically or endoscopically than it is by the pathologist. However, there are some stigmata of chronic recurrent obstruction that can be observed by the pathologist.

Strictures may also be responsible for chronic recurrent obstruction and the pathologist may be able to help if there is histological evidence of carcinoma or Crohn's disease. Frequently, however, biopsies are not diagnostic and the diagnosis can only be made by inference as, for example in ischaemic stricture.

Neurological disorders

These may be associated with gross constipation. The best known and possibly the most important of these is Hirschsprung's disease. In this disease the histopathological diagnosis is vitally important as is the delineation of the extent of the disease. In the assessment of this condition the closest possible collaboration is necessary between surgeon and the pathologist; they should plan before operation the site and the depth of biopsies which will provide maximum information. Other neurological disorders include neuronal dysplasia and adynamic bowel syndrome. Silver impregnation studies or immunocytochemical studies of the myenteric plexus are rewarding in the diagnosis.

Hirschsprung's disease

Cases of suspected Hirschsprung's disease require serial section study of rectal biopsies which must include the submucosa. A strip of mucosa and submucosa at least 2 cm in length, starting 1 cm above the anal canal is necessary so as to be above the area normally free of ganglion cells. However, most pathologists prefer a full thickness biopsy taken 1–2 cm above the pectineal line to include both Auerbach's and Meissner's plexuses. Absence of ganglion cells and hypertrophy of nerve bundles occur in the aganglionic segment. It has recently been claimed that histochemical acetyl cholinesterase estimation on suction biopsies provides a highly accurate diagnosis of Hirschsprung's disease. A minimum of two or three biopsies are taken 1–2 cm above the anal margin at various distances to consist of mucosa, muscularis mucosa and submucosa. The specimens are properly orientated and fresh frozen in liquid nitrogen. The technique reveals absence of ganglion cells and thick tortuous nerve fibres in the lamina propria, muscularis mucosae and submucosa which are acetyl cholinesterase positive.

Other causes of chronic recurrent obstruction include adynamic bowel syndrome and neuronal dysplasia.

In parts of Southern and Central America acquired megacolon may also be due to Chagas' disease. It may also occur through damage to the colonic myenteric plexus by drugs. Special argyrophil techniques (Smith) or methods to demonstrate peptidergic fibres (Polak) can also be utilized.

Intestinal pseudo-obstruction is also a feature of scleroderma associated with disappearance of smooth muscle from the muscularis propria.

Disordered bowel habit may be associated with degenerative conditions of the large gut such as pneumatosis coli, and the solitary rectal ulcer syndrome. In each of these, biopsy material is essential to the diagnosis and the histological picture is characteristic. It is always important that the surgeon knows from which part of the lesion to take the biopsy; particularly so in the solitary rectal ulcer syndrome.

Pneumatosis cystoides intestinalis (Pneumatosis coli)

Gas containing cysts lined with histiocytes and Langhans giant cells are encountered in the mucosa and submucosa and occasionally in other layers. They are usually readily recognizable as bullae on endoscopy but the cobblestone pattern in the rectal mucosa is occasionally mistaken for carcinoma or polyposis. Therefore a diagnostic rectal biopsy is mandatory before excision of the rectum.

The histological features are characteristic. The aetiology is unknown but there are associations with chronic chest disease and peptic ulcer disease. Production of cysts by gas producing bacteria is one of the popular theories of pathogenesis.

Solitary rectal ulcer syndrome (See Chapter 10, p. 124)

A simple chronic solitary rectal ulcer usually exhibits characteristic histological features. These include proliferation and extension of smooth muscle bundles into the lamina propria of the mucosa, dysplasia associated with fibrosis, buried islands of regenerating mucin secreting epithelium and ischaemic changes. Aetiological factors include prolapse of rectal mucosa during defaecation, trauma and ischaemia.

Other causes of ulceration in the rectum include the primary chancre of syphilis, Behçet's syndrome and polyarteritis nodosa.

Inflammatory bowel disease

There is hardly any aspect of gastro-intestinal surgery where collaboration between surgeon and pathologist is more important than in the diagnosis and the assessment of inflammatory bowel disease. The acute inflammatory bowel diseases have been discussed in the previous section on diarrhoea. The chronic inflammatory bowel diseases are even more common as diagnostic problems.

The suspicion of tuberculosis, bilharzia, Chagas' disease or actinomycosis will depend largely on which part of the world the patient comes from or in which country the disease is being investigated. In temperate and sub-tropical areas, particularly in the developed parts of the world, the diagnosis of chronic inflammatory bowel disease tends to rest between Crohn's disease and chronic mucosal ulcerative colitis. Most of the discussion in this section is concerned with their differentiation in that it affects therapy, prognosis and possible cancer risk.

Clinical presentations and the place of pathology

When a patient presents with bowel disease, which is obviously not acute bacterial or viral the clinician has to decide whether the disease is neoplastic, degenerative or inflammatory. Clinical examination often gives little clue to the differentiation, though occasionally a localized lesion can be felt on abdominal or rectal examination.

Endoscopy

Sigmoidoscopy is the first major step in the differential diagnosis; it tells the clinician whether the disease is localized or generalized. If localized then the differentiation between a neoplasm, or solitary rectal ulcer or a localized patch of Crohn's disease can usually be made on the biopsy material. If the disease is generalized and the diagnosis of pneumatosis has been ruled out on biopsy, the differentiation of generalized chronic inflammatory bowel disease is between the specific and the nonspecific.

Endoscopic mucosal biopsies are vitally important in determining the diagnosis of mucosal ulcerative colitis and in determining its extent. Biopsies are also of great value in determining the degree of dysplasia that may indicate the risk of malignant degeneration. However, it must be remembered that one does not necessarily find advanced dysplasia in the mucosal biopsies of the rectum of even those patients with chronic ulcerative colitis who have already developed large bowel carcinoma. Furthermore, not every patient with advanced dysplasia develops a neoplasm. Nonetheless, the careful evaluation of proper biopsies gives by far the best indication as to when prophylactic bowel resection should be performed in chronic ulcerative colitis. Conversely, the absence of dysplastic change on multiple biopsies is a good reassurance for clinicians who are wishing to preserve the large bowel in patients with a long history of colitis.

It is important to remember that many patients who were diagnosed initially as having ulcerative colitis and who had a proctocolectomy on the basis of such a diagnosis, have had to be re-diagnosed as Crohn's disease when typical granulomatous lesions have appeared later in the small bowel. Such humbling experiences have occurred to many of us interested in this field and teach us all to avoid being too dogmatic.

Careful histological examination of resected specimens in ulcerative colitis is important for two reasons: small areas of malignant change may not have been obvious macroscopically and backwash ileitis may be difficult to differentiate on macroscopical grounds from Crohn's ileitis.

Ulcerative colitis

The disease usually begins spontaneously and insiduously in the rectum or rectosigmoid but occasionally it follows an attack of infective diarrhoea. It may affect the whole large bowel *ab initio*. It is advantageous to subdivide ulcerative colitis according to its extent: proctitis, distal proctocolitis, subtotal colitis and total colitis.

Rectal biopsy in the early stages of the disease may reveal crypt abscesses (Fig. 9.2), ulceration, epithelial regenerative changes and chronic inflammatory cellular infiltration of the lamina propria. None of the features are specific but if bacteriological investigation is negative and no parasites are visible in the biopsy then the histological changes indicate active inflammatory bowel disease. However, it must be remembered that bacteriological proof of chronic infective diarrhoea may be elusive.

Cytology smears of the mucosa in the early stages show numerous eosinophils and they are frequently prominent in the lamina propria. Ulceration and crypt abscesses represent the most convincing evidence of proctitis. Epithelial regenerative changes can follow mechanical trauma or infective diarrhoea. The pathologist should avoid making a diagnosis of ulcerative colitis on the basis of an apparent increase in lymphocytes and plasma cells in the mucosa, since cell populations can be increased in other chronic infective states. Except during remission established chronic disease is easier to diagnose than acute disease.

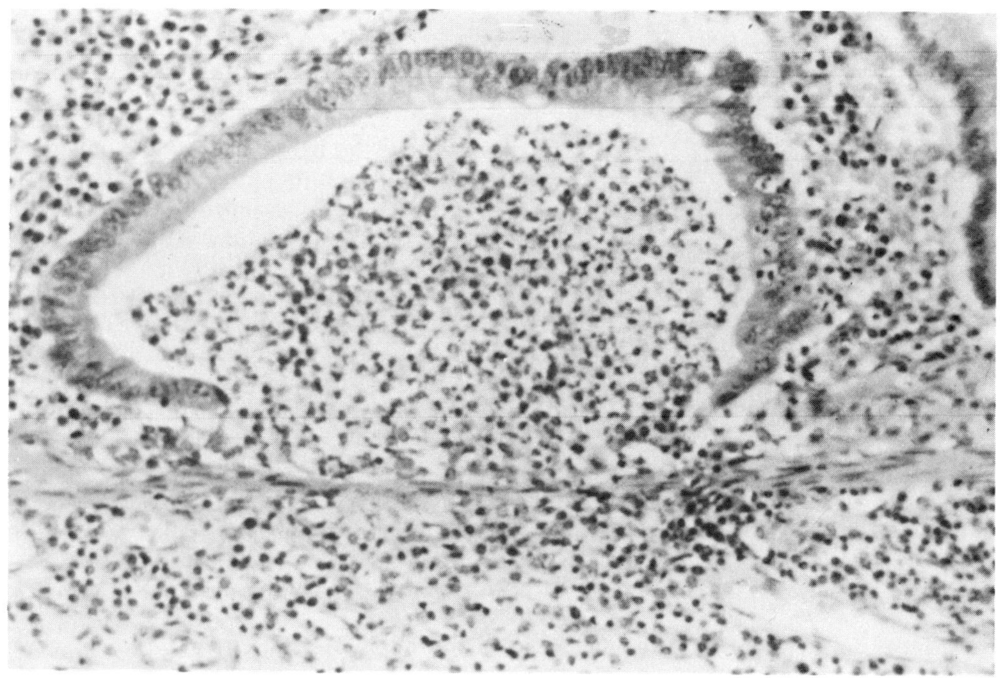

Fig. 9.2 Crypt abscess in ulcerative colitis.

Proctitis and distal proctocolitis

It is convenient to discuss these together. In both conditions approximately half the patients suffer from constipation rather than diarrhoea, also in both there is no statistical proof of an increased cancer risk.

The endoscopic features include inflammatory hyperaemia, granularity and friability of the mucosa, ulceration and, in chronic disease, pseudopolyposis. Characteristically the changes end a few centrimetres above the dentate line and the upper reaches of the sigmoidoscopy are entirely normal. Perianal disease occurs in only a small proportion of cases and there is a low incidence of strictures. Histologically crypt abscesses are breaches in the crypt epithelium with neutrophils from the lamina propria streaming into and collecting in the crypt lumen. Occasional Langhans giant cells may be seen around the crypt simulating granuloma. Crypt abscesses and inflammatory erosions coalesce to form ulcers. In active disease, epithelial regenerative changes are accompanied by mucin depletion. Exuberant epithelial regenerative changes may mimic mild dysplasia. In longstanding disease, Paneth cell metaplasia is a feature and in quiescent disease there is also atrophy of the mucosa.

The chronic inflammatory cellular infiltrate includes plasma cells, lymphocytes, neutrophils, eosinophils, mast cells, macrophages and occasional Langhans giant cells. There is an increased population of IgA and IgM plasma cells but reports of increased numbers of IgE cells have not been confirmed; it is probable that IgE antisera were' unreliable. Mast cells are increased in number but there is no relationship between this increase and activity of disease. Frei and Morson claim that ulcerative colitis can be diagnosed correctly in 70 per cent of cases simply by assessment of the histological features in rectal biopsy material; in approximately 10 per cent of patients, proctitis extends to involve the rest of the colon. Buried crypts are occasionally identified in the submucosa but they are so well differentiated that there is no serious risk of confusion with carcinoma. Vascular changes include angiitis, endarteritis obliterans and thrombosis.

Subtotal and total proctocolitis

Diarrhoea with the passage of blood and mucus is a characteristic feature although the course of disease is punctuated by remissions or response to treatment. There is a wide range in the severity of symptoms ranging from profuse diarrhoea and prostration to low grade chronic diarrhoea.

Total colitis is often associated with changes in the terminal ileum—the so-called backwash ileitis. The gross features of total colitis are similar to those of proctitis and distal proctocolitis but in longstanding disease, carcinoma is a more likely complication. The colon is often shorter than normal due to contracture and this tends to facilitate colonoscopic examination. Occasionally ulceration and inflammatory hyperaemia are patchy particularly in the ascending colon and caecum. Quiescent colitis may assume the features of colitis polyposa in which large numbers of villous pseudopolypi are present.

Backwash ileitis is a superficial inflammation of the mucosa and is usually mild. The appendix mucosa is frequently involved and diverticular disease may coexist. Toxic dilatation can develop, as a dangerous complication associated with the risk of perforation.

The histological features are similar to proctitis and distal proctocolitis but dysplasia and neoplasia are more common. Ulcerative colitis is a mucosal and not a transmural disease. Ulceration, crypt abscesses, epithelial regenerative changes, lymphoid hyperplasia are usually present in active disease.

Dysplasia

In longstanding disease foci of dysplasia may develop; these are characterized by nuclear hyperchromatism, disorderly arrangement of the crypts, nuclear pleomorphism and mitoses. The histological changes can be graded as mild, moderate or severe and are comparable to similar changes that occur in tubular and villous adenoma. Although dysplasia can be classified on naked eye appearances as villous or polypoid type it can also occur in the flat mucosa. Severe dysplasia (Fig. 9.3) can progress to invasive carcinoma. The identification of moderate or severe dysplasia represents a warning signal that the patient could develop invasive carcinoma and will alert the clinician to consider prophylactive colectomy or at least regular total colonoscopic biopsy surveillance.

Hepatic and cholangitic complications

The hepatic and cholangitic complications of mucosal ulcerative colitis often require histopathological investigation to establish the diagnosis

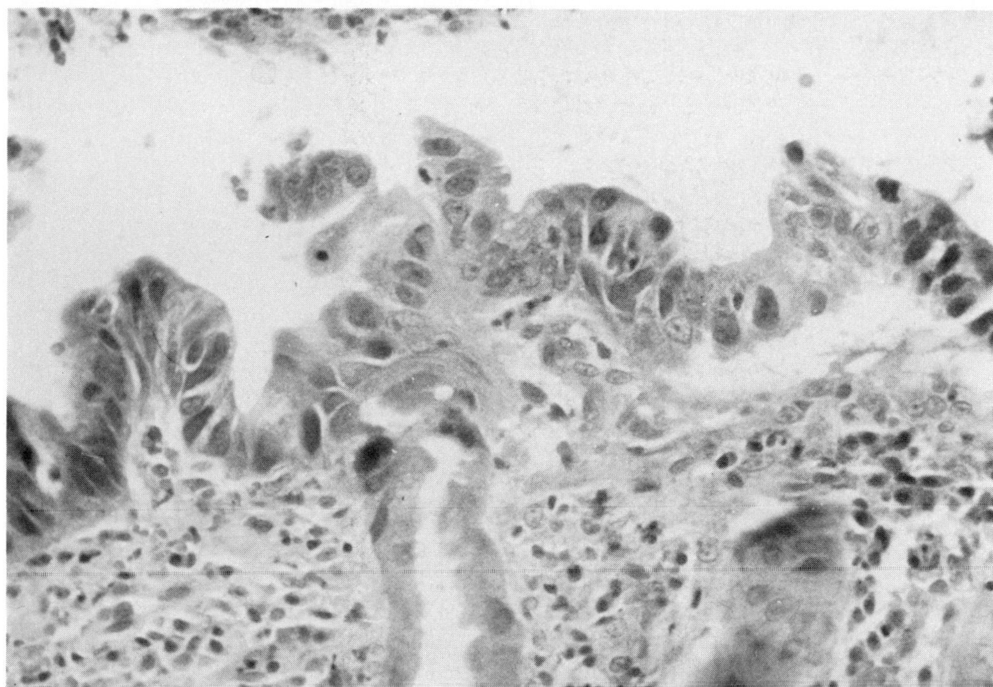

Fig. 9.3 Severe dysplasia in ulcerative colitis.

and to assess the severity and the risks of complications.

The incidence of cirrhosis complicating ulcerative colitis is about 1.1 per cent. The picture is usually one of portal triaditis (Chronic pericholangitis) associated with elevation of the serum alkaline phosphatase level but occasional cases progress through chronic aggressive hepatitis to cirrhosis. Malignant hepatoma can occur. In liver biopsies, portal triaditis and fatty change are frequently observed. Less commonly seen are amyloidosis and liver abscess. Sclerosing cholangitis and biliary tract carcinoma are well recognized complications of ulcerative colitis and they can develop after colectomy. Intrahepatic or endoscopic cholangiography are invaluable but sometimes the final diagnosis may only be reached at necropsy.

Extracolonic manifestations

Occasionally histopathological examination is necessary also for the evaluation of supposed extracolonic manifestations of ulcerative colitis. Pyoderma gangrenosum and oral ulceration are occasional complications, and rare associations are cutaneous angiitis, disseminated intravascular coagulation, arteritis and Takayasu's disease. Arthritis is a well-known, serious and disabling complication; coexistent adult coeliac disease is a recognized association.

When the differentiation is between Crohn's disease and ulcerative colitis, the histopathologic findings are of even greater importance than the endoscopic and radiological. However, many pitfalls in the diagnosis exist and the surgeon and the pathologist must co-operate in obtaining the most appropriate biopsy material and in knowing when it is necessary to repeat the examination. The clinician may be able to provide the best chance of a histological diagnosis by biopsying the smallest or earliest lesions, rather than taking a biopsy from the most grossly affected area when secondary changes may cloud the histological picture.

Crohn's disease

In the understanding of the natural history of Crohn's disease and on planning the execution of medical and surgical treatment the clinician and pathologist both play a part. In the understanding-of the nature of the disease it is important to remember that biopsies from the mouth, the oesophagus, the stomach, the duodenum and the rectum can all prove abnormal in a patient with Crohn's disease whose only gross clinical manifestation may be, for example, a limited ileo-caecal lesion.

In patients in whom the differential diagnosis between Crohn's disease and tuberculosis is difficult, it is important that operative specimens and biopsies are examined and re-examined for the presence of tubercle bacilli and that fresh material is sent for bacteriological examination.

In the guidance as to the extent of surgical resection in Crohn's disease the role of the histopathologist has probably been exaggerated. If we believe that the disease affects the whole of the alimentary tract, then it is naive to expect that one should always resect to a level of histological normality before making an anastomosis or a stoma.

In a research field the collaboration of the surgeon and the pathologist is important in attempts to decide whether it is better policy to resect little or large for isolated areas of Crohn's disease.

Crohn's disease of terminal ileum

Crohn's disease most frequently affects the terminal ileum. Clinical presentation can be variable with subacute intestinal obstruction, diarrhoea, malabsorption syndrome, appendicitis etc. The gross features include ulceration, fissures, sinuses, cobblestone mucosa and hosepipe thickening of the bowel wall. In the early stages, aphthoid ulceration is characteristic and in the later stages more diffuse or linear ulceration occurs along the mesenteric border.

Skip lesions develop proximally in the small intestine, fibrous strictures are common and pseudopolypi occasionally appear in the diseased segment. Ulceration and oedema extend into the adjacent caecum in 20 per cent of cases. Oedema also extends into the attached mesentery and tubercles may be visible on the peritoneal surface. "Fatwrapping" is a common feature in the affected segment. Fistulae, usually entero-enteric or ileocolic, complicate the disease in 10–20 per cent of operated cases. The ileo-caecal lymph nodes enlarge and abscesses may develop together but adhesions are noticeable by their absence. It is unusual to have dense adhesions even in someone who has had many and complicated operations.

The histological changes are variable and patchy and include the same ulceration, fissures, sinuses, submucosal and subserosal oedema and fibrosis seen on gross inspection. In addition the microscope reveals lymphoid hyperplasia, thickening of the muscularis mucosa, dilatation of lymphatic channels and proliferation of nerve bundles. Non caseating granulomata (Fig. 9.4) are found in

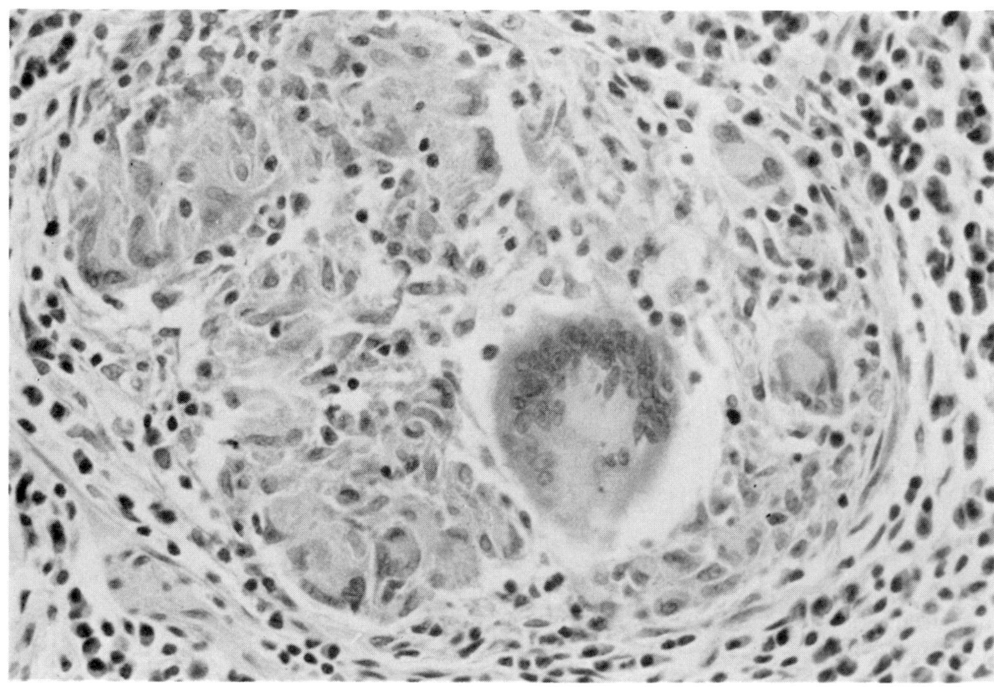

Fig. 9.4 Granuloma with epithelioid cells and Langhan's cells in Crohn's disease.

approximately 50 per cent of cases and consist of epithelioid cells with occasional Langhans giant cells The granulomas are distributed in all layers of the gut wall and tend to appear in relation to lymphatics and blood vessels. More diffuse granulomatous inflammation is noted round fissures and sinuses. Foreign body giant cells are also encountered. Angiitis, which can be inflammatory, necrotizing or granulomatous, is found in 9.5 per cent of cases. Vascular changes also include endarteritis obliterans and occasionally telangiectasia or thrombosis. Granulomata may also be identified in lymph nodes in 29.5 per cent of cases, but the lymph node enlargement is usually due to reactive hyperplasia and sinus catarrh.

Crohn's disease of the colon and rectum

This may occur synchronously or metachronously with regional ileitis or it may present as primary disease in the colon. The clinical features may be indistinguishable from ulcerative colitis but appearances that suggest Crohn's disease are the presence of perianal lesions, the pattern of ulceration, strictures, rectal sparing and skip lesions.

On endoscopy, foci of aphthoid ulceration are often seen and they represent the earliest stage and may disappear without trace. Discrete ulceration, more diffuse ulceration or linear ulceration appear as the disease progresses associated with cobblestone mucosa.

There is a high incidence of perianal disease with fissures, sinuses, fistulae and abscesses. Ulceration may also extend over the genitalia. Internal and external fistulae can occur and ileo-sigmoid communications are not uncommon. The lymph nodes enlarge along the mesenteric attachment.

Hosepipe thickening and stenosis occur in long-standing disease and the distribution is often patchy rather than continuous. Pseudopolyposis and occasional mucosal bridges develop in 12–20 per cent of cases.

The histological features are similar to those found in regional ileitis but microgranulomata tend to be more common in the rectum and colon than in the small bowel and their presence is useful in biopsy diagnosis. The incidence of non caseating granulomata is approximately 70 per cent. Paneth cell metaplasia, buried crypts and dysplasia can occur in Crohn's disease as they do in ulcerative colitis but mucin depletion of the surface and crypt epithelium is a less striking feature. The mucosa between the lesions may show a relatively normal appearance but occasionally there is mucin depletion and other features which are indistinguishable from ulcerative colitis. Crohn's disease is transmural and inflammatory changes extend to involve the submucosa, muscle and subserosa or perirectal tissues. Frei and Morson quote a 40 per cent diagnostic accuracy rate in the assessment of rectal biopsies from patients with Crohn's disease. The histological diagnosis of Crohn's disease during the state of toxic dilatation can be extremely difficult or even impossible in the resected specimen.

Crohn's disease in other sites

The vermiform appendix, Meckel's diverticulum, jejunum, duodenum, stomach and, rarely, the buccal cavity and oesophagus can be involved by Crohn's disease. This can occur in conjunction with regional ileitis or Crohn's disease of the colon or as primary disease in these sites. Identification of granulomata in multiple sections of the appendix may be the first indication of Crohn's disease. There are also rare reports of granulomatous lesions in the skin, joints, and liver in patients with Crohn's disease.

Jejunal biopsies may show villous abnormalities ranging from mild morphological abnormality to convolutions or flat mosaic biopsy. Crohn's disease and coeliac disease are occasionally diagnosed in the same patient. Granulomata may be identified in jejunal, gastric, or oesophageal biopsies. In such cases lamina propria cell counts may be increased contributing to the diagnosis of Crohn's disease.

Specific disease

The diagnosis of specific chronic inflammatory bowel disease will depend largely on such important clinical data as the race and country of origin of the patient and a possible exposure to the appropriate bacteria or parasites. In the tropics, the possibility of specific bowel disease is always uppermost in the clinician's mind and suitable material is then taken for appropriate diagnostic tests. We must remember that even when the clinical index of suspicion is high it may be very difficult to differentiate between tuberculosis and Crohn's disease as it is not always easy to isolate the tubercle bacillus from tuberculous lesions and the presence of acid fast bacillus is an ulcerated lesion of the bowel does not necessarily mean that tuberculosis is the primary cause of the disease.

Tuberculous enteritis

The incidence of intestinal tuberculosis is low in the United Kingdom compared to that in India, Pakistan, Middle East, Japan, etc. There is also an increased incidence amongst Asians in the United Kingdom. Tuberculous ulcers may complicate the course of pulmonary tuberculosis due to swallowed sputum containing tubercle bacilli. Ulcers can develop in the stomach, small intestine, colon or rectum. In the small intestine, they tend to encircle the bowel wall and they may be multiple. Strictures can occur following healing of the ulcers. Ulcers of this kind can be diagnosed with confidence, although rarely similar ulcers may be encountered in Crohn's disease.

Tuberculosis of the terminal ileum can mimic regional ielitis with diffuse ulceration, hosepipe thickening, stenosis and stricture. Histological examination reveals caseating granulomata or a suspicion of caseation necrosis in some of the lesions. Examination of the lymph nodes is extremely valuable in this context since in this location conglomerate tubercles and caseation tend to be more prominent than they are in Crohn's disease. If there is any suspicion of tuberculosis the surgeon should send an adequate portion of an ulcerated area and fresh swabs to the microbiology department. The pathologist will scrutinize sections stained with the Ziehl Neelsen technique for acid fast bacilli. Unfortunately tubercle bacilli tend to be scanty in the lesions of intestinal tuberculosis and it can take up to 4 hours to find a single organism. Immunofluorescent staining may be helpful to facilitate identification. Although the histological search for bacilli is tedious it is extremely valuable if the surgeon has not submitted material to the department of Microbiology or if no bacilli could be grown. Furthermore, there is a risk that, if the diagnosis of tuberculosis is overlooked and the lesion regarded as Crohn's disease, steroid therapy will be instituted and dissemination of tuberculosis could occur.

Among the Asian Community in Britain either Crohn's disease or tuberculosis can occur in different patients and it is therefore important to establish the correct diagnosis.

Hyperplastic caecal tuberculosis (Fig. 9.5) can also simulate Crohn's disease with a mass in the right iliac fossa and gross and histological features indistinguishable from Crohn's disease including pseudopolyposis. Segmental tuberculosis can also occur in other sites such as the duodenum, small intestine and rectosigmoid region.

The Mantoux reaction may be positive although there may be no clinical evidence of active pulmonary tuberculosis. If a diagnosis of ileocaecal tuberculosis is established on radiological grounds for example in an Asian then there is no need to carry out surgical resection since anti-tuberculous

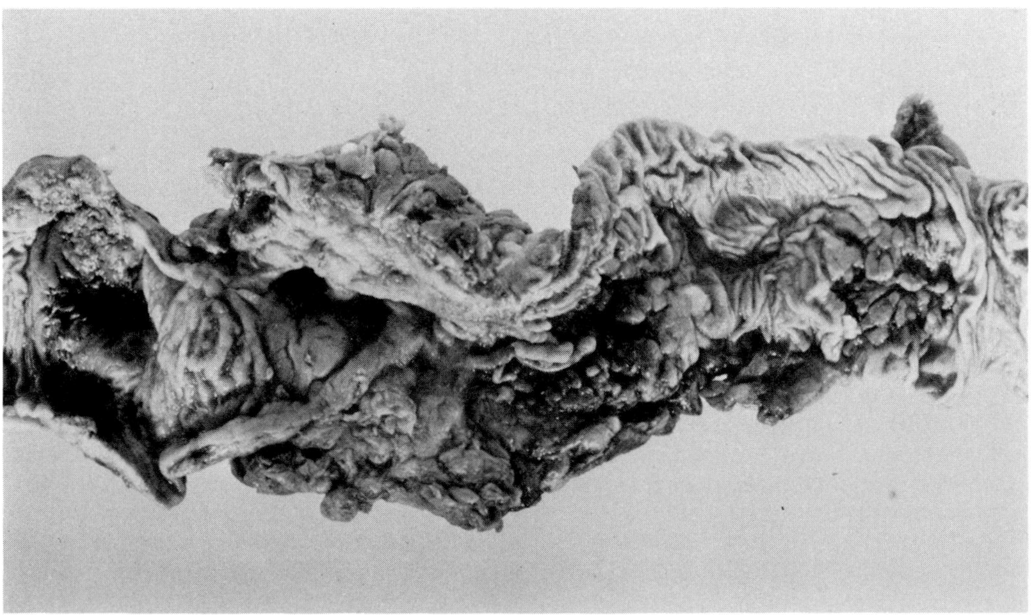

Fig. 9.5 Hyperplastic caecal tuberculosis.

therapy is adequate. If obstructive symptoms persist after treatment, stricturoplasty may be required.

Further reading

Allan RN, Keighley MRB, Alexander-Williams J, Hawkins C. *Inflammatory Bowel Diseases.* Edinburgh, London: Churchill Livingstone, 1983.

Claireaux A. *Recent Advances in Paediatric Surgery* p. 99, (edited by AW Wilkinson). Edinburgh, London: Churchill Livingstone, 1969.

Dew MJ, Thompson H, Allan RN. The spectrum of hepatic dysfunction in inflammatory bowel disease. *Quart J Med New Series XLVIII* 1979; **189:** 113–35.

Frei JV, Morson BC. Medical audit of rectal biopsy diagnosis of inflammatory bowel disease. *J Clin Pathol* 1982; **35**:341–4.

Harland NA, Lee FD. Intestinal spirochaetosis. *Br Med J* 1967; **iii**:718–19.

Kitis G, Holmes, GKT, Cooper, BT, Thompson H, Allan RN. Association of coeliac disease and inflammatory bowel disease. *Gut* 1980; **21**:636–41.

Morson BC, Dawson IMP. *Gastro-intestinal Pathology.* Oxford, London: Blackwell Scientific Publications, 1979.

Polak JM, Bishop AE, Low GRG *et al.* Pathology of the gut peptidergic system. *Gut* 1979; **20**:A. 942.

Smith B. *The Neuropathology of the Alimentary Tract*, p. 68. London: Edward Arnold, 1972.

Thompson H, Bonser RS. Granuloma, arteritis and inflammatory cell counts in Crohn's disease. In: *Recent Advances in Crohn's Disease*, edited by AS Penna, IT Weterman, CC Booth, W Strober in Developments in Gastroenterology, Vol. 1, p. 80. Martinus NIJHOFF Publishers, 1981.

10

The Complaint of Piles and Anal Incontinence

M M Henry and B C Morson

Introduction

When a patient complains of piles, the surgeon should consider a list of differential diagnoses of which haemorrhoids is the most common. The clinician sometimes needs to be particularly adept in excluding less common and sometimes potentially more sinister pathology.

Haemorrhoids

Aetiopathology

Haemorrhoidal prolapse is almost certainly not due to a localized venous varicosity, a traditional view extending back to Hippocrates. Thomson found from post-mortem dissections and latex infusion techniques that venous dilatation in this region is a universal finding in normal individuals.

It is now reasonably established that haemorrhoids are related to straining and to inadequate dietary roughage. It is probable that abnormal patterns of defaecation result in degeneration of the supportive tissue surrounding the veins in the submucosa of the anal canal so permitting the rectal mucosa to slide downwards into the anal canal. The fact that such prolapse tends to occur in constant positions around the circumference of the anal canal has been explained by Thomson on the basis of a "cushion" theory. From a series of post-mortem dissections, including one of an infant, it was found that cushions of submucosal tissue comprising pads of thickened submucosa containing veins and arteriovenous shunts were present in constant positions in the anal canal of all normal subjects. These positions are identical to those observed in patients with haemorrhoids. In some patients, haemorrhoids are associated with overactivity of the internal anal sphincter. It is possible that when the rectal mucosa prolapses into the anal canal in these patients the venous return becomes obstructed so leading to engorgement and many of the symptoms associated with haemorrhoids (*see below*).

In contrast, there is a second group in which the internal sphincter is deficient perhaps because mucosa which has been prolapsing over a prolonged period causes dilatation damage; as occurs in full thickness rectal prolapse.

The role of the external anal sphincter and pelvic floor muscles in haemorrhoids is as yet not fully understood. There is strong evidence to suggest that patients with a full thickness rectal prolapse (p. 123) have abnormal pelvic floor muscles resulting probably from a localized neuropathy. In some patients with haemorrhoids a similar neuropathic change can be demonstrated in these muscles, although usually to a lesser degree.

Symptoms

While some controversy surrounds the aetiology of this condition there is general agreement on the related clinical features.

The most important symptoms are listed in Table 10.1. The bleeding is usually arterial, associated with defaecation and may be either profuse or sufficient only to cause staining of underwear or lavatory paper. Haemorrhoidal prolapse is classified according to whether the prolapse remains within the confines of the anal canal (*first degree*); prolapses outside the anal canal, but reduces spontaneously at the completion of defaecation (*second*

Table 10.1 Rectal symptoms associated with haemorrhoids.

Bleeding
Prolapse
Mucous discharge
Pruritus ani
Discomfort/Pain
Faecal soiling

degree); or remains extruded and requires digital replacement (*third degree*). It is of greater importance to establish whether the prolapse is of mucosa alone or of full thickness since the treatment of the two conditions differs.

Rectal mucosa contains mucus secreting glands hence prolapse may cause a clear discharge which soils underwear and may be a factor in the pruritus many of these patients describe.

Pain, other than a slight dull ache, is unusual unless the complication of thrombosis develops.

Clinical findings

The clinical evaluation is based on the routine adopted for any patient with anorectal symptoms. Following abdominal examination inspection of the anus and perineum is carried out. Third degree haemorrhoidal prolapse will be immediately apparent. If no obvious overt prolapse is observed examination should then proceed with the patient straining down as if preparing for defaecation. Skin tags may form as a secondary development of haemorrhoids and as such may need to be distinguished from other pathologies which can mimic this situation (*see below*).

Digital examination of the anal canal is usually non-contributory since haemorrhoids are rarely palpable. Similarly, sigmoidoscopy has limited value except in the exclusion of other pathology. Proctoscopic examination may reveal haemorrhoidal prolapse in the resting state. If, however, prolapse is not observed, the patient should be instructed to strain; the prolapsing mucosa may then be observed obtruding into the lumen of the instrument. The mucosal cushion situated in the right anterior position (with the patient in the lithotomy position) is most commonly affected. Less commonly in cases of pelvic floor descent hemicircumferential prolapse of the anterior rectal wall mucosa may be seen.

Perianal haematoma

Frequently patients confuse piles with the common condition of perianal haematoma. The principal clinical distinction is that the latter condition is acutely painful. The haematoma arises from rupture and thrombosis of a perianal vein probably in response to excessive straining. Examination reveals an acutely tender swelling at the anal margin. A blue colour is imparted because of the retained blood and there may be considerable oedema of the underlying skin.

Full thickness rectal prolapse

This is a condition occurring most commonly at the extremes of life whereas haemorrhoids occur throughout adult life and rarely in childhood. The prolapse is circumferential and is inclusive of both mucosa and muscle wall.

Aetiopathology

This is far from clear; almost certainly some intussusception of the rectal wall into the lumen of the rectum occurs and subsequently is extruded through the anus. Why this process occurs has not been fully explained. Many of these patients exhibit a myopathy of the pelvic floor which in turn may be the result of localized nerve damage. There is also a relationship between lower motor neurone lesions and rectal prolapse which is endemic in such patients. The possible mechanisms whereby the damage may arise are discussed in the section on incontinence. however, not all patients with prolapse have any evidence of a neurological lesion, the aetiology in this group remains unexplained.

Clinical features

Depending on the stage of presentation, the prolapse may be coincident with defaecation and subsequently reduce at its completion or alternatively may be permanent. Faecal incontinence of varying degrees may develop and is sometimes the presenting symptom. Irregularity of bowel function, particularly constipation, is commonly associated.

The examination of the patient usually takes place with the patient in the left lateral position, but if difficulty is encountered in eliciting the prolapse, the patient should be examined in the squatting position. Prolapse is circumferential and may extend several centimetres below the plane of the perineum. Sphincter function is frequently abnormal in that both the internal and external anal sphincters may be deficient. On sigmoidoscopy the changes consistent with traumatic proctitis sometimes are seen. There is a danger that such appearances are confused with those arising from inflammatory bowel disease and inappropriate treatment provided. Wherever this dilemma occurs histological examination of a representative biopsy can be immensely helpful in discriminating between the two.

Solitary ulcer syndrome and descending perineum syndrome

These two conditions are allied to rectal prolapse in the sense that they frequently co-exist. Both problems are strongly related to abnormal patterns of defaecation, principally one of excessive straining. In the solitary ulcer syndrome this becomes associated with a zonal proctitis situated anteriorly, sometimes a demarcated shallow ulcer, and indurated polypoid changes which mimic carcinoma. In the descending perineum syndrome abnormal degrees of descent of the pelvic floor in relation to the bony outlet of the pelvis occurs.

Histopathology

There may be only an area of zonal proctitis on the anterior or antero-lateral walls of the lower rectum. When an ulcer is also present it has an irregular shape and can vary in size from 0.5 cm to 5.0 cm in diameter. They are usually rather flat, well-demarcated lesions, often covered by a white slough. In addition, to the surrounding proctitis the rectal mucosa often has a lumpy appearance.

Although defaecation difficulties are strongly implicated in the generation of the descending perineum syndrome, there is evidence to suggest that in these patients the muscles have been denervated. Whether this is primary or secondary to a nerve stretch is not known.

Biopsy of the lesion reveals characteristic appearances. The earliest and most significant change is obliteration of the lamina propria by fibrosis and smooth muscle fibres growing towards the lumen from a thickened muscularis mucosae, and this change may be present without ulceration, or in the mucosa away from the immediate vicinity of the ulcer. In a tangentially cut biopsy, the appearance of mucosal glands surrounded by muscle can give the false impression of invasive carcinoma. Additional features include superficial mucosal ulceration, irregularity of the crypts and hyperplastic changes in the epithelium with depletion of goblet cells. When an ulcer is present it is invariably superficial and never penetrates beyond the submucosa. Its floor is covered by necrotic cells overlying organising granulation tissue. In some cases there is misplacement of mucus-filled glands lined by normal colonic epithelium into the submucosa at the edge of the ulcer, another feature which may be mistaken for adenocarcinoma. This appearance has been described under a variety of names such as "localized colitis cystica profunda", hamartomatous inverted polyp of the rectum, and enterogenous cyst. Finally, in resection specimens, histological examination may reveal fibrosis of the submucosa and thickening of the muscularis propria.

These histological features commonly occur in other clinical situations (e.g. at the apex of a complete rectal prolapse, the apex of a prolapsing haemorrhoid and at the tip of a colostomy or ileostomy). Hence it would seem that prolapse itself is responsible for some of these pathological features. The aetiology of ulceration may be ischaemia, particularly if the submucosal vessels either rupture or become obliterated by the fibrous and muscular tissue infiltration of the lamina propria. Electromyographically many of these patients fail to relax the puborectalis muscle during defaecation. In such cases ulceration may be caused by traumatic damage to the prolapsing anterior rectal mucosa caused by a tight unyielding puborectalis muscle during the act of defaecation.

Clinical features

The symptom complex in both syndromes differs little from that associated with piles. A solitary ulcer may give rise to bleeding which can be profuse. In perineal descent increased obliquity of the anorectal angle (*see* below) permits the anterior rectal wall to prolapse into the anal canal. Like haemorrhoidal prolapse this may also give rise to bleeding. Unlike haemorrhoidal prolapse, however, the hemi-circumferential prolapse may form a plug which can obstruct the passage of faeces and so intensify the defaecation difficulties. Intense problems with defaecation thus characterize both conditions. Sometimes perineal pain is a feature, the reason for which is not understood.

On examination a solitary ulcer may be palpable and be associated with some induration. Abnormal descent is defined as being present when the plane of the perineum descends below that of the ischial tuberosities during a straining effort. Digital examination of the anus in perineal descent may detect some diminished sphincter function. A solitary ulcer is usually diagnosed on sigmoidoscopy where it is usually apparent on the anterior rectal wall at a level 4 to 15 cm from the anal verge. Occasionally, polypoid forms occur and can be mistaken for carcinoma. Where doubt exists biopsy is essential. On proctoscopy prolapse of the anterior rectal mucosa occurs in both syndromes.

Anal fissure

This is a small laceration in the epithelium of the lower anal canal occurring in either the posterior or, less commonly, anterior midline positions.

From the clinical history the distinction from piles can be made on the basis that pain is the predominant symptom. Some bleeding may be associated, but this is usually of a minor nature. Mucosal prolapse does not occur, but a small "sentinel" tag of oedematous skin at the lower end of the fissure may prolapse with defaecation and give rise to some confusion.

On examination, the fissure is usually seen in one of the midline positions, particularly if the internal anal sphincter is gently retracted laterally. A sentinel tag is indicative of an underlying fissure. Digital examination of the anus is attended by intense spasm of the internal sphincter and pain. Signoidoscopy and proctoscopy are only of value in the exclusion of co-existent pathology and in particular inflammatory bowel disease (*see below*).

Histopathology

A typical anal fissure forms an elongated triangular ulcer in the squamous membrane of the lower anal canal. The pathogenesis is not clear. Predisposing causes include loss of the normal elasticity and mobility of the mucosa due to fibrosis accompanying infection; it is probable that trauma by the passage of hard faeces may be a precipitating factor. Superficial tissues may heal spontaneously, but more often the condition becomes chronic probably because associated muscle spasm and constant exposure to infection interfere with healing. Microscopic appearances are those of non-specific inflammation. The edges of chronic fissures are thickened and somewhat undermined, and the tissues immediately adjacent are oedematous and heavily infiltrated by lympocytes and plasma cells. The oedematous edge at the lower end of a fissure may form a little polypoid projection, the "sentinel tag". Non-specific acute fissure is a common condition, but must be distinguished from other causes of anal ulceration such as Crohn's disease, tuberculosis, primary syphilis or a squamous cell carcinoma.

Anal fistula and abscess

Aetiopathology

In the past, the most widely accepted theory of the cause of anal fistula was that the wall of the anal canal became infected through a fissure or wound and that faecal contamination prevented the condition from healing. However, other evidence suggests that infection of the anal glands is probably the commonest cause. Various authors have demonstrated infection in and around the glands in cases of fistula and have suggested that the chronicity of the condition is due to persistence of the anal gland epithelium in the part of the track adjoining the internal opening: the presence of this persisting epithelium keeps the opening patent and healing cannot take place.

The anal glands provide a channel between the lumen of the anal canal and connective tissues around the terminal part of the bowel including the ischiorectal space. In many cases the branching of the anal glands takes place wholly within the submucosa of the anal canal and it is infection of this superficial variety of gland that would seem to be the cause of the subcutaneous and submucosal types of fistula. Sometimes, however, the glands penetrate the internal sphincter: several branches of a single gland may pierce the muscle at different levels and then terminate abruptly within the connective tissues external to the muscle.

The anal glands may be regarded as diverticula of the anal canal. As in the case of any diverticula of the alimentary tract the contents of the glands are subject to stasis and secondary infection. Thus bacteria will multiply in a gland that has been obstructed by faecal material, foreign bodies or trauma. Those glands that pass right through the internal sphincter, moreover, will not be able to discharge their contents so readily for the tone of the muscle will tend to compress their lumen. Thus cystic dilatation of the gland occurs. In fact a fistula-in-ano is virtually a sinus secondary to disease of an anal gland and this view fits with the practical observation that there is no clinically detectable internal opening in about half the cases: in fact, the condition in such cases is a sinus rather than a true fistula. It seems likely that stasis and secondary infection of the gland are generally due to obstruction resulting from inflammation: the commonest cause is probably an anal fissure.

The ducts of normal anal glands are often surrounded by well-developed lymphoid tissue, forming the so-called "anal tonsils". It is believed that this lymphoid tissue may become the focus of inflammation, specific or non-specific and of local or blood-borne origin. Certainly the mid-portion of the anal canal shows a special liability to intramural hyperplasia of the lymphoid tissue comparable to the hyperplasia of the lymphoid tissues of the oropharyngeal and ileocaecal regions.

Clinical features

The principal symptom, unlike haemorrhoids, is acute pain often attended by swelling and the subsequent discharge of pus. With a fistula these symptoms have a recurring pattern.

Where an abscess alone occurs, clinical examination reveals a tender swelling at the anal verge or alternatively it may only be revealed by digital examination of the anal canal. Infection of one of the anal glands situated in the intersphincteric plane can give rise to a well localized abscess which is usually situated posteriorly and is readily palpable as a tender nodule.

Once a fistulous track has been established a sinus opening on the perineal skin is apparent and may discharge either pus or faeces. Digital examination will establish the course taken by the track in the pelvis or anal canal. Induration may be palpable above the plane of the levator musculature if the fistula has a high "supralevator" extension or more commonly the track lies below this plane ("infralevator extension"). The track may be localized within the intersphincteric plane in which case the external opening will be close to the anus. Alternatively, the track may extend laterally through the external sphincter ("transphincteric extension") in which case the external opening will be sited more lateral to the anus. In all types of fistula circumferential extension can occur in any of the horizontal anatomical planes of the anorectum. Digital examination may also reveal a small pit at the level of the dentate line which is the internal opening of the fistula. This can be confirmed by proctoscopic examination. Sigmoidoscopy should be performed to exclude inflammatory bowel disease.

Histology

Representative samples of tissue should always be referred for histological examination. This is partly to exclude Crohn's disease and rarely tuberculosis. The latter is sometimes difficult to distinguish from Crohn's disease and may ultimately depend on the demonstration of the tubercle bacillus.

In the great majority of cases sections will show an ordinary pyogenic type of inflammatory reaction. Giant cells of the foreign body type are frequently encountered; presumably they are a reaction to the presence within the fistulous track of material derived from the faeces. An oleogranulomatous reaction is occasionally present and is probably due to treatment of the condition with vaseline impregnated gauze or to the escape of oily substances used for softening the faeces from the rectum into the fistulous track. The spread of infection in and around fistulous tracks can provoke tissue damage such as fat necrosis, secondary vasculitis and degenerative changes in striated muscle with the formation of giant hyperchromatic nuclei.

Pilonidal sinus

This common condition is predominant in the young adult male and is probably caused by puncture of the skin of the natal cleft by ingrowing hair shafts. This subsequently institutes an inflammatory reaction with the formation of subcutaneous abscess tracks. Microscopic examination reveals a track lined by squamous epithelium with the changes of chronic inflammation and containing hair shafts which frequently incite a foreign body giant cell reaction. Clinically, they are readily recognizable by the presence of tell-tale single or multiple pits in the skin of the natal cleft. In the acute phase an abscess may develop at this site.

Faecal incontinence

Faecal incontinence is commonly reported in the elderly, but may also develop in younger age groups.

Aetiopathology

Incontinence can occur in the presence of normal anal sphincter function if these should become overwhelmed by copious liquid stool. This situation may arise following infestation of the gut with certain micro-organisms or as a consequence of inflammatory bowel disease for example. Minor degrees of dysfunction can be the consequence of decreased internal anal sphincter function. Such may follow certain surgical procedures (e.g. manual dilatation of the anus, sphincterotomy) or may develop secondary to full thickness rectal prolapse, where the sphincter is stretched by the prolapsing bowel. In the elderly, faecal soiling is often the result of faecal impaction. The latter leads to over-activation of a locally conducted reflex whereby rectal distension (by faeces) results in relaxation of the internal sphincter and subsequent leakage of semi-solid stool.

Major incontinence (i.e. to fully formed stool) usually results from abnormal neuromuscular function in the pelvic floor musculature. Electrophysiological and histochemical studies have revealed evidence to suggest that in the majority some localized damage to the nerves supplying these muscles has taken place. It is possible that the source of the neuronal damage in some women may be the result of traumatic childbirth in which undue compression of the pelvic nerves (which lie in the side wall of the pelvis) by the fetal head can occur in prolonged labour or transverse arrest. Alternatively, in cases of perineal descent the nerves may be subjected to a stretch injury or be subject to entrapment in the pudendal canal; a syndrome analgous to the carpal tunnel syndrome.

Less commonly incontinence can develop if the integrity of the puborectalis sling is disrupted by trauma or if the muscle fails to develop as a consequence of rectal atresia. Lower motor neurone lesions from cauda equina tumour or trauma are rare. the incontinence which attends generalized neurological disease (e.g. multiple sclerosis) is usually the result of faecal impaction.

Clinical features

The distinction between an incontinent patient and one with haemorrhoids should be straight forward. Some confusion may arise if the patient with piles complains of a mucous discharge or faecal soiling since both are fairly common features of this condition. The patient with rectal prolapse as discussed above may be affected by incontinence of varying degrees of severity.

Patients with normal neuromuscular function of the somatic muscles of this region, but who have abnormal internal anal sphincter function usually report only minor disability limited to loss of control to flatus and liquid stool. Sometimes there is a history of previous anal surgery and on examination the resting tone on digital examination is diminished and there may be co-existent haemorrhoids or rectal prolapse.

Those patients who present with an inability to withhold the inadvertent passage of fully formed stool per anum usually have been subject either to previous traumatic damage to this region or pathology related to the nerve supply of the pelvic floor musculature as outlined above. Pads often have to be worn throughout the day and a sense of alienation is strongly present in this group of patients. Where trauma is responsible, a history of previous fistula surgery or of road traffic accident may exist. In the remainder, there may be a history of traumatic childbirth or of defaecation difficulties causing either rectal prolapse or the descending perineum syndrome. In the rare case of congenital defects, incontinence is clearly likely to have been extant from birth.

Examination of the patient may reveal scar tissue from previous surgery or injury. If a rectal prolapse is present the anus is lax and abnormal degrees of perineal descent may be displayed. In patients with a neuropathy in addition the anal reflex is often diminished or absent and on digital examination a poor response from the external sphincter is elicited when the individual is requested to tighten this muscle. All patients should be subjected to sigmoidoscopy and proctoscopy again to exclude co-existent disease.

Inflammatory disorders

In comparison with haemorrhoids, these disorders are comparatively rare. In most cases there is little confusion in diagnosis provided sigmoidoscopy complemented by biopsy is considered.

Crohn's disease

Confusion in diagnosis may exist when Crohn's disease affects the anus, a situation developing in approximately 75 per cent of patients with large bowel involvement. Fleshy skin tags may develop which can resemble the skin tags which form secondary to haemorrhoids. However, in Crohn's disease the macroscopic appearances tend to be exaggerated – the lesions may have a dusky blue "cyanotic" colour and can be markedly oedematous. In addition, in Crohn's disease of the anus, chronic fissure, anal fistula (often anatomically complex) and ulceration may occur in any combination. In a few patients the ulceration may lead to severe destruction of the anal sphincter muscles and ischiorectal fat.

In view of this complex manifestation the symptomatology is variable. Pain with recurrent purulent discharge is the principal symptom. Unlike the patient who presents with piles, rectal bleeding is unusual. If the disease is more widespread, constitutional symptoms, diarrhoea and abdominal pain may suggest this diagnosis. On sigmoidoscopy, a proctitis of varying degrees of severity may be apparent. Biopsy of the rectal mucosa should always be considered in this situation and occasionally a skin tag should be excised for histology. This is partly to facilitate the diagnosis of Crohn's disease and partly to exclude squamous carcinoma.

Histology

The diagnosis can be made by biopsy during surgical treatment of the anal lesion. However, it will only be helpful in those 60 per cent of cases of Crohn's disease in which sarcoid granulomas are present. In the patients without such a tissue response the diagnosis rests on the clinical appearance of the anal lesion, together with any evidence of intestinal involvement. Because the clinical features are not always distinctive and a granulomatous histology is absent in some 40 per cent of cases, it is probable that anal lesions due to Crohn's disease will continue to remain unrecognized until the abdominal disease becomes manifest. Apart from lack of the characteristic clinical and histological features the failure to biopsy all anal lesions at the time of surgical treatment must be a frequent cause of failure to recognize the pathology.

A sarcoid reaction is a purely descriptive term applicable to any collection of epithelioid cells, sometimes with giant cells, without central caseation, although a little central necrosis with preservation of the reticulin pattern is permissable. In some cases of Crohn's disease of the anus the granulomas are few in number and very sparsely distributed. In other cases the tissues of the dermis, subcutaneous fat and fistulous track are riddled with lesions. The chances of finding granulomas are dependent on the amount of tissue available for examination. For this reason small biopsies are often inadequate.

A confident distinction between a sarcoid reaction due to Crohn's disease, sarcoidosis or tuberculosis is impossible on histological evidence alone. The presence of caseation is suggestive of tuberculosis, but examination by Ziehl-Neelsen staining is often negative, in which case culture or guinea pig inoculation of fresh tissue is required.

Giant cells of the foreign body type are commonly seen in tissue removed from anal fistulae. They usually appear spherical with a tendency for their many nuclei to be centrally placed, in contrast to the peripheral position of the nuclei in Langhans' giant cells. They are isolated or grouped in small numbers, and may be placed around foreign matter such as vegetable material derived from the faeces. However, many seem to be formed from striated muscle cells which have been broken up and destroyed by inflammation and fibrosis. The appearances are reminiscent of the giant cells derived from muscle in myocardial fibrosis. Epithelioid cells are not a feature of an ordinary foreign body reaction. Their absence is a useful, if arbitrary, distinction from the sarcoid type of tissue response.

Anorectal tuberculosis

Tuberculosis of the anorectal region is now a rare disease in Great Britain, having steadily declined over the last 50 years. However, it still seems to be common in those countries where pulmonary and intestinal tuberculosis are still common. There are two different clinical types. First, there are those presenting with anal ulceration who always have active pulmonary tuberculosis; tubercle bacilli can be readily demonstrated in smears from the surface of the ulcer or in biopsy material. Second, there are those who have anal fistulae or chronic anorectal abscesses. The fistulae are often anatomically complex, clinically unsuspected, and may be associated with stricture of the lower rectum. There is a history of pulmonary tuberculosis in most cases, but this is often of a mild or chronic character. The only certain way is by demonstrating the tubercle bacillus in biopsy material or by using guinea-pig inoculation or culture of fresh tissue from the anal lesion.

Ulcerative colitis

Clinically, ulcerative colitis can be confused with haemorrhoids only for the reason that both conditions cause rectal bleeding. In the former, however, the diarrhoea is usually accompanied by diarrhoea which is a combination of mucous and stool of loose consistency. The diagnosis usually rests on the macroscopic appearances of the rectum at sigmoidoscopy.

Pathology

Although anal lesions do occur in patients with ulcerative colitis, they are less frequent than and have a different character from the anal lesions of Crohn's disease. Ordinary anal and rectovaginal fistulae are seen, but the inflammatory changes in the anal canal and anal margin are usually more superficial presenting as acute anal fissure or excoriation of the skin around the anus whereas chronic anal lesions are more characteristic of Crohn's disease. The histology shows no specific features.

Hidradenitis suppurativa

This is a chronic inflammatory condition which affects the skin and subcutaneous tissues of the parts of the integument where apocrine sweat glands are found, namely the axilla, areola of the breast, umbilicus, genitalia and peri-anal area. Peri-anal hidradenitis is an uncommon condition which is more frequent in males than females. The affected area of skin has a red and white blotchy appearance, is thickened and oedematous with watery pus draining from multiple openings of sinus tracks. The persistent chronic nature of the disease leads to ulceration and scarring. Lesions can be localized or involve large areas of peri-anal skin extending into the buttocks. Microscopic examination of excised specimens shows an inflammatory exudate consisting of plasma cells, lymphocytes and occasional giant cells of the foreign-body type, with the formation of sinus tracks. The latter become lined by squamous epithelium by downgrowth from the surface. Ordinary sweat glands are present in normal numbers, but apocrine glands are usually absent. This has led to the view that hidradenitis suppurativa is a primary infection of apocrine glands. More recent studies, however, indicate that these glands are infected secondarily rather than primarily and that hidradenitis can affect skin in sites other than apocrine gland bearing areas. The cause of the disease is not understood, but like acne, it seems to have some relationship to endocrine activity. Other aetiological factors suggested include excessive local moisture in apposing skin surfaces and the difficulty of maintaining cleanliness in the regions involved. Malignant change has been reported.

Venereal infection

Sexually transmitted diseases are becoming increasingly common.

Syphilis

This disease occurs most commonly in the homosexual male and clinically presents as a superficial ulcer (primary chancre) developing 4–6 weeks after contact. The primary lesion can be easily confused with anal lesions due to other causes in particular anal fissure. The clinical distinction from epithelioma, anal lesions of Crohn's disease and tuberculous ulcer can also be difficult.

If an anal lesion gives rise to suspicion of primary syphilis the surface of the ulcer must not be exposed to any lubricant until relevant examinations have been completed. The diagnosis is made either by demonstration of the organism from tissue in the ulcer or by serology.

Manifestations of secondary syphilis can also be seen in the anal region. They include dermatitis of the peri-anal skin and, at a later stage, condyloma lata. The latter are moist, reddened hypertrophic papules and are distinguishable clinically from condyloma accuminata, although both types can be present together.

Granuloma venereum

This condition, which is not to be confused with lympho-granuloma inguinale, is a venereal disease characterized by a slowly progressive ulceration of the tissues in the genital region. It is widespread in the tropics, but very rare in Great Britain. Intracellular bodies, regarded as relatives of the pasteurellae, have been described in smears from the ulcerated lesions.

Macroscopically there are ulcerated areas of varying size. On microscopic examination a well-circumscribed mass of chronic inflammatory cells is seen, mainly polymorphs and plasma cells, a few lymphocytes, and occasional large round macrophages in which the Donovan bodies can be demonstrated by Leishman's method or the stains of Giemsa or Wright.

Lymphogranuloma inguinale

The anal manifestations include confluent nodules with fissuring, multiple anal fistulae and peri-anal elephantiasis. In addition enlargement of the inguinal lymph nodes occurs and sometimes a mild proctitis is observed sigmoidoscopically.

Gonorrhoea

This disease affects the mucous membrane only, hence lesions are only seen in the upper anal canal and rectum. In the majority no symptoms occur, the diagnosis being suggested by a proctitis observed during sigmoidoscopy or proctoscopy.

Confirmation of the disease is made by gram staining of a specimen of rectal mucosa and by subsequent culture.

Condyloma accuminata

The papilloma virus is responsible for this condition which is sexually transmitted in the majority of cases (*see below*).

Anorectal tumours

The symptomatology of a patient who complains of piles is very similar to that of a patient with a tumour of this region. Rectal bleeding is a common form of presentation and occasionally polypoid tumours may prolapse with defaecation. The patient with a rectal tumour may report an alteration in bowel habit and constitutional symptoms related to weight loss and anaemia. An anal tumour may give rise to a sensation of a lump accompanied by pain and bleeding with defaecation. At a later stage a mucous discharge or faecal incontinence from destruction of the sphincters may occur.

The diagnosis of anorectal tumour is made by digital examination complemented by sigmoidoscopy. An early anal carcinoma presents usually either as a localized ulcer or as a small raised warty lesion. At a later stage a more pronounced ulceration with tissue destruction and raised warty edges may become apparent. Digital examination may become impossible because of pain and stenosis. In all cases of anorectal neoplasia sigmoidoscopy should be attempted to determine the precise anatomical site of the lesion (which dictates surgical management) and more importantly to acquire tissue for histological examination.

Pathology

Epithelial tumours of the anal canal are all uncommon and represent a motley collection of histological types; this is a reflection of the many different varieties of epithelium seen in this area. A detailed knowledge of the histology of the epithelial lining of the anorectal region is an essential pre-requisite to the classification of anorectal tumours.

It is important to distinguish between tumours of the anal canal and tumours of the anal margin. The former are mostly variants of squamous carcinomas arising from mucous membrane, whereas the latter are epidermoid tumours of the skin which behave differently and require different methods of treatment. Apart from the exceptional occurrence of lymphomas and connective tissue tumours in the anorectal region consideration must also be given to tumours of the ischiorectal fossae and to presacral tumours.

Benign epithelial tumours and precancerous conditions of the anal canal

Leukoplakia

There are two entirely different circumstances to which the term leukoplakia may be applied in the anal region. First, white plaques of tissue may be present over the lower pole of prolapsing internal haemorrhoids as a result of squamous metaplasia with hyperkeratosis of the transitional zone of the anal canal; alternatively leukoplakia may result from upgrowth of thickened squamous mucosa from the anal canal over ulcerating haemorrhoids. There is no evidence that this type of leukoplakia is precancerous. Second, the term can be applied to a white, thickened peri-anal skin which microscopically shows thickening of the epidermis, with hyperkeratosis, acanthosis and an underlying chronic inflammatory cell infiltration. In contrast to the first type leukoplakia of the peri-anal area seems to be uncommon.

Carcinoma in situ

Carcinoma in situ of the anal canal is found in the transitional epithelium above the dentate line, including the anal crypts, more frequently than in the squamous mucous membrane of the lower anal canal. This observation corresponds with the relative incidence of invasive carcinomas above and below the dentate line. It seems certain that an *in situ* stage commonly exists for anal canal cancer.

Benign epithelial tumours and precancerous conditions of the anal margin

Viral warts (condyloma acuminata)

These red, papilliferous and warty growths are found in the peri-anal region as well as other parts of the perineum, the vulva and penis. They are usually multiple and can cover a wide area of peri-anal skin. Exceptionally, they extend up the anal canal and can be found in the transitional zone, but are rarely seen in rectal mucosa. Condyloma acuminata are due to an auto-inoculable and transmissable virus which is apparently identical or closely related to the virus causing the common skin wart (verruca vulgaris). It can be demonstrated by electron microscopy.

Microscopically anal warts show marked acanthosis of the epidermis with hyperplasia of prickle cells, parakeratosis and an underlying chronic inflammatory cell infiltration. They are noted for the vacuolation of cells in the upper layers of the epidermis. Malignant change is rare.

Giant condylomas

These are huge tumours resembling giant viral warts which are clinically aggressive yet histologically benign. Cases have been described in which there has been extensive erosion of the soft tissues around the anus with invasion of the ischiorectal fossae, perirectal tissues and even the pelvic cavity. The relentless nature of the process is typical of a low grade carcinoma yet repeated histological examination fails to show the characteristics of a malignant tumour. Fortunately giant condylomata are rare.

Verrucous carcinoma

This rare lesion could represent one possible final outcome of viral warts. In such cases evidence of invasion by well differentiated squamous cell carcinoma is found and metastases to inguinal nodes can occur, sometimes many years after the primary tumour has been treated.

Extramammary Paget's disease

Paget's disease of the peri-anal skin is an extremely rare condition which presents clinically as a slightly raised, soft, scaly and moist area with a red and grey colour. The presence of induration usually indicates that an underlying invasive carcinoma is already present. The condition is most commonly found in elderly persons of either sex and is histopathologically identical with Paget's disease of the breast. The diagnosis is established by biopsy with reveals the characteristic Paget cells in the epidemis and sometimes in the ducts of underlying apocrine glands. These are large cells with foamy vacuolated cytoplasm and a vesicular nucleus which is often displaced to the periphery of the cell, giving a signet-ring appearance.

Electron microscopic studies suggest that Paget cells originate from the epithelium of apocrine gland ducts and migrate into the epidermis. If many sections are taken during the examination of surgical specimens evidence of intraduct carcinoma will often be found. Paget's disease of the perianal skin has a long pre-invasive phase, but if the patient lives for long enough an adenocarcinoma of apocrine gland type will develop. Sometimes, however, secondary deposits in the inguinal glands will be found when only intraduct carcinoma can be demonstrated at the primary site.

Malignant epithelial tumours of the anal canal

Squamous cell carcinoma

Cancer of the anal region is uncommon in England and Wales. There are probably no more than 100 deaths per annum from it, but it is impossible to be precise because cancer of the anal margin is registered with other malignant neoplasms of the skin and many deaths from anal canal carcinoma are probably registered under rectal cancer. A better picture of the incidence is obtained from the study of surgical patients in whom anal cancer as a whole comprises only 3 per cent of adenocarcinomas of the rectum. However, epidermoid cancer of the anal margin is much more common in those parts of the world such as north-east Brazil and some areas of the Indian continent, where conditions of extreme poverty are found. Under these circumstances carcinoma of the penis, vulva and cervix as well as the anus have a relatively high incidence, at least partly due to extremely poor personal hygiene. The practice of anal intercourse and the materials with which cleansing of the perineal area is carried out could also be significant in the aetiology.

The importance of distinguishing between squamous carcinoma of the anal canal and anal margin must be emphasized. They should be considered as two quite separate types of cancer, differing in their pathology, treatment and behaviour. Anal canal carcinoma is nearly three times more common than cancer of the anal margin in the population of England and Wales. The age incidence is the same (average 57 years), but anal canal cancer is more common in women than men (3:2) whereas anal margin carcinoma is more frequent in men (4:1).

Site

It is not sufficiently well known that the majority of squamous carcinomas of the anal canal arise above, or mainly above, the dentate line, that is from the region of the transitional zone. Probably only about one quarter arise from the squamous mucous membrane of the lower anal canal. Moreover, direct spread in continuity is preferentially upwards in the submucosal plane because downward spread is limited by the way in which the dentate line is tethered down to the underlying internal sphincter thus obliterating the submucosal layer. this also explains why most anal canal carcinomas present clinically as tumours of the lower rectum.

Histology

Ordinary squamous cell carcinoma of varying degrees of differentiation closely resembling histologically cancer of the cervix accounts for about one third of all cases. These do not show intercellular cystoplasmic bridges or prickle-cell formation and generally produce less keratin than is seen in typical skin cancers such as those arising from the anal margin. However, prickle-cell carcinomas are seen uncommonly in the anal canal, particularly when there has been a long history of benign ano-rectal disease, leukoplakia or lymphogranuloma venereum. The most common type of squamous carcinoma of the anal canal is the so-called basaloid or cloacogenic carcinoma. The term basaloid is used because of the histological resemblance to basal cell carcinoma or rodent ulcer of hair-bearing skin.

Spread and prognosis

Squamous cell carcinoma of the anal canal shows preferential direct spread upwards into the lower third of the rectum, which explains why many squamous cell carcinomas of the anal canal present clinically as tumours of the rectum. Anal canal carcinoma also spreads to the superior haemorrhoidal lymph nodes and to nodes of the lateral walls of the pelvis as well as to the inguinal glands. Haemorrhoidal gland involvement is found in about 43 per cent of major operation cases of anal canal cancer and clinical and pathological evidence of inguinal gland metastases in about 36 per cent of cases. There is clinical evidence that in anal canal cancer the inguinal nodes are involved at a later stage than the haemorrhoidal glands, the malignant cells possibly spreading backwards from within the pelvis.

Malignant melanoma

Approximately one malignant melanoma of the anal canal will be seen for every eight squamous cell carcinomas of the anal region, and for every 250 adenocarcinomas of the rectum. The age incidence is about the same as for cancer of the rectum and the sex incidence seems to show a preponderance of men in some series though in others there has been no sex preponderance. Patients present clinically with a protuberant or polypoid mass in the lower rectum, often very large, which can resemble thrombosed "piles" particularly if the tumour is pigmented. The diagnosis is made by biopsy, but the distinction from undifferentiated adenocarcinoma of the rectum or undifferentiated squamous cell carcinoma of the anal canal can be very difficult unless obvious pigmentation is present.

Malignant melanoma invariably arises from the transitional zone above the dentate line of the anal canal and is therefore classified among the malignant melanomas of mucous membranes. Pigment is not always obviously present on macroscopic observation. As with squamous cell carcinomas of the anal canal malignant melanomas show preferential upwards submucous spread, which is one reason why they present clinically as growths of the rectum.

Malignant melanoma of the anal canal spreads rapidly in the anorectal tissues and may even ulcerate onto the perianal skin through the ischiorectal fossae. The superior haemorrhoidal group of lymph nodes are involved early in the course of the disease; later the glands on the lateral wall of the pelvis, the para-aortic nodes and the inguinal glands are affected. Death occurs from widespread blood-borne deposits mostly in the liver and lungs. The survival rate after surgical excision of the rectum is measured in months rather than years.

Adenocarcinoma in anorectal fistulae

In this condition the patient present with anorectal fistulae or recurrent abscesses around the anus. Colloid material can sometimes be clearly seen within the abscesses or fistulous tracks, but there is no visible mucosal lesion in the rectum or anal canal. Microscopic examination of biopsies obtained during surgical treatment of the fistulae show mucinous adenocarcinoma. It has been suggested that these colloid carcinomas arise in duplications of the lower end of the hindgut. Support for this view is provided by the fact that some of the fistulous tracks in such cases are lined by normal rectal mucosa including muscularis mucosae. Indeed, it may be possible to demonstrate that rectal mucosa lines the upper part of the track only and gives way to squamous epithelium about the line of the anal valves. We have also seen cases of anal fistula in which it has been possible to demonstrate by biopsy that the track is lined by rectal mucosa without any evidence of carcinoma. Since this aberrant rectal mucosa can mimic invasive carcinoma should it become misplaced into the wall of the fistulous track by inflammation causing retention of mucus secretion which is then forced into surrounding tissue spaces, it is obviously important to establish a correct diagnosis of invasive mucinous carcinoma, because this will require treatment by excision of the whole rectum and anal region with a permanent colostomy.

Malignant epithelial tumours of the anal margin

Squamous cell carcinoma

Squamous cell carcinomas of the anal margin mostly arise at the junction of the squamous mucous membrane of the lower end of the anal canal with the hair-bearing peri-anal skin. This junctional origin, the appearance of the tumours, their histology and behaviour suggest a comparison with squamous carcinoma of the lip. At both sites we are usually dealing with a slowly growing squamous cell carcinoma which metastasises to regional nodes at a late stage in its natural history.

Squamous carcinoma of the anal margin is about one-third as frequent as anal canal carcinoma. It is more common in men than women (4:1) but there is no significant difference in age incidence compared with adenocarcinoma of the rectum or squamous cell carcioma of the anal canal. Macroscopically, it presents as a typical epitheliomatous ulcer or as a cauliflower or verrucous carcinoma. Microscopically, it is usually a keratinizing, prickle-cell type of carcinoma which is well-differentiated and of relatively low grade of malignancy. Poorly-differentiated tumours are very rare.

Inguinal lymphatic metastases are found in about 40 per cent of cases. The majority of anal margin cancers are treated by local excision of the primary tumour, but in cases which are so extensive as to require radical removal of the rectum involvement of the haemorrhoidal group of lymphatic glands is rare.

The 5-year-survival figures for anal margin cancer show that the prognosis is more favourable than for disease of the anal canal; survival for anal margin cancer is about 50 per cent and for anal canal cancer about 35 per cent. Moreover this better 5-year-survival occurs despite the fact that most anal margin tumours are treated by local excision, whereas the majority of anal canal cancers have excision of the rectum which allows removal of the haemorrhoidal lymphatic glands.

In at least 75 per cent of cases of anal margin and anal canal cancer there is no treatment directed towards the inguinal gland route of spread either by surgery or radiotherapy. It is possible that the prognosis of anal cancer could be improved if an effective method of removing inguinal lymph nodes were devised which did not carry the morbidity of present procedures. The latter is a potent factor inhibiting prophylactic lymph node clearance.

Miscellaneous tumours

Leiomyomas and leiomyosarcomas arising from the internal sphincter are very rare. Peri-anal rhabdomyosarcoma has been reported. Benign lymphoid polyps are not infrequently found in the upper anal canal just above the dentate line though they are more common in rectal mucosa. Malignant lymphoma involving the anus is very rare, but it is not uncommon for peri-anal abscess to be a presenting sign of leukaemia. Lipoma, liposarcoma and fibrosarcoma are seen in the ischiorectal fossa. Secondary carcinoma can occasionally present in the anal canal as a manifestation of spread by implantation from an adenocarcinoma of the colon or rectum.

A wide variety of conditions can present as a presacral tumour. Most of them fall into one of four categories; congenital anomalies, bone tumours, neurogenic tumours and a miscellaneous group of lesions including secondary carcinoma and connective tissue tumours. Among the congenital anomalies dermoid cysts, teratomas, meningocoele and pelvic kidney can be included. Among tumours found at this site are chordomas, osteochondroma, giant cell tumour, sarcoma and myeloma – neurofibroma and ependymona are also seen. Cystic hamartomas composed of multiple cysts embedded in smooth muscle, so-called anal gland cyst – hamartoma, are probably inclusion cysts of anal glands on an inflammatory basis.

Further Reading

Henry MM, Parks AG, Swash M. The anal reflex in idiopathic faecal incontinence; an electrophysiological study, *Br J Surg* 1980; **67**:781–3.

Morson BC, Dawson IMP. *Gastrointestinal Pathology* Second Edition, Oxford, Blackwell Scientific Publications, 1979.

Morson BC. *Systemic Pathology* Second Edition, Edited by W St C Symmers, Vol III, Chapter 18. Edinburgh, London and New York: Churchill Livingstone, 1978.

Parks AG, Swash M, Urich H. Sphincter denervation in anorectal incontinence and rectal prolapse, *Gut* 1977; **18**:656–65.

Thomson WHF. The nature of haemorrhoids, *Br J Surg* 1975; **62**:542–52.

11

Bile Ducts, Liver, Pancreas

J L Dawson and K L Arulambalam

Bile ducts

Primary lesions of the bile ducts are uncommon, most pathology is related to the obstruction of bile flow due to stones or tumour. Patients commonly present with:

(a) *obstructive jaundice*;
or
(b) *cholangitis*.

Rarely gross dilatation of the bile ducts (choledochal cyst) may present as an abdominal mass in childhood.

Emergency operation is occasionally required to deal with biliary peritonitis which follows damage to the bile ducts as a result of operation, penetrating wounds or spontaneous rupture of a choledochal cyst.

Obstructive jaundice

Neonatal period

The investigation of neonatal jaundice is difficult but early and accurate diagnosis is important so that duct obstruction due to atresia can be corrected. Unless early exploration is undertaken the chances of surgical success are poor.

The use of the Rose Bengal test, radio nucleide scans and liver biopsy are the mainstays of making the diagnosis.

Congenital biliary atresia

Biliary atresia is a condition in which the lumen of the bile ducts is obliterated; whether this is a failure of canalization or due to intra-uterine damage is not clear. Bile is absent in the extrahepatic ducts and the gall bladder is often collapsed.

The obliteration is confined to the extrahepatic bile ducts in the first few weeks of life and histological examination of the affected segments usually reveals the presence of small duct-like structures. These communicate with the intrahepatic ducts which are progressively destroyed if surgical drainage is not established. The main complications of biliary atresia include portal hypertension, ascending bacterial cholangitis (after operation) and rickets which may be prevented by supplements of vitamin D.

The liver appears greenish and the ducts may be absent or appear as fibrous cords. If the condition is not corrected by three months it will probably proceed to secondary biliary cirrhosis, portal hypertension and associated splenomegaly.

Needle biopsy of the liver in a suspected case of biliary atresia usually shows features of a cholestatic jaundice. The portal tracts are dilated with oedema and fibrosis, there are acute and chronic inflammatory cells and proliferation of the bile ducts. There may be multinucleated giant cells which may make differentiation from neonatal hepatitis difficult.

Uncorrected the process proceeds to cirrhosis.

Adults and children

Investigation

Cholestatic jaundice is not usually difficult to diagnose in adults or children. The patient has pale stools, dark urine and frequently complains of itching. Biochemical tests give some guidance as to the nature of the jaundice. Cholestasis is produced either by (a) *cell damage* (drugs, virus etc); or (b) *duct obstruction*. The latter is treatable, so early recognition is of paramount importance.

The simplest and safest investigation is an ultrasound examination which in competent hands will demonstrate the presence of dilated ducts and will often localise the site of the causal lesion and distinguish between stone and tumour. If ultrasound shows no dilatation of the duct system a needle biopsy of the liver is done providing the prothrombin time is not more than 4 seconds prolonged.

Liver biopsies are sometimes difficult to interpret and will merely show cholestatic jaundice. If the patient does not improve, then repeat of the ultrasound in one to two weeks is necessary as dilatation of the duct system takes time to develope in some patients. Cholangiography (PTC or ERCP) will confirm the exact site of the obstruction and the need for surgical exploration. If there is a mass suggestive of carcinoma then fine needle aspiration cytology under ultra-sound control will frequently give a tissue diagnosis.

Common bile ducts

Causes

Although common duct stones may present with pure obstructive jaundice there is usually evidence of cholangitis (see p. 137). Primary tumours of the bile ducts are uncommon. Involvement by carcinoma of the pancreas is the commonest single cause of malignant duct obstruction.

Primary tumours

Benign tumours of the large bile ducts are very uncommon. Patients usually present with obstructive jaundice. At operation they may be easily mistaken for carcinoma. Fibromas, leiomyomas and lipomas have been described and appear as firm nodules.

1. *Papillomas* of the ducts may be sessile or pedunculated, they are soft and project into the lumen of the duct.
2. *Adenomas* are firm, well-circumscribed lesions which may occur in any part of the biliary tree (*see* Liver).
3. *Neuromas* which may be seen following division and ligation of the cystic duct after cholecystectomy are probably symptomless.

Biochemical investigations do not distinguish between a benign or malignant neoplasm. The serum bilirubin may be high or may fluctuate if the obstruction is incomplete.

The serum pyruvic transaminases and the alanine transaminases are usually unaffected. The alkaline phosphatase is elevated and the mitochondrial antibody is negative.

Needle biopsy of the liver shows features of duct obstruction. There may be bile thrombi in the canaliculi, bile lakes, bile infarcts and feathery degeneration of the hepatocytes (depending on the duration of the obstruction).

Carcinomas of the extrahepatic bile duct

Malignant tumours of the bile ducts are much commoner than benign lesions of the bile duct. Gallstones and inflammation have a predisposing influence. Incidence is higher in ulcerative colitis, choledochal cysts, Caroli's disease and polycystic disease. In the East liver fluke infestation is a common association.

An early feature is progressive obstructive jaundice and pruritus (unless only one hepatic duct is involved when these symptoms may be delayed). The serum bilirubin and alkaline phosphatase are raised but the mitochrondrial antibody is absent. Weight loss is common.

Site of origin Tumours may begin anywhere in the biliary tree viz:

(a) Right or left main hepatic ducts or bifurcation
(b) Cystic duct with main hepatic duct
(c) Common bile duct
(d) Peri-ampullary region (*see* Carcinoma of the head of pancreas)

Bile duct carcinoma may appear as a small sclerotic lesion in the wall of the bile ducts, which may be virtually impalpable. It is greyish white on cut section and causes narrowing of the lumen. In a second variety there is a definite mass present and the presence of the tumour is obvious. The third variety is uncommon. The duct is expanded by a proliferative lesion filling the lumen and extending right up to the intrahepatic bile ducts.

Before ultrasound and cholangiography were readily available, small fibrotic tumours at the hilum were easily missed at laparotomy. They cause complete obstruction of the extrahepatic duct with intrahepatic dilation of the ducts and enlargement of the liver. The gall bladder is collapsed. Small sclerotic carcinomas are slow growing, metastatise late and generally have a better prognosis than the other two varieties.

All tumours are invariably adenocarcinomas composed of acini with low cuboidal or columnar epithelium in abundant fibrous stroma. Tumours may show variable amounts of mucin secretion. Even microscopically it may sometimes be very difficult to distinguish between a carcinoma and an inflammatory fibrosis.

On section the small tumours show a dense fibrotic stroma with comparatively few cells. This makes diagnosis from a small biopsy specimen difficult.

Tumours developing at the ampulla are often polypoidal. They may occlude the pancreatic duct causing chronic pancreatitis and atrophy of the exocrine pancreas. The proximal biliary tree is dilated. Although usually much less aggressive than carcinoma of the pancreas they spread in a similar manner to regional nodes and liver.

Secondary tumours

Secondary involvement by tumours growing in adjacent organs is common especially in tumours arising from the pancreas (*see* p. 148). Occasionally lymph nodes in the portahepatis or primary tumours in the duodenum can cause bile duct obstruction.

Cholangitis

Cholangitis may present "de novo" or may develop during the investigation of a patient with obstructive jaundice. The introduction of preoperative cholangiography either endoscopically or transhepatically has resulted in a great increase in frequency of cholangitis seen in hospital practice. Cholangitis is an inflammation of the bile ducts which rarely develops unless there is an obstruction to bile flow. In the patient presenting de novo the obstruction is most commonly due to a stone which has migrated from the gall bladder. Cholangitis is usually present in bile duct stricture following operative trauma. It is unusual for tumours to present with cholangitis unless the biliary tract has been punctured during investigation.

Cholangitis produces a spectrum of clinical presentations depending upon the virulence of the infection and the completeness of the obstruction. Severe cholangitis may produce scarring in the biliary tree which on cholangiography may resemble idiopathic sclerosing cholangitis.

Lowgrade infection with incomplete obstruction may present as a pyrexia of unknown origin with little or no rise in bilirubin but a disproportionately high alkaline phosphatase. Severe infection associated with obstruction may produce septicaemia and a life threatening illness with deepening jaundice and threat of acute renal failure. The patient presents with rigors, fever and jaundice (Charcot's Triad). Bacteraemia is common and blood cultures are frequently positive if taken during the time the patient is experiencing rigors. Urgent operative decompression of the biliary obstruction may be life saving in very ill patients.

In an established case the bile ducts are thickened and dilated. The bile is opaque and may form greenish-black concretions. Sometimes the bile ducts are full of pus. Infection of the intrahepatic ducts may result in multiple abscesses. The ducts are oedematous and vascular. The wall is infiltrated by polymorphs and the lining of the duct may be replaced by granulation tissue which is very friable and bleeds readily when the duct is explored. Within the liver the bile ducts are surrounded by a polymorpho-nuclear infiltrate so that liver biopsy may suggest the diagnosis. The commonest infecting organisms are *E. coli* or *Klebsiella*.

Choledochal cyst

The commonest variety of choledochal cyst is a segmental dilatation of the common duct which may be associated with segmental dilatation of ducts within the liver.

The cyst presents in infancy or childhood with either pain, jaundice or a mass. Aetiology is not understood but a common finding is that the pancreatic duct drains into the bile duct well above the ampulla. Pancreatic juice in the bile duct may possibly weaken the wall and cause dilatation.

The wall of the cyst is fibrotic and may contain inflammatory cells; the epithelial lining may be absent. There is a considerable risk of carcinoma developing in the biliary tree, occasionally spontaneous rupture may occur.

Caroli's disease

This is a rare congenital saccular segmental dilatation of the intrahepatic bile ducts. It usually presents as recurrent cholangitis. It may be associated with other congenital abnormalities such as hepatic fibrosis and medullary sponge kidney.

Stricture

The majority of traumatic strictures follow duct injury at cholecystectomy. They usually involve the common hepatic duct or the right hepatic duct: those related to duodenal or pancreatic disease involve the distal bile duct.

Following inadvertent division of the bile duct at operation, the proximal stump retracts up into the hilum of the liver leaving little patent extrahepatic biliary apparatus. This remnant is usually found to connect by a fistulous tract to the distal bile duct or to a viscus if stricturing has developed despite reconstruction. There is much surrounding fibrosis. The lumen is narrowed and lined by granulation tissue. The biliary tree above the stricture is dilated and may contain stones and biliary mud. The term biliary stricture is a misnomer; it is really a fistula.

The damaged part of the duct becomes fibrotic and thickened and there are islands of trapped epithelium in the scar tissue which can easily be mistaken for a scirrhous carcinoma and the pathologist may be misled, particularly in a frozen section. But the history of previous surgery usually makes the diagnosis clear. If the obstruction is not relieved, a secondary biliary cirrhosis may develop.

Sclerosing cholangitis

Primary sclerosing cholangitis is a rare condition of unknown aetiology. The whole biliary tree is usually involved and the commonest associated disease is ulcerative colitis. The biliary disease follows the colitis but once established treatment of the colonic disease does not seem to influence the progress of the biliary disease. Frequently once the biliary disease is established the colonic disease decreases in intensity; it may even be burnt out.

Rarely sclerosing disease involves only the extrahepatic ducts and it is in this type of disease that improvement by biliary-intestinal anastomosis (e.g. choledocho-jejunostomy) may be obtained.

Occasionally, diffuse biliary sclerosis may follow recovery from suppurative cholangitis, the damage to the ducts being sustained during the healing process after the infection. Rarely sclerosis of the intrahepatic ducts may follow the use of formalin as a scolicide in a communicating hepatic hydatid cyst.

In chronic diffuse disease the whole of the biliary tree undergoes a progressive narrowing with ulceration of the mucosa, which may involve the gall bladder.

The duct is found to be white and thickened and when exploration is attempted it may be quite difficult to find the lumen. The appearance is rather that of an atheromatous vessel. The clinical course varies from patient to patient. In some the disease progresses rapidly and the patient usually dies of recurrent cholangitis and septicaemia. In others it runs a more indolent course and the patient may survive for years.

Oriental cholangio-hepatitis

A condition almost exclusively seen in South East Asians of Chinese origin. The exact aetiology of the condition is not known, but infection with *Clornochis Sinensis* and use of opium derivatives are thought to be contributory factors in some, but not all patients. The condition presents as an acute abdominal pain which may vary from mild to severe and is often associated with fever, hepatomegaly, vomiting and jaundice.

The biochemical tests show a raised alkaline phosphatase and raised serum bilirubin. The IgM fraction of the immunoglobulins is raised but the mitochondrial antibodies are absent.

ERCP is diagnostic. There is irregular stricturing of the intra and extrahepatic ducts.

The liver is enlarged, the gall bladder is dilated and tense. The intra and extra hepatic ducts are dilated with thick inspissated bile and may contain friable stones. Periductular abscesses in the liver may develop and sometimes coalesce to form multilocular cavities.

If, however, the inflammation is low grade, the liver tissue may show atrophy with stones within the ducts.

The bile ducts show oedema and thickening of the wall. The epithelium may show hyperplasia in the early stages, but later may be replaced by granulation tissue.

Needle biopsy of the liver often shows a portal zone infiltration with lymphocytes, polymorphs and occasionally macrophages. There is often periductular inflammation. There is periductular fibrosis: the portal tracts have a characteristic stellate appearance.

Liver disease

Liver disease presents to the surgeon electively as

(a) a mass and/or pain;
(b) complications of portal hypertension.

Emergency surgery may be required for

(c) liver trauma;

and very rarely for

(d) peritonitis due to pathological rupture of tumour, cyst or abscess.

Liver mass

The patient may present with, or be found to have, an enlarged liver. The enlargement may be *Diffuse* or *Focal*.

Enlargement of liver is often associated with other symptoms which themselves may cause the patient to seek advice and lead to the discovery of a mass. The most common presenting symptoms are listed below.

Pain Usually in the right upper quadrant sometimes radiating to the right scapular region. The pain is probably due to capsular stretching. It is common in expanding focal lesions as well as acute diffuse swelling e.g. hepatitis or congestive heart failure.

Jaundice Hepatocyte dysfunction leads to jaundice. Liver function tests usually reflect evidence of cell damage or death as well as impairment of normal protein synthesis.

Constitutional non-specific symptoms Poor appetite, reduction in stamina and loss of a sense of well being are common in extensive lesions of the liver, e.g. metastatic carcinoma after previous cancer surgery.

Pyrexia Fever and vague ill health may be the presenting features.

Encephalopathy Impaired hepatocyte function associated with shunting of portal blood into the systemic circulation through collateral channels leads to impaired cerebral function varying from subtle personality change to profound coma. Clinical examination usually reveals signs of chronic liver disease; spider naevi, liver palms, foetor, breast enlargement and testicular atrophy. Liver function tests reflect impaired synthesis and cell damage.

Ascites Persistent ascites may be the presenting symptoms of chronic liver disease. The signs of liver disease and muscle wasting are usually present.

Heart failure Rarely in childhood large A-V shunts present as high output cardiac failure.

Inappropriate endocrine secretion Tumours may produce a systemic disturbance due to the production of abnormal metabolites e.g. carcinoid deposits producing 5-Hydroxy-tryptophan.

Investigation of a liver mass

This is done using imaging techniques, examination of histological or cytological specimen and biochemical tests.

Imaging techniques

Modern imaging techniques have greatly simplified the assessment of patients with liver disease.

Ultrasound

This simple cheap and safe examination readily establishes the presence or absence of structural liver disease. Furthermore it accurately demonstrates the lesion to be diffuse or focal. It will also demonstrate whether the consistency is *solid* or *cystic*.

Thus four varieties of liver disease are defined:

Diffuse	Cystic (1)
	Solid (2)
Focal	Cystic (3)
	Solid (4)

C T Scanning This investigation is expensive and will provide the same information as ultrasound. In addition it provides the clinician with a more detailed permanent record of the scans performed which are much easier to interpret than ultrasound.

Isotope scans Isotope scans may be of some help in isolating focal lesions in the liver but the resolution is not very good and normal appearances are surprisingly variable. The surgeon learns to beware of reports such as possible filling defects at the hilum. Tumours, cysts and abscesses show up as filling defects on ^{99}m Techneium sulphur colloid scans. However, some hepato-cellular tumours take up ^{75}Se Methionine and these show an area of increased or normal uptake compared with the colloid scan.

Angiography Selective arteriography is a particularly helpful investigation for the surgeon contemplating exploring a patient with a focal lesion. It establishes the vascular anatomy of the liver; it is helpful in deciding on operability; it may be diagnostic, e.g. tumour circulation and; it may demonstrate areas of devitalized liver tissue in patients with complicated trauma.

Biopsy of the liver

Open biopsy

Biopsy of the liver may be open (at laparotomy) or percutaneous. At laparotomy a wedge of liver tissue may be taken from a focal lesion or when the biopsy is done for diffuse parenchymal disease it should be taken from the convex surface of the liver as biopsies taken from the liver edge may be difficult to interpret as there is normally a good deal of fibrosis at this site which can mimic cirrhosis. These changes extend only a few millimetres into the parenchyma.

There are often artefactual changes in operative samples—haemorrhage and diffuse polymorph infiltration.

Percutaneous needle biopsy

Percutaneous needle biopsy of the liver has brought tremendous advances in the diagnosis and management of liver disease; although the interpretation is usually straightforward, occasional cases do require considerable experience on the part of the pathologist for the correct interpretation. Focal disease of course can never be excluded on such samples. The platelet count and clotting studies should be checked before biopsy is undertaken.

The biopsied tissue is approximately 1–4 cm. long and is immediately fixed in 10 per cent formol saline. The operator can make observations on the biopsied tissue; cirrhotic liver tissue tends to fragment, the fatty liver tends to be yellowish and float in the formol saline.

The biopsy in a cholestatic jaundice appears greenish in the centre and paler at the periphery. In the chronic congestive liver there are darker centres. In secondary carcinoma whitish nodules may be seen.

Cytology

Cytological examination for malignant cells may be done on aspirated bile or pancreatic fluid as well as from brushings from suspicious lesions obtained at ERCP. The best yield for cytology comes from fluid aspirated from tumours under ultrasound or CAT control. The material is immediately smeared onto a glass slide and either air dried or wet fixed in cytofix. It is best if the cytologist is present to confirm that the specimens obtained are diagnostic and no further aspirates are necessary.

Biochemical tests

Biochemical tests are sensitive indicators of a diffuse disturbance of liver function but they are often normal in focal lesions. A raised conjugated bilirubin and alkaline phosphatase suggest cholestasis, hepatic or post hepatic. Defects in synthesis are reflected by a low serum albumin and a prolonged prothrombin time which is not corrected by the administration of vitamin K.

Cell damage or death causes release of enzymes into the circulation. Raised levels of transaminases SGPT and ALT are common. The glutamyl transferase is raised in cholestasis and is also a sensitive marker of recent excess alcohol intake.

An auto-antibody screen should be done in chronic liver disease. Mitochondrial antibodies are found in most patients with primary biliary cirrhosis. Smooth muscle antibodies and antinuclear factor are raised in chronic active hepatitis.

Portal hypertension

Portal hypertension presents as either haemorrhage from varices or as splenomegaly (especially in childhood). Haemorrhage may be torrential and require urgent treatment.

The normal portal venous pressure is 5 mm/Hg. If there is impedence to portal flow the pressure rises up to 20 mm/Hg and causes the spleen to enlarge (congestive splenomegaly).

A collateral circulation develops at the sites of porto-systemic anastomoses. The most important of these is the lower oesophagus where the local venous anatomy together with the abrupt pressure gradient between intra abdominal and intra thoracic pressure leads to the development of submucosal varices which are the usual site of gastro intestinal haemorrhage in these patients. Similar varices are sometimes seen around ileostomies or colostomies in patients with portal hypertension. Haemorrhoids are not more common in these patients.

Diagnosis

Oesophageal varices are readily demonstrated by endoscopy or barium studies. The venous phase of an aortoportogram gives good views of the anatomy of the portal circulation and collaterals.

The obstruction to portal blood flow may be

(a) extrahepatic; or
(b) intrahepatic.

Extrahepatic

The obstruction is due to occlusion of the main portal vein. Causes are neonatal sepsis, blood disorders predisposing to thrombosis, e.g. polycythaemia, thrombotic thrombocythaemia and tumours of the pancreas or other organs that involve the portal vein. Sometimes no cause is found for the thrombosis. The portal vein and often the splenic veins are replaced by tortuous collaterals (portal cavernoma).

Intrahepatic

Intrahepatic pathology may cause obstruction to the portal flow at the pre-sinusoidal, sinusoidal or post-sinusoidal location.

Intrahepatic—pre-sinusoidal The obstruction is in the smaller branches of the portal veins and the portal tracts. In Schistosomiasis it is due to ova causing fibrosis of the small venous radicals and thrombophlebitis of the venules. In biliary cirrhosis it may occur before the cirrhosis due to cellular infiltration of portal zones. Exposure to toxins, e.g. inorganic arsenic, methotrexate, vinyl chloride, cause portal sclerosis and hence portal hypertension.

Intrahepatic—sinusoidal The intrahepatic type is associated with hepatocellular disease. Cirrhosis due to whatever cause leads to portal hypertension; this is the result of fibrosis and regenerating nodules. Obstruction to portal venous blood is mainly sinusoidal.

Intrahepatic—post sinusoidal: Budd Chiari syndrome Clinically the Budd Chiari syndrome is characterised by intractable ascites. It develops when there is obstruction of hepatic veins at any site from the efferent vein of a lobule to the entry of the inferior vena cava in the right atrium.

Causes vary depending upon the site of obstruction viz: congenital caval webs, thrombosis of hepatic veins and infiltration by tumour. The liver is enlarged, tender, purplish and smooth. There is venous congestion and appears as advanced nutmeg change.

Microscopically there is marked centrizonal venous dilatation, haemorrhagic necrosis of liver cells in the centrizonal areas with sinusoidal congestion.

Haemodynamic effects of portal hypertension

As obstruction to portal flow increases, the amount of portal blood reaching the liver decreases; indeed in some patients with severe disease the portal vein acts as an outflow tract i.e. blood actually flows away from the liver.

The combination of decreased portal flow, impaired hepatocyte function and direct shunting of portal blood into the systemic circulation are thought to be responsible for encephalopathy. Various neuropsychiatric disturbances may be seen but the commonest are mental and range from disturbances of behaviour to the development of coma. The creation of a surgical shunt undoubtedly increases the risk of encephalopathy and hastens the development of hepatic failure. For this reason shunt surgery has lost favour in the UK in the past few years.

Diffuse enlargement: cystic

Fibropolycystic disease

Fibropolycystic disease is a group of inherited disorders of the biliary tract and liver. They may be associated with a renal disorder, but vary from patient to patient.

Adult polycystic This is an autosomal dominant disorder.

The liver may be normal or enlarged, depending on the number and size of the cysts. The largest cysts may reach up to 1 cm and the smaller ones appear as speckled spots. The surface of the liver may be smooth or deformed.

The hepatocytes are normal and the liver cell architecture is maintained. The cysts are related to the bile ducts and are lined by columnar epithelium. The cut surface of the liver may appear honeycomb; cysts are thin-walled and contain clear or bloodstained fluid. Bile is never found (for *Caroli's disease* and *Choleclochal cyst see* the section on Bile Ducts, p. 135.).

Diffuse liver disease: solid

Hepatic fibrosis

Hepatic fibrosis may appear sporadically or be inherited as an autosomal recessive disorder. Patients present in childhood or early adulthood either with splenomegaly, secondary to portal hypertension, or with bleeding oesophageal varices. Liver function is normal apart from alkaline phosphatase. It is sometimes associated with Caroli's disease (see p. 137). Liver biopsy confirms the diagnosis: normal architecture is disturbed by intersecting serpiginous bands of tissue between which the normal lobular architecture is maintained. There may be occasional islands of trapped parenchyma but true hyperplastic areas are never found.

The dense fibrous bands may contain bile ducts; they may be dilated to microcysts.

Appearance of liver in cirrhosis

Cirrhosis is a diffuse process involving the entire liver and consists of areas of fibrosis with parenchymal nodules. The gross appearance varies from an enlarged organ to a small, shrunken organ weighing a few hundred grams. On morphological grounds cirrhosis has been described as micronodular when the nodules are less than 3 mm and macronodular when the nodules exceed 3 mm and may reach up to 2–3 cm. On the other hand there may be a mixed picture of micro- and marconodular cirrhosis.

Cirrhosis of the liver may present in many ways but commonly either with signs of liver failure, jaundice, ascites, encephalopathy, or because of bleeding from oesophageal varices secondary to the raised portal pressure. Laboratory tests reflect the deterioration in hepatocyte function such as abnormal serum albumen and prothrombin time. The liver SGPT and ALT are also raised reflecting the activity of the disease process. Ultrasound examination will usually show dilatation of the portal veins and an aorto-portogram will confirm the presence of portal hypertension in the venous phase with evidence of collateral formation. The arterial phase shows abnormalities in the arterial circulation with spiralled vessels supplying the parenchyma.

The aetiology is not evident from the morphological appearance of the liver. In the West alcohol is the most important aetiological agent and in the developing countries, viral hepatitis. In chronic alcoholism, long-standing biliary disease and haemochromatosis the cirrhosis is often of the micronodular type. In chronic alcoholism the liver is yellowish due to fatty change, appears greasy and is often associated with Mallory's hyaline. In biliary cirrhosis the liver is greenish and in haemochromatosis the liver may appear dark; the excess iron may be demonstrated by the Prussian blue reaction. The older post-necrotic cirrhosis or that following a severe attack of viral hepatitis is often macronodular.

The diagnosis may be established by wedge biopsy or by needle biopsy, though this is not always easy. There are shortcomings in both.

If the biopsies are taken from a large macronodule the biopsy material may have the semblance of normal architecture, and the diagnosis thus missed. But an experienced pathologist quite often is able to suggest the diagnosis from attention to minor changes.

In a needle biopsy there are other features which may indicate cirrhosis, such as fragmentation of the biopsy during the procedure or during processing. Fibrosis, regenerating nodules, liver cell dysplasia, twin liver cell plates or abnormally small portal tracts.

Biliary cirrhosis

Primary biliary cirrhosis is an autoimmune disorder which is commoner in females. The initial presentation is frequently pruritus which may precede the jaundice by months or even years. The liver is enlarged and the presence of xanthelasma around the eye is common.

Clinically the jaundice is cholestatic. The alkaline phosphatase level is grossly elevated compared with the serum bilirubin. There is elevated gamma globulin IgM with a high mitochrondial antibody. The liver is enlarged and green in the early stages.

Needle biopsy is often helpful. Four stages have been described for the progress of the disease; the florid duct lesion in which there is focal damage to septal and interlobular ducts, ductular proliferation, scarring and cirrhossis. There is, however, considerable overlap and all four stages may coexist. Often well defined granulomata and lymphoid follicles with germinal centres are seen. The condition may be associated with other autoimmune disease. The patient may develop steatorrhoea which can cause loss of fat soluble vitamins and hence cause osteomalacia.

Secondary biliary cirrhosis occurs infrequently in long-standing duct obstruction. The common findings are nodules separated by serpiginous bands of fibrous tissue showing no compression of the liver cells.

Chronic active hepatitis

This invariably progresses to cirrhosis. The term chronic active hepatitis implies a mode of progression of hepatocellular disease, rather than a single disease entity. This may occur as an autoimmune disorder, follow an episode of Australia antigen positive viral hepatitis or other types of chronic liver disease, such as Wilson's disease, drugs or alcoholism. These patients may present with jaundice but the jaundice is associated with the presence of autoantibodies, particularly anti-smooth muscle and antinuclear antibody, and biochemical changes of hepatocellular disease. The liver is enlarged initially but with the development of cirrhosis it becomes smaller. Needle biopsy is often helpful. The characteristic features are piecemeal necrosis, very marked portal tract inflammation with a high proportion of plasma cells, bridging fibrosis connecting portal tracts and central veins. In that associated with hepatitis B, ground glass cells are seen in the liver. These stain with orcein or with specific immunological markers.

The precise diagnosis of the type of cirrhosis is important both in assessing correct treatment, withdrawal of the causative agent and in giving some guide to prognosis. Cirrhosis once established is irreversible but deterioration may be slowed or prevented in certain varieties.

Parasitic infestation

Schistosomiasis

Schistosomiasis in the liver is the result of infestation by the flat worm Schistosoma (*S. Mansoni* and *S. Japonicum* commonly infest the liver). It is endemic in many parts of the world especially in the Middle East and South America, the infection occurring from contaminated fresh water lakes.

The ova that enter the portal venous radicles may lodge in the larger branches of the portal veins and produce coarse fibrosis, or in the smaller branches a fine diffuse fibrosis.

In the acute phase there may be hepatomegaly but late stage of the disease results in an enlarged spleen and a small scarred liver.

Initially there is a chronic granulomatous reaction with giant cells and large numbers of eosinophils around the Schistosoma ova. The inflammation is thought to be due to antigens released by the ova. This is followed by fibrosis which may be extensive and referred to as "pipe stem" fibrosis; this is pathognomic, and though the hepatic architecture is disturbed, cirrhosis never occurs. However, the contracting fibrotic bands cause vascular occlusion and hence portal hypertension develops; thrombosis of some of the veins is a contributory factor.

Diffuse enlargement: infiltrations

Fatty infiltration

Fatty infiltration is an asymptomatic benign condition which is reversible. It is commonly associated with alcoholism, diabetes, malnutrition following jejunal by-pass operation, obesity, poisoning, e.g. carbon tetrachloride. It may present as a diffuse smooth enlargement of the liver. The liver is yellowish and pale. Biopsy tissue may feel greasy and often floats in the formalin. Abdominal injury is more likely to cause rupture of the abnormal liver and may be complicated further by fat embolism.

In the alcoholic, fatty infiltration may indicate serious liver damage and liver failure not infrequently follows abdominal surgery.

Amyloidosis

Hepatic involvement in amyloidosis is usually asymptomatic. Rarely portal hypertension may be produced, and ascites, if present, is usually the result of the nephrotic syndrome, due to amyloid involvement of the kidney, rather than to liver disease.

The liver is involved in both primary and secondary amyloidosis. In the past, primary amyloidosis was regarded as amyloidosis occurring without any co-existing disease, secondary amyloidosis as occurring with an antecedent cause such as long standing suppurative disorders or rheumatoid arthritis. With electron microscopy the structure of amyloid has been resolved. Structurally, primary amyloid is found to be composed of aminoacids, the sequence of which is similar to the light chain component of immunoglobulins and is similar to amyloid seen in myeloma. In contrast, secondary amyloid is composed of a new protein referred to as Protein A and its aminoacid sequence is different from any other protein described hitherto.

The liver may be pale, enlarged, smooth and waxy in appearance. There may be no functional abnormality in the liver, apart from hepatomegaly. Rarely there may be pressure atrophy of the hepatocytes, particularly those of the midzonal region.

Deposition of amyloid in the liver may occur in (a) blood vessels in the portal tract; and (b) the space of Disse—between the hepatocytes and the endothelial lining of the sinusoids.

Focal disease: cystic

Simple cysts

Simple cysts of the liver occasionally occur and are often large and single. They have to be differentiated from parasitic cysts.

Parasitic: hydatid disease

Uncomplicated hydatid disease may present with pain in the region of the cyst or the patient may notice an abdominal swelling. Clinical examination reveals enlargement of the liver and a straight abdominal X-ray may show calcification in the wall of the cyst. The diagnosis of a cystic lesion is readily made by ultrasound examination which may also show the presence of daughter cysts within. Immunofluorescent techniques replace the other methods of recognising a challenge by hydatid protein. It is contraindicated to attempt to aspirate or biopsy any cystic lesion if there is the slighest possibility of it being hydatid in origin.

Hydatid disease in the human occurs by ingestion of the larva passed in dog excreta, either by contamination of the food or by handling infected dogs. The embryos liberated in the intestines pass through the mucosa into the portal blood stream. The majority of the embryos encyst in the liver, the rest pass into the systemic circulation to the lungs, spleen, kidney, skeletal muscle or brain to produce hydatid cysts in these organs.

Echinococcus granulosus which causes the human infection in the UK produces a unilocular cyst. The cyst wall consists of an innermost germinal layer giving rise to scolices, brood capsules and daughter cysts and contains a clear fluid. The germinal layer is surrounded by an outer chitinous layer and external to this is granulation tissue and a fibrous capsule. The surrounding liver parenchyma may show pressure atrophy with an intense portal infiltrate with eosinophils. Calcification may occur in the ectocyst. Frequently the complications of hydatid disease lead to clinical presentation.

Rupture of a hydatid cyst into the peritoneum may cause intestinal obstruction. Rupture into the intrahepatic ducts may cause cholangitis and obstructive jaundice. Rupture through the diaphragm into the lungs may cause the daughter cysts to be coughed up in the sputum and sometimes rupture into the colon may allow the daughter cysts to be passed per rectum. Rupture of a hydatid cyst into the peritoneum may give rise to anaphylactic shock which sometimes may be fatal.

Infection of a cyst by a pyogenic organism may result in a liver abscess following which the cyst may undergo spontaneous regression with death of the parasite. In any patient with hepatic abscess who has lived in an endemic area of hydatid disease, the hydatid origin for the cavity in the liver should be considered. It leads to difficulties in surgical management as resolution of the cavity following drainage of the abscess may not occur readily, because the wall is composed of a rigid adventitia.

In the UK hydatid disease is rare apart from some parts of Wales. It is prevalent in the Mediterranean, e.g. Greece, South America and parts of Africa, but the incidence has been greatly reduced in Australia and New Zealand by an energetic programme to control the spread of adult worms in the dog.

Pyogenic liver abscess

Pyogenic liver abscess is an uncommon condition and diagnosis may be difficult. Clinically, liver abscess may complicate any infective lesion of the large bowel (e.g. appendix or diverticulitis) or of the biliary tree (cholangitis or severe cholecystitis). However, in a proportion of patients there is no antecedent illness and the abscess arises de novo with non-specific symptoms. The abscess may be single or multiple.

The patients usually present with pyrexia but few localizing signs; the pain over the liver is often mild if present. Jaundice is present in less than half the patients and the presence of a high white count and a very high sedimentation rate in such a patient should raise the possibility of encapsulated pus somewhere in the body. Usually ultrasound examination of the liver, isotope scan or a CAT scan of the liver will show the lesion quite readily although there may be false negatives. Sometimes necrotic tumours may masquerade as abscess; and in difficult patients an arteriogram may show tumour circulation at the periphery of such a lesion, which makes the diagnosis easier.

In the majority of patients the bacteriology of the abscess shows more than one organism growing. Common ones found are *E. coli*, *Klebsiella*, and anaerobic organisms; in recent years *Streptococcus milleri* has been recognized with increasing frequency. Sometimes patients with liver abscess present with metastatic abscesses in the lung or brain before the hepatic abscess is diagnosed. Abscess formation may follow injuries of the liver when encapsulated haematoma or devitalized liver becomes secondarily infected.

Amoebic abscess

The patients present with malaise, fever, abdominal pain with weight loss and night sweats, very similar to the picture seen in pyogenic abscess. However, the history of possible exposure to amoebae in an endemic area should suggest the diagnosis and serological tests will usually confirm it. Ultrasound examination of the liver will confirm the presence of a fluid-containing cavity. Metronidazole is so effective in the treatment that a therapeutic trial of this drug is often used in endemic areas on clinical grounds alone.

Needle aspiration may show amoebae in the necrotic debris. It is important to be certain that the patient is not suffering from hydatid disease as needling of a hydatid cyst may produce fatal complications. Serological tests for amoebiasis may remain elevated after the clinical control of the disease. The trophozoites may be seen when an immunofluorescent stain is used.

Focal lesions: solid

Benign tumours

Bile duct adenomas are found incidentally at laparotomy.

They are seen as small subcapsular nodules, both on gross appearance and frozen section and may be mistaken for metastatic disease, especially if multiple.

These nodules show well-formed bile ducts embedded in a fibrous stroma (*synonyms*: microhamartomas and von Meyenberg complexes).

Liver cell adenoma

Liver cell adenomas are now recognised to develop most commonly in women who are taking the contraceptive pill. They may present as a mass or sometimes as an acute abdomen following spontaneous rupture of a previously asymptomatic lesion. Rupture leads to serious haemoperitoneum. Sometimes the lesions are multifocal.

Grossly the lesions are smooth, soft yellow or tan coloured and poorly encapsulated. They are composed of cords of mature hepatocytes with no portal tracts or bile ducts. They are very vascular and haemorrhage may occur into the substance of the tumour. It may be difficult to distinguish an adenoma from a well differentiated malignant liver cell tumour. The vascularity of the lesion is well shown on angiogram. Pill tumours are often associated with a widespread abnormality of the intrahepatic vasculature (peliosis) which is readily seen on selective angiography.

Focal nodular hyperplasia

This is usually an asymptomatic lesion.

It is often solitary, found by chance at operation. Larger lesions may present as a dark red to brown solid mass, sometimes pedunculated. Cut sections reveal a fibrotic area with stellate radiating bands. Many abnormal dilated vessels are present in the lesion. Fibrotic bands with bridging fibrosis may be mistakenly diagnosed as cirrhosis but the morphology of the hepatocytes and their relationship to bile ducts is that of normal tissue. Angiography confirms the vascularity of the tumour with a characteristic centrifugal filling pattern.

Mesenchymal hamartoma

This lesion occurs in infancy and is often asymptomatic.

It may present as a palpable abdominal mass and is composed of loose fibrous tissue with branching bile ducts.

Haemangiomas

These are rare tumours and present in infancy. They enlarge rapidly during the first few months of life and are often associated with cutaneous haemangiomas which grow during the first few months of life. The main clinical importance of hepatic haemangiomas is they produce a large arterio-venous communication which is of sufficient size to produce high output cardiac failure. An audible bruit over the palpable liver makes the diagnosis. Angiograms confirm the arterio-venous communication with early filling of the hepatic veins. These lesions tend to regress after the first few months of life.

Primary malignant tumours

Most focal solid lesions of the liver are secondary tumours.

Hepatomas and cholangiocarcinomas

Primary tumours of the liver which hitherto have been thought to be uncommon are on the increase: (a) hepatomas arise from hepatic parenchymal cells; and (b) cholangiocarcinomas arise from ductular epithelium. The incidence of these tumours is higher in the cirrhotic liver, hence if there is a sudden deterioration in the health of a well compensated cirrhotic patient, a hepatoma should be suspected.

Primary tumours developing in an otherwise healthy person present with a mass or pain due to capsular stretching or infiltration of adjacent structures. There is usually loss of weight. Some patients present with fever and this is usually associated with a massive tumour. Other systemic symptoms may include lassitude, anorexia and weakness, or sudden onset of ascites. Occasionally, pathological rupture of the tumour occurs, producing haemoperitoneum and the patient presents as an acute abdominal emergency.

Both the hepatoma and the cholangiocarcinoma may have the following *macroscopic appearance*: some present as a solitary, massive tumour, sometimes replacing one lobe; others as multiple nodules throughout the liver which may be difficult to distinguish from secondary tumour. Occasionally, a diffuse type is seen which may look like a cirrhotic liver. The tumour varies from yellow to greenish in colour. The hepatocarcinomas are more likely to be greenish as the tumour cells may excrete bile. These tumours also show early invasion of the hepatic veins.

Primary tumours are not always easy to differentiate from secondary ones. Seventy per cent of hepatocellular tumours produce alpha fetoprotein which is diagnostic; a sudden leucocytosis as opposed to a leukopenia seen in a cirrhotic patient or a sustained elevation of alkaline phosphatase is suspicious. Needle biopsy is an established method of making the diagnosis although the possibility of seeding tumour along the needle tract is a real one. The site of the biopsy may be guided by ultrasound localization of the tumour.

The well-differentiated hepatoma may be difficult to distinguish from liver tissue. Anaplastic variants may show giant cell and acinar structures. The tumour cells may contain bile.

Cholangiocarcinomas are adenocarcinomas and may be difficult to distinguish from metastatic tumour of the gastrointestinal tract. Angiograms show a tumour "blush" which confirms the vascular nature of the hepatoma and the appearance of the malignant circulation is diagnostic, but in contrast a cholangiocarcinoma is a comparatively avascular tumour.

Fibrolamellar carcinoma

A tumour of the liver in young adults; it has been described with a very distinctive macroscopic and microscopic picture.

This tumour arises as a solitary mass in a non-cirrhotic liver. Sometimes there may be multiple nodules. In the majority the tumour is in the left lobe, and the tumour may have a central depressed fibrous scar rather like focal nodular hyperplasia.

Two distinctive features have been described. Deeply eosinophilic plump hepatocytes with abundant fibrous stroma arranged in parallel bands round the tumour cells. In some cases the tumour cells contained well-defined, pale eosinophilic hyaline intracytoplasmic globules.

Prognosis The justification for identifying these tumours as a distinct entity is based on slow clinical progression, the patient's age and its potential surgical cure. The gross and histological features of the tumour have been confused both with hepatocellular adenomas and focal nodular hyperplasia. Unlike the malignant hepatomas, the alpha fetoprotein is negative.

Hepatoblastoma

This tumour is rare and occurs before the age of three. The epithelial elements may resemble normal foetal tissue and haemopoiesis may be seen in sinusoidal channels. The mesenchymal elements are fibrous tissue, cartilage, osteoid or bone.

Haemangiosarcoma

This is a rare tumour but it is of special interest because of its association with exposure to thorotrast and also as an occupational disease in workers exposed to vinyl chloride. It sometimes develops in cirrhotic livers.

Secondary malignant tumours

Metastatic spread to the liver is the commonest cause of hepatic enlargement. It may be discovered on routine follow up examination after resection for a tumour somewhere in the gastrointestinal tract or the patient may notice pain or non-specific symptoms such as anorexia, or lethargy. If the tumour is near the hilum of the liver, then jaundice may follow obstruction of the bile ducts. Investigation by scanning shows the tumour to have no uptake of colloid; the venous phase of an angiogram of the liver again shows filling defects within the liver, and ultrasound examination and CAT scanning will demonstrate lesions of different density within the liver. The blood supply of the deposits is derived almost exclusively from the hepatic artery. They are usually relatively avascular except for deposits from carcinoid tumours.

The appearance varies enormously. Frequently as the deposits enlarge the centre undergoes necrosis producing a characteristic umbilication on the surface of the tumour. Metastatic spread to the liver is usually multiple. Confirmation of the cell type or origin may be useful in some patients in deciding management, and liver biopsy may be taken by needle, or under direct vision at peritoneoscopy. Biochemical tests have little part to play in making the diagnosis apart from when there is some duct obstruction and there is an elevated alkaline phosphatase with a high γ glutamyl transferase. Quite extensive metastatic disease may be present with no biochemical disturbance. Secondary deposits from patients with argentaffinomas may produce carcinoid syndrome because of production of 5 hydroxytryptamine by tumour cells in the liver. The attacks of flushing, dyspnoea, diarrhoea and bowel colic are usually readily recognized. Confirmation of the diagnosis is made by measurement of the excessive excretion of 5 hydroxy-indole-acetic acid in the urine.

Acute problems

The commonest acute surgical problem involving the liver is undoubtedly trauma. In the UK this is almost always blunt trauma. Penetrating wounds from knife or bullet are rare but liver biopsy occasionally produces haemoperitoneum.

Blunt injury

Blunt injury of the liver is most commonly produced by road traffic accidents. Another common cause in Britain is the kick of a horse. Damage to the liver varies enormously depending upon the mechanism of injury and ranges from minor surface lacerations, stellate fractures, pulping of the liver tissue or sometimes complete avulsion of the liver from the vena cava. Sometimes haemorrhage beneath the capsule produces a large haematoma which may slowly enlarge over the next few days causing increasing pain and swelling. Patients with liver injury may have associated tears of the hepatic vein at the point where they join the vena cava; this is a very difficult surgical problem to deal with.

There seems little doubt that tight suturing of the hepatic capsule in an attempt to stop arterial haemorrhage in the depth of the liver may result in increased disruption of liver tissue as the haemorrhage occurs into a closed space. Sometimes in such circumstances the rupture of the blood under pressure may occur into the biliary tree resulting in haemobilia some days after the initial injury. Liver injury should be suspected in all patients who have abdominal trauma with haemoperitoneum, it is frequently associated with other visceral injuries which must be looked for before the abdomen is closed. If devitalized liver is left *in situ* post operative sepsis is almost inevitable.

Penetrating injury

Stab wounds and gunshot injuries are the commonest in this category. Most superficial stab injuries produce little damage and the wounds tend to be linear.

Occasionally liver biopsy leads to severe and life-threatening haemorrhage. Patients who have cirrhosis with deranged clotting factors and a lowered platelet count are at increased risk. The bleeding point is usually recognised by following the direction of the needle track. Despite the large amounts of blood in the peritoneum it is not usually difficult to stop the bleeding point with one or two sutures.

Gunshot injuries

The damage produced depends upon the bullet size and its velocity. Small calibre, low velocity bullets may produce surprisingly little damage unless they transect a major vessel. In contrast, high velocity bullets produce extensive parenchymal damage due to the shock wave produced by the dissipation of energy within the tissues.

Other acute problems

Occasionally rupture of an hepatic tumour gives rise to haemoperitoneum and may be the presenting symptoms of the disease in adenomas related to the contraceptive pill. Rupture of an hydatid cyst may occasionally occur producing severe anaphylaxis which may prove fatal. Intra peritoneal dissemination is likely if the patient survives.

Pancreas

Disease of the pancreas becomes symtomatic either because of (a) Disturbance of structure (pain and/or mass); or because of (b) Disturbance of function.

In clinical practice patients present with

(a) an acute abdomen—usually acute pancreatitis;
(b) obstructive jaundice—usually carcinoma (*see* p. 135);
(c) chronic abdominal pain—carcinoma or chronic pancreatitis;
(d) a mass;
(e) a malabsorption syndrome; } usually to a
(f) unusual endocrine disturbances } Physician.

The two commonest pancreatic diseases are acute pancreatitis and carcinoma of the pancreas.

Symptoms due to structural disturbance

Acute pain

The pain of acute pancreatic disease is usually severe; typically it is epigastric and radiates into the back and is associated with retching. However atypical symptoms are common so that the pancreatic origin is not always easy to diagnose. Exudation from the pancreas leads to peritonitis in the lesser and usually the greater sac and so presents as an acute abdomen.

Chronic pain

In chronic lesions of the pancreas pain is difficult to diagnose accurately when it begins. It is usually felt in the upper abdomen, radiating to the back: sometimes in lesions of the head, it is worse on the right and in lesions beginning in the body and tail, worse on the left side. Pain may be made worse by lying down and relieved by sitting up. Even powerful analgesics have remarkably little effect. The mechanism of pain production is not clear but it may be due to ductal distension as well as infiltration of the surrounding tissues which in cancer includes the nerve sheaths.

Mass

Sometimes pancreatic pathology may present with a palpable and/or visible epigastric mass. The diagnosis of disturbance of pancreatic structure is usually made by an ultrasound examination or CAT scanning. Retrograde cannulation of the pancreatic duct is usually abnormal in widespread parenchymal involvement (tumour/chronic pancreatitis).

Functional disturbance

Pancreas Exocrine insufficiency follows pancreatic duct obstruction or severe parenchymal disease and results in steatorrhoea. The patient notices pale, foul-smelling bulky stools, which are difficult to flush away. It is usually accompanied by weight loss. Steatorrhoea is not usually a presenting symptom in surgical patients.

Inappropriate endocrine secretion (endocrine excess) Some rare pancreatic tumours manifest themselves by inappropriate hormone secretion e.g. insulin producing hypoglycaemic attacks, or gastrin, causing intractable peptic ulcer disease.

Endocrine insufficiency This follows destruction of islet cell tissue by recurrent bouts of pancreatitis and results in hyperclycaemia and glycosuria.

Duodenum Advanced pancreatic disease may obstruct the duodenal lumen and cause vomiting. Clinical presentation of these patients is similar to pyloric stenosis except that the vomitus may contain bile.

Bleeding Ulceration of tumours into the duodenum may cause chronic blood loss and give rise to anaemia.

Bile duct Pancreatic tumours frequently involve the distal end of the bile duct and cause obstruction to bile flow; the patient then develops cholestatic jaundice (*see* p. 135).

The acute abdomen: Acute pancreatitis

Within the normal pancreas the enzymes are in the form of inactive precursors and any activated enzymes are neutralized by endogenous inhibitors.

In acute pancreatitis, this protective mechanism

is lost, but the manner in which the enzymes are activated, within the gland, to cause tissue destruction is not understood.

Acute pancreatitis is a common cause of acute abdominal pain but the diagnosis is not always straightforward.

The pain is usually epigastric and sudden in onset: radiation to the back is common. Nausea and repeated retching are also common. Physical examination may show a tinge of jaundice, tenderness and rigidity in the epigastrium. The peritoneal signs may be less dramatic than expected, because the main effusion initially occurs into the lesser sac and does not always immediately impinge on the parietal peritoneum of the anterior abdominal wall.

Systemic disturbance depends upon the severity of the pancreatic involvement. In severe cases, shock, renal insufficiency and disturbances of gaseous exchange are seen.

The diagnosis is made by thinking of it and confirming by serum amylase, serum lipase and peritoneal tap. It has to be differentiated from perforated ulcer, acute cholecystitis and myocardial infarction. The serum amylase may only rise above normal levels for 36 hours, so the timing of the blood sample is important in interpretation. Serum lipase, however, remains elevated for longer. False positive results are found particularly in perforated ulcer and high intestinal obstruction. Examination of peritoneal fluid helps to exclude a perforated viscus (the fluid in pancreatitis is not bile-stained, it is odourless, contains no organisms, but has polymorphs and a high amylase content). The colour is of prognostic value; the darker the colour, the worse the outlook.

The serum bilirubin and alkaline phosphatase may rise. Serum calcium may fall, particularly if fat necrosis is extensive and the fall reflects the severity of the disease.

The macroscopic changes vary from a mild serous form, to an acute haemorrhagic or even pancreatic necrosis. In mild cases there is no visible abnormality of the gland to the naked eye. In more acute cases the gland is congested and swollen but the lobular architecture is maintained.

In acute haemorrhagic pancreatitis the peritoneal cavity contains blood-stained fluid and in very severe cases, there may be frank blood. The pancreas is swollen, appears greyish-black with soft necrotic areas. The peripancreatic adipose tissue may contain creamy-white chalky areas. Similar areas may be seen in the adipose tissue of the omentum mesentery and abdominal wall. In severe cases the entire pancreas may appear as a haemorrhagic, necrotic mass.

Microscopical appearances in acute pancreatitis depend on the severity of the lesion. In mild cases there is oedema with a scanty inflammatory cell infiltration of the tissue. In severe cases there is necrosis of the pancreatic parenchyma with haemorrhage and an intense inflammatory cell infiltration, with areas of fat necrosis and calcification. Secondary bacterial infection may result in a suppurative pancreatitis with abscess formation.

The acute haemorrhagic form may present to the surgeon as an abdominal emergency with acute pain and profound shock. Occasionally patients die in the acute phase with refractory shock.

The majority of cases of acute pancreatitis are associated with cholelithiasis or alcoholism, particularly an alcoholic debauch after a very heavy meals. Many other aetiological factors are recognized, among which are hyperparathyroidism, hyperlipidaemia, viral infection (mumps) diabetes mellitus, trauma (including operative), iatrogenic (post-ERCP), post-cardiac bypass after renal transplantation, renal and hepatic failure. Drugs may also cause acute pancreatitis for example, an immunosuppressive such as Azothiaprine and steroids, thiazamide, diuretics, antibacterial drugs e.g. sulphonamides and tetracycline, cimetidine and oestrogens.

Prognosis

The most important factor in assessing the prognosis is the age of the patient (mortality rises above the age of 55 years) the presence of dark or blood-stained peritoneal exudate and an arterial oxygen saturation of less than 60 mmHg.

The other factors which are associated with a bad prognosis are: blood glucose of more than 200 mg per cent; white cell count of more than 16 000/cu.mm; serum calcium of less than 2.0 mmol/litre; haematocrit—a drop of more than 10 per cent base deficit of more than 4 mEq/litre; LDH levels of greater than 700 IU/litre; SGOT levels of greater than 250 units/litre.

Generalized: non-septic complications

Shock is probably the most serious complication of acute haemorrhagic pancreatitis and is the main cause of death in these patients. Shock is the result of gross reduction of circulating volume due to haemorrhage and leakage of exudate into the pancreas and retroperitoneal tissues as well as the peritoneal cavity.

Shock lung This is a well-known, though infrequent complication. It is thought to be due to circulating phospholipases which damage the capillary endothelium and the phospholipid surfactant and produce pulmonary oedema. Other respiratory complications such as pleural effusion and bronchopneumonia are also seen.

Renal failure Rarely, acute renal failure may dominate the clinical picture. It occurs in severe cases; acute tubular necrosis is due to shock and peripheral circulatory collapse. The prognosis is grim; the mortality rate being over 50 per cent.

Haemorrhagic complications Haemorrhagic complications occur usually as a result of disseminated intra-vascular coagulation.

Hyperglycaemia and glycosuria Hyperglycaemia follows disturbance of islet cell function with severe disease.

Tetany Extensive fat necrosis can cause lowering of the serum calcium and hence tetany.

Septic complications of pancreatitis

Secondary bacterial infection of the pancreas or peritoneum may occur. It usually follows operation undertaken to deal with severe disease.

Pyelophlebitis or thrombosis of arteries or veins may cause infarction of the small or large intestines.

Obstruction of the bile ducts may cause obstructive jaundice.

Non-septic complications

Pseudocyst Sometimes a large pseudocyst develops following acute pancreatitis. It is usually the result of loculation of exudate within the lesser sac: the contents are rich in amylase.

The walls may be thin, or thick and fibrous, depending on their duration. Within the cysts there is necrotic debris and brownish fibrinous material from altered blood. Secondary bacterial infection will cause an abscess.

There is no epithelial lining but the dense fibrous tissue wall shows an intense inflammatory reaction.

These cysts can present some weeks or months after an acute attack as an epigastric mass and be mistaken for carcinoma.

Other acute pancreatic presentations

Trauma

Penetrating or blunt injuries These may damage the surface of the gland and lead to an escape of enzymes into the surrounding adipose tissue, which can result in pancreatitis and subsequent fistula formation. The latter is occasionally a problem after surgical biopsy of the pancreas at laparotomy. Pancreatitis may follow any operative trauma especially operations on the ampulla of Vater.

Inflammation

Viral infection Generalized viral infection can affect the pancreas and mumps virus is one of the best known; glandular fever and Coxsackie B viruses too have been implicated. The inflammation generally passes unnoticed, or with transient abdominal pain, and rarely may proceed to acute pancreatitis.

Pancreatic disease: obstructive jaundice

Carcinoma of the pancreas

Carcinoma of the pancreas is an aggressive tumour which is usually advanced when diagnosed, and has a very poor prognosis; the incidence is rising. The most common presenting symptoms are pain, jaundice and weight loss, much less commonly late onset diabetes, duodenal obstruction and steatorrhoea.

The clinical differentiation from carcinoma of the ampulla of Vater, distal bile duct and duodenum is important because these less common tumours have a much better prognosis and surgical excision is well worth while. The presence of occult blood in stools is suggestive of carcinoma of the ampulla of Vater. The advent of ultrasound, percutaneous fine needle cytology and endoscopic cannulation of the biliary and pancreatic system and percutaneous cholangiography allow an accurate anatomical and tissue diagnosis to be made before operation.

Diagnosis is most difficult in patients with carcinoma arising in the body and tail of the gland who present with weight loss and abdominal pain. The sedimentation rate is often raised. The GTT is abnormal and ERCP, ultrasound and CAT scans usually demonstrate the lesion.

Cytology

Tumours of the pancreatic, duodenal and biliary system can be diagnosed on exfoliative cytology of the duodenal secretion, but accuracy is not very high.

Aspiration of pancreatic juice during ERCP examination has produced better results.

Frozen sections are indicated; however, both the surgeon and the pathologist must be aware that chronic pancreatitis is common in the pancreatic tissue around carcinomas. Well-differentiated carcinomas can be difficult to distinguish from normal pancreatic tissue. Pancreatic tumours show a predilection for perineural invasion, so if this is seen in frozen material it would be a helpful guide. Eighty to ninety per cent of pancreatic carcinomas are tumours of duct origin. About two-thirds begin in the head of the pancreas and the rest in the body and tail.

Because tumours developing in the head of the pancreas are closely related to the bile ducts, the first symptom is frequently progressive obstructive jaundice. At least 50 per cent of the patients will have significant abdominal pain associated with this. Tumours of the body and tail often present late. They tend to infiltrate the surrounding organs and present with intractable pain.

Pancreatic tumours are poorly delineated and may not be visible on the surface. On cut section the tumour appears yellowish-grey and does not have the lobular pattern of the normal gland. In tumours of the pancreatic head the remainder of the gland may feel hard and swollen because of duct obstruction.

The pancreatic tissue surrounding the tumour frequently shows chronic pancreatitis, and as already mentioned may lead to difficulty in the interpretation of biopsy specimens.

The majority of tumours are well differentiated adenocarcinomas arising from duct epithelium with a variable amount of fibrous tissue, hence close attention must be given to cytological details to identify features of malignancy such as cellular and nuclear pleomorphism, mitoses, loss of polarity. There is a significant degree of fibrosis. The tumours cause duct obstruction and there may be gross duct dilatation in areas away from the tumour. Some of the tumours may contain abundant mucin and hence may feel soft. Other histological variants, such as undifferentiated tumours, pleomorphic tumours and tumours composed of small round cells similar to a lymphoma, have all been described. Rarely, squamous carcinomatous areas may be seen. There may be extensive loss of acinar tissue due to compression or obstruction, but the islet cells are usually well preserved.

Direct spread

Direct extension of pancreatic tumours is common and takes place into the stomach, duodenum, portal vein and bile ducts. Tumours of the body and tail infiltrate directly in the retroperitoneum. Perineural spread is commonly seen on section.

Metastatic spread

Pancreatic tumours commonly spread to the regional lymph nodes and the liver. Transcoelomic spread may also result in omental deposits, but spread outside the abdominal cavity is seen less often.

Prognosis

The outlook in carcinoma of the pancreas is grim; the overall 5 year survival rate is about 0.5 per cent. Prognosis is related to nodal spread. In Stage I (disease within the gland capsule) or Stage II (local direct invasion only), resection does seem to prolong survival, but in Stage III (nodal spread) or Stage IV (distant spread) resection of the primary tumour confers no benefit.

Associated features

Carcinoma of the pancreas is sometimes associated with:

1. Migratory thrombophlebitis;
2. A peculiar syndrome of polyarthritis, panniculitis and eosinophilia syndrome;
3. Diabetes.

Other carcinomas of the periampullary region

Tumours of the periampullary region may also arise in the ampulla of Vater, the distal third of the bile duct or the mucosa of the duodenum or Brunner's glands. They are less aggressive than pancretic cancer and 5-year-survival rates of around 25 per cent are usual after resection.

Clinically and macroscopically it may be difficult to distinguish these and tumours of the head of the pancreas as they all present and spread in a similar way.

Tumours of the ampulla and duodenal mucosa are papillary. Because of their softness, they may not be readily palpable through the duodenal wall. If they are biopsied, the surgeon should make sure he has got the full thickness of the base, otherwise the deeper malignant parts may be missed.

Carcinomas of the distal third of the bile duct may produce very little in the way of a mass, merely a thickening of the duct wall with a granular appearance in the mucosal surface.

These tumours are often well differentiated adenocarcinomas.

Chronic abdominal pain

Chronic abdominal pain due to pancreatic disease when due to carcinoma increases in severity within weeks or months so that the diagnosis becomes more obvious. The other common cause of persistent abdominal pain due to pancreatic disease is chronic pancreatitis.

Chronic pancreatitis

This disease is often preceded by recurrent attacks of acute pancreatitis. Progression to chronic disease is usually a feature of alcoholic pancreatitis. The gland is firm and fibrous with focal whitish specks of fat necrosis and calcification. If the previous attacks of pancreatitis have caused extensive damage to the glandular parenchyma, the gland feels very hard, so that at laparotomy it may be mistaken for carcinoma. In some cases of carcinoma of the pancreas, the surrounding parenchyma may show features of chronic pancreatitis possibly due to tumour causing obstruction of the ducts.

Pancreas divisum

Abnormalities in the fusion of the ventral and dorsal outgrowths during pancreatic development may result in various abnormal arrangements of the pancreatic duct drainage. When the glands are entirely separate and drain by individual ducts, this is called pancreas divisum. Sometimes this may be associated with recurrent acute pancreatitis, especially in young patients. They present with repeated bouts of abdominal pain which is sometimes not easy to diagnose at first. The other abnormality of pancreatic development which is sometimes seen, is an annular pancreas which causes obstruction of the duodenum and presents with persistent bouts of vomiting. As the pancreatic tissue surrounding the duodenum is functioning, division of the gland substance to relieve the obstruction leads to pancreatitis, fistula formation and proper management is a gastro-jejunostomy to by-pass the obstruction.

Pancreatic disease: mass

Neoplastic lesions of the pancreas/mass

Cystadenomas

These are very rare benign cystic lesions of the pancreas and are thought to arise from the ducts. They develop at an earlier age than malignant tumours and 90 per cent occur in women. They are more common in the body and tail of the pancreas and are often asymptomatic, being found incidentially at laparotomy.

Larger cystadenomas may present as a palpable abdominal mass, or abdominal pain. Rarely they may be a source of massive haemorrhage into the intestinal tract and may cause diabetes due to pressure atrophy of the islet tissue.

They are multilocular, cystic tumours and the surface may be lobulated.

Two distinct types are seen:

The mucinous tumours are composed of large locules containing thick viscid mucin and are lined by tall columnar mucin-secreting epithelium. At times they appear as papillary fronds.

The serous tumours are lined by a very flat cuboidal epithelium. The connective tissue stroma may show myxomatous degeneration. The locules are smaller and cut surface may have a honeycomb appearance. The epithelium contains glycogen.

Malignant cystadenocarcinomas

These have been described: the diagnosis is based on the presence of invasion of the gland by the neoplastic epithelium. The distinction between the benign and malignant may be very difficult, and extensive sampling may be necessary.

Conclusion

The practice of hepato-biliary surgery has been revoluntionized by modern imaging techniques.

A clear understanding of surgical pathology is required to get the maximum information from these investigations as well as to appreciate their limitations.

Laparotomy is now rarely required for diagnosis. An accurate histological (or cytological) diagnosis is possible pre-operatively in most patients in addition the precise anatomical extent of mass lesions can be established but in a few patients the resectability of a lesion is only established at operation.

Further reading

Ackerman's Surgical Pathology, 6th Edition, Volume 1 Chapters 12, 13, 14. New York: C. V. Mosby & Co., 1981.

Scheuer Peter J. *Liver Biopsy Interpretation*. 3rd edition. London: Baillière Tindall, 1980.

Wright R. *Liver & Biliary Disease*. WB Saunders, Co. Ltd., 1979.

Sherlock Dame Sheila, *Diseases of the Liver & Biliary System*. London: 6th edition, Blackwell Scientific Publications, 1981.

MacSween RNM, Primary Sclerosing Cholangitis. *Recent Advances in Histopathology*, No. 12, pages 158–65.

Foulis, AK, Acute Pancreatitis. *Recent Advances in Histopathology* No. 12, pages 188–95. London and Edinburgh: Churchill Livingstone, 1984.

Sleisinger Marvin H, Fordham John S, *Gastrointestinal Disease*. 3rd edition, Volume II Section D & Section E.

Longmire WP, Tompkinis RK, *Manual of Liver Surgery*. Springer-Verlag, 1983.

12

The Lymphoreticular System

W S Shand, A G Stansfeld and J S Malpas

Introduction

What is the lymphoreticular system?

Distributed throughout much of the body there are aggregated masses of lymphoid cells intermingled with reticulum (reticular) cells of the mononuclear phagocyte system. Now that the immunological function of lymphoid cells is more clearly understood, the necessity for an intimate association of reticulum cells and lymphoid cells becomes more apparent. In the simplest terms, the phagocytic reticulum cells (macrophages) engulf microorganisms or other antigenic foreign material from the lymph or blood streams and then the "processed" information is passed on to the lymphocytes to initiate the immune process. Not all the varieties of reticulum cell now recognized are phagocytic, but all are probably concerned in some way with the handling of antigen and its presentation in suitable form to the lymphoid cells. Thus these two main types of cell act in concert to bring about an immunological response, either at a local level or on a more widespread scale, according to the nature and extent of the immunogenic stimulus. The concept of the lymphoreticular system (LR system), here briefly outlined, has broadened and largely superseded Aschoff's earlier concept of the reticuloendothelial system.

Origin and functions of lymphoid cells

A detailed account of the development of the LR system is out of place, but it is helpful to an understanding of the different types of immune response to appreciate that, although all small lymphocytes look alike under the microscope, there are in fact two distinct populations of these cells which inhabit broadly different areas within the lymphoreticular tissues and which have different, though complementary, functions. Throughout most of prenatal development and in post-natal life, all lymphoid cells in mammalian species appear to be derived from a single bone marrow precursor, but on leaving the marrow, the hitherto uncommitted cells either undergo a process of "initiation" in the thymus to become "T" lymphocytes or else receive instruction in the bone marrow or possibly elsewhere (e.g. the bursa of Fabricius in birds) to become "B" lymphocytes. The T-lymphocytes are concerned primarily in cell-mediated immunity, while the B-lymphocytes are concerned in the production of antibodies (immunoglobulins). Alas! the situation is far more complicated than appears at first sight and sub-sets of T-lymphocytes, having differing functional characteristics, are now distinguished (helper, suppressor and killer cells). Likewise, in the maturation process of B-lymphocytes which culminates in the production of mature plasma cells, the cells pass through various stages of immunoglobulin synthesis, switching from the production of one class of immunoglobulin to another. However, these details need not concern us here. Suffice it to say that collaboration between different populations of lymphocytes is necessary to achieve normal immune responses and although many bacterial infections, for instance, excite predominantly an antibody response, and most viral infections tend to excite predominantly a cell-mediated response, in many immunological reactions there is evidence of both types of response. The effect of antigenic exposure on a previously "committed" lymphocyte (whether T or B) is to cause that cell to transform into a large 'blast' type cell (immunoblast) capable of dividing and giving rise to a "clone" of similarly committed cells. As the immune reaction declines, surviving lymphoid cells revert to the resting phase and some may persist to become long-lived "memory cells". It is thought to be survival of such cells that determines the much more rapid development of the 'secondary immune response' when the body is exposed again to the same antigen.

Distribution of lymphoreticular tissues

In the course of development, lymphocytes from the primary lymphoid organs (bone marrow and thymus) migrate to and colonize the scattered areas of lymphoreticular tissue throughout the body (secondary lymphoid organs). These organs are the lymph nodes, the lymphatic tissue of Waldeyer's ring and similar tissue dispersed throughout the gut and lungs, and the white pulp of the spleen. Whilst the lymph nodes serve as filters of the lymph stream, the spleen and bone marrow subserve a similar function in respect of the blood stream. Likewise the lymphatic tissue of the pharynx, gut and lungs is strategically placed beneath a "contaminated" epithelial surface, no doubt to exercise a similar "filtration" function. In each of these sites, whilst the microanatomy differs in detail, filtration of micro-organisms etc. is largely achieved by the high concentration of macrophages present and if the ingested material carries antigenic determinants, then the immunocompetent cells will respond accordingly.

Microanatomy of lymph nodes

The disposition of the main lymph node groups is of such importance to the practice of surgery that it is deemed unnecessary to remind readers of such essential facts. The microscopical anatomy of individual lymph nodes may not be so well known. In studying a microscopical section of a lymph node, it is necessary constantly to remind oneself that the picture is "frozen" at a single moment of time, the moment when the excised node was dropped into fixative. In life, however, the picture is constantly changing with the continued recirculation of many of the lymphocytes, especially the T-cells, which make up the larger percentage of the lymphocytes in central lymph and in the peripheral blood. The lymphocytes pass from the blood, through the walls of the specialized post-capillary venules, into the pulp of the node and many leave the node again in the efferent lymph. This constant traffic of lymphocytes ensures that there will be cells of the appropriate clone available when a fresh immunogenic stimulus arrives and rapid "recruitment" of cells of that clone is one of the main factors responsible for the rapid enlargement of the regional lymph nodes draining, for example, a focus of staphylococcal infection. Not only lymphocytes, but macrophages too are motile cells and their numbers within the node may also fluctuate.

Two further factors must be borne in mind when assessing whether a given lymph node is to be judged "normal" or not. First, the age of the subject and secondly the site of the lymph node. The activity of the lymphoid tissue progressively declines after puberty (*see* p. 158) and there are often many more lymphocytes packed into the nodes of children than are generally to be seen in adult life. The relatively minor variations in the structure of lymph nodes from different parts of the body need not concern us here and the structure of a "typical" lymph node is shown in semidiagramatic form in Fig. 12.1.

Lymph enters the node by way of a number of afferent lymphatics which penetrate the capsule on the outer, convex surface. With a quiet lymph flow much of the lymph passes through the peripheral (marginal) lymph sinus to gain the single efferent lymphatic at the hilum. When lymph flow is increased, however, the deep cortical and medullary sinuses dilate and may be very conspicuous. The lymph sinuses do not have continuous walls like blood and lymph vessels and no doubt some fluid percolates through the dense pulp of the node as well. Carcinoma cells carried in the afferent lymph commonly become arrested in the lymph sinuses which are traversed by slender trabeculae of reticulin continuous with the structural framework of the node and invasion of the dense pulp may follow, with the establishment of an enlarging lymph node metastasis. Anchored to the walls and trabeculae of the lymph sinuses, there is the largest concentration of histiocytes (macrophages) to be found within the node. Proliferation of these sinus-lining histiocytes (littoral cells) often results from the repeated presence of red cells or other particulate matter in the afferent lymph, to produce the picture of "reactive sinus histiocytosis". Histiocytes are also present in smaller numbers throughout the node and in certain circumstances these too may increase by cell division and recruitment, sometimes turning into epithelioid cells and forming "granulomata" as in Mycobacterial infections and sarcoidosis.

As already indicated, most of the lymphocytes

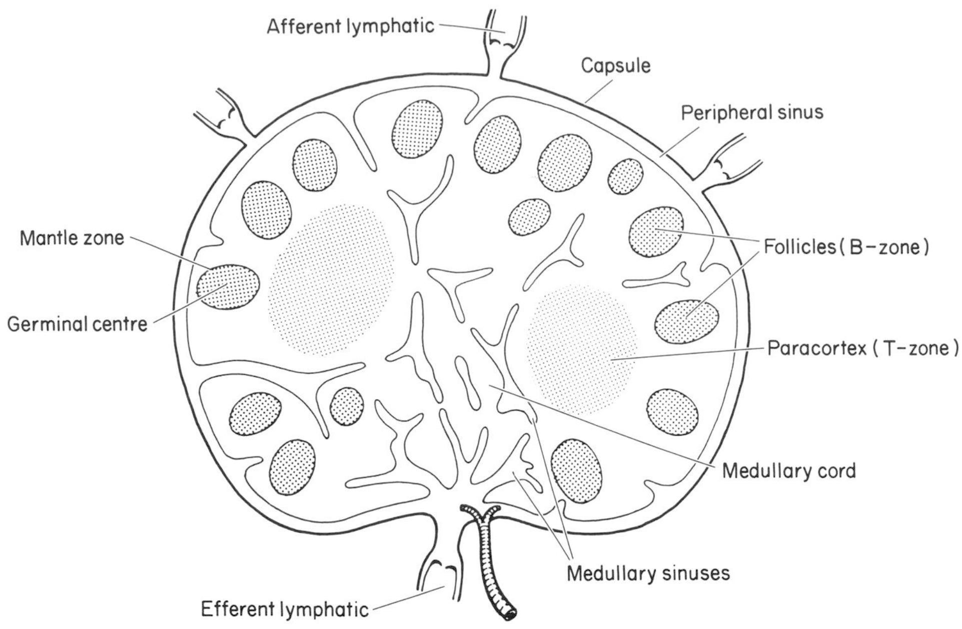

Fig. 12.1 Semidiagramatic representation of a lymph node.

reach the lymph node by way of the post-capillary venules which are a special feature of the paracortex (deep cortex or 'thymic dependent' zone). Although the cortical follicles (germinal centres and lymphocyte "mantles") are inhabited largely by B-lymphocytes, whilst the paracortex is mostly filled with T-lymphocytes, this territorial subdivision is far from absolute and some T-lymphocytes are regularly to be found within the follicles, just as some B-lymphocytes are always seen in the paracortex. Immunological stimulation of the node by an antigen which excites antibody production results in increased activity of the follicles—follicular hyperplasia, which is often accompanied by the appearance of plasma cells in the medullary cords. In extreme cases, the node may become filled with large reactive follicles and confusion may then occur with follicular lymphoma. Alternatively, the follicles may remain comparatively inactive and the paracortex may expand in cell-mediated immune reactions. As implied above, there is often evidence of lymphoid hyperplasia in both B and T regions.

Since throughout life we are all continuously exposed to foreign antigens of one kind or another, it follows that the lymphoreticular system is constantly undergoing "stimulation". The appearances seen in a "normal" node reflect this and it is only when the stimulus evokes a particularly violent reaction that the node enlarges to a degree which warrants a clinical description of "lymphadenopathy".

From the facts cited above—the constant traffic of cells through the node, the rapid alterations which may take place in response to injurious or immunogenic stimuli and especially the transformation of resting lymphocytes into large, mitotically active, "blast" cells, the difficulty sometimes encountered in the interpretation of lymph node biopsy sections may be better understood. There is probably no other tissue in the body to rival lymphoreticular tissue for the problems it may present in histopathological diagnosis.

Clinical presentation of lymphoreticular disease and indications for biopsy

Introduction

Disease of the LR system will often be manifest clinically by local or generalized lymphadenopathy, sometimes accompanied by hepato-splenomegaly. There is considerable variation in the amount of lymphoid tissue present during life, so that the significance of lymphadenopathy will vary with the age of the patient. The newborn infant enters life with only a small amount of lymphoid tissue, but this rapidly increases, so that from approximately six years of age to puberty the body contains more lymphoid tissue than an adult, and at this age palpable lymph nodes, especially in the cervical region, are the rule rather than the exception. From puberty onwards the lymphoreticular tissue starts to atrophy, and is also less reactive. Consequently, persistent enlargement of the lymph nodes at this age has more significance than earlier in life.

Persistent local or generalized lymphadenopathy must, at any age, give rise to concern that primary or secondary neoplastic change has occurred in the glands, and the surgical and histological techniques appropriate to the elucidation of these problems will be dealt with in detail later. Although the histology of the lymph nodes or spleen must be the final arbiter, a careful clinical history and examination may suggest a differential diagnosis with a less serious prognosis and invoke ancillary haematological or immunological tests which can establish the diagnosis without recourse to surgery.

Diseases other than lymphomas which cause lympadenopathy

Reactive conditions

Lymph nodes enlarge as a response to bacterial, viral, fungal or protozoal infection. Local lymph node enlargement in the region of the head and neck may have an obvious cause in pharyngitis, tonsillitis, sinusitis, but occasionally the infective source may be occult, such as an apical dental abscess or chronic dental sepsis, and this may be overlooked. In children, especially boys, inguinal lymphadenopathy subsequent to infected cuts and abrasions is quite common.

Chronic infections that give rise to lymphadenopathy include secondary syphilitic disease, while tuberculosis seems particularly to provoke a marked lymphadenopathy in West Indian and Asian immigrants. A history of exposure to these infections and appropriate serological tests and Mantoux skin test respectively will be confirmatory evidence.

Acquired toxoplasmosis infections are now being recognized more frequently in the young. Such patients are usually in households where there is contact with pets. Symptoms are usually mild, but a frequent finding is a lymphocytosis. Serological tests are available for the confirmation of the diagnosis. Other illnesses which are accompanied by marked lymphadenopathy and may be associated with animal bites or scratches include cat-scratch disease. In this there is a history of being bitten or scratched by a cat some days previously to the onset of fever, skin rash, headache, conjunctivitis and marked lymphadenopathy, usually in the site draining the abrasion. The disease is self-limiting; skin testing may be diagnostic.

Because of their profoundly stimulating effect on the lymphoreticular system, many viruses produce marked lymphadenopathy and possibly splenomegaly. Infectious mononucleosis caused by the Epstein Barr virus results in a florid increase in lymphoid tissue, which may spill over into the blood, where atypical lymphoid or infectious mononucleosis cells may be seen. The monospot and Paul Bunnell tests are positive. Patients who present with the clinical features of infectious mononucleosis but are Paul Bunnell negative should be considered as possibly having cytomegalovirus infection. In this condition, fever and hepatitis may occur, but lymphadenopathy with atypical mononucleosis is not uncommon. Diagnosis can be made serologically, or sometimes on urine samples some four weeks after the onset of the illness. Other viruses, including those of the childhood illnesses measles, rubella, chicken-pox, may give mild symptoms but produce lymphadenopathy. Lymphadenopathy in the neck, axilla or groin may precede or accompany the florid and painful segmental lesions of herpes zoster. Immunization procedures may induce lymphadenopathy. In the past, vaccinations for smallpox produced lymph node enlargement, but this can now be seen with measles, diphtheria, pertussis, influenza and poliomyelitis innoculation. Recent immunization or vaccination procedures should be inquired into.

It would be impossible to mention all the conditions which are associated with lymphadenopathy, but some which present with quite florid lymph node enlargement may be presented occasionally to the surgeon for biopsy, and the necessity can be reconsidered if the underlying clinical condition is recognized.

In rheumatoid arthritis, large fleshy nodes develop frequently in the axilla and inguinal regions. They are often associated with the development of skin nodules, and are usually seen in seropositive disease. Subcutaneous nodule or synovial biopsy are more helpful if the diagnosis is in doubt. Lymph node excision is rarely helpful. Lupus erythematosus is another member of this group of diseases where lymphadenopathy may be prominent, but if this is recognized, the demonstration of lupus erythematosus cells or a positive antinuclear factor will relieve the necessity for biopsy. Enlarged nodes are quite common in patients suffering from chronic skin diseases, and may complicate chronic eczema, particularly when there is excoriation and infection. Dermatopathic changes are readily detected in the lymph node, but under normal circumstances there is no need for a lymph node biopsy.

A history of drug exposure may give a cause for lymph node enlargement. A good example is the lymphadenopathy secondary to the regular medication with phenytoin for epilepsy. Many patients in epileptic colonies who are on continuous and heavy medication develop these physical signs.

Rheumatoid disease, lupus erythematosus and extensive skin lesions with associated lymphadenopathy probably do not require lymph node biopsy. On the other hand, there are three conditions in which lymph node biopsy may make a helpful contribution. These are "sinus histiocytosis with massive lympadenopathy" (SHML), histiocytosis X, and angioimmunoblastic lymphadenopathy. In these conditions there may be very close simulation of lymphomas and the diagnosis will ultimately rest on the histological picture.

SHML is a benign disorder occurring most frequently in black children and characterized by painless cervical lymphadenopathy of sometimes massive proportions. The lymphadenopathy is associated with fever, malaise, anorexia and loss of weight. There is polymorphonucleocytosis, a polyclonal increase in plasma protein, and an elevated erythrocyte sedimentation rate. The course may be prolonged over several months or years and eventually spontaneous regression occurs with complete recovery. The few patients ever to have been reported to die from this condition were mostly those in which a mistaken diagnosis of lymphoma was made, and who had been treated by intensive combination chemotherapy.

A second disorder of childhood, the so-called histiocytosis X, presents as three main clinical entities: Letterer-Siwe disease, Hand-Schüller-Christian syndrome, and eosinophilic granuloma of bone. The latter two have pathognomonic features which should give rise to little difficulty in their diagnosis, but Letterer-Siwe disease may be more difficult to distinguish from, for example, non-Hodgkin's lymphoma. It usually occurs in the very young, and is characterized by malaise, failure to thrive, fever, sweating, lymphadenopathy, hepato-splenomegaly, the presence of a seborrhoeic rash on the scalp and back, where it is distributed in a triangular shape with the apex over the lower part of the back. Occasionally an aural discharge of eosinophilic granulomatous material is seen, and cytology of this discharge may render a lymph node biopsy unnecessary. Without treatment, the disease progresses, and a fatal outcome is frequent.

The other disease which may simulate lymphoma and which is now recognized as a distinct entity is angioimmunoblastic lymphadenopathy (AIL). This is a disease of late middle age and the elderly, and it is distinctly rare in children. The condition is characterized by fever, lymphadenopathy, hepatosplenomegaly, loss of weight and, in particular, a non-specific maculopapular erythematous rash which is sometimes accompanied by pruritus. Occasionally, purpura or urticaria appear to be present alone. In patients who do not respond, the course of the disease may be complicated by infection, malignant lymphoma, haemorrhage or, less often, by acute renal failure, hepatic necrosis, pancreatitis and pulmonary embolism. An elderly person presenting with malaise and lymphadenopathy who is troubled by a persistent, irritating rash similar to a drug-sensitivity rash, should be considered as possibly having AIL.

Secondary neoplasms

These call for little comment here. It is only nodal metastases from unknown or occult primary tumours (nearly always carcinomas) that demand a lymph node biopsy to establish the diagnosis. Clues to the probable site of the primary tumour may be given by (a) clinical history; (b) the distribution of metastases; and (c) the morphology of the tumour (if biopsy is undertaken). Unfortunately it is only in a minority of cases that the histological structure of the growth is sufficiently specific to pinpoint exactly the site of the primary. Sometimes a primary growth is never found. In such cases, particularly, the possibility of malignant melanoma should be borne in mind.

Lymphadenopathy as a presentation of lymphoma

When a patient presents with lymphadenopathy, the possibility of it being due to lymphoma has to be considered if the conditions described above have been excluded. The node swelling may have been present only a few weeks, or may have been there for many months. It may have fluctuated in size, or even have disappeared. It may apparently respond to antibiotics. None of these features should lead to a diagnosis of lymphoma being discounted.

It is reasonable, after a full clinical history and examination, to arrange for blood count, serology and radiology, and to observe the lymphadenopathy. If at the end of six weeks the nodes are still present, and there is no explanation for their causation, then a biopsy is indicated.

In Hodgkin's disease, most patients presenting with lymph nodes develop them in the neck in the early stage of the disease, and there is generally an orderly spread to contiguous glands so that axillary, mediastinal, para-aortic and inguinal lymph nodes are involved, then the spleen, and finally, the liver. Extranodal presentations are uncommon. This is in contrast to the non-Hodgkin lymphomas, where extranodal presentations are much more frequent, the disease appearing in the skin, in Waldeyer's ring, the thyroid, salivary glands, gastrointestinal tract, retroperitoneum and pelvis, and some other sites.

Surgery in lymphoreticular disease

Introduction

Pathological investigation of resected lymph nodes is of course a daily occurrence in the histopathology laboratory and this applies particularly to surgical resections for cancer in any site where the draining lymph nodes are removed, either concurrently with, or subsequent to, the resection of the primary tumour. The determination of the degree of involvement of the regional nodes is an essential part of many staging procedures.

There are two other principal indications for surgery in the investigation or treatment of lymphoreticular disorders, which are:

1. Lymph node biopsy in the investigation of the cause of lymphadenopathy. Although there may be occasions when the needle aspiration is more appropriate than surgical biopsy, the results may be unhelpful or even misleading.
2. Splenectomy, either as a primarily diagnostic procedure in cases of splenomegaly of undetermined cause, or for a variety of other indications, including staging laparotomy to determine the extent of a malignant lymphoma (usually Hodgkin's disease).

There are, of course, other situations in which surgeon and pathologist may be jointly involved in the investigation and treatment of lymphoreticular disease, ranging from tonsillectomies to the surgical resection of extranodal tumours which are known to be, or prove to be, malignant lymphomas.

Dealing with specimens of lymphoreticular tissue

Before considering these issues in greater detail, some general remarks on the handling of specimens of this nature may not be out of place. The importance of gentle handling and prompt fixation of biopsy tissue, already stressed in the introductory chapter of this book, is nowhere more pertinent than in the case of the lymphoreticular tissues. Lymphoid cells are especially fragile and are notoriously prone to "stringy artefact" when roughly handled. This artefact—particularly liable to occur in small biopsies—results not only from crushing of tissue by biopsy forceps, but also from tension on the tissues at the time of biopsy. It may render the biopsy quite uninterpretable and is thus to be avoided at all costs.

In hospitals where lymph node biopsy is a common procedure, special arrangements are often made by agreement between the surgical team and the pathological laboratory, whereby the biopsy tissue is placed in a dry sterile jar and delivered immediately to the laboratory. This is ideal, for it enables the pathologist to inspect and cleanly incise the fresh lymph node and to make imprints (touch preparations) for cytological and cytochemical study. Further, the appearances seen in the incised node may indicate the need for culture or other bacteriological investigations. Fresh, unfixed tissue is also required for frozen sections, necessary for the performance of many histochemical and immunohistochemical investigations. Minute samples (less than 2 mm in diameter) may be taken at this stage for electron microscopy and placed directly in small bottles of glutaraldehyde fixative. In many laboratories today, facilities exist for the resin embedding of larger blocks of tissue (up to 1 cm in diameter). By this technique semi-thin sections (1–2 microns in thickness) can be prepared for study with the light microscope. These sections are thinner than can generally be cut with paraffin wax embedded tissue and, in the case of highly cellular tissues such as lymph nodes, they have the advantage of showing the details of cellular morphology more clearly, although the overall topography is often less clearly shown, than in conventional 4–5 micron sections. If sufficient tissue is available, a portion of the fresh node may be used for the preparation of cell-suspensions for phenotyping, in laboratories where the necessary expertise is available. More important, however, than any of these things is that an adequate sized piece of the node should be put promptly into neutral, or buffered, formol saline, or whatever other fixative is preferred by the pathologist for routine processing. This is the overriding consideration which must take precedence over all the more sophisticated investigations, for it is upon the histological appearances (and sometimes bacteriological culture) that the diagnosis will ultimately rest. If no special arrangement exists for the immediate collection of fresh tissue from the operating theatre, it is better that the node biopsy should be put into fixative solution without delay (NOT into *normal* saline). If it is thought likely that the node may be tuberculous, then the node should be divided and one half placed in a dry sterile container for bacteriological study, while the remainder is put into fixative. In any event, if the node is enlarged (1 cm or more in diameter) it should be cleanly divided with a sharp knife before being put into fixative to ensure proper, even fixation throughout. All too often, the histopathological diagnosis of lymph node biopsies is jeopardized by inadequate fixation of the tissue.

Remarks concerning inadequate fixation apply with even greater force to resected spleens. The penetration of fixative solutions into the spleen is very slow, not only on account of the tough capsule and large bulk of the organ, but even more because of the large amount of blood which it contains. For this reason, it is imperative that any spleen should be sliced open before being put into fixative. Again the ideal arrangement is for all resected spleens to be delivered immediately to the laboratory where steps can be taken to ensure adequate fixation and the pathologist can take note of the macroscopic appearances of the fresh organ.

Lymph node biopsy

Any lymph node, or part of a lymph node, removed for diagnostic purposes must be representative of the clinical picture, adequate for histological interpretation and must reach the laboratory in a state fit for study. Provided these criteria are fulfilled the actual technique of removal is unimportant, but there are various details which must be considered.

Which lymph node should be removed? Often, as in Hodgkin's disease, there is no choice as only one node may be palpable. If lymphadenopathy is generalized, however, then it is better to choose a cervical node rather than axillary or inguinal, since at the latter two sites nodes may consist largely of hilar fat with only a thin rim of nodal tissue present for histological study.

Unless the node is very superficial and mobile, general rather than local anaesthesia is to be preferred. Excessive handling of the node as a result of inadequate exposure or excessive diathermy control of troublesome bleeding, may render it unsuitable for study. Ideally a whole node should be removed, since incision of a node mass often results in troublesome bleeding from the capsule, and the nodal pulp is often so soft that the architecture is destroyed when excision is attempted. Sometimes this may mean choosing for excision a smaller discrete node beside a more obviously pathological gland mass.

It is of paramount importance that the node is manipulated as little as possible during removal, tissue holding forceps of the Babcock pattern being very helpful for gentle handling.

In some cases more aggressive biopsy has to be undertaken, for example by mediastinoscopy, thoracotomy, or by laparotomy, but the above principles still apply. Very occasionally, assessment of a nodal mass requires frozen section study, but this can often do no more than distinguish lymphoma from carcinoma or sarcoma. Under these circumstances the surgical management of the case may rest on the macroscopic findings and it is then very important to have all the clinicians involved in the management of the patient in the operating theatre for a joint consultation.

Re-biopsy of nodes after diagnosis and treatment is frequently required. In a small percentage of cases of Hodgkin's disease the disease may recur as a different histological type. The disease may de-differentiate from a lymphocyte predominant pattern through a mixed cellularity pattern to a lymphocyte depleted pattern while nodular sclerosing disease usually tends to recur as nodular sclerosing disease. Occasionally a case of Hodgkin's disease recurs as a non-Hodgkin's lymphoma and vice versa.

Pathological interpretation of lymph node biopsies

Details of histopathology are beyond the scope of this book, but it is important for the surgeon to appreciate that the pathologist's task is sometimes easy, sometimes very difficult, in interpreting the changes in a lymph node biopsy. It is essential that his task is made as easy as possible by the surgeon supplying him with a good biopsy (an *intact* node if possible) and all relevant information about the patient. Most important are the age of the patient, the exact site of the excised lymph node, the duration of lymphadenopathy and its extent, the presence or absence of hepatosplenomegaly and the results of other relevant investigations (e.g. blood count, Paul Bunnell test). Possible causative factors and any relevant previous history should be mentioned on the request form.

The single, most important step in diagnosis is in discriminating between benign, reactive conditions and malignant ones, especially malignant lymphomas. From the point of view of prognosis and treatment, this is generally of much greater importance than, for example, deciding between different types of malignant lymphoma. There is, as yet, no generally agreed classification of the lymphomas other than Hodgkin's disease, but it is sufficient to recognize that, broadly speaking, the non-Hodgkin's lymphomas (NHL) can be divided into two categories—low grade and high grade. The low grade lymphomas are composed mainly of lymphoid cells in the resting phase, whilst the high grade lymphomas are composed mainly of transformed or 'blast' cells. In the absence of effective treatment, survival in the first group is measurable in years, whilst the second group are liable to die in a matter of months. Paradoxically, however, many of the 'high grade' lymphomas now hold out a better prospect of cure than the "low grade" lymphomas owing to the greater vulnerability of lymphoid cells in the dividing phase and the introduction of effective combination chemotherapy.

Splenectomy

Indications

Splenectomy may be undertaken for mechanical reasons such as traumatic rupture or because of an abnormally long pedicle leading to torsion. The spleen may also be removed incidentally during operations for cancer of the lower oesophagus, stomach, pancreas or splenic flexure of the colon allowing radical clearance of the appropriate glandular field. Occasionally, rupture of an aneurysm of the splenic artery requires splenectomy. In all these circumstances the spleen is removed and histological examination adds nothing to the management of the patient.

Occasionally, a patient presents with an enlarged spleen for which no cause can be found and splenectomy may be undertaken as a diagnostic procedure. Under these circumstances it is important that all the abdominal contents are examined to look for clinically undetectable disease. Such spleens can be enlarged due to a lipid storage disorder such as Gaucher's disease, the presence of simple cysts which may be single or multiple, parasitic cysts due to echinococcal infestation, rarely due to secondary neoplasia, or even more rarely due to primary neoplasia such as cavernous haemangioma or fibrosarcoma. Splenomegaly may also be due to lymphomatous infiltration although a clinically palpable spleen in these conditions is not necessarily involved with lymphoma. In Hodgkin's disease granulomata may be found in the spleen which are certainly not typical of lymphomatous tissue but the aetiology of which is at present unknown. The place of splenectomy in the pathological staging of the lymphomas is discussed below. In all these conditions histological examination of the spleen is essential and may be the only means of achieving a diagnosis. It should be remembered that a spleen which is enlarged for any reason may give rise to pain, either simply due to its size or because of peri-splenitis or of infarction. Splenectomy may be indicated under such circumstances but must be undertaken only in the light of the underlying disease, if known.

A large group of haematological conditions may call for splenectomy. The first of these is hypersplenism, a syndrome which consists of (a) splenomegaly; (b) anaemia, leukopenia, neutropenia or thrombocytopenia; (c) normal or hypocellular marrow; and (d) absence of immature cells in the peripheral blood. Hypersplenism can be "primary" (idiopathic) if no cause is known, or "secondary" to another condition such as infection, parasitic infestation, lipid storage disease or lymphoma. Many factors may contribute to the various blood features in an individual patient and hence the effect of splenectomy on the peripheral blood picture is often unpredictable. Haemolytic anaemia may occur as a result of specific abnormality in the red cells e.g. hereditary spherocytosis, haemolytic variant of hereditary elliptocytosis and warm antibody auto-immune haemolytic anaemia. Splenectomy may be helpful in the hereditary disorders but is less commonly so in auto-immune haemolytic anaemia. Thrombocytopenia may be "primary" (idiopathic) and if relapses continue in spite of adequate steroid therapy splenectomy is indicated. Where thrombocytopenia is "secondary" to marrow replacement or depression, splenectomy is only indicated if hypersplenism supervenes. Neutropenia can occur with splenomegaly for example in primary splenic neutropenia, or in Felty's syndrome (rheumatoid arthritis with hypersplenism) and splenectomy may well be beneficial. In all these cases close co-operation between physician, surgeon and pathologist is essential in deciding the appropriate time for surgery and also in managing the complicated haematological picture during and after surgery. The accurate and regular monitoring of the peripheral blood picture, with appropriate transfusion of one or more peripheral blood elements as necessary, calls for haematological and transfusion expertise throughout.

Approach

Again the exact technique of splenectomy is unimportant. In trauma cases a rapid approach is required and a left paramedian incision is appropriate. This allows access to the rest of the abdomen if evidence of additional trauma is found. Removal of a small spleen, for example for idiopathic thrombocytopenic purpura, may be done through a sub-costal incision. For a very large spleen or where the diagnosis is not known a long mid-line incision offers the best access. It is customary to drain the splenic bed as there is a danger of haematoma formation and consequent development of sub-phrenic abscess if it becomes infected.

Staging of lymphomas

Indications

It is very important that the pathologist, surgeon and oncologist should be aware of the reason for staging procedures, including abdominal laparotomy. If the result of any procedure including laparotomy does not influence the patient's treatment, then there is no point in performing it.

In Hodgkin's disease staging laparotomy is necessary if radiotherapy is the sole modality of treatment to be employed, and it is then undertaken to define the geographical extent of the disease so that adequate radiotherapy may be given. Lymphangiography or computerized axial tomography (CAT) scanning and indeed all the other modalities of clinical assessment have not replaced the need for laparotomy, as histological examination of lymph nodes and the spleen in particular is vital. At the present time all patients with B symptoms receive chemotherapy as primary treatment as do patients with Stage III and IV disease. This leaves clinical stages Ia and IIa patients for consideration of radiotherapy and therefore pre-treatment laparotomy.

In non-Hodgkin's lymphoma a laparotomy may be necessary in order to make the diagnosis. The use of *staging* laparotomy now has no place in the management of this disease as it does not influence therapy, and in the case of the high-grade lymphomas may seriously delay the beginning of therapy and prejudice the patient's recovery.

Controversy exists about exclusions from staging laparotomy as a procedure. It has been suggested that, since chemotherapy is so effective in relapsed Hodgkin's disease, it is justifiable to avoid laparotomy in patients, both adult and children, where the only evidence of disease is in the high cervical chain of nodes. The risk of relapse is less than 10 per cent in this group, and in those who do, survivals of 80 to 90 per cent may be seen following chemotherapy. The argument against staging laparotomy is particularly strong in children, where splenectomy is associated with a high mortality subsequently from overwhelming infection. Death rates of between 3 per cent and 10 per cent are recorded in large series of children who have had splenectomy as part of their staging procedure. Where the death rate from the disease itself in the early stages is now less than 5 per cent, this of course is totally unacceptable. Moreover, the treatment with mantle or inverted Y radiotherapy fields, which would logically follow the use of staging laparotomy in children, gives rise to grave problems with regard to growth and development.

Partial splenectomy has been advocated, but does not seem very reasonable on theoretical or practical grounds, and the latest trend in the management of Hodgkin's disease in children and adolescents is to avoid staging laparotomy altogether.

The principle of 'second-look' surgery to remove residual disease or define the extent of residual disease after therapy is now established as useful in a number of tumours, and research programmes investigating post-treatment laparotomy in Hodgkin's disease have been of great interest. Some patients can be shown to have had disease in the abdomen which has been eliminated by chemotherapy while about 15 per cent show what appears to be viable disease still present. Post-treatment laparotomy should only be done at the present time as part of a research programme, or where there is difficulty in defining a complete response by any other method.

Technique of staging laparotomy

The technique of staging laparotomy is theoretically simple but in practice there may be considerable difficulty, not only in assessing whether disease is present in the abdomen, but also in presenting the material in a suitable condition for pathological study.

A long mid-line incision is suitable. Basically the operation is not a confirmation of what is already known clinically but a search for clinically undetectable disease and this must include an assessment of organs other than the lymphoreticular system. The spleen, which is an organ impossible to assess macroscopically, impossible to biopsy and difficult to irradiate is removed together with spleniculi if present. It is convenient to take a splenic hilar lymph node at the same time. Perhaps the most important lymph node group to assess however is that around the coeliac axis, particularly if mediastinal disease is present, and a node is removed from this area for study. If the liver appears macroscopically abnormal a biopsy is taken of that area but in the absence of abnormality a wedge biopsy of the left lobe is taken. A wedge rather than a drill biopsy gives a much more satisfactory piece of tissue to examine histologically. An assessment of all other intra-abdominal lymph node areas is made and if any macroscopic abnormality is apparent then the appropriate node is removed. It is particularly important to assess lymph nodes in the porta hepatis, para-colic and mesenteric areas which do not show up on bipedal lymphangiograms. Although the pre-operative lymphangiographic assessment of the iliac or para-aortic nodes is accurate, these areas are nevertheless examined carefully. It is the removal of these nodes which calls for particular care especially after chemotherapy and in particular if the nodes have been involved in disease, for the whole retro-peritoneal area becomes very 'woody' making assessment of nodes difficult and atraumatic removal both difficult and hazardous. The site of each lymph node which is removed is marked with a tantalum clip. This allows one to assess on the pre-operative lymphangiogram which nodes have been removed. In the presence of massive lymphatic disease the extent is delineated by tantalum clips which may help the planning of subsequent radiotherapy. The appendix is removed but this is not part of the lymphoma assessment. After pre-treatment laparotomy if disease is present below the diaphragm, inverted Y radiotherapy to all gland fields below the diaphragm is required in addition to mantle radiotherapy to all gland fields above the diaphragm. If active untreated disease is found at post-treatment laparotomy then further chemotherapy is essential.

Conclusion

In conclusion, it can be seen that the closest co-operation is necessary between the oncologist, the surgeon and the pathologist if they are to use their skills to the maximum benefit of the patient. Not only will a careful clinical history and examination often give a clue to the diagnosis and sometimes render lymph node biopsy unnecessary, but when lymph node biopsy or laparotomy is done, discussions between the surgeon and pathologist may allow the material that is obtained to be used effectively and so avoid the need for subsequent re-biopsy. Discussions of the treatment programme between the oncologist and his surgical colleague may render the use of staging laparotomy unnecessary and thus avoid possible morbidity from this procedure.

Further reading

Carbone, PP, Kaplan HS, Musshof K, Smithers DW,

Tubiana M. Report of the Committee on Hodgkin's Disease staging classification. *Cancer Research* 1971; **31**:1860.

Dorfman RF, Warnke R. Lymphadenopathy simulating the malignant lymphomas. *Human Pathology* 1974; **5**:519.

Lennert K. *Malignant Lymphomas other than Hodgkin's Disease*. New York, Berlin: Springer-Verlag, 1978.

13

Surgical Pathology of the Thyroid Gland

J H S Wade and E D Williams

Introduction

The five basic clinical situations that confront a surgeon dealing with thyroid patients are those of:

(a) Solitary nodule
(b) Hyperthyroidism
(c) Goitrous hypothyroidism
(d) Multinodular goitre
(e) Hard, possibly infiltrating, thyroid lesion

We will deal with each of these problems in turn, and will add a final section concerned with two other less commonly encountered situations:

(f) Unexpected thyroid carcinoma
(g) Presentation of thyroid carcinoma by metastasis

We would stress at the outset the need for good communication between surgeon and pathologist at all times. The surgeon must remember that the pathologist needs adequate clinical information with the specimen; that is to say, not only the age and sex of the patient, but also information on the thyroid functional status, the family history, a description of the goitre and a differential diagnosis—particularly if malignancy is suspected. The pathologist must remember that the surgeon needs a clear statement of opinion on the lesion on which he can base his management of the case. Conclusions such as "this should be regarded as a borderline lesion" are not in themselves helpful; the surgeon needs to know whether the sample was adequate, whether the lesion was completely removed, and whether further sections or a second opinion are likely to be of assistance. A statement such as "this is a follicular tumour of borderline malignancy. Adequate numbers of capsular sections have been taken, and as only one site of possible vascular invasion is present, metastasis is unlikely" enables the surgeon to plan future care with more confidence.

Communication is particularly important over the use of frozen sections. We consider that discussion between surgeon and pathologist over frozen sections is of such importance that an "intercom" system between theatre and laboratory is essential. Good management of patients with thyroid problems depends upon the joint efforts of surgeons and pathologists, and is helped by the establishment of a good working relationship between them.

It is also essential that both surgeon and pathologist use the same classification of thyroid tumours, and understand its uses and its difficulties. The current standard classification is that of the World Health Organization. The major types of thyroid carcinoma are papillary, follicular, medullary and anaplastic carcinoma. Papillary and follicular carcinomas are sometimes jointly referred to as "differentiated carcinomas", to contrast with undifferentiated carcinoma, a synonym for anaplastic carcinoma. The commonest source of confusion lies in the use of the words "papillary" and "follicular". Many of the difficulties can be avoided if it is remembered that these words can be used either as descriptive or as diagnostic terms. As descriptive terms, they refer to the microscopic architectural arrangement. As diagnostic terms, they refer to two reasonably well defined tumour entities, which differ in a number of characteristics. To emphasize this distinction in usage in the discussion that follows, the diagnostic terms are always capitalized. Papillary Carcinoma is typically multifocal, unencapsulated, invades lymphatics, and characteristically metastasizes to lymph nodes, while Follicular Carcinoma is typically solitary, encapsulated, invades veins and characteristically metastasizes to bones. Papillary Carcinomas usually show wholly or in part a papillary architecture, but neoplastic follicles are common; occasionally, the tumour may lack any papillary pattern. These "pure follicular variants of Papillary Carcinoma" show the biologic behaviour expected of Papillary Carcinomas generally, and usually show the cytologic features of the cells of a Papillary Carcinoma. Follicular Carcinomas do not contain any papillary architecture, but may show well differentiated follicles, or a less well differentiated or trabecular architecture. In addition, either type of tumour may be made up of mitochondrial rich cells, variously referred to as oxyphil, Hurthle, or Askanazy cells. While these are sometimes referred to as Hurthle cell carcinomas, it is more correct to regard them as either Papillary Carcinomas (Hurthle cell type) or Follicular Carcinomas (Hurthle cell type). Tumours made up of these cells do not in general show significant radioiodide concentration; evidence that their prognosis differs from non-oxyphil tumours is conflicting. Some of the features of the major types of thyroid carcinoma are shown in Table 13.1.

Table 13.1 Some features of the major types of thyroid carcinoma

Cell of origin	*Diagnostic type of tumour*	*Architectural variants*	*Cytological variants*	*Other features*	*Immuno-localization*	*Typical pattern of spread*
Follicular cell	Papillary Carcinoma	Pure papillary Mixed papillary/ follicular Pure follicular	Oxyphil/non-oxyphil	Psammoma bodies Clear nuclei Intranuclear cytoplasmic inclusions	Thyroglobulin +ve Calcitonin & CEA* −ve Keratin +ve	Lymphatic invasion, intrathyroid spread, cervical lymph nodes. Distant metastases especially to lung
	Follicular Carcinoma	Well differentiated. Trabecular (less well differentiated)	Oxyphil/non-oxyphil		Thyroglobulin +ve Calcitonin & CEA −ve	Venous invasion. Distant metastases especially to bones
	Anaplastic Carcinoma		Spindle cell Spindle & giant cell Giant cell Clear cell		Usually −ve for thyroglobulin, calcitonin, CEA	Direct local invasion, venous invasion, wide distant metastases, especially to lung
C cell	Medullary Carcinoma	Solid Papillary Tubular	Spindle cell Anaplastic	Amyloid Calcification	Thyroglobulin −ve Calcitonin, CEA, histaminase +ve	Lymphatic and venous invasion. Lymph node involvement in neck and upper mediastinum. Distant metastases to bone and liver

*CEA = carcinoembryonic antigen

Solitary nodule

The management of the patient with a clinically solitary nodule in the thyroid is one of the commonest problems facing the surgeon with an interest in the thyroid, and the diagnosis of the solitary nodule is a common and occasionally a very difficult problem for the pathologist. The nature of the problem has altered over the last few years, partly because of the use of more sophisticated scanning techniques, and partly because of the introduction of aspiration biopsy of the thyroid.

The clinically solitary nodule may, of course, represent an asymmetrical multinodular goitre; it may be a truly solitary follicular lesion, or it may be a Papillary or Medullary Carcinoma. Rarely, other lesions may present in this way; for example, a Hashimoto's thyroiditis or a virus thyroiditis is occasionally asymmetrical and may appear as a hard single nodule. Metastatic tumours, notably from renal carcinomas, do very rarely present as thyroid nodules.

The most important initial step in the investigation of a patient with a solitary nodule is to ascertain the thyroid status. If the patient is found to be hyperthyroid with raised serum hormone levels and the nodule is shown by scan to be "hot", the chance of malignancy is so small that, for the purposes of practical management, it can be ignored. If the patient has hyperthyroidism and is found on scanning to have a "cold" nodule in a diffuse overactive goitre, the clinical management must take into account both the "cold" nodule and the diffuse toxic goitre; the nodule must be treated on its merits as a cold nodule.

We have set out in Fig. 13.1 a summary of the management of a cold nodule.

knowledge of Follicular Carcinoma is dependent upon diagnoses based on the identification of capsular and vascular invasion in sections. In the absence of vascular invasion after adequate sampling of the capsule in a follicular lesion, metastasis is extremely unlikely, whatever the histology of the lesion itself, as long as no focus of Anaplastic Carcinoma is present. The diagnosis of Follicular Carcinoma on cytology alone is therefore at present unjustified. The presence of colloid rich follicles, lined by flattened follicular cells, and often accompanied by many histiocytes—in other words the features of a colloid nodule—is, however, a good indication of the benign nature of a follicular lesion. When these features are seen, resection is not required unless there are other overriding reasons. We would stress that at present ABC should still be regarded as providing a guide to therapy rather than a final tissue diagnosis.

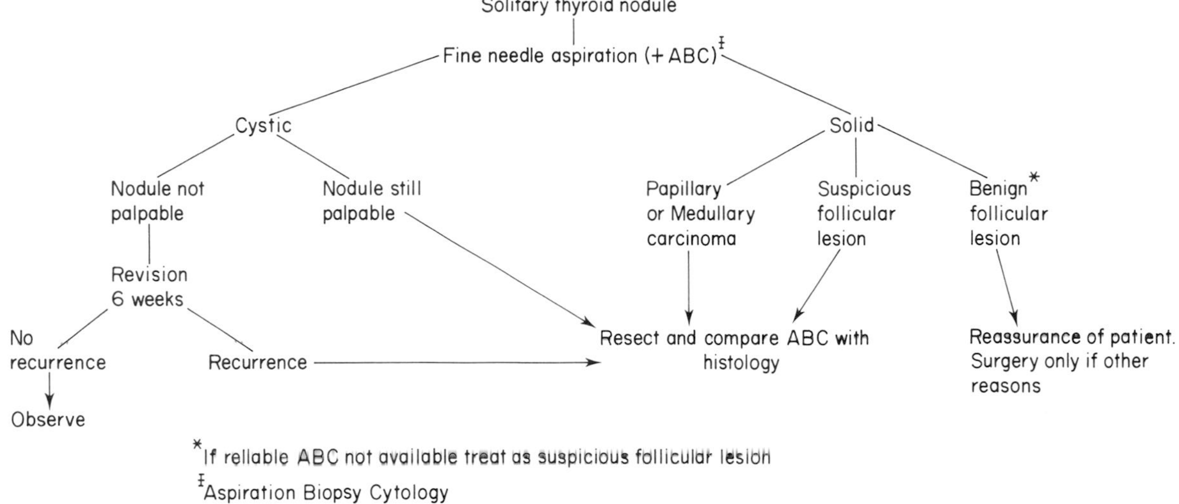

Fig. 13.1 The management of a cold nodule.

Cold nodule – preoperative management

The use of aspiration biopsy cytology (ABC) has extended greatly recently, although some centres use "thick" needle biopsy in place of the fine needle of ABC. While thick needle biopsy is best performed by a surgeon, aspiration biopsy cytology is performed using a fine needle, with very few attendant hazards, and may be carried out either by surgeon or pathologist. There are advantages in both surgeon and pathologist becoming skilled in its use, and collaborating in an ABC clinic, where both see the patients, carry out biopsies, and discuss the results.

This is not the place to discuss either the performance or the detail of the interpretation of the biopsies, but it is important for certain problems to be jointly understood by both surgeon and pathologist. Firstly, as with all biopsies, it is essential that the smear be adequately prepared. Secondly, the recognition by the pathologist of Medullary or Papillary Carcinoma enables a definitive plan of operation to be prepared. However, we do not believe that it is wise for the pathologist to make an outright diagnosis of Follicular Carcinoma on ABC. The whole complex of our

Another value of ABC is the opportunity it provides for aspiration of a cystic lesion (*see* Fig. 13.1). Neoplasms, particularly Papillary Carcinomas, may be partially cystic, and when a palpable nodule remains at the end of the aspiration of a cyst, it should be reaspirated, or, if this fails, resected.

The extent of the thyroid surgery that should be undertaken when a diagnosis of thyroid carcinomas has been made is still a controversial subject. Our own view is that differentiated thyroid carcinomas are of such a varied prognosis that a rigid treatment plan for all types is not justified.

Cold nodule – intraoperative management

The next point of contact between the surgeon and the pathologist is in the use of the frozen section during operation. Frozen section should be carried out on any suspicious lesion found during thyroid surgery whether or not ABC has been performed. The interpretation of a frozen section of a cold nodule is subject to the same general constraints as is the interpretation of ABC.

The diagnosis of Medullary or Papillary Carcinoma enables the surgeon to plan the operation accordingly. When the diagnosis of Papillary Carcinoma is made on frozen section of a nodule, either subtotal thyroidectomy or total thyroidectomy should be performed. When the diagnosis of Medullary Carcinoma is made, total thyroidectomy should be performed because of the possible presence of bilateral primary tumours.

A follicular lesion may be recognized as being benign, but the diagnosis of Follicular Carcinoma is seldom possible on frozen section. A cellular follicular nodule with an apparently intact capsule is best reported on frozen section as "suspicious", because the absence of extracapsular invasion in the relatively small sample available is not adequate evidence that the nodule is benign. Where obvious extra-capsular invasion is seen, and the diagnosis of Follicular Carcinoma is made, the surgeon may wish to proceed to total thyroidectomy, so that a whole body scan and radioiodine therapy for any distant metastases can subsequently be carried out. If the frozen section shows a suspicious follicular lesion, and no other factor is present to suggest that it is a carcinoma, then we would consider a lobectomy to be an adequate operation. A lobectomy is the minimum operation which should ever be performed on a solitary cold nodule, and the lobe is the specimen which should be sent—unfixed—by the surgeon to the pathologist for frozen section examination.

Discussion of the frozen section findings between surgeon and pathologist is often invaluable in making the quick decisions needed in the theatre, that is to say whether to regard lobectomy as adequate surgical treatment, or to proceed to subtotal or total thyroidectomy. The prognosis of thyroid carcinoma is related to many factors: for example, a small Papillary Carcinoma (less than 1.5 cm in diameter), not involving the capsule of the thyroid gland and presenting in a young woman, has an extremely good prognosis, even if cervical lymph nodes are involved. On the other hand a large Papillary Carcinoma involving extrathyroid tissue and presenting in an old man, has a relatively poor prognosis.

Even though pathological studies show that the opposite lobe of the thyroid is frequently the site of intrathyroid deposits of Papillary Carcinoma, clinical recurrence of tumour in the residual thyroid tissue after lobectomy is rare in cases with a favourable prognosis, perhaps this tumour may be extremely slowly growing, and may undergo spontaneous death. Psammoma bodies, one of the features of Papillary Carcinoma, are regarded as the gravestones of dead papillae.

In this thyroid cancer which behaves in such an unusual fashion, we believe that management should be based on clinical experience rather than on dogma. It may be that in the future lobectomy will be shown to be adequate surgery for the Papillary Carcinoma with a good prognosis. Currently, many surgeons believe that the risks of total thyroidectomy do not justify its largely theoretical benefits for the small Papillary Carcinoma in a young patient.

The situation with Medullary Carcinoma is very different. When the tumour is bilateral, it is more often due to a second primary tumour than to intraglandular spread. The purpose of advising total thyroidectomy is not only to remove a possible second primary tumour, but also to provide the pathologist with the material needed to establish whether or not C cell hyperplasia or bilateral tumours exist, so that decisions on family studies can be made.

Cold nodule – postoperative management

The postoperative management of the patient with a cold nodule is largely determined by the pathological findings. The pathologist's task is helped if the specimen is not sliced in the theatre merely to satisfy curiosity; the thyroid tends to become distorted when fixed, and the normal anatomy is much easier to determine in an intact than a shredded lobe. It is good practice for the surgeon to identify and send each lobe separately, and to mark the upper pole with a loose stitch because anatomy that is obvious in the unfixed newly resected thyroid is not so obvious in the fixed specimen. Any lymph node resected should also be sent separately and any that are particularly unusual because of site or appearance should be separately identified. Obviously the lymph nodes from the two sides of the neck should also be separated.

The pathologist should weigh all thyroid tissue sent, and as well as the normal description, should measure the size of the main lesion, and record whether it involved the gland capsule and perithyroid tissues. The presence of multiple lesions will, of course, be recorded, and blocks taken from the various lesions should be separately numbered. A block including an adequate sample of non-neoplastic thyroid tissue must always be taken, and samples must obviously be taken of both lobes where both have been resected.

In follicular lesions the main diagnostic criterion of malignancy is the presence of invasion of pericapsular veins, usually accompanied by breaching of the capsule. Adequate sampling of the capsular region is, therefore, essential; indeed, in the case of a follicular tumour of suspicious histology, it has been recommended that up to 10 capsular blocks should be taken to exclude malignancy. The actual number will, of course, depend on the size of the tumour; in a small, encapsulated tumour up to 2 cm in diameter, it may be difficult to obtain more than 4 adequate blocks. Normally, one to four blocks would be taken initially, depending on the size of the tumour, with additional blocks as needed. In small tumours, all blocks should include the capsule. In large tumours, central blocks are needed to study any particular features of note, but most blocks should include tumour, an adequate length of capsule, and a rim of pericapsular tissue.

In Papillary Carcinoma, usually seen macroscopically as an irregular, unencapsulated firm tumour, the need for such careful sampling is normally much less. As well as the usual sampling of tumour, of apparently uninvolved thyroid tissue, and of any resected lymph node, it is wise to take a block where the tumour approaches most nearly to the capsule of the thyroid gland.

In Medullary Carcinoma, the position is much the same as Papillary Carcinoma in relation to establishing the diagnosis. However, it is usually also necessary to look for evidence of a possible genetic basis for the disease. This requires the study of the presence or absence of C cell hyperplasia or of bilateral tumours. Multiple blocks should be taken around the periphery of the primary tumour, and the opposite lobe should be adequately sampled. C cells normally lie in the centre or just above the centre of the lobes but, if the lobe is of no more than normal size, it is wise to block the whole of it, taking serial blocks from the upper pole down. These should then be studied for C cell hyperplasia or microscopic foci of Medullary Carcinoma. If these are present, it is usually necessary to undertake family studies.

Hyperthyroidism

The three major causes of hyperthyroidism, Graves' disease, toxic multinodular goitre, and toxic adenoma, are all frequently treated surgically. The first two usually require subtotal thyroidectomy, and the third lobectomy. The need for close collaboration between surgeon and pathologist in the management of such patients is much less than in that of cold nodule, and in most cases, the pathologist's role is confirmatory. While in some centres ABC is performed, this is not essential. A frozen section is also of little value, unless there is an unexpected intraoperative finding. As has been mentioned, malignancy in a hot nodule is exceptionally rare. Thyrotoxicosis may rarely be caused by a thyroid cancer, but these unusual cases generally have a large bulk of poorly functioning tumour tissue, often with widespread metastases. The problem of the unexpected postoperative histological finding will be dealt with later.

In Graves' disease, the pathologist should take at least one block from each lobe, with additional blocks taken from any unusual structures found on slicing all thyroid tissue at approximately 2–3 mm intervals. The combination of epithelial hyperplasia and lymphoid infiltration may allow Graves' disease to be suspected by the pathologist without knowledge of the history, but the diagnosis cannot with present techniques be established by histopathological examination alone. The degree of lymphoid infiltration should be commented on in the pathological report, as extensive lymphoid infiltration is associated with an increased likelihood of the development of postoperative hypothyroidism.

In toxic multinodular goitre, the pathologist should make multiple slices through both lobes, and take at least one block from each lobe. He should also sample any unusual nodules—particularly those which are more solid or fleshy. Microscopically, he should attempt to distinguish Graves' disease occurring coincidentally in a multinodular goitre, from the multinodular goitre with one or more hot nodules. In the former, there is background internodular hyperplasia and a lymphoid infiltrate; in the latter, there is epithelial hyperplasia in the nodule(s) and suppressed thyroid tissue in the background. The distinction may be made difficult by preoperative antithyroid therapy, which may lead to background hyperplasia, and also by the fact that epithelial hyperplasia in a nodule or tumour does not necessarily correlate with hormone production; for example, some tumours have been shown to have various metabolic defects.

Goitrous hypothyroidism

A hypothyroid patient with a goitre most commonly has Hashimoto's thyroiditis; dyshormonogenesis is a rare but important cause. Diagnosis of these conditions can often be made by non-invasive investigation, although ABC may play a useful confirmatory role. These patients may come to surgery for cosmetic reasons, obstructive symptoms or occasionally because of suspicion of malignancy; but the majority are treated medically. The preoperative diagnosis of either Hashimoto's thyroiditis or dyshormonogenesis does not, of course, exclude malignancy. Hashimoto's thyroiditis may rarely be complicated by the development of a Malignant Lymphoma. The great majority of Malignant Lymphomas of the thyroid arise in glands with a severe thyroiditis, and malignancy occurring in a hypothyroid patient is most commonly due to a lymphoma. However, Hashimoto's thyroiditis is relatively common, whereas Malignant Lymphoma is relatively rare. Although this complication should be borne in mind, it is not an indication for surgery for a Hashimoto goitre unless there are suspicious clinical features.

In dyshormonogenesis, malignancy is liable to be overdiagnosed, both by clinician and pathologist, but carcinoma does occur rarely, and is usually follicular in type. The surgeon may suspect malignancy in a case of dyshormonogenesis because of a large, often asymmetrical goitre; the pathologist may suspect malignancy because of marked nuclear atypia in the thyroid nodule, although it should be noted that this alone is a poor guide to malignancy in thyroid tumours.

Untreated dyshormonogenesis is associated with a long-standing elevated TSH level, and this causes diffuse hyperplasia and nuclear pleomorphism of the thyroid follicular cells together with multiple nodule formation. The changes are variable, depending on whether the enzyme defect is complete or partial, and on the extent of preoperative therapy. As in endocrine pathology in general, it is necessary for the pathologist to ensure that blocks taken sample the background thyroid tissue adequately as well as the nodules.

The pathological diagnosis of a Follicular Carcinoma in dyshormonogenesis requires the same criteria as any Follicular Carcinoma; however, needless suspicion is still aroused because of the variability of appearances. In a few cases, the cellular disorder and nuclear pleomorphism of the severe generalized hyperplasia has been so gross that a diffuse carcinoma has been suspected.

It is important to recognize dyshormonogenesis both clinically and pathologically in order that appropriate hormone replacement treatment can be instituted for the patient, that further unnecessary surgery is avoided, and that the necessary family studies can be carried out on this autosomal recessive group of conditions.

Multinodular goitre

The patient with a euthyroid multinodular goitre will usually come to operation on account of obstructive symptoms or for cosmetic reasons, and the operation most commonly performed is subtotal thyroidectomy. ABC or frozen section is not usually required. The pathologist is faced with the problem of which nodules to sample in a gland which may contain too many nodules to allow each to be studied microscopically. A reasonable working rule is to regard the minimum requirement as one section from each lobe. This section should include the edge of a representative nodule and an adequate sample of uninvolved thyroid tissue. In addition, any nodule which lacks the typical appearance of a colloid nodule should be sampled; again, the interface of the nodule and the adjacent tissue should always be included. The pathological diagnosis rarely possess any particular problem, although there are, of course, occasional unexpected findings.

The pathologist must always check the background thyroid tissue and comment on any severe thyroiditis which may alert the surgeon to the possibility of the development of hypothyroidism. He must also bear in mind that dyshormonogenesis with partial enzyme deficiency may present as a euthyroid multinodular goitre and check that there are not hyperplastic changes in the background thyroid, with tall epithelial cells and marked nuclear variation.

Hard, possibly infiltrating, thyroid lesion

The management of a patient with a lesion that is clinically thought to be malignant is one in which the closest co-operation between surgeon and pathologist is required. The major lesions to be considered are Anaplastic Carcinoma, Malignant Lymphoma, and Riedel's thyroiditis; occasionally, a Papillary or Follicular Carcinoma will present with direct extra-thyroid invasion. Rarely, a primary carcinoma of the larynx or oesophagus may extend directly into the gland. Both Hashimoto's and viral thyroiditis may also rarely present as hard, possibly infiltrating lesions.

As with a cold nodule, it is common practice for the diagnosis to be established either pre-operatively by ABC, or by frozen section at operation. When there is a rapidly expanding mass in the neck in an old person, clinically considered to be an Anaplastic Carcinoma, ABC is of particular value, as a definite confirmation of the diagnosis may spare the patient surgery, and allow palliative radiotherapy or chemotherapy to be started as early as possible in the treatment of this rapidly lethal malignancy. In the other malignant tumours, ABC or frozen section should enable a diagnosis of Papillary Carcinoma, Medullary Carcinoma, or Malignant Lymphoma to be established in most instances so that the appropriate operation can be planned.

If the tumour is resectable, then, in general, the same procedure should be undertaken as discussed under the section on cold nodules, with, of course, wide resection of the local infiltration, where possible, When ABC or frozen section of an infiltrating tumour shows a follicular neoplasm, then total thyroidectomy is required, as the clinical presentation of the tumour shows that it is more aggressive than most Follicular Carcinomas, and total thyroidectomy permits further investigation by whole body scan for metastatic tumour.

The recognition of Riedel's thyroiditis by ABC is difficult, both because of the problem of obtaining samples from the densely fibrous lesion, and because the basis of the pathological diagnosis is anatomical and architectural rather than cytological. The diagnosis may also be difficult on frozen section, and in the presence of a unilateral infiltrating lesion, lobectomy is usually justified if no firm diagnosis can be obtained. If the lesion is bilateral and no firm diagnosis is available, the decision as to whether to proceed to a total thyroidectomy requires careful consultation between surgeon and pathologist.

The unexpected thyroid carcinoma

A common problem in the management of patients with thyroid disease is the recognition of a thyroid carcinoma only after the initial operation, either lobectomy or subtotal thyroidectomy, has been carried out. These cases can be considered in two groups:

(a) the diagnosis of an "occult" thyroid carcinoma removed for some other reason;
(b) the recognition after lobectomy that a cold nodule is in a reality a carcinoma.

Occult carcinoma

Occult thyroid carcinomas are generally small, unencapsulated Papillary Carcinomas, often with a densely fibrous stroma. They are relatively common autopsy findings if the thyroid is carefully studied and are not uncommonly found in thyroidectomy specimens, particularly if these are examined with great care, and every little white spot is sectioned. The present evidence suggests that such Papillary Carcinomas, of less than 1.5 cm in diameter, have an excellent prognosis, and further surgery is not required if such a lesion is discovered accidentally.

Post-operative diagnosis

The single nodule, which was not considered to be malignant preoperatively or by intraoperative frozen section, may nevertheless be discovered to be malignant in the definitive histological examination. Usually these are Follicular Carcinomas of low grade malignancy. Sometimes, other types of tumour present in this way—for example, a pure follicular variant of Papillary Carcinoma.

The Follicular Carcinomas pose a particular problem of judgement. It is known that the prognosis is linked to the extent of vascular invasion present; metastasis is likely in a tumour with extensive vascular involvement, but is unlikely in a tumour with minimal vascular involvement. Other factors are known to be correlated with the prognosis, namely that males in general do worse than females, that old patients do worse than younger patients, and that trabecular tumours have a poorer prognosis than well differentiated Follicular Carcinomas.

A similar problem is posed with the unexpected Papillary Carcinoma in a lobectomy specimen, but here again the risk factors are known, the size of the tumour, involvement of the thyroid capsule, and the age and sex of the patient being the most important.

In both cases, the small but nevertheless real risk of further treatment by surgery or by radioiodine ablation, followed by whole body scan, and perhaps by radioiodine therapy, must be weighed against the risk of not treating a metastatic lesion at its most vulnerable time. When all the risk factors are favourable, as, for example, a minimally invasive well-differentiated Follicular Carcinoma in a young woman, we believe that thyroid hormone therapy and careful follow-up is adequate therapy. When the risk factors are unfavourable, as in an older man with a trabecular type of Follicular Carcinoma with extensive vascular invasion, further surgical or radioiodine ablation of the residual lobe is recommended, provided that there is reasonable evidence to support the possibility of radioiodine uptake by the tumour. Currently, this is judged histologically by the presence of follicular differentiation and colloid secretion; however, in the future, demonstration that the tumour contains thyroglobulin, using immunological techniques on tissue sections, may well prove to be very useful. Inevitably, there will be a number of cases which fall between these guidelines, but we do not believe that it is wise to propose a uniform treatment policy for all patients with a tumour which varies so widely in its clinical behaviour.

If a Medullary Carcinoma is discovered unexpectedly in a lobectomy specimen, we believe that a total thyroidectomy should be carried out, because of the risk of a second primary in the opposite lobe.

Presentation of thyroid carcinoma by metastasis

The management of thyroid carcinoma presenting by metastasis rarely causes difficulty.

Cervical lymph node metastasis

Commonly, the first indication of a thyroid problem arises when a lymph node is resected from the neck and is shown to contain a Papillary Carcinoma of the thyroid. Under these circumstances, it is advisable, if the tumour is impalpable and the lymph node confined to one side of the neck, to do a total lobectomy on that side, and to carry out a total or subtotal lobectomy on the opposite side, together with removal of any enlarged lymph nodes. The thyroid will, of course, require very careful examination to reveal the presence of a particularly small papillary carcinoma.

Occasionally, the lymph node may contain a Medullary Carcinoma. Although the primary tumour is usually palpable, cases have occurred when metastasis was found and the primary could not be detected clinically. Whether or not this is the case, a total thyroidectomy should be performed, so that both lobes can be carefully studied for the presence of both tumour and C cell hyperplasia.

A particularly difficult problem may arise where the tissue removed, clinically considered to be a lymph node, is found to be made up entirely of thyroid follicles of apparently normal histology. In this event, the differential diagnosis lies between a metastasis of a thyroid carcinoma replacing a lymph node, or a portion of normal thyroid separated from the main gland. The distinction between these two is usually possible on pathological grounds, but metastases of thyroid carcinomas may on occasion be so well differentiated as to be difficult to separate from normal thyroid tissue on histology; particularly on frozen section. The surgeon should therefore always note carefully the exact anatomical location of the "lymph node" removed.

A second problem may arise when the tissue removed contains a mixture of thyroid follicles, not obviously malignant, and lymphoid tissue. The usual criteria for the histological recognition of thyroid carcinoma apply, but it must be remembered that a severe thyroiditis will affect sequestered portions of thyroid tissue as well as the main gland, and this combination can be mistaken for a lymph node metastasis.

Small groups of apparently normal thyroid follicles are occasionally found in the peripheral sinus region of true lymph nodes removed from the neck for some other reason. The histogenesis of these is uncertain; they may represent developmental abnormalities. The commonest cause of the presence of thyroid follicles in a cervical lymph node is, of course, thyroid carcinoma, almost always Papillary Carcinoma. Follicular Carcinoma only rarely metastasizes to cervical lymph nodes, but the metastases of a Papillary Carcinoma may be made up in part or completely of neoplastic follicles.

Distant metastasis

Presentation with distant metastasis may occur with any type of thyroid tumour, but is particularly common with Follicular Carcinoma. Bone is the commonest site for a distant metastasis in Follicular Carcinoma, and this may present as a pathological fracture. The decision about further thyroid surgery if the primary has not already been removed is dependent on the general appraisal of the patient. In general, if the primary tumour is removable, a total thyroidectomy is indicated in order to reduce the risk of further metastases and to allow effective treatment with radioiodine of metastases already present.

Medullary Carcinoma may also present with a distant metastasis; under these circumstances, thyroidectomy would normally only be advised if there were local reasons such as a huge goitre or tracheal obstruction due to pressure. However, resection of a considerable portion of a tumour which is otherwise inoperable, whether primary or secondary, may be justified in the treatment of humoral manifestations of Medullary Carcinoma, for example, intractable diarrhoea or, more rarely Cushing's syndrome.

Papillary Carcinoma occasionally presents with multiple lung metastases and Malignant Lymphoma of the thyroid is particularly associated with lymphomatous deposits in stomach or small intestine.

Surgical pathology of the parathyroid glands

The surgery of parathyroid disease is essentially the surgery of hyperparathyroidism. Parathyroid pathology in hyperparathyroidism is basically that of six separate diseases; some features of these, together with secondary hyperparathyroidism, are shown in Table 13.2. In the established case of severe hyperparathyroidism, the separation of these entities is usually simple—except that the distinction of parathyroid adenoma from carcinoma may be difficult. The earlier in its natural history the disease process is diagnosed, the more difficult may be both the surgery and the pathology. The widespread use of biochemical screening for hypercalcaemia has led to the diagnosis of hyperparathyroidism at a much earlier stage, and also to the recognition that the disease is much more common than was once thought. Although it is not strictly within the remit of this chapter, we feel we must point out that, in the management of hyperparathyroidism, it is essential to recognise that the interpretation of serum parathyroid hormone (PTH) assays is entirely dependent on the level of the serum calcium. A raised PTH level in a patient with hypocalcaemia is usually a normal response; a PTH level within the normal range in a patient with hypercalcaemia is usually regarded as evidence of hyperparathyroidism. It may be difficult to accept that a "normal" PTH level is evidence of hyperparathyroidism, and perhaps it is a pity that the term "normal range" is used in this context. It may be better simply to regard the level of parathyroid hormone as appropriate or inappropriate.

The problems in the co-operation between surgeon and pathologist in the management of parathyroid disease are easily defined as follows:

(a) Is the disease process an adenoma?
(b) Is the disease process basically hyperplasia, requiring resection of either three and two-thirds or all four glands?
(c) Is the disease process a carcinoma?
(d) Can primary hyperparathyroidism be excluded by biopsy of four normal glands?

Intra-operative management

A diligent search for all four parathyroid glands is essential in all operations for hyperparathyroidism, because more than one adenoma may be present and because parathyroid hyperplasia involves all four glands.

The experienced surgeon will almost invariably recognize parathyroid tissue macroscopically at operation, but biopsy with a frozen section must be done for confirmation. It is, therefore, essential that parathyroid surgery be accompanied by a frozen section service with telephonic communication between the surgeon in the theatre and pathologist. Both must appreciate that the purpose of the frozen section is to provide a guide to operative management rather than a definitive diagnosis. The role of the pathologist, put at its simplest, is to confirm that the tissue removed for biopsy is parathyroid: he cannot with certainty differentiate between an adenoma and hyperplasia on frozen section.

At operation, a suspected parathyroid adenoma

Table 13.2 Some features of the major types of parathyroid disease.

	Macroscopic	*Microscopic architecture*	*Cytology*	*Associated clinical features*
Parathyroid adenoma	One enlarged and three small glands	Tumour, sometimes with rim of parathyroid tissue. Other glands and 'rim' show variable degrees of suppression	Adenoma may contain any proportion of chief or oxyphil cells. Mitosis rare, pleomorphism common	Hyperparathyroidism. Pure oxyphil cell tumours may be non-functional
1^{Y} Nodular (chief cell) hyperplasia	Four enlarged glands, upper glands often bigger than lower glands. May not involve all glands macroscopically	Multiple nodule formation throughout affected gland	Nodules may be made up of chief or oxyphil cells	Hyperparathyroidism. Often part of MEN I,* less often of MEN II.* May be familial
1^{Y} Waterclear cell hyperplasia	Four enlarged glands, 'milk chocolate' colour. Upper glands often bigger than lower glands	Unusually uniform pattern throughout all glands	Large cells with water-clear cytoplasm and diagnostic inclusions on electron microscopy	Hyperparathyroidism. Not associated with other endocrine disease
Parathyroid carcinoma	One enlarged gland, usually tethered to surrounding tissue. and three small glands	Tumour, sometimes with rim of parathyroid tissue. Other glands usually show suppression, as carcinomas tend to be bigger and associated with a greater degree of hypercalcaemia than adenoma. Vascular and soft tissue invasion may be seen	Chief or oxyphil cells, relatively uniform nuclei, with prominent nucleoli and mitotic activity. Fibrous strands may be prominent in this tumour	Hyperparathyroidism. Rarely familial
2^{Y} Hyperplasia	Four enlarged glands, lower glands often larger than upper glands	Usually uniform pattern throughout glands	Usually chief cells	Hypocalcaemia with high PTH levels. Commonly secondary to renal failure
3^{Y} Hyperplasia	Variable enlargement of all glands	Variable picture from a single tumour to multiple nodules throughout all glands	Variable	Hypercalcaemia with high PTH levels. Commonly a consequence of prolonged renal failure
Lipoadenoma	One lipoma-like enlarged (usually huge) and three small glands	Yellow tumour composed of strands of parathyroid cells embedded in fat	Usually chief cells	Hyperparathyroidism, may be non-functional

* Multiple Endocrine Neoplasia Type I (pituitary, parathyroid, pancreatic islets and adrenal cortex) or Type II (medullary carcinoma of thyroid, phaeochromocytoma, with variable parathyroid involvement)

must be removed completely for biopsy; incisional biopsy is unacceptable because of the risk of seeding tumour cells in the wound. Incisional biopsy is, however, an accepted procedure for parathyroid hyperplasia if part of one gland is to be left in situ. The biopsy of a normal parathyroid gland entails a small but adequate sample which is taken from its tip in order to avoid damage to the vascular pedicle at the hilum.

If one enlarged parathyroid is found and removed, and the other identified glands are of normal or small size, and all are confirmed as parathyroid tissue by frozen section, the surgeon is almost certainly dealing with an adenoma and an adequate operation has probably been performed.

If four enlarged glands are confirmed as parathyroid tissue, the surgeon is dealing with parathyroid hyperplasia; in this case, it is necessary either to remove 3 and two-third glands or remove all four and reimplant a portion of one gland in muscle.

Occasionally, the surgeon is faced with the operative findings of two enlarged parathyroid glands and two of normal size. The incidence of two parathyroid adenomas being present is far less frequent than used to be thought. Many of the reported cases have proved in the course of time to be due to parathyroid hyperplasia with initial unequal enlargement of glands. When the surgeon finds two enlarged and two normal glands he may well be dealing with hyperplasia, but because there may be difficutly in proving this, we believe that the two enlarged glands should be removed and at least one of the other glands biopsied.

It is not usually possible for the pathologist to be certain of the diagnosis of carcinoma of the parathyroid on frozen section. However, the surgeon will probably suspect malignancy because of adherence of or infiltration by the tumour. He must then ensure a wide local removal of the lesion if this is possible.

The pathological recognition of suppression of parathyroid tissue is of interest, but rarely of crucial importance in intraoperative decisions.

Post-operative management

The pathologist, in his study of the paraffin sections, will be able to make a much more certain distinction of the relevant entities of adenoma, carcinoma, primary nodular (chief cell) and primary waterclear cell hyperplasia and of parathyroid suppression. Lipoadenoma is an interesting but extremely rare entity. A major clinical consequence that stems from these diagnoses is the study of the patient and his relatives for multiple endocrine disease, if primary nodular hyperplasia is discovered.

The finding of only 2 or 3 normal parathyroid glands in the neck after a painstaking dissection together with transcervical thymectomy is highly suggestive that an intra thyroid or mediastinal tumour is present. Under these circumstances thyroid lobectomy should normally be carried out on the side of the missing gland, particularly if any thyroid nodularity is present. The pathologist should examine this carefully at frozen section, and bear in mind that parathyroid adenomas may occasionally show a follicular pattern, this may be associated with intraluminal amyloid but is never associated with intraluminal oxalate crystals which are frequent in follicular adenomas. If no intrathyroid parathyroid tumour is found, an intramediastinal tumour is possible. This is an indication for careful reassessment and probably for exploration of the mediastinum at a second operation.

Very infrequently, neither a tumour nor hyperplasia can be discovered at operation in an apparently clear-cut case of primary hyperparathyroidism. The number of parathyroid glands in man is variable, and the finding of four glands of normal or reduced size does not exclude the presence of an adenoma in a fifth gland. "Ectopic" hypercalcaemia associated with non-parathyroid tumours is, of course, well described; whether this is mediated by ectopic production of parathyroid hormone or by other factors, it may be associated with suppression of the normal parathyroid glands.

Parathyroid surgery is occasionally necessary for tertiary hyperparathyroidism. In these patients, the hypercalcaemia is commonly associated with renal failure, and the diagnosis is already established prior to operation. The nature of the operation is planned in advance and is the same as that for primary hyperplasia. The role of the pathologist is to confirm by frozen section during the operation that the tissue being removed is parathyroid.

Further reading

Thyroid

Hedinger Ch, Sobin LH (eds): *Histological Typing of Thyroid Tumours*. International Histological Classification of Tumours, No 11, Geneva: WHO, 1974.

Taylor S (ed): Progress in the treatment of thyroid cancer. *World Journal of Surgery* **5**, 1981.

Williams ED (ed): *Pathology and Management of Thyroid Disease*. Clinics in Endocrinology and Metabolism, Vol 10, London: WB Saunders Co Ltd, 1981.

Woolner LB, Beahrs OH, Black BM, McConamey WM, Keating RK Jr: Classification and prognosis of thyroid carcinoma, a study of 885 cases observed in a thirty years period. *Amer J Surg* 1961; **102**:354–87.

Parathyroid

Castleman B, Roth SI: *Tumors of the Parathyroid Glands*. Atlas of Tumor Pathology, Second Series Fascicle 14. Washington: Armed Forces Institute of Pathology, 1978.

Scantz A, Castleman B: Parathyroid carcinoma. A study of 70 cases. *Cancer* 1973; **31:** 600-605.

Wang CA: Hyperfunctioning intrathyroid parathyroid gland: a potential cause of failure in parathyroid surgery. *J Roy Soc Med* 1981; **74**:49–52.

Wells S A Jr, Leight G S, Ross A J III: Primary Hyperparathyroidism. *Current Problems in Surgery* 1980; **17**:398–463.

Williams ED, Siebenmann R, Sobin LH (eds): Histological Typing of Endocrine Tumours. *International Histological Classification of Tumours*, No. 23, Geneva: WHO, 1980.

14

Non-Thyroid Cervical Swellings

M Hobsley and A C Thackray

Introduction

Figure 14.1 schematically presents the regions of the neck. It is important to remember that the parotid region encroaches on the neck (Chapter 2) and that the superficial lobe of the submandibular salivary gland lies in the suprahyoid part of the anterior triangle. Note that the anterior triangle is posteriorly bounded by the *anterior* border of the sternomastoid.

We do not find the concept of the *midline* very useful in the present context, because a lump cannot by definition lie in a line, and because individual examples of many conventionally "midline" lesions such as goitres and thyroglossal cysts eccentrically straddle the midline, and a few even lie to one side of it. We therefore consider both anterior triangles together as a single area.

This chapter excludes lumps in the skin (*see* Chapter 17) and subcutaneous tissue (Chapter 18).

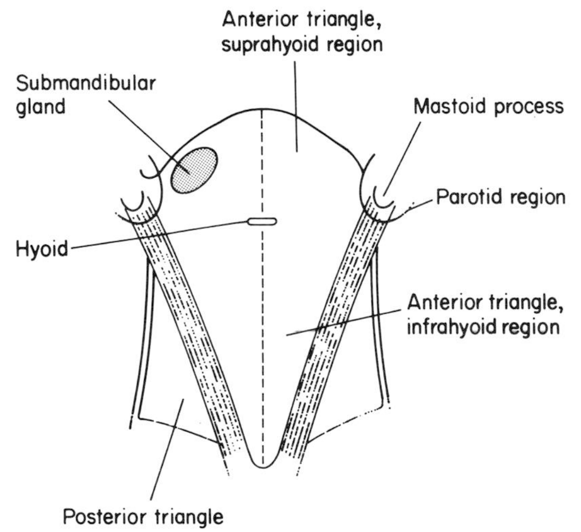

Fig. 14.1 Schematic drawing of the regions of the neck. The anatomical location of a lesion is a powerful guide to management.

Anterior triangles

Movement on swallowing

Lumps which move upwards when the patient swallows are either thyroid or thyroglossal in origin. If the lump does not move when the patient protrudes the tongue, its origin must be assumed to be the thyroid gland itself (see Chapter 13). Those lumps which do move with the tongue are derived from the thyroglossal tract.

Thyroglossal cysts, sinuses and fistulas

The first sign of the future thyroid is seen at the fourth week of fetal development as a diverticulum of the floor of the primitive pharynx between the first and second branchial arches. Its site of origin is still identifiable in the adult at the junction of the anterior two-thirds and posterior third of the tongue where there is a small depression, the foramen caecum. From its point of origin the thyroid rudiment migrates caudally, keeping in front of the pharynx and the developing hyoid, to reach the front of the larynx and the definitive site of the thyroid gland. As it descends it leaves in its wake a column of cells which hollows out to form a tube, the thyroglossal duct.

The thyroglossal duct normally begins to disintegrate at about the eighth week, but a few microscopic remnants of it can often be identified in adults if specifically sought. Rarely, long enough stretches of the duct escape disintegration to give rise to cysts if fluid accumulates in them. Such cysts may be found anywhere along a line which passes down through the substance of the tongue in the midline and is then closely applied to the front of the body of the hyoid, beneath which it usually hooks to reach the back of the bone before continuing down to the thyroid isthmus, diverging a little to one side in front of the thyroid cartilage.

Thyroglossal cysts present as round or ovoid

swellings, usually between 2 and 3 cm diameter, close to the midline. They vary in consistency from soft to firm depending on the tension of the fluid within. Some 10 per cent of all cysts are found in young children, but the great majority are first noticed between the ages of 15 and 25, though a few first appear in later life. There is no significant difference between the sexes. About 80 per cent are found at or a little below the level of the hyoid, the remainder being in or just below the tongue.

Normally they are painless, but may be tender in mild inflammatory episodes, or acutely painful if an abscess develops. Often it is not clear how they become infected, or, for that matter, why they form, perhaps quite suddenly, in the first place. The thyroglossal duct does not normally open onto the skin surface at any point, but if an abscess spontaneously ruptures or is incised a sinus may persist, as it may after incision into and incomplete removal of an uninfected cyst. If the tract between the cyst and the tongue remains patent and an opening from the cyst onto the skin surface develops, a fistula will result.

The thyroglossal duct has a fibrous wall lined by epithelium, most often pseudostratified columnar epithelium which may be ciliated, but also in some places by squamous epithelium, particularly in the region of the tongue. More than one type of epithelium may be found lining a cyst. Mucous goblet cells may be present in the epithelial lining and mucous glands may be found in the wall of the cyst or tract, as also may foci of ectopic thyroid tissue and aggregates of lymphoid tissue.

The fluid in cysts is usually clear and often mucoid, though it may be turbid and shimmer with cholesterol crystals. If there is a sinus opening onto the skin fluid will drain from it, or into the mouth if the upper part of the tract has remained patent.

Malignant change in cysts is extremely rare; the few recorded examples have been papillary adenocarcinomas, possibly arising in foci of thyroid tissue.

Treatment Infected lesions containing pus are drained by incision, but evacuation of the abscess and the institution of efficient drainage only tide the patient over the inflammatory episode without curing the lesion. Recurrence is inevitable unless the whole of the embryological remnant is excised.

If the lesion is a cyst, evidence of the tract must be carefully sought at the upper and lower poles of the lump. Palpation is usually more reliable than vision because the tract usually contains so much firm fibrous tissue. In patients with a sinus opening low in the neck, the opening is circumcized with a margin of skin (to ensure no vestige of the tract remains at that site) and followed pertinaciously upwards. The central portion of the hyoid bone is usually strongly adherent to the tract, but even if it is not, a central segment of the bone at least one centimetre across must be excised in continuity with the tract.

Above the hyoid bone, the continuation of the tract upwards may be palpable right up to the mucous membrane of the tongue. However, even if the tract is not to palpable in this region, a core of tissue should be excised in continuity with the rest of the dissection, extending upwards and at 45 degrees backwards through the muscles of the tongue towards the foramen caecum.

No movement on swallowing

It is convenient to consider separately lumps above and below the hyoid bone.

Suprahyoid (submental) region

For lumps arising from the mandible see Chapter 3; and remember that a lump in the region of the submandibular salivary gland must be treated as a tumour of the gland unless there is evidence of calculous disease.

The two chief clinically diagnosable lesions are the *ranula* and the *dermoid cyst.* If the lesion is clinically not diagnosable as one of these, it is statistically most likely to be an enlarged lymph node and dealt with as in Chapter 12. If the lesion does not feel like a lymph node, it is usually best dealt with by excision-biopsy or biopsy.

Ranula

A ranula is a soft, glistening, bluish, translucent swelling in the floor of the mouth beneath the tongue, to one or other side of the midline. The swelling has been likened to a little frog seen belly-side uppermost, hence the name, a diminutive of Rana. Its situation and the nature of its mucoid contents suggest that the swelling is an extravasation cyst of the sublingual gland, and this is confirmed by the cure that regularly follows complete removal of the gland. There is often a history of trauma to the region a short time before the swelling first appeared. The injury may have actually divided one or more of the several ducts of the gland, or perhaps only blocked them, for the sublingual gland is a persistent secretor, despite opposition to its outflow, and if a duct is blocked it may well rupture from the pressure which builds up within it. Sometimes the damage has occurred in the course of surgery in the neighbourhood, such as the removal of a stone from the nearby submandibular duct.

Treatment If the ranula is aspirated or incised it soon refills, and if excision of the cyst is attempted it nearly always slowly reforms. If the cyst wall is removed and sectioned it will be seen to have an outer fibrous coat which merges into a vascular zone of fibroblastic proliferation and an innermost layer of histiocytes, some of which, in contact with the mucoid cyst contents, have a foamy cytoplasm. There is no epithelial lining.

Later, perhaps after unsuccessful attempts to deal with the oral swelling, the extravasation may extend down through gaps in the mylohyoid muscle to form a visible swelling in the submaxillary region of the upper neck. In time, this cervical swelling may extend, still mainly on the same side, as far as the root of the neck, the base of the skull, or around the pharynx. A ranula which extends in this way is called a cervical, plunging, or burrowing ranula. Any connective tissue space into which the mucoid fluid forces its way develops a granulation tissue reaction similar to that described above. Although a communication between the oral and cervical swellings can usually be demonstrated it has been claimed that the cervical ranula is an independent coincidental branchiogenic cyst, a claim possibly based on a misinterpretation of the lining flattened layer of histiocytes as epithelium, though it is quite unlike the lining of a branchial cyst with its intimately associated lymphoid tissue.

Most writers now accept that the burrowing ranula is an extension of an oral ranula, and like it will be cured by removal of the sublingual gland. Several cases are on record where the submandibular gland has been removed in an attempt to cure the condition without success, a cure being subsequently achieved by removing the sublingual gland. Operations on the ramifying and intercommunicating cavities in the neck are ineffectual and unnecessary; when the source of the mucoid fluid is removed they gradually collapse.

Dermoid cysts and teratomas

A rounded, fluctuant swelling, usually (but not always) fairly symmetrically disposed about the midline) and either subcutaneous or attached on its deep aspect to the mylohyoid muscle is clinically a dermoid cyst.

The midline of the neck, particularly that part above the level of the hyoid, is one of the regions of the body where dermoid cysts may be encountered. In this situation they are believed to arise from groups of cells from the surface layers of the embryo sequestrated during fusion of the mandibular and hyoid branchial arches in the midline. The relationship of the buried cell rest to the mylohyoid and geniohyoid muscles determines whether the dermoid cyst which may subsequently develop will bulge into the floor of the mouth or present as a submental swelling. Such cysts are occasionally noticed at an early age but are more likely to present in adolescents or young adults.

The cysts have a lining of squamous epithelium lying on a layer of fibrous tissue, corresponding to the dermis, in which there are usually some hair follicles, sebaceous and sweat glands. These accessory skin structures add their products to the shed and degenerating squamous cells in the cavity of the cyst, and depending on their number and activity the cyst varies in consistency from firm to soft and fluctuant.

Teratomas—firm, lobulated polycystic structures—are very rare in the neck. The cysts are lined by epithelia of various kinds, and the solid areas contain cartilage, bone and other assorted tissues sometimes including nervous elements. They are nearly always present at birth, and may be large enough to obstruct labour. Cervical teratomas are usually situated in the neighbourhood of the hyoid or thyroid isthmus, and have occasionally seemed to arise in and replace the thyroid gland. Though they may cause death from their size, position and pressure effects, they are nearly always benign in the pathological sense. The very few malignant teratomas in this region have been in adults, and it has been suggested that they represent malignant change in small unnoticed teratomas present since birth.

Treatment The treatment of a dermoid cyst is complete excision, since if a portion of its lining epithelium is left in situ a recurrence is likely. Great care should therefore be taken to preserve the lesion intact during the dissection which should if possible be pursued in a layer of connective tissue around the cyst rather than along its wall.

The differentiation by the clinician between a dermoid and a thyroglossal cyst depends solely on the physical signs of movement on swallowing and with the tongue. Should there be the slightest doubt about whether the lesion does move with the tongue, a careful search should be made during the dissection for evidence of the thyroglossal tract (p. 177).

Infrahyoid region

Some authorities refer to the infrahyoid region of the anterior triangles as *the* anterior triangles themselves. We prefer the classification described here.

The commonest clinical swelling in this region, as elsewhere in the neck, is an enlarged lymph node, and such nodes may occur anywhere. There is however one site in which lesions that are clinically diagnosable occur reasonably frequently —the junction of the upper and middle thirds of the anterior border of the sternomastoid muscle. Lesions at this "typical" site lie mainly deep to the sternomastoid but project forwards beyond its anterior border to be palpable easily in this region. They therefore become fixed when the patient contracts the sternomastoid. A good initial clinical differentiation of these lesions is into *solid* and *cystic*.

The "typical" site—solid lesions

Is the lump *pulsatile*? This is the most important question for the clinician to ask himself. The site is close to the common carotid artery at its bifurcation into the external and internal carotid arteries: any lump overlying these major vessels may transmit pulsation. However, if the lesion exhibits *expansile* pulsation, it is either an aneurysm (rather uncommon; see Chapter 19) or a *carotid body tumour*.

Carotid body tumours

The carotid bodies are small solid structures close to the carotid bifurcation, from which they receive a copious blood supply. The chief cells of the carotid body are of neuroectodermal origin and are chemoreceptors, being sensitive to alterations in the chemical composition of the blood flowing around them. Carotid body tumours, also known as chemodectomas or paragangliomas, are very rare, though less so in dwellers at high altitudes in whom the carotid bodies normally hypertrophy. The tumours are occasionally bilateral, and several examples of familial occurrence are on record. Occasionally, too, in the same patient there may be other paragangliomas, such as tumours of the glomus jugulare or of the aortic body.

Carotid body tumours grow slowly and have often been present for several years before the patient, of either sex and usually between 30 and 60 years old, seeks advice. The tumour is situated deep to the anterior edge of the sternomastoid at the level of the carotid bifurcation, and as it slowly enlarges it splays the bifurcation, extending a variable distance up the internal and external carotids, particularly the latter. The tumour, lying mainly medial to the vessels is usually adherent to their adventitia, is grooved by them and even, rarely, surrounds one or the other. The tumours transmit the carotid pulsation, and as they are very vascular may even be pulsatile.

Carotid body tumours are round or ovoid, and may be lobulated or grooved by the carotids. Although circumscribed they have only a thin and sometimes incomplete capsule of condensed connective tissue. Some tumours are firm or even hard enough to justify the old name "potato tumour" from their consistency and shape, but many are rubbery or even soft. The cut surface is solid, and the colour varies from pink to reddish brown. Microscopically they show some resemblance to the normal carotid body, consisting of a rich network of vascular channels in a fibrous stroma surrounding alveolar groups or nests of epithelioid tumour cells proper. The amount of fibrous stroma varies; sometimes, in the potato-like tumours it is abundant. The epithelioid so-called chief cells are quite large, with abundant pale eosinophilic cytoplasm which may be finely granular or vacuolated. The cell boundaries are often indistinct, so that some of the cell groups have a syncytial appearance. Mitoses are rare, but tumours showing cellular pleomorphism and nuclear hyperchromatism are not uncommon.

There is no doubt that some carotid body tumours prove malignant and metastasize, but estimates of the percentage that do so vary widely. The figures most often quoted lie between 5 and 10 per cent, but the metastases often grow as slowly as the primary and some series followed up for very many years suggest that the malignancy of these tumours has been underestimated. It is generally conceded that the usual histological criteria of malignancy are no guide in this matter, whilst some writers also fail to find any correlation between local invasiveness, either demonstrated histologically or suspected clinically, and prognosis. Local recurrence will follow incomplete removal and does not necessarily indicate malignancy. The first metastasis is likely to be in a nearby lymph node, and in at least one reported case a secondary deposit in a cervical lymph node was so vascular that it was shown up in the arteriogram which so clearly demonstrated the primary carotid body tumour. Later, more distant metastases appear, often in bone.

Treatment The surgeon should maintain a high index of suspicion for this diagnosis. The vascularity of the tumour and its intimate anatomical relationship with the carotid bifurcation make surgical exploration without due precautions a hazardous undertaking—both because of blood loss and because of possible interruption of the blood supply to the brain via the internal carotid artery.

The least suspicion of expansile pulsation should lead therefore to the performance of carotid angiography, an investigation requiring a general anaesthetic. If a carotid body tumour is present, the lateral view shows the characteristic splaying apart of the external and internal carotid arteries.

Once the diagnosis has been confirmed, the operation should, in ideal circumstances, be undertaken by a surgeon with experience of arterial, including carotid, surgery. Usually, it is found to be possible to dissect the tumour free of the arteries without interrupting their channels. However, occasionally it is necessary to insert a temporary, or even a permanent by-pass between the common and internal carotid arteries.

Malignancy is a difficult problem, the individual patient being treated according to the extent of spread.

Other solid lesions

A large variety of other solid lesions may be encountered. They are diagnosed by biopsy or excision-biopsy, and further treatment depends on the histopathological findings.

The "typical" site—cystic lesions

If the lump is spherical, and fluctuant (although the latter sign cannot be detected where the lesion is covered by thick muscle), there are three important diagnoses to consider—pharyngeal pouch, branchial cyst, or a tuberculous cold abscess.

Pharyngeal pouch

Clinical features suggesting this diagnosis are that the patient is middle-aged or elderly, has a long history of mild but gradually increasing dysphagia, that the dysphagia worsens during the progress of a meal, that the lump is in the left side of the neck (a right-sided pharyngeal pouch is most unusual though the reason for this is not known), and that any measure that empties the pouch (such as self-induced retching) relieves the dysphagia.

If palpation of the lump produces a squelching sound because the contents are a mixture of solid, liquid and air, there is scarcely any need for radiology, but a barium swallow series demonstrates that the lump arises at the level of the junction between pharynx and oesophagus, and as it fills it enlarges and presses on the upper oesophagus, thereby producing an increasing interference with swallowing.

In the region where the pharynx and oesophagus merge the arrangement of the muscle fibres of the two parts of the inferior constrictor of the pharynx is such that there is a small area of weakness in the mid-line posteriorly, immediately above the circular fibres of the cricopharyngeus. At this point a backward protrusion of the mucosa may develop, due, it is generally believed, to increased intrapharyngeal pressure resulting from failure of the cricopharyngeus to relax at the appropriate moment in the act of swallowing. No fibrosis or other histological abnormality is apparent in the muscle and the cause of the condition would seem to be spasm or achalasia.

The diverticulum as it forms presses on the vertebral bodies, and to enlarge it must protrude to one side, usually the left. As it fills with food at each meal it gravitates and becomes flask-shaped, sometimes elongating to the full length of the neck The pouch or diverticulum is lined by the squamous epithelium normal to the region, with a submucosa and sometimes a muscularis mucosae. At first there may be a thin outer muscle layer derived from the inferior constrictor bordering the gap through which the mucosa herniated, but this is soon lost, and at most it forms a ring round the neck of the sac. If food stagnates in the sac the lining epithelium may thicken and show white leukoplakic patches, and there may be ulceration, inflammation and even perforation. Carcinoma is a possible, but extremely rare, sequel.

Treatment Excision of the mucosal diverticulum in its entirety, including its neck where it originates through the deficiency in the muscle wall of the pharyngo-oesophagus, is usually effective. There is, however, said to be an incidence of recurrence because the cricopharyngeus muscle is still in spasm and may re-initiate the obstruction that originally caused the lesion. It is therefore wise to divide the cricopharyngeus, when the sac has been excised.

Branchial cyst

The rounded, fluctuant lesion has usually appeared suddenly and recently, in a child or young adult. If there are no clinical features suggestive of a pharyngeal pouch or a tuberculous cold abscess (p. 183), such a lesion is nearly always a branchial cyst (but see *Treatment* below).

Most branchial cysts are situated beneath the anterior border of the sternomastoid, lying on the carotid sheath below the angle of the mandible. They usually remain small and comparatively superficial, but a few enlarge and track upwards towards the base of the skull or inwards towards the pharynx.

The cysts are at first rounded, but they may become ovoid or elongated if they extend among the structures of the neck. Most cysts are lined by stratified squamous epithelium, many fewer by ciliated or non-ciliated pseudo-stratified columnar epithelium, and a few by simple cuboidal or flattened epithelium. Even the apparently squamous-lined cysts may be shown to have patches of other types of epithelium if enough sections are examined. The squamous lining is typically intimately related to a zone of lymphoid tissue, with lymphoid follicles, immediately beneath it. Outside the lymphoid tissue there is an external thin fibrous coat to the cyst. The cavity of the cyst contains shed epithelial cells, glairy fluid and cholesterol crystals. Branchial cysts are liable to attacks of inflammation, which may leave areas of ulceration of their walls, and occasionally there may be actual abscess formation. It is debatable whether carcinoma ever arises from a branchial cyst; usually what is thought to be an example of this phenomenon proves to be a cervical lymph node containing cavitated metastatic squamous carcinoma from an unrecognized primary site.

Similar cysts with a wall of lymphoid tissue and a squamous lining found a little higher up in the immediate neighbourhood of the parotid probably result from cystic dilatation and squamous metaplasia of the ectopic salivary tissue that is not uncommonly found in lymph nodes there. Indeed, it has been suggested that all so-called branchial cysts arise in this way, and would be better called by the non-committal term "lympho-epithelial cysts". The majority view, however, remains that branchial cysts originate from persistent remains of the ectoderm of the second branchial cleft or cervical sinus.

Branchial fistulae are less common than cysts, but whereas branchial cysts are nearly always unilateral, fistulae are not infrequently bilateral, and tend to run in families. The commonest type of fistula opens onto the skin somewhere along the line of the anterior border of the sternomastoid, usually between 4 and 6 cm above the sterno-clavicular joint. The opening, from which a viscid secretion escapes, may be marked by a tag of skin, occasionally containing a nodule of cartilage. The opening leads into a very narrow passage, which may end blindly as a sinus, or continue upwards on a sinuous course to open into the pharynx as a fistula. The track is usually palpable as a cord, and has a little muscle in its wall as well as a layer of lymphoid tissue as in the cyst. The epithelial lining is stratified squamous for the most part, but a ciliated columnar epithelial lining is more likely in the upper reaches.

Treatment The treatment for this anomaly, whether expressed simply as a cyst, or whether part of the tract remains as a sinus or fistula, can be summarized as *complete* excision.

If there is no clinical evidence of a congenital tract, there can be no certainty that the rounded cystic lesion is of branchial origin. The most important implication of this fact is that if the swelling is large enough to encroach upon the parotid region, it could be a neoplasm arising in the parotid salivary gland and therefore require excision with a wide margin of normal tissue and exposure and preservation of the facial nerve (Chapter 2). This is a possibility even if the lesion is obviously fluctuant. The surgical exploration should therefore start with the making of the cervical and mastoid parts of the full parotid cervicomastoid-facial incision. Mobilization off the anterior border of the sternomastoid of the lump and the lower pole of the parotid then permits the surgeon to expose the posterior belly of the digastric muscle, and demonstrate whether this muscle is above the lesion (branchial cyst) or below it (parotid tumour).

If there is a sinus (or fistula) opening on the skin at the junction of the middle and lower thirds of the sternomastoid muscle, an ellipse of skin around it is incised and the whole tract excised just as in the case of the thyroglossal tract (p. 178). An upper opening of the tract (in the pharynx) is less rare than in the case of the thyroglossal tract, and it is wise to pursue the upper end of the tract through the middle constrictor muscle so as to be able to excise a small portion of the pharyngeal mucosa. Leaving any remnant of the tract invites a recurrence.

Tuberculous ('cold'') abscess (see Chapters 28 and 30)

Infra-hyoid region—other sites

For the most part, it is impossible to make a confident clinical diagnosis: the exact nature of the lesion will be determined by biopsy or excision-biopsy, treatment will depend on diagnosis and extent of spread. However, there is one clinically characteristic lesion—the cystic hygroma.

Cystic hygroma or lymphatic cyst

The neck is one of the regions where cystic hygromas or lymphatic cysts may be found. These soft, ill-defined swellings are usually apparent at birth, though they may only be noticed later. The anterior triangle on one or both sides is the usual site of the swelling, which may extend from the supra-sternal notch to the level of the hyoid or even higher. Rarely, there is an associated similar swelling in the axilla or mediastinum. The condition is the result of an abnormal hamartomatous proliferation of the lymphatics of the area, the sprouting lymphatic channels ramifying in amongst the muscles, nerves and blood vessels of the neck, and producing a network of intercommunicating channels and a honeycomb of small cysts. As fluid accumulates in the cysts they progressively enlarge and coalesce to form fewer and larger cysts, so that very impressive swellings may result. The fluid within is clear and limpid so that, with the skin stretched over it, the swelling is translucent and was once known as "hydrocele of the neck". Microscopically, the spaces have thin fibrous walls and flattened endothelial linings, with some smooth muscle in the walls of the larger channels. Here and there haemangiomatous foci may be seen, and it is possibly from these that sudden haemorrhage into the cysts occurs. Cystic hygromas are also liable to attacks of inflammatory swelling, when they become hot and tender, after which they characteristically shrink and disappear. By the time of puberty the hamartomatous proliferation has long ceased and the cystic lesions have usually shrivelled and fibrosed.

Posterior triangles

Here again, the commonest swelling is an enlarged lymph node (Chapter 12), but biopsy may well reveal that the true diagnosis is different, and one of a huge range of possibilities.

Further reading

Ranula

Roediger WEW, Lloyd P, Lawson HH. Mucous extravasation theory as a cause of plunging ranulas. *Br J Surg* 1973; **60**:720–22.
Van den Akker HP, Bays RA, Becker AE. Plunging cervical ranula. *J Maxillofacial Surg* 1978; **6**:286–293.

Thyroglossal cysts and fistulae

MacDonald DM. Thyroglossal cysts and fistulae. *Int J Oral Surg* 1974; **3**:342–6.
Wampler HW, Krolls SO, Johnson RP. Thyroglossal-tract cyst. *Oral Surg* 1978; **45**:32–8.

Branchial cyst

Wilson CP. Lateral cysts and fistulae of neck of development origin. *Ann Roy Col Surg Engl* 1955; **17**:1–26.
Rickles NH, Little JW. The histogenesis of the branchial cyst. *Am J Path* 1967; **50**:533–47.

Carotid body tumour

Van Asperen de Boer RS, Terpstra JL, Vink M. Diagnosis, treatment and operative complications of carotid body tumours. *Br J Surg* 1981; **68**:433–38.

15

Ear, Nose and Throat

P D M Ellis and D G D Wight

Introduction

In this chapter we shall discuss the pathology of the major conditions which bring patients into the care of ear, nose and throat surgeons. Space will not permit detailed discussion of rarities or exhaustive lists of differential diagnoses, but throughout emphasis will be placed upon the ways in which an understanding of pathology and the pathologists needs can contribute to the successful management of the most important diseases.

We shall now consider in turn each of the three areas within this discipline and the major symptoms which bring patients to the ENT clinic. These are the nose and nasal obstruction, the larynx and hoarseness and the ear and deafness.

The nose

Rhinitis

The major symptom which draws attention to disease in the nasal cavity, nasopharynx and paranasal sinuses is nasal obstruction, which is one of the commonest symptoms encountered in the ENT clinic.

Nasal obstruction may be the consequence of a great variety of different conditions ranging from the simple and trivial to aggressive malignant disease. By far the commonest cause of nasal obstruction is acute inflammation of the nasal passages due to the common cold which is primarily a viral infection, but it may also be found in the prodromal phase of other viral infections such as measles. Less commonly it can be attributed to occupational exposure to irritants such as chemical fumes or to dusts. Acute allergic rhinitis is also common, particularly as a symptom of hay-fever.

In any of these conditions the inflammation may be confined to the nasal cavities or it may extend to involve the paranasal sinuses and the nasopharynx. Although acute rhinitis of this type is often complicated by bacterial secondary infection, rapid recovery is the rule. In a minority, however, symptoms may persist. When nasal examination reveals no more than an oedematous mucous membrane, especially over the turbinate bones, the condition may be an expression of allergic or vasomotor rhinitis.

In a proportion of patients the symptoms will be directly attributable to frank allergy to a wide variety of different antigens, of which grass pollen is the best known. Skin testing may be necessary to determine the antigens to which the patient is reacting, but a biopsy of the nasal mucous membrane may help to identify this group. In addition to oedema and vascular engorgement seen in all types of rhinitis, an excess of eosinophils is virtually pathognomonic of an allergic cause.

When no allergic cause can be found the symptoms may be associated with changes in temperature of atmospheric pressure, infection, hormonal factors or even psychological disturbances. This rather ill-defined condition is known as vasomotor or non-specific rhinitis.

Nasal polyps

Persistent acute inflammation, whatever the cause, will lead to hypertrophy of the mucosa and eventually to the formation of polyps. These are common lesions and although the majority occur in the fifth, sixth and seventh decades they may be found in all age groups. They may be unilateral or, more commonly, bilateral and they arise most often in the ethmoid region. As they enlarge they fill first the air cells and then the nasal cavity and may even present at the external nares.

Polyps are mobile, shiny and appear oedematous, even waterlogged. Traditionally, they are divided into two principal categories, allergic and non-allergic or inflammatory. Histologically, both are composed of very oedematous fibrous tissue, covered by ciliated respiratory epithelium which often shows goblet cell hyperplasia. Ulceration is rare but focal squamous metaplasia is common, especially if they present at the external nares. Hyaline condensation or thickening of the basement membrane is characteristic. There are very variable numbers of chronic inflammatory cells in the stroma, usually most numerous in the subepithelial zone. The only major difference between allergic and non-allergic polyps is that the former are said to contain significant numbers of eosinophils in the stroma. However, a recent multidisciplinary study in 37 patients was unable to distinguish between atopic and non-atopic individuals on histological examination alone. Polyps from all patients contained large quantities of immunoglobulin E (IgE) in the stroma, suggesting that it may play a role in the pathogenesis of all polyps.

Rarely, stromal fibroblasts may appear bizarre and atypical, so that they may be confused histologically with sarcomatous transformation and can, for example, resemble the strap cells of a rhabdomyosarcoma. They should probably be regarded as a pitfall for the unwary rather than an expression of malignancy, since true malignant transformation in nasal polyps is excessively rare.

When typical and bilateral, nasal polyps are highly distinctive and many surgeons feel that histological examination is not obligatory. However, it is important to remember that all the granulomatous and neoplastic diseases described below may also present as polypoid lesions and thus histological examination of all polyps, particularly when unilateral, might be the wisest course.

Persistent rhinitis and nasal polyps are much the most common cause of nasal obstruction at all ages. However, different age groups tend to suffer from different diseases and thus children, young adults and the middle-aged and elderly will now each be considered separately.

Young children

The main causes of nasal obstruction in this age-group are listed in Table 15.1.

Table 15.1 Main causes of nasal obstruction in children.

Adenoidal hypertrophy	
Nasal polyps:	antrochoanal
	simple
	cystic fibrosis
Choanal atresia	

Adenoidal hypertrophy

Much the most common cause of nasal obstruction in young children is adenoidal hypertrophy. The adenoids or nasopharyngeal tonsils are part of the lymphoid tissue of Waldeyer's ring, all of which tends to be relatively inconspicuous at birth and then gradually hypertrophies during the first few years of life. In a few children the hypertrophy is excessive and may give rise to enormous pharyngeal and/or adenoidal tonsils. The latter are associated not only with nasal obstruction and a characteristic "adenoidal facies", but, because of their position, they frequently also obstruct the Eustachian tube and thus lead to recurrent ear infections and "glue-ear". Hypertrophied tonsils and adenoids may thus need to be surgically excised. Histological examintion reveals abundant lymphoid tissue with germinal centres beneath a normal respiratory epithelium. However, since microscopy rarely is informative it is not usually considered necessary in the clinically straightforward case.

Nasal polyps

Nasal polyps are not as common in children as in older patients but they are nevertheless probably the most common nasal mass in children. Apart from the simple nasal polyps already described, which may be unilateral or bilateral, children are liable to two other forms of polyp.

Antrochoanal polyps Antrochoanal polyps, which account for some 5 per cent of all nasal polyps, may occur at any age but are especially common in children and young adults. Ninety per cent are unilateral and single. They arise in the wall of the maxillary sinus and enter the nasal cavity through the osteum or through an accessory osteum in the middle meatus. They then tend to expand backwards to enter the nasopharynx through the choana. Protrusion through the relatively narrow osteum frequently produces a waisted or "hour-glass" profile to the polyp. They appear to arise as the result of chronic bacterial infection and this is probably why about a third will recur unless the antrum is cleared in a Caldwell–Luc procedure. Histologically, they are identical to simple inflammatory nasal polyps.

Cystic fibrosis Nasal polyps are common in cystic fibrosis which may account for up to 20–30 per cent of all nasal polyps in this age-group. Rarely, patients with cystic fibrosis may even present with nasal polyps and thus it is important that the true diagnosis is suspected. Fortunately, although they have many features in common with those of inflammatory polyps, there are a number of distinctive microscopic appearances. Basement membrane thickening and eosinophil infiltration, which are so common in inflammatory polyps, are not seen in cystic fibrosis, but the most striking difference is in the nature of the mucin. In inflammatory polyps the mucin in glands and mucous cysts is predominantly neutral, and thus does not stain with Alcian blue, whereas in cystic fibrosis it is predominantly acidic and thus is Alcian blue positive.

Congenital masses Rarely, particularly in very young children and neonates, a meningocele or encephalocele may present intranasally. Most congenital masses, for example dermoid cysts, haemangiomas and nasal gliomas, however, are extranasal and thus do not cause nasal obstruction. Choanal atresia is a developmental defect and may be unilateral as well as bilateral.

Young adults

Juvenile angiofibroma

Teenagers are as susceptible to antrochoanal polyps as young children, but the most characteristic lesion in this age group is the juvenile angiofibroma. This lesion accounted for one quarter of the benign lesions in a large series of non-epithelial tumours of the nasal region but is nevertheless rare. It occurs almost exclusively in males at or near puberty. It probably arises from periosteum near to the choanae and may extend both forwards into the nasal cavity and backwards into the nasopharynx, both of which may be filled by new growth. Indeed it may even prise apart sutures in the base of the skull causing separation of the orbits and the so-called "frog-face deformity".

It is composed of numerous vascular channels embedded in fibrous tissue which may be dense and hyaline or loose and granulation-tissue-like. Most of the vessels are composed of an endothelial lining only, but others have a partial or complete muscular wall, suggesting that it may be a malformation of nasal erectile tissue rather than a true neoplasm. The reason for the marked preponderance of males remains uncertain but there is recent evidence that it may have specific androgen receptors.

Formal surgical excision is the treatment of choice although not always possible. The lesion responds well to radiotherapy when surgery is impracticable but there appears to be a definite if small risk of late malignant transformation in these cases. More recently embolization has been successfully employed.

Middle-aged and elderly

In older patients nasal obstruction may be the first symptom of granulomatous or neoplastic disease (Tables 15.2 and 15.3).

Table 15.2 Granulomatous disease of the nose.

Specific infections:	tuberculosis
	leprosy
	syphilis
	scleroma
	phycomycosis
	aspergillus
	rhinosporidiosis
	leishmania
Sarcoidosis	
Non-healing granulomas	

Granulomatous disease

Specific infections A great variety of specific infections may affect the nose (Table 15.2). They are all uniformly rare in the United Kingdom and Western Europe, but with rapid air travel continually increasing, it is necessary to be aware of their existence since most are quite common in certain parts of the world, particularly in underdeveloped countries. They all may present as polypoid or tumour-like masses. Fortunately, in most cases the histological appearances are fairly distinctive, and any organism can usually be demonstrated relatively easily, especially with appropriate special stains. If any of these conditions is suspected on clinical grounds, a portion of the unfixed tissue should always be sent to the microbiological department for culture and, since many of the organisms require special culture methods, it is essential that the differential diagnosis is clearly stated on the request form.

Sarcoidosis Sarcoidosis occasionally presents with upper respiratory tract symptoms. Histologically, it is identical to that elsewhere and consists of well-formed, non-caseating epithelioid and giant-cell granulomata, in which no organisms can be demonstrated. In the vast majority of cases there is already evidence of multisystem disease at the time of presentation, especially hilar lymph node enlargement and skin lesions, and thus confirmation of the diagnosis should present no problems.

Non-healing granulomas Necrotizing lesions of the upper airway continue to frustrate pathologists, exasperate clinicians and spawn a considerable literary effort. Patients in this group usually present with an ulcerated indurated swelling of some part of the nose, such as the vestibule or septum, associated with nasal obstruction or a foul discharge which may be blood-stained. Although diagnosis depends upon biopsy, there are often considerable problems because any ulcerating lesion in the nose is often complicated by a marked inflammatory reaction which may obscure the underlying pathology. Multiple biopsies are thus often required before the diagnosis can be confirmed. Secondly, some of the infective disorders described above may present in a similar fashion and thus special stains and culture methods are mandatory in all cases. Similarly, malignant disorders, especially malignant lymphomas, may present in a very similar fashion. Having eliminated other conditions there remain two diseases, Wegener's granulomatosis and idiopathic midline granuloma (Stewart's type). Although both have some features in common it is essential that the disease is precisely defined because of marked differences in responses to therapy.

Wegener's granulomatosis Wegener's granulomatosis is a systemic disease in which a generalized hypersensitivity-like syndrome classically involves the kidneys, lungs and other organs as well as the upper respiratory tract. Although in the majority of patients the disease is clearly systemic from the start, there does appear to be a limited form of the disease which only involves the upper respiratory tract and thus it cannot be excluded because other organs are not involved. Nevertheless, any patient in whom the diagnosis is suspected should always have a full blood count, chest X-ray and renal function tests as an absolute minimum.

Histologically the diagnosis of Wegener's granulomatosis is dependent upon the presence of a necrotizing vasculitis, epithelioid and giant cell granulomas and a chronic inflammatory cell infiltrate. More than one biopsy may be necessary in order to obtain the characteristic findings, but once the diagnosis has been made, a good response to immunosuppressive drugs can be expected.

Idiopathic midline granuloma Idiopathic midline granuloma, is much less easy to define. Some authors believe that it is related to Wegener's, others that it is a variety of malignant lymphoma, a polymorphic reticulosis. There is recent evidence that some cases at least may represent a true malignant histiocytosis associated with jejunal villous atrophy, in other words an unusual presenting manifestation of the type of malignant lymphoma which occasionally complicates gluten-sensitive enteropathy.

In contrast to Wegener's granulomatosis, the disease appears predominantly to be localized and consists of a progressive destructive ulceration of the nose which may extend to involve the sinuses, the face, the hard palate and related structures. Untreated, it may eventually lead to the patient's death through cachexia, haemorrhage or intercurrent infection. Microscopically there is a pleomorphic cellular infiltrate, composed of lymphocytes, plasma cells and a variable proportion of large histiocytic cells, some of which may be atypical and immature. The infiltrate shows a distinct tendency to be related to blood vessels. The cellular infiltrate is accompanied by varying quantities of non-specific granulation tissue, fibrosis and necrosis, the last not necessarily related to ulceration. This histological picture tends to be much less distinctive than Wegener's granulomatosis and the diagnosis therefore tends to be confirmed by the clinical context and by exclusion. It is not yet clear whether jejunal villous atrophy (see above) is present in all cases and thus the role of jejunal biopsy has yet to be defined.

The differential diagnosis includes non-Hodgkin's lymphoma of B-cell origin—in which the infiltrate is much more uniform—and lymphomatoid granulomatosis—another rare systemic disease which is also characterized by an angiocentric destructive condition associated with a vasculitis involving both arteries and veins—which primarily affects the lungs. Midline granuloma does not respond to immunosuppressive therapy and the correct treatment is external radiation, which nevertheless is not always successful.

Tumours of the nose, nasopharynx and paranasal sinuses

Epithelial tumours of the nose and paranasal sinuses

These are listed in Table 15.3. Benign tumours in the nose apart from the unique transitional papilloma, resemble their counterparts in other tissues and thus will not be further considered here.

Table 15.3 Epithelial tumours of the nose and paranasal sinuses.

TUMOURS OF SQUAMOUS EPITHELIUM		
Benign	Squamous papilloma	
	Transitional papilloma	
malignant	Squamous carcinoma	
	Variants:	transitional
		verrucous
		spindle
TUMOURS OF SEROMUCINOUS GLANDS		
Benign	Adenoma	
	Oxyphil adenoma	
	Pleomorphic adenoma	
Malignant	Adenocarcinoma	
	Mucinous adenocarcinoma	
	Adenoid cystic carcinoma	
	Others	

Transitional papilloma The transitional or inverted papilloma, also known as the Ringertz tumour, is a polypoid neoplasm which may resemble simple inflammatory polyps, although it is usually firmer in consistency and nearly always unilateral. There is a wide age-range, but the majority occur in the fifth and sixth decades and there is a marked male preponderance.

Transitional tumours are covered by epithelium which may be columnar, or fully keratinized squamous, or an intermediate type which resembles urothelium (hence the term "transitional"). The overgrowth of the epithelium, which may contain many mitoses, is accommodated by progressive infolding into the stroma giving rise to nests of epithelium, which, in section, may have a superficial resemblance to stromal invasion but the basement membrane remains smooth and intact. Since true malignant transformation undoubtedly occurs in a few cases, but probably in less than 5 per cent, follow-up is necessary. On the other hand, recurrence after primary excision is common, occurring in over 50 per cent in most series and thus more radical excisive surgery may then be required.

Malignant tumours Carcinoma of the nose or sinuses is a relatively unusual neoplasm, accounting for less than 1 per cent of all cancers. Over half are squamous cell carcinomas which occur most commonly in the sixth decade. Most arise in the nasal cavity, but they also occur in the maxillary and ethmoidal sinuses. Histologically, squamous carcinomas resemble those in other sites, although most are well differentiated, which may explain why they remain localized for long periods.

The other types of carcinoma in the nose are more likely to arise in the posterior part of the nasal cavity. The transitional cell carcinoma resembles the epithelium of the transitional cell papilloma, although true stromal infiltration in the form of breaches of the basement membrane is always found. The majority are almost certainly malignant *ab initio* and the prognosis is somewhat better than in other forms of carcinoma with about 35 per cent surviving for five years. Anaplastic carcinoma is important because it may be confused with malignant melanoma or myeloma. Adenocarcinomas presumably arise from the mucosal glands of the nose or sinuses, especially in the ethmoid region, and a proportion are attributable to chronic occupational exposure to hardwood dusts in cabinet makers. They may be well or poorly differentiated, but there is evidence that the well differentiated tumours may have a much better prognosis than the other malignant tumours in this region.

Malignant melanomas are second only to squamous carcinoma in frequency, accounting for about a quarter of nasal malignant tumours, but are much less common in the sinuses. They are usually polypoid and may or may not be pigmented. Curiously, the normal nasal mucosa adjacent to a malignant melanoma may contain conspicuous pigmented melanocytes, but they are extremely rare in the normal population. Naevi, so common in the skin, have not been recognized in the nose. The prognosis of malignant melanoma is bad, although some patients may survive for years before finally succumbing.

Tumours resembling those in the salivary glands may also arise in the nasal mucosal glands, and once again these behave in a similar fashion to their counterparts elsewhere. It is also important to remember that tumours arising in other organs may occasionally present as metastases to the nose or sinuses, including for example the ubiquitous renal carcinoma.

Epithelial tumours of the nasopharynx

Apart from nasal obstruction, tumours of the nasopharynx may also present with Eustachian tube obstruction, cranial nerve palsy or cervical node metastases. At least 90 per cent are malignant and since surgical excision is impracticable, the principal role of the surgeon is to provide the pathologist with adequate tissue for diagnosis. The inevitable normal presence of lymphoid tissue and secondary changes attributable to ulceration, together with the difficulties experienced in biopsy of this site mean that diagnosis is not always straightforward.

About three-quarters of all tumours at this site are carcinomas. Their classification remains a matter for controversy, but that most widely used defines three subgroups: squamous carcinoma (keratinizing), non-keratinizing (transitional) and undifferentiated (lymphoepithelioma).

Squamous carcinoma and non-keratizing carcinoma resemble their counterparts in the nasal cavity and sinuses, but the undifferentiated carcinoma or lymphoepithelioma is distinctive. This tumour is composed of sheets (Regaud type) or small groups (Schmincke type) of undifferentiated cells, often with a large open or vacuolated nucleus and scanty cytoplasm, embedded in a dense lymphoid stroma. Arguments raged for many years over whether the lymphocytic component was truly neoplastic, but it is now generally accepted that the tumour is basically a variant of squamous carcinoma showing only minimal differentiation, with a pronounced lymphocytic stromal reaction. This is perhaps comparable to the medullary carcinoma with lymphoid stroma of the breast, and both tumours may retain their lymphoid stroma in metastases.

All nasopharyngeal carcinomas show a striking geographic variation in incidence. Although rare in the West (accounting for only 1 per cent of all carcinomas), in certain parts of China and South-East Asia they account for over 50 per cent of all cancers. This has been linked with high titres of antibodies to the EB virus in these populations, and thus the virus may well have an aetiological role in this neoplasm as well as Burkitt's lymphoma.

More than 50 per cent of patients may present with unilateral or bilateral cervical node enlargement, which is often mistaken for a branchial cleft cyst. Thus any patient who presents with a lump in the neck should have a full examination of the nasopharynx. In a proportion, the nasopharynx may not look abnormal and thus blind biopsies should be taken, especially from the fossa of Rosenmuller.

There are definite epidemiological differences between undifferentiated tumours and the others. They tend to occur at a younger age and show more extensive cervical node involvement, yet are more radiosensitive. Furthermore, recurrence, especially in nodes, may occur beyond four years whilst in the other tumours recurrence tends to be at the primary site and is rare beyond four years.

Staging of nose and nasopharyngeal cancer

In practice this remains essentially a clinical assessment, despite the fact that many studies have shown that histological examination of nodes provides a much better guide to prognosis.

Non-epithelial tumours of the nose, nasopharynx and paranasal sinsuses

Apart from the juvenile angiofibroma already discussed, the commonest non-epithelial tumour is the benign haemangioma, which usually presents with haemorrhage but is identical to that seen elsewhere in the body. The commonest malignant non-epithelial tumours are the non-Hodgkin's lymphomas, which may arise primarily in this region. These, too, are identical to those elsewhere and pose the same problems of classification. Also they must be distinguished histologically from the necrotizing granulomas as well as the infective lesions and lymphoepithelioma as described above.

It is important to remember that this region also contains an abundance of connective tissues, all of which may, from time to time, give rise to benign or malignant neoplasms. In general they are identical to those in other sites and should cause no particular diagnostic problems. It is also important to remember that the nose and nasopharynx may be invaded from without, craniopharyngioma and chordoma being perhaps the most important of these neoplasms.

The larynx

Hoarseness

Every patient with hoarseness of the voice for three weeks or longer has carcinoma of the larynx until proved otherwise. Three weeks is considered to be the critical period because most unimportant lesions, for example acute laryngitis and acute trauma following vocal abuse, will have resolved by then. Of course, when hoarseness lasts longer than three weeks malignancy is only one of a variety of possible causes but mirror examination of the larynx (indirect laryngoscopy) is then mandatory. Abnormalities of phonation fall into two distinct groups.

1. *A failure of the mechanics.* This may be the result of neurological disease affecting the brainstem or any part of the recurrent layrngeal nerve; of primary muscular disease, for example myasthenia laryngis; or of disturbance of the laryngeal joints, for example fixation of the crico-arytenoid joints in rheumatoid arthritis.

2. *Mucosal abnormality or mass in the larynx.* When a focal abnormality is detected in the larynx a more detailed examination by direct laryngoscopy will be necessary to establish the anatomical extent of the lesion as well as to obtain a biopsy for histological examination. Apart from true neoplasms a wide variety of other processes may present as apparent tumours of the larynx (Table 15.4).

Table 15.4 Tumour-like lesions of the larynx.

Pseudoepitheliomatous hyperplasia		
Epithelial proliferation	(a) without atypia	
	(b) with atypia	
Oncocytic lesions		
Cysts		
Intubation injury		
Polyps		
Amyloid		
Granulomas	(a) Infective	
	(b) Non-infective	(i) sarcoid
		(ii) plasma-cell
	(c) Non-healing	(i) midline
		(ii) Wegener's

Vocal cord polyps

These are amongst the commonest causes of hoarseness and are also amongst the commonest lesions in the larynx. It has long been recognized that polyps are associated with faulty voice production, hence the popular name of "singer's node". Mechanical injury to the vocal fold, following for example attempts to vocalize after full exhalation, results in vascular engorgement and oedema which are then followed by repair. The internal structure of the polyp seems to depend upon the fate of the initial exudate and the extent of new injury, but most contain dilated thin-walled vessels and hyaline stroma in variable proportions, whilst connective tissue predominates in others. They are always covered by normal respiratory or metaplastic squamous epithelium.

Macroscopically as well as microscopically they are fairly distinctive, but, rarely, other lesions such as neoplasms may masquerade as polyps and thus they should always be sent for histological examination. The main histological differential diagnoses are between granulation tissue polyps, nearly always associated with intubation or other history of trauma which should thus always be sought, and amyloidosis. Amyloid is sometimes an isolated finding in the larynx, without systemic significance, and is histologically indistinguishable from the hyaline material seen in vocal cord polyps unless special stains are used.

Laryngeal epithelial proliferation

It has long been known that benign epithelial proliferation of the larynx may subsequently be followed by the development of cancer in 3–4 per cent of cases. For a long time, as in other mucous membranes, the malignant potential was related by clinicians to the degree of keratinization present and it is keratin that causes affected mucosae to appear white, hence the term "leukoplakia". "Keratosis" is the histological counterpart of leukoplakia but neither term takes any account of the degree of dysplasia of the underlying squamous epithelium. Since keratinization, and thus leukoplakia, may occur in almost any condition from inflammatory processes to invasive malignancy, the term should probably no longer be used. The same arguments apply with equal force to the term "keratosis", but most clinicians and pathologists prefer to retain it as a non-committal term for potentially pre-malignant epithelial proliferation.

In 1963 Kleinsasser introduced a classification based solely on the degree of differentiation of the epithelium, which thus requires histological examination in all cases. The operating microscope may help to identify the correct area to biopsy, perhaps aided by toluidine blue staining, but some surgeons prefer to strip both vocal cords and submit them all to histology whenever they see any mucosal abnormality, however localized.

There are three grades of dysplasia, currently named mild, moderate and severe. These three grades are entirely comparable to those seen in the uterine cervix, and here too there is probably no fundamental difference between severe dysplasia and carcinoma-in-situ.

Mild dysplasia shows only minimal atypia and it is often not at all certain in an individual case whether the appearances represent early neoplasia or merely a reactive change. At the other end of the spectrum, the atypia is extensive with a complete (carcinoma-in-situ) or near complete (severe dysplasia) failure of the epithelium to mature towards the surface, coupled with disorderliness and loss of polarity of the prickle cells.

Many authors have shown that the risk of malignant transformation increases with the degree of dysplasia but, somewhat unexpectedly, in those cases with the severest atypia the malignant potential appears to be highest in those in which keratinization is prominent (i.e. severe dysplasia, termed "well differentiated severe dysplasia" by Hellquist and his colleagues) compared to those in which there is no maturation at all (carcinoma-in-situ).

It is important to remember that there may be severe sampling problems with lesions of this type. The pathologist can only report upon the material that he receives and thus if the clinician chooses to biopsy only part of the vocal fold it remains possible that more advanced disease is present elsewhere. Cytological examination of smears made from brushings or scrapings of the larynx (in addition to, not instead of, biopsy) may improve the accuracy of diagnosis although there are real problems in interpretation of this type of material.

The management of laryngeal dysplasia (as of cervical dysplasia) remains controversial. The traditional approach has been either radiotherapy, especially for severe dysplasia, or surgical excision of the whole abnormal area. The latter technique has the advantage of providing a conclusive biopsy for diagnosis, although it is usually not possible for the pathologist to give any indication of the completeness of the excision, however desirable that might appear on theoretical grounds. Radiotherapy has a high failure rate for non-invasive lesions but there is recent evidence that the laser is more successful and so may well prove to be the treatment of choice.

Squamous carcinoma of the larynx

This tumour accounts for about 1–2 per cent of all cancers and over 90 per cent of all laryngeal cancer. Most patients are male smokers and there appears to be a linear relationship between tobacco consumption and cancer risk, heavy smokers having 30 times the risk of non-smokers. There may also be some interaction between tobacco and alcohol, and certain occupations have a higher than expected prevalence of laryngeal cancer. Asbestos exposure is certainly the most important of these factors, but nickel may also be carcinogenic. A few patients give a history of a pre-existing proliferative lesion or keratosis, much less commonly of a papilloma or even tuberculous infection.

The old terminology of "intrinsic and extrinsic cancer" has now been abandoned in favour of a classification based upon the level of the tumour. Sixty per cent of tumours are glottic, that is to say they arise from the vocal folds and commissures. These have the most favourable prognosis for a number of reasons. Clearly, any lesion arising in the vocal fold will cause irregularity and thus present early with hoarseness. Secondly, there is no lymphatic drainage of the vocal fold, and thirdly, glottic tumours are more likely to be well differentiated. Radiotherapy can be expected to cure about 90 per cent of these early lesions.

Supraglottic and subglottic tumours are less common but have a much less favourable prognosis. This is partly because they tend to present later in their natural history, and partly because they are less well differentiated. Ulceration and excavation of these tumours is common, often leading to secondary invasion by bacteria or fungi.

Spread of all laryngeal tumours takes place by direct extension within the mucosa and submucosa. Involvement of the anterior commissure may be followed by invasion of the laryngeal cartilages, the thyro-artenoid muscles and even the skin of the neck. Tumours are particularly liable to enter the post-hyoid space, hence the necessity for removal of the hyoid bone at laryngectomy. Supra and subglottic tumours also metastasize early in lymphatics to cervical lymph nodes.

In most cases the diagnosis is quite straightforward, especially if direct laryngoscopy shows typical changes in the form of thickening, induration and ulceration of the cords, or fungating or excavating lesions elsewhere. However, the following four conditions may sometimes cause diagnostic problems.

Pseudoepitheliomatous hyperplasia This represents an irregular overgrowth of squamous epithelium with tumour-like downward extensions into the stroma, but which is nevertheless entirely benign. It may cause some problems for the pathologist, but the epithelium is always fully mature with no dysplasia, and it should usually be possible to detect the underlying cause. It is a well known response to granular cell tumours in any part of the body, including the larynx, but may also be seen in chronic inflammatory conditions, including, for example, fungal infections.

Squamous cell papilloma Two forms of squamous cell papilloma are recognized clinically, the juvenile form which is often multiple and an adult type that is usually single. They may well have a viral aetiology although this has been difficult to prove. When typical with a branching fibrovascular stalk covered by mature squamous epithelium showing focal parakeratosis, they are easily recognized. Local recurrence, often many times, is common, particularly with juvenile papillomas, but true malignant transformation is extremely rare (except following irradiation). Thus cytological atypia is not necessarily a bad prognostic sign.

Verrucous carcinoma This interesting lesion may arise on any mucosal surface covered by squamous epithelium, most commonly in the mouth, but about 10 per cent occur in the larynx. Although it only accounts for 2–3 per cent of all laryngeal cancers, it is of considerable importance because of diagnostic difficulties, especially when there is poor communication between clinicians and pathologists. To the clinician it appears as an exophytic broadly implanted fungating tumour, an appearance which is virtually diagnostic. However, especially if the biopsy is superficial, the pathologist, confronted with apparently benign keratinizing squamous epithelium, may merely diagnose keratosis or papilloma unless he is fully informed on the request form of the clinician's suspicions. With an adequate sample the histological appearances are, in fact, distinctive, often with a suprabasal palely staining band akin to that in a keratoacanthoma, covered by a thick keratin layer arranged in deeply invaginated folds, the latter being the key to the diagnosis. There is often a very well developed chronic inflammatory cell infiltrate in the underlying stroma. This tumour is locally invasive on a broad front, and thus liable to recurrence, but does not metastasize. The lesion is usually found on the vocal folds, but a histologically and behaviourally very similar tumour arising in the ventricles and typically extending into the laryngeal saccule is probably much commoner than generally appreciated, accounting for 11 of 76 unselected excised laryngeal carcinomas in a recent study. Excision is the treatment of choice since there is evidence that irradiation may actually encourage metastasis.

Spindle cell carcinoma Sometimes called a pseudosarcoma this is an unusual variant of squamous carcinoma which has a biphasic growth pattern. In addition to the ordinary squamous carcinoma component, there is a spindle cell component which closely resembles a sarcoma. When this phase is dominant the true nature of the lesion may not be apparent. However, examination of multiple sections always reveals a transition between the two elements. Despite a very anaplastic appearance, these tumours, particularly when polypoid as is often the case, have a better than expected prognosis which compares favourably with other laryngeal carcinomas. As in verrucous carcinoma, excision is the treatment of choice since radiation therapy is associated with a high local recurrence rate.

Other laryngeal lesions

Most other conditions in the larynx are rare; however it is important to be aware of their existence in order that they may be considered in the appropriate circumstances. These include the remaining non-neoplastic conditions listed in Table 15.4. Many of the granulomatous conditions are very similar to those already described in the nose. Similarly, the larynx also contains seromucinous glands and a range of connective tissues, all of which may from time to time give rise to neoplasms which may be benign or malignant as may those arising in other parts of the body.

The ear

Systematic histopathological study of whole temporal bones has led to great advances in our understanding of many diseases of the ear. However, apart from skin disease affecting the pinna, pathology plays a relatively much smaller part in the day-to-day management of disease of the ear than in the nose and throat. The main symptom is deafness, which may or may not be accompanied by pain or discharge.

Deafness

Deafness can be classified on the basis of tuning fork and audiometric tests into two fairly distinct groups.

1. *Sensorineural deafness* is due to damage to the cochlea, to the eighth cranial nerve or to the auditory pathways in the central nervous system. With the exception of nerve sheath tumours of the eighth nerve (acoustic neuroma), pathology plays almost no part in its diagnosis and management and thus it will not be considered further.

2. *Conductive deafness* is due to interruption of the passage of sound up to and including the stapedo-vestibular joint. It can usefully be subclassified into diseases of the external auditory meatus (EAM), and of the middle ear and tympanic membrane.

Wax, the normal secretion of the ceruminous glands, when produced to excess can occlude the

EAM and, indeed, is much the commonest cause of deafness in clinical practice. Foreign bodies may have an identical effect as may infection or otitis externa. The latter may be caused by a range of bacteria or fungi and thus it is important to take a specimen for culture before embarking upon specific therapy.

Aural polyps

Less commonly the patient may present with a polypoid mass in the EAM which is often accompanied by a discharge. Aural polyps may arise not only from the EAM, but may also be a consequence of middle ear disease associated with a perforation of the tympanic membrane (see below). Any condition associated with ulceration of the EAM may be followed by the development of a granulation tissue polyp. Thus impacted wax, foreign bodies or infection may all be implicated.

Tumours of the ear

Neoplasms are relatively rare, and most are of epithelial origin. As at other sites, histological section is essential for tumour diagnosis and thus all tissue removed from the ear must be sent for section. The EAM is lined by skin and thus is subject to squamous tumours and basal cell carcinomas which do not differ from those of the pinna. Squamous carcinoma is also very rarely encountered in the middle ear. When it does so it is almost always in an old mastoid cavity.

The EAM contains the wax-secreting ceruminous glands which are modified apocrine sweat glands. Tumours are rare, accounting for less than 1 in 6 of all ear tumours, and, as might be expected, have the same range of behaviour and histogenesis as salivary tumours. Since four main types can be distinguished, namely adenoma and pleomorphic adenoma, adenoidcystic carcinoma and adenocarcinoma, all of which differ greatly in their natural history, the generic term "ceruminoma" should not be used.

Chemodectoma

As with the larynx, there are a number of paraganglia related to the ear. The most constant is situated just beneath the floor of the tympanic cavity in relation to the jugular bulb, but they are also found in relation to the tympanic branch of the glossopharyngeal nerve. Any paraganglia may give rise to vascular tumours histologically identical to those seen in the larynx. Here too they are essentially benign, but they may spread extensively through pre-existing anatomical pathways, the most important of which appear to be the air-cell tracts within the temporal bone. They frequently protrude into the EAM as a reddish polypoid mass which bleeds readily, and they may also extend down the Eustachian tube even as far as the nasopharynx. In most cases, therefore, the tumour tends to grow along the line of least resistance without showing any sign of invasion of the surrounding structures. Even although they often present relatively late, the key to successful treatment is wide local excision.

Acute suppurative otitis media

Acute bacterial infection of the middle ear is a common condition in young children. The infection is most often due to pyogenic cocci and usually gains access to the middle ear along the Eustachian tube, following similar infection in the nasopharynx, for example following coryza, itself nearly always associated with negative pressure in the middle ear. Since the resulting inflammation invariably leads to occlusion of the Eustachian tube, the exudate causes a build-up of pressure within the middle ear. Untreated, this may be followed by rupture of the tympanic membrane and/or spread of the infection to neighbouring structures.

Glue-ear

The relationship of acute suppurative otitis media to glue-ear (chronic serous and mucoid otitis media) remains a matter of controversy. There is no doubt that occlusion of the Eustachian tube alone in germ-free animals can lead to goblet cell metaplasia of the mucosa, and effusion in the middle ear cleft and this is also a constant finding in patients with glue-ear. Patients with mucoid otitis media have more goblet cells than those with serous otitis media. Impaired aeration of the middle ear is thus a common factor in all patients, but the relative importance of persistent infection and diminished resistance of the patient is much less certain.

Chronic suppurative otitis media (tubo-tympanic type)

In this type of disease, which usually follows acute

suppurative otitis media, there is a large central perforation of the tympanic membrane. In some cases the mucosa becomes polypoid and may protrude through the perforation and even present at the concha. Histologically, the polyps are usually composed of chronic inflammatory granulation tissue only, but occasionally they contain cholesterol granulomas which are probably no more than an expression of previous haemorrhage in the presence of tubal obstruction.

Chronic suppurative otitis media with cholesteatoma (attico-antral type)

Cholesteatoma is a term which refers to an epidermoid cyst of the middle ear which is found most often in the attic and usually accompanied by a superior (pars flaccida) or postero-superior perforation. Histologically, it is composed of normal squamous epithelium covered by laminated keratin. The pathogenesis is another area of controversy, at least partly because diagnosis is traditionally based upon naked-eye examination only. Although secondary infection becomes a problem, it is not at all certain that infection is the cause of cholesteatoma. Thus it should probably not be regarded as a variety of otitis media although often called the attico-antral type of chronic suppurative otitis media by some clinicians. The most popular theory states that the squamous epithelium enters the middle ear by migration from the external ear. Late appearance of the perforation in many patients, however, would seem to provide support for the alternative suggestion that the epithelium arises as a result of metaplasia. Like chronic otitis media, cholesteatoma undoubtedly is correlated with tubal obstruction. Perhaps the normally flat attic epithelium is prone to squamous metaplasia as a response to injury, as distinct from the mucociliary epithelium of the meso- and hypotympanium which is prone to goblet cell metaplasia.

In addition to secondary infection, cholesteatoma is often complicated by the same type of aural polyps seen in chronic otitis media. A more serious complication is erosion of bone, mainly of the ossicular chain, which thus makes an important contribution to deafness. Most authors believe that ossicular damage is caused primarily by the accompanying subepithelial chronic inflammation, although others have experimentally produced bone resorption with squamous implants in the absence of significant inflammation.

Other inflammatory conditions of the middle ear

It is important to remember that Wegener's granuloma also involves the middle ear, again stressing the importance of sending all excised tissue for histological examination.

Otosclerosis

Otosclerosis is a common cause of conductive deafness which principally affects young adults. It has excited considerable interest because of its susceptibility to cure by surgical means. It is a disease which may affect any part of the otic capsule, but its site of predilection is the wall of the labyrinthine capsule just in front of the oval window. Nearly 10 per cent of the population can be shown at autopsy to have evidence of disease, but, fortunately, it only causes symptoms in about one tenth of these. Otosclerosis becomes significant when it extends to involve the stapes, the end result of which is nearly always ankylosis of the stapedo-vestibular joint.

Histologically, the normal compact lamellar bone is replaced by disorganized basophilic woven bone. It is initially an active process which commences with active osteoclastic resorption followed by the formation of new woven bone. The new bone completely lacks structural organization and has numerous well vascularized marrow spaces giving a sponge-like appearance on section (hence the alternative term "otospongiosis"). There is usually a sharp demarcation line between diseased and normal bone.

The aetiology and pathogenesis of otosclerosis are quite unknown. However, there are very strong similarities between the sequence of events outlined above with those encountered in Paget's disease. This too is a focal disease of bone in which subclinical involvement is much more common than overt and which causes disorganization of bone by a process of osteoclastic resorption followed by the appearance of new woven bone. Both conditions eventually enter a quiescent phase with the affected bone now thicker than before. In contrast to Paget's disease, however, otosclerosis is associated with a strong family history.

Conclusion

Histological examination or, less commonly, microbiological methods, ultimately affect the clinical outcome in comparatively few ENT patients. Nevertheless, since entities with widely diverse aetiological, pathogenetic, therapeutic and prognostic implications may be clinically indistinguishable from the common benign conditions, it is vital that the laboratory is correctly used at all times.

Further reading

Ballantyne J, Groves J (eds). *Scott-Brown's Diseases of the Ear, Nose and Throat.* London: Butterworths, 1969.

Friedmann I. *Pathology of the Ear.* Oxford: Blackwell, 1974.

Friedman I, Osborn DA. *Pathology of Granulomas and Neoplasms of the Nose and Paranasal Sinuses.* Edinburgh: Churchil-Livingstone, 1982.

Hinchcliffe R, Harrison D. *Scientific Foundations of Otolaryngology.* London: Heinemann, 1976.

Stell PM, Maran AGD. *Head and Neck Surgery.* London: Heinemann, 1978.

16

Central Nervous System

J G Brice, J S Garfield and R O Weller

Introduction

Anatomical and functional considerations preclude major resective surgery of the nervous system. This puts certain constraints upon the surgeon and pathologist and makes close clinico–pathological co-operation an essential part of daily routine. Tumours and other lesions removed from inside the skull or spinal canal are usually resected piecemeal, and it may be impossible for the pathologist to establish firm anatomical relationships between normal and abnormal tissue. It is essential, therefore, that information about the site and position of any lesion should be relayed to the pathologist together with a clear and precise clinical history. A firm understanding between pathologist and surgeon should be established so that the pathologist is aware of the requirements in speed and exactitude of diagnosis required by the surgeon, particularly during an operative procedure. The surgeon should be aware of the techniques used by the pathologist to arrive at such a diagnosis and should take care to supply tissue in an appropriately fixed or unfixed state for histological examination.

In general, neurosurgical practice is concerned with expanding or space-occupying lesions within the cranial cavity or spinal canal. The requirement for pathological opinion differs according to the nature of the lesion being treated. The histological identity of a tumour is essential for postoperative management of the patient and often for the planning of the neurosurgical procedure. Microbiological and histopathological evaluation of pus and tissue removed from infected lesions such as abscesses and encephalitic brain may also be essential for management of the patient. In some cases, however, the major role of pathology is in the post-mortem evaluation of nervous system damage as in cases of hydrocephalus, intracranial haemorrhage, head injuries and a number of spinal disorders. The experience gained by pathologist and surgeon in correlating the pathological changes in these cases with the observed clinical course is invaluable for planning the management of future cases.

This chapter concentrates first upon the general effects on the brain of space-occupying lesions trapped within the rigid confines of the skull, and secondly, reviews the clinical and pathological aspects of the major disorders which result in raised intracranial pressure. The third section covers spinal cord disorders. Finally, diagnostic procedures in non-surgical disorders are briefly mentioned; cerebral biopsy for the diagnosis of hereditary and infective disorders, or dementia, may play an important role in clinical management. Muscle and peripheral nerve biopsies are more common procedures and the precautions to be taken during these surgical operations will be covered in this section.

Raised intracranial pressure and brain displacement

Many intracranial disorders present to the surgeon because of their space-occupying nature which causes a local and general rise in intracranial pressure. The local effects of the lesion will disturb neurological function both by pressure and by the induction of oedema and vascular changes in the surrounding tissues. As the intracranial and spinal cavities are closed spaces, this local rise in pressure is rapidly transmitted to the whole cavity. The speed with which the pressure rises and the effects become clinically apparent, depends upon the nature of the lesion. Haemorrhage and haematoma formation result in a rapid rise in intracranial pressure, whereas compensatory mechanisms may operate to allow a slowly growing tumour, such as a meningioma, to reach a considerable size until ultimately these mechanisms fail and the patient develops symptoms of intracranial hypertension.

Clinical features suggesting incracranial hypertension may be any of the following:

(a) *Headache* of a novel nature, often described as vice-like, bifrontal or characteristically in the sub-occipital region.
(b) *Vomiting* which is effortless and projectile and occurs in the early morning.
(c) *Blurring of vision* due to the development of papilloedema and loss of oculomotor balance.
(d) *Deterioration in level of consciousness.* This has serious implications and if the intracranial hypertension is not effectively treated, the patient will die.

These symptoms appear with varying degrees of rapidity depending upon the basic pathology of the mass lesions, some of which will be further discussed in subsequent sections of this chapter. However, there are a number of important general pathological features of space-occupying lesions which should be discussed before specific disease processes are considered.

Once a lesion has reached a significant size and compensatory mechanisms such as displacement of cerebrospinal fluid and blood have failed, the brain itself will be displaced away from the space-occupying lesion and its surrounding oedema. A number of secondary clinical signs and symptoms may develop due to the effects of brain distortion upon parts of the brain remote from the primary pathological lesion. Many of the secondary effects are related to the anatomical arrangement within the skull whereby the intracranial cavity is divided into three compartments by folds of dura mater. The falx cerebri is in the midline and partly separates the cerebral hemispheres, whereas the tentorium cerebelli is a tent-like structure disposed in a horizontal plane separating the posterior fossa from the supratentorial region of the skull. Inferiorly, the posterior fossa is continuous with the spinal canal through the foramen magnum. A mass lesion in the left or right half of the supratentorial compartment, or in the posterior fossa, results in brain displacement into an adjacent compartment. Notably, an expanding lesion in the superior aspect of one cerebral hemisphere will produce herniation of brain tissue under the falx cerebri (subfalcine herniation of the cingulate gyrus). Large lesions, particularly in the lower parts of the cerebral hemispheres, result in the herniation of the medial portion of the temporal lobe (parahippocampal gyrus) (Fig. 16.1) through the opening in the tentorium cerebelli, a hemicircular gap which usually only admits the brain stem and a few associated structures. Such transtentorial herniation results in serious clinical manifestations, particularly as the herniation causes brain stem compression with venous infarction and haemorrhage into the sensitive midbrain region. Change in the patient's level of consciousness, and dilatation of the pupil on the same side as the mass lesion, are indicators of transtentorial herniation and midbrain compression. The pupillary signs are due to compression of the oculomotor nerve which is also compressed as it passes from the posterior fossa into the supratentorial compartment. Imaging techniques, such as arteriography, ultrasonography, CAT scanning, and ventriculography, demonstrate brain displacement, and an analysis of the degree and direction of brain shifts may be of great value in localizing and characterizing a space-occupying lesion.

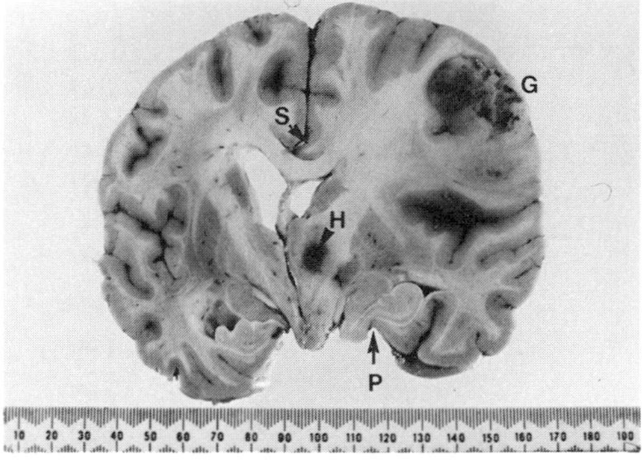

Fig. 16.1 Brain shift and herniation: A fronto-parietal glioblastoma (G) and its surrounding oedema has caused subfalcine herniation (S) and parahippocampal herniation with prominent grooving of that gyrus (P). There is mid-line shift and thalamic haemorrhage (H).

The full extent of brain damage associated with transtentorial herniation may be seen in fixed autopsy brains. Prominent grooving of the parahippocampal gyrus will be seen on the side of the expanding cerebral hemisphere lesion (Fig. 16.1) and the gyrus itself may be necrotic and infarcted. Compression of the midbrain with associated flame-shaped haemorrhages is thought to be responsible for the deterioration in conscious level. The oculomotor nerves may show haemorrhagic bands at sites where they are compressed against the edge of the tentorium during displacement of the midbrain. Another complication which is perhaps more significant if the patient survives the transtentorial herniation is compression of branches of the posterior cerebral artery as they pass over the surface of the herniated gyrus. Such compression frequently results in infarction of the temporal and occipital lobe, supplied by the posterior cerebral artery, and, most importantly, of the visual cortex on the medial aspect of the occipital lobe, resulting in an homonymous hemianopia.

An expanding lesion such as a tumour, haemorrhage or abscess in the posterior fossa may result in herniation of the cerebellar tonsils through the foramen magnum causing compression of the medulla and respiratory failure. Herniation, or coning, at the foramen magnum is a particularly severe complication of withdrawing cerebrospinal fluid at lumbar puncture in a patient who has a space-occupying lesion in the cranial cavity.

In addition to the general clinical signs and symptoms associated with the major displacement effects of space-occupying lesions, local disturbances of the brain function give rise to a variety of focal neurological signs which depend upon the position of the pathological lesion. Classical syndromes are described; for example, a meningioma arising in the floor of the anterior fossa of the skull may compress the olfactory tracts and cause bilateral anosmia; and a cerebellar abscess associated with chronic suppuration of the middle ear or mastoid may present with the rapid onset of ataxia and nystagmus. There are many other examples which depend upon the nature and the site of the lesion.

Major displacement with its accompanying complications may result from a number of intracranial lesions; these will be covered under the following headings:

(a) Intracranial tumours
(b) Intracranial abscesses
(c) Encephalitis
(d) Hydrocephalus
(e) Intracranial haemorrhage
(f) Head injury

In some cases there may be a combination of these lesions in the same patient; for example, a metastatic tumour deposit in the cerebellum and its associated oedema may be large enough in volume to obstruct the fourth ventricle, impede the flow of cerebrospinal fluid and cause hydrocephalus which then may become the major problem requiring treatment.

Intracranial tumours

Tumours arising from tissues within the cranial cavity are the sixth most common form of cancer in adults and the second commonest in children. In adults, primary tumours occur four times more frequently in the cerebral hemispheres than in the posterior fossa, whereas the ratio is reversed in children in whom primary tumours are found most commonly in the cerebellum and brain stem. Primary intracranial tumours may be classified as follows:

(a) *Tumours of neuroectodermal origin:* These include the various forms of glioma such as astrocytoma, oligodendroglioma, ependymoma, glioblastoma and medulloblastoma; they account for half of all primary intracranial tumours.
(b) *Tumours of nerve sheaths cells:* The majority are Schwannomas (neurilemmomas) that arise most commonly on the eighth cranial nerve; they account for approximately 10 per cent of primary intracranial tumours.
(c) *Tumours of meningeal origin:* Meningiomas arise from arachnoid but are usually firmly attached to dura; they account for 15 per cent of primary intracranial tumours.
(d) *Tumours of pituitary origin:* Adenomas of the anterior pituitary and craniopharyngiomas comprise 10 per cent of primary intracranial tumours.
(e) *Blood vessel tumours:* This group includes haemangioblastomas which are true tumours and arteriovenous malformations which are developmental anomalies and not tumours, although they are frequently referred to as "angiomas". Arteriovenous malformations will be discussed in relation to intracranial haemorrhage.
(f) *Pineal tumours:* These are very rare.

Many cancers metastasize to the central nervous system, notably those arising from bronchus, breast and kidney. Secondary deposits from malignant melanoma are also commonly found in the brain, and leukaemias and lymphomas are notorious for their central nervous system complications. It is difficult to estimate the true incidence of metastatic tumours in the brain, as the clinical effects of intracranial secondary deposits are often overshadowed by the complications of the primary tumour.

All the tumours listed above are of special interest to the neurosurgeon. The more common types will be described in this chapter but the major textbooks on neuropathology listed at the end of the chapter should be consulted for information regarding the less common tumours.

Glioblastoma multiforme and anaplastic astrocytoma

These tumours are often grouped together under the term "malignant glioma", and are the most frequent primary tumours encountered in the brain. They usually arise in patients over the age of 40 years and are found most commonly in the frontal and temporal lobes of the cerebral hemispheres. The cerebellum is an infrequent site for these tumours. With their rapid growth, they follow a truly malignant course, although like other neuroectodermal tumours, they very rarely metastasize or extend outside the central nervous system.

Clinically, patients present with a history of progressive neurological deficit, intellectual impairment, personality change, or epilepsy of increasing frequency over a period of six months or less. The symptomatology depends upon the site of the lesion, but eventually patients may develop the signs of raised intracranial pressure discussed previously in this chapter. Glioblastomas and anaplastic astrocytomas not only grow rapidly, but also infiltrate the surrounding brain in which they induce extensive cerebral oedema. Enlargement of the tumour and deterioration in the patient's clinical state may also occur following infarction, necrosis, and haemorrhage within the tumour. At surgery, the edges of the tumour are difficult to define as tumour cells infiltrate the surrounding brain beyond the region which is macroscopically recognizable as tumour. Infiltration along fibre pathways in the nervous system may give rise to satellite lesions and give the impression that the tumour has a multicentric origin. Frequently these tumours form an irregular grey or brown necrotic mass occupying the white and grey matter deep in the brain; the lack of a distinct margin to the tumour and its involvement of vital areas in the brain, usually preclude complete surgical extirpation. Surgical management is therefore largely palliative and directed towards relieving intracranial hypertension by partial removal of the tumour and reducing oedema by the administration of steroids such as dexamethasone. Irradiation may marginally prolong life, but even so, less than five per cent of patients survive one year after surgical treatment. This poor prognosis has led to extensive trials of chemotherapy and immunotherapy but, as yet, no effective treatment is known.

Histologically, these tumours show a wide variety of appearance. The tumour tissue is much more cellular than normal brain and many mitoses may be present. Extensive tumour cell pleomorphism may be observed; cells are bizarre in shape with large densely staining nuclei. However, in many tumours there are small rod-shaped cells which avidly infiltrate and spread through the brain tissue surrounding the tumour. Necrosis is almost always present within tumours of this group, and many abnormal blood vessels are seen. One of the most striking features is the abundant endothelial cell proliferation with redundant capillary loops forming glomeruloid structures within the tumour.

A rapid histological diagnosis can be made on smear preparations or cryostat sections of tissue removed through a burr hole biopsy or at craniotomy. Smears may be prepared by squashing a small piece of tumour between two microscope slides, fixing briefly in alcohol, and staining for a few minutes in one per cent toluidine blue. Not only can the abnormal blood vessels, so characteristic of a malignant glioma, be readily seen in this type of preparation, but detailed cytological examination of the tumour can be valuable in establishing the diagnosis within a few minutes of surgical removal of tissue from the brain.

The site of a malignant glioma may be apparent from the clinical history and from shift of a calcified pineal on skull X-ray, or from distortion of the vascular pattern on a cerebral angiogram. However, CAT scanning shows most readily the site of a malignant glial tumour, the low density area of its surrounding oedema and cystic change within the tumour. Injection of iodine-containing radio-opaque preparations, such as Conray, before the CAT scan, not only allows greater accuracy of localization of the tumour but also enhances areas within the tumour in which the blood vessels are abnormal. Conray does not enter normal brain tissue from the blood due to the presence of the blood–brain barrier. However, the abnormal blood vessels which are so prominent in histological preparations allow not only oedema fluid but also Conray to leak into the tumour and thus produce CAT scan enhancement.

Patients with malignant gliomas ultimately suffer the problems of raised intracranial pressure, brain displacement and death due to enlargement of the tumour mass, an increase in the extent of associated oedema, and cyst formation or haemorrhage within the tumour.

'Benign' astrocytoma, oligodendroglioma and ependymoma

These slowly growing tumours arise in the cerebral hemispheres of young adults, or in the brain stem and cerebellum of children. Patients present with a long history of progressive neurological deficit, epilepsy, or with a progressive rise in intracranial pressure. Histologically, the tumours are well differentiated with moderately uniform cellular populations, no necrosis, and none of the abnormal blood vessels and capillary endothelial proliferation seen in glioblastomas, or anaplastic astrocytomas. Some tumours are calcified and may be visible on skull X-ray but, in the absence of grossly abnormal blood vessels, they do not show enhancement on CAT scan. Although these tumours are often labelled as benign, they frequently give rise to fatal complications. Either they are in an inoperable position in the brain stem or deep regions of the cerebral hemispheres, or even if they are accessible to surgery, their margins cannot be defined, as the tumour cells diffusely infiltrate the surrounding brain tissues. In many cases, astrocytomas and oligodendrogliomas undergo malignant or anaplastic change, and then behave in a similar way to glioblastoma multiforme or anaplastic astrocytoma. Such malignant evolution may take ten years, or more, during which time the patient may survive following partial removal of the tumour. Ependymomas frequently arise within the cerebral ventricular system and may be complicated by obstructive hydrocephalus.

Medulloblastoma

Although these tumours only represent three per cent of all primary intracranial tumours they are of great interest to the surgeon as they are one of the most common types of malignant tumour in childhood. Medulloblastomas arise almost exclusively in the midline of the cerebellum and as they enlarge they obstruct the outflow of the cerebrospinal fluid from the fourth ventricle and hydrocephalus ensues. Local effects of the tumour produce ataxia of the lower limbs and disturbances of gait. As highly malignant tumours, medulloblastomas tend to seed widely throughout the cerebrospinal fluid pathways, and tumour cells can often be identified in cytological preparations of lumbar cerebrospinal fluid.

Histologically, medulloblastomas are composed of small cells with densely staining, slightly elongated nuclei and little cytoplasm. These tumour cells are extremely sensitive to irradiation, and treatment of medulloblastomas consists of removal of as much tumour as possible, combined with irradiation locally; irradiation of the entire neuroaxis is usually carried out at the same time to eliminate tumour that has spread away from the primary site of origin in the cerebellum. Chemotherapy has been used particularly in the management of recurrence. Five-year survival rates of 30–40 per cent have been achieved by these techniques but the outlook is poor if there is extensive tumour spread before treatment is initiated.

Schwannoma (neurilemmoma)

Schwannomas are benign tumours which probably arise from Schwan cells, and the majority grow on the eighth (acoustic) cranial nerve; they are thus frequently known as acoustic neuromas. Clinically, patients present with deafness and tinnitus, although vestibular signs and symptoms may also occur. Acoustic neuromas often cause enlargement of the internal auditory meatus, which can be detected on skull X-ray. Schwannomas are also found on the fifth, ninth and tenth cranial nerves.

At surgery, acoustic Schwannomas are firm well circumscribed tumours, occupying the cerebellopontine angle, and frequently protruding from the internal auditory meatus. Larger tumours compress the cerebellum, the middle cerebellar peduncle, and the pons, and by distorting the fourth ventricle and the basal cisterns, Schwannomas may obstruct cerebrospinal fluid flow, giving rise to hydrocephalus. The fifth cranial nerve is often stretched over the upper pole of the tumour, and the seventh (facial) nerve is usually elongated and displaced, but it may also spread out as a fan of nerve fibres over the superior and medial aspects of the Schwannoma. At this site, the facial nerve is easily damaged during surgical removal of the tumour, and preservation of this nerve presents a major challenge to the neurosurgeon.

Histologically, Schwannomas are benign tumours composed of sheets of spindle cells with elongated nuclei forming characteristic palisades (Antoni type A pattern), and loosely packed areas within the tumour (Antoni type B). Malignant change is very rare in these tumours, and surgical excision results in cure, although postoperative neurological disability may be a problem if the tumour is large.

Meningioma

Meningiomas are rarely seen in patients before the age of 30 years and, although they occur in both sexes, they are more common in older women. The clinical presentation depends upon the site of the tumour. Focal neurological deficit may be a local effect of the tumour or, in the case of large meningiomas, the patient may show signs of raised intracranial pressure. An exostosis may be seen in the bone overlying the site of the meningioma.

Essentially benign well circumscribed tumours, meningiomas arise from arachnoid cells but are usually adherent to the dura. They are found in relation to the dural venous sinuses, the falx cerebri, and on the base of the skull; as they enlarge they compress the surface of the brain, but usually remain well demarcated (Fig. 16.2).

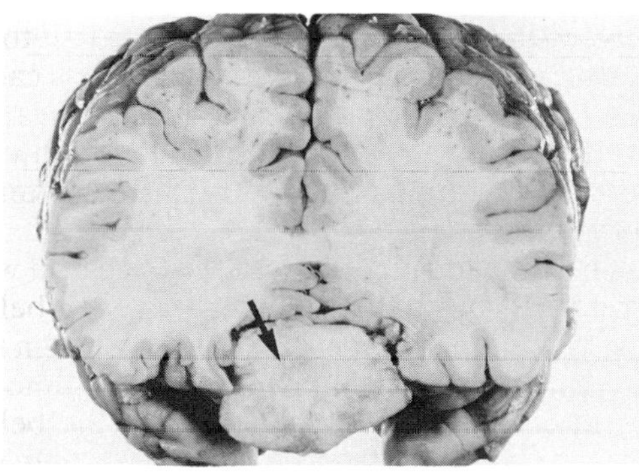

Fig. 16.2 A large subfrontal meningioma: The tumour remains well demarcated from the overlying brain although some damage to cerebral tissue has occurred due to compression by the tumour.

Although they are almost all benign in nature, meningiomas do tend to locally invade bone and induce exostoses, and they also invade the dural venous sinuses. These tendencies limit surgical excision of some of these tumours so that recurrences may occur. Most meningiomas are globular in shape, but occasionally they grow as a thick carpet of tumour on the inner aspect of the dura, particularly in relation to the lesser wing of the sphenoid bone. Such tumours are described as "meningioma en plaque".

In CAT scans, meningiomas can be localized as enhancing tumours, which may sometimes be confused with gliomas, or metastatic tumours. Histologically, meningiomas are composed of sheets or whorls of spindle-shaped cells often forming calcospherites or psammoma bodies; if gross, the calcification may be detected on radiological examination or CAT scanning. Despite their probable common origin, there is a wide degree of variation in the histology of meningiomas. These tumours can usually be distinguished from gliomas on frozen section or in smear preparations, by the presence of collagenous bands of connective tissue; a feature which is seen only in a minority of gliomas.

The majority of meningiomas can be excised completely, with a good prospect of cure, but when there is extensive invasion of bone and the venous sinuses in the dura, fragments of tumour are inevitably left in the skull. Local adherence to underlying brain tissue may cause problems in removal of the tumour and, very rarely, meningiomas show extensive invasion of brain and they even metastasize; in these latter cases the prognosis is poor.

Pituitary tumours

Adenomas and craniopharyngiomas are the two major types of tumour which arise from the pituitary, or in association with this endocrine gland in the base of the skull.

Pituitary adenomas are derived from cells in the anterior pituitary (adenohypophysis). They present, either with the effects of excessive hormone secretion or, in the case of larger tumours, with disturbance of vision due to compression of the optic nerves and chiasm overlying the pituitary fossa. Adenomas may also extend laterally into the cavernous sinuses and damage the oculomotor nerves.

Some adenomas are extremely small (microadenomas) and are hardly visible to the naked eye but, nevertheless, they may secrete excessive amounts of growth hormone to produce acromegaly, or excessive adrenocorticotrophic hormone with resulting Cushing's disease. Many adenomas secrete high levels of prolactin and patients present with infertility, amenorrhoea and galactorrhoea.

Small adenomas producing excessive amounts of hormone may not be accompanied by any enlargement of the pituitary fossa, but raised hormone levels in the serum are detected by radioimmune assay techniques and confirm the presence of pituitary abnormality. Trans-sphenoidal hypophysectomy or partial removal of a portion of the gland containing the adenoma, is a very effective way of treating hormone-producing tumours.

Large adenomas, expanding from the sella turcica and compressing the optic chiasm, result in enlargement of the sella, which can be identified radiologically. Such tumours may or may not produce excessive amounts of hormone. Surgical decompression of the optic pathways, followed by irradiation, to prevent recurrence of tumour, is the preferred treatment in these cases, as total removal of the larger tumour is rarely achieved. At operation, pituitary adenomas are soft and vascular; on rare occasions they may become infarcted, and the consequent haemorrhage and necrosis causes the mass to expand rapidly with a drastic deterioration in vision and endocrine function. This catastrophic event is known as "pituitary apoplexy" and requires urgent surgical decompression.

Histologically, pituitary adenomas are composed of cells with moderate amounts of cytoplasm, usually containing at least some secretory granules, which can be recognized either by light microscopy or by electron microscopy. In some tumours the cells are uniform in shape and size and arranged in diffuse sheets, whereas in others the cells are more variable and are arranged in groups around blood vessels. Tumour tissue can be distinguished from normal pituitary in which acidophil, basophil and chromophobe cells are gathered in small clumps. Adenoma cells are usually of only one type and their hormone secretory activity can be assessed partly by their cytoplasmic staining (either acidophil or basophil) in routine stains, or, much more reliably by immunocytochemical (immunoperoxidase) techniques which stain specifically for each hormone. The terms eosinophil, basophil, and chromophobe adenoma, do not accurately reflect hormonal secretion by these tumours.

Smear preparations may be used to rapidly identify tumour or normal pituitary tissue excised during trans-sphenoidal hypophysectomy, and may enable the surgeon to selectively remove a microadenoma.

Craniopharyngiomas are rare tumours associated with the pituitary gland, and are composed of sheets of squamous epithelial cells, possibly derived from Rathke's pouch. They are usually situated above the sella turcica and produce symptoms due to compression of the optic chiasm, in the same way as a pituitary adenoma. Compression of the hypothalamus may lead to endocrine deficiencies, obstruction of the third ventricle, and hydrocephalus. Craniopharyngiomas occur at any age, but they characteristically affect children, in whom they may produce failure of maturation and hypogonadism due to their effect on the hypothalamus. As they frequently contain foci of calcium, these tumours may be detected radiologically, and their cystic nature is often obvious on CAT scan.

Many of the tumours are cystic and are found at operation to contain an oily yellow or brown fluid rich in cholesterol crystals. The cysts are lined by squamous epithelium which resembles that seen in skin and in certain tumours of the jaw. Some craniopharyngiomas or suprasellar cysts, are lined by stratified squamous epithelium, and contain large amounts of keratin; they thus resemble epidermoid cysts. Diagnosis of craniopharyngioma is suspected if birefringent cholesterol crystals are detected in the cyst fluid, and the nature of the tumour can be confirmed, either on frozen section, or paraffin section, by the presence of the squamous element.

Total excision of craniopharyngiomas may be achieved, but may result in serious endocrine and neurological deficit. Many tumours locally invade the brain tissue of the hypothalamus. Their clinical course is variable and at times they appear to be extremely benign, but in other patients there is early recurrence and further extirpation may be difficult. There is little evidence to suggest that craniopharyngiomas are radio-sensitive.

Metastatic tumour

Most secondary tumour deposits are well circumscribed lesions which can occur anywhere in the brain. On rare occasions, metastatic tumour cells are widely distributed throughout the cerebrospinal fluid, producing "carcinomatous meningitis". Frequently metastatic deposits are multiple and may be the terminal event in carcinomatosis. In some cases, however, a solitary metastasis may be found in the subcortical white matter of the cerebral or cerebellar hemispheres, and these surgically accessible lesions may present before the site of the primary cancer has been identified.

Clinically, patients with metastatic deposits in the brain may present with epilepsy, focal neurological signs, hydrocephalus or raised intracranial pressure, due to the mass effect of the metastasis. Before embarking upon the removal, even of a solitary metastasis, it is advisable to look carefully for a primary neoplasm. Metastatic tumours enhance on CAT scan due to their lack of blood–brain barrier, and the associated brain oedema may be extensive. Steroid therapy produces dramatic relief of symptoms through reduction of peritumoral oedema.

Excision of a solitary metastasis is occasionally worthwhile in the absence of widespread neoplastic disease. The operation is relatively easy, as the tumour separates readily from the surrounding brain, and has surprisingly few vascular connections. Malignant melanoma is an exception to this last statement; it is a vascular tumour and may produce severe haemorrhage into the brain, either spontaneously or during surgical removal. CAT scans show that malignant melanoma deposits are usually multiple.

Histologic examination of post-mortem, and biopsy specimens has confirmed the sharp demarcation between tumour and the surrounding brain in most cases. In patients who have solitary metastasis and no known primary, the origin of the tumour in lung, breast, kidney, or a much less common site, may be obvious from the histology of the tumour. Not infrequently, however, the metastasis may be too poorly differentiated for a primary site to be definitely identified. Examination of the cerebrospinal fluid in cases of carcinomatous meningitis, presenting with cranial nerve root or spinal nerve root lesions, frequently reveals metastatic tumour cells whose cytological characteristics may be useful in identifying the origin of the primary tumour.

Intracranial abscesses

Pyogenic organisms may enter the cranial cavity by direct spread from infected sites in the skull, such as the middle ear cavity or paranasal sinuses, or the infection may spread from elsewhere in the body via the bloodstream. On rare occasions there may be direct implantation of organisms, particularly in penetrating head injuries. In many patients, infection results in leptomeningitis, with a diffuse spread of pus throughout the subarachnoid space. But in other cases, often depending upon the site of origin of the infection and the organisms involved, the infection is more localized and forms an abscess. Pus may collect between the dura and the skull (extradural abscess), between the dura and the arachnoid (subdural abscess), or within the cerebrum, or cerebellum, as a brain abscess.

Extradural abscess

Collection of pus at this site is uncommon and it is associated with osteomyelitis of the skull following frontal sinusitis or middle ear infection. The classical signs of osteomyelitis may be present producing the appearance known as "Pott's puffy tumour" on the surface of the head.

Subdural abscess

Pus accumulates in the subdural space over a wide area of cerebral hemisphere surface, usually as a complication of acute frontal sinusitis. Streptococci, or staphylococci, are the common organisms involved in this infection, and the pus is frequently loculated and associated with venous thrombosis and superficial infarction of cortex. Patients with this condition are severely ill with a high fever, epilepsy and often a hemiplegia. The clinical picture may be modified by previous antibiotic therapy, so that the florid clinical picture is masked and the diagnosis difficult. Drainage of pus from the subdural space may involve multiple burr holes or an extensive craniotomy. Prognosis is often poor due to the underlying cerebral oedema and venous infarction.

Brain abscess

Abscess formation within the substance of the brain occurs more frequently than subdural abscess and results from spread of infection from frontal sinuses of from sites of chronic ear suppuration. The location of the abscess is usually a good indication of the origin of the infection. Frontal abscesses are associated with sinusitis, whereas abscesses of the temporal lobe and cerebellum may complicate chronic suppurative otitis media. Blood-borne infection frequently results in multiple cerebral abscesses, often in the distribution of the middle cerebral arteries and particularly within the parietal lobes. Lung infections, particularly bronchiectasis, lung abscess, or chronic empyema, may be the origin of the infection, or septic emboli may arise from sites of bacterial endocarditis. Cyanotic congenital heart disease with a left to right shunt may allow septic emboli to bypass the lungs, and lodge in the brain, giving rise to a chronic, and often very large, brain abscess. Improved treatment of the primary sites of infection in the lung and heart, in recent times, has reduced the incidence of brain abscess arising from haematogenous spread of infected material.

Clinically, brain abscesses may present as space-occupying lesions with progressive focal neurological deficit, epilepsy and signs of raised intracranial pressure. Abscesses in the brain may be complicated by meningitis due to spread of infection to the subarachnoid space.

Pathological studies have shown that, initially, an abscess is an area of septic encephalitis and, in patients who show poor resistance to the infection, the process may spread throughout the brain. Frequently, however, the early stages of abscess formation pass unnoticed, and masked by the general illness. If the infection remains localized, and the organisms survive, pus accumulates in the area of brain necrosis, which is frequently located in the white matter. Over the succeeding two or three weeks, a fibrotic capsule forms from fibrous tissue and granulation tissue, heavily infiltrated by inflammatory cells, and starts to wall off the abscess cavity. The tough fibrous capsule of a chronic abscess, several weeks old, may be several millimetres thick and, together with its area of surrounding oedema, it is readily identified by CAT scan. With progressive enlargement of the abscess and progressive cerebral oedema, the patient may suffer brain shift and raised intracranial pressure and death may ensue. Rupture of a brain abscess into the ventricle, or on to the surface of the brain, is another serious complication; death may follow rapidly from spread of meningitis or septic ventriculitis and hydrocephalus.

Brain abscesses should be treated early, by initial drainage of the pus and by excision of the abscess capsule, to prevent the severe and fatal complications mentioned above. Frequently, brain abscesses are multilocular so that care must be taken to ensure that all pockets of pus are drained. The bacteriology of brain abscesses is very important as it provides the key to successful antibiotic therapy. Almost any organism may be found within a brain abscess cavity, but most frequently the organisms are anaerobic and include *Bacteroides fragilis* and streptococci; other organisms in abscesses may be the common inhabitants of the upper respiratory tract. Treatment with large doses of penicillin and related antibiotics form the intial therapy until the results of aerobic and anaerobic bacteriological cultures of the pus can be obtained.

Early diagnosis, drainage and intensive antibiotic therapy have reduced the mortality of this dangerous disorder.

Encephalitis

Until recently, this group of diseases was not considered to be in the province of the surgeon. However, in some cases of acute necrotizing encephalitis such as herpes simplex encephalitis, patients may present not only with seizures and focal signs of neurological disturbance, but they may exhibit drowsiness and other signs of raised intracranial pressure. With the introduction of imaging techniques such as the CAT scan, oedematous necrotic areas of encephalitic brain can be identified. They may be localized to specific areas of brain as, for example, herpes encephalitis is to the temporal lobes. The surgeon may become involved either in the biopsy of cerebral tissues for virological investigations or in a more extensive operation of decompression to relieve the raised intracranial pressure arising from widespread necrosis and oedema of the encephalitic brain.

It is essential in all cases of encephalitis in which surgical intervention is planned, that the pathologists and virologists are informed well in advance of the surgical procedure. Frozen sections of temporal lobe in herpes encephalitis will show widespread necrosis and extensive perivascular cuffing by lymphocytes and plasma cells. Viral inclusions may be detected within nuclei of neurons or glial cells, and viral antigen can be identified by immunfluorescence within the infected brain cells. Virus may be isolated from the infected brain tissue and visualized by electron-microscopy or characterized in cell culture.

Firm identification of the virus causing the encephalitis is most desirable, as anti-viral drugs such as Acyclovir are now available, especially for the treatment of herpes simplex encephalitis.

Hydrocephalus

Cerebrospinal fluid is constantly produced by the choroid plexuses in the cerebral ventricles; fluid circulates through the ventricular system and passes out into cisterns in the posterior fossa and thence over the surface of the brain, to drain mainly through the arachnoid granulations into the superior sagittal venous sinus. Impedence of the flow of cerebrospinal fluid results in hydrocephalus and dilatation of the cerebral ventricles (Fig. 16.3).

When hydrocephalus occurs in infants before the sutures of the skull have fused, the ventricles may become enormously dilated and the head enlarges. This is seen particularly in untreated children with congenital aqueduct stenosis or the Arnold–Chiari malformation associated with myelomeningocele.

Acute hydrocephalus occurs in adults when the

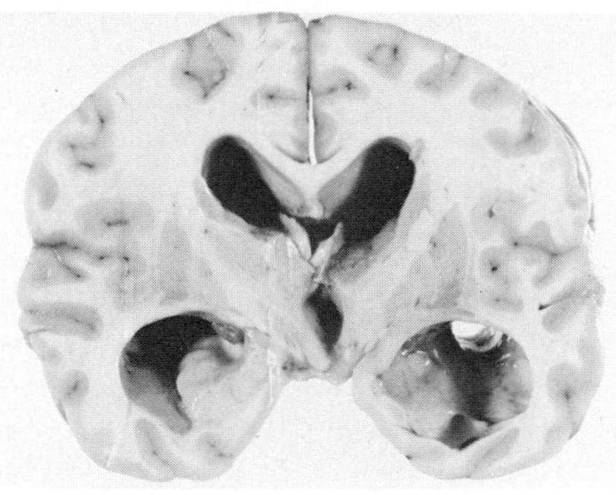

Fig. 16.3 Hydrocephalus in a 17 year-old boy following meningitis in childhood. The lateral ventricles and their temporal horns are widely dilated.

circulation of cerebrospinal fluid is blocked, particularly by tumour involving the third or fourth ventricle or the aqueduct. Such patients may present with the clinical signs of raised intracranial pressure, in addition to the neurological signs due to the local effect of such a tumour. Meningitis may also cause acute high-pressure hydrocephalus.

Low-pressure (intermittently raised pressure) hydrocephalus is a late complication which may follow head injury, subarachnoid haemorrhage or meningitis. Cerebrospinal fluid circulation is impaired by fibrosis and scarring of the subarachnoid space and of the arachnoid granulations. Patients present, clinically, with progressive dementia, incontinence and ataxia.

Pathological studies have shown that there is oedema of the periventricular white matter in the acute stages of hydrocephalus, as cerebrospinal fluid is forced into the brain tissue from the ventricles. At a later stage, the affected white matter becomes atrophic and gliotic. Intellectual function is frequently impaired in children with hydrocephalus.

CAT scanning demonstrates not only ventricular dilatation, but also periventricular oedema. Treatment of hydrocephalus by the insertion of a valve and shunt from a cerebral ventricle into the right side of the heart, or peritoneum, will be a life-saving operation in acute high-pressure hydrocephalus and a curative procedure for low-pressure hydrocephalus.

Cerebral vascular disease

Stroke

Stroke can be defined as a sudden event in which there is disturbance of central nervous system function, such as paralysis, and which is due to vascular disease. The term "cerebrovascular accident" is inappropriate and should be avoided. Although most patients with strokes are managed medically, surgical procedures may be used to prevent strokes and to treat those evolving strokes which are due to intracerebral haemorrhage. About 75 per cent of strokes are due to brain infarction, the rest are mainly due to haemorrhage into the cerebral hemispheres, brain stem or cerebellum.

oedema may result in the patient's death from raised intracranial pressure. If the infarct is in a vital area, such as the midbrain or medulla, the patient may also die soon after infarction.

Brain infarction may be due to the occlusion of a vessel by an embolus, to local thrombosis associated with an atherosclerotic plaque, or it may be due to poor perfusion during periods of hypotension, particularly in the elderly patient in shock or prolonged anaesthesia. Emboli entering the cerebral circulation may arise from thrombus in a fibrillating left atrium, on a damaged heart valve, or associated with a myocardial infarct of the left ventricle (mural thrombus). Necrotic debris or thrombus from an ulcerated athersclerotic plaque, particularly in the carotid arteries, may also form emboli giving rise to cerebral infarction. Numerous small infarcts from emboli in the cerebral circulation may produce no focal neurological signs, but may be associated with multi-infarct dementia.

In strokes, the neurological disability lasts for more than 24 hours, but in transient ischaemic attacks, the impairment of neurological function may be present for only a few minutes and has recovered by the end of the 24-hour period. Such transient ischaemic attacks are probably due to small emboli entering the cerebral circulation and occluding small vessels within the brain. An atherosclerotic carotid artery with its adherent thrombus may be the source of the emboli, and may be amenable to surgical endarterectomy or replacement of the artery by a graft. Bypass operations have also been tried whereby branches of the external carotid artery have been anastomosed with branches of the middle cerebral artery on the surface of the brain.

Intracerebral haemorrhage

Haemorrhage into the brain stem, cerebellum and cerebral hemispheres, must all be included under this heading. Frequently associated with hypertension, intracerebral haemorrhages are often the most dramatic. Clinically, the patients may present with sudden loss of consciousness due to a massive haemorrhage into the centre of one cerebral hemisphere. Neurological problems arise from the gross disruption of tissue, particularly the internal capsule and basal ganglia. The haematoma may expand into the frontal, temporal or parietal lobes and may even burst on to the surface or into the ventricles. In many cases, the haematoma acts as a massive space-occupying lesion and there is raised intracranial pressure and brain distortion with all the consequences of transtentorial herniation, brain-stem compression and death of the patient.

If the patient survives, the haemorrhage is slowly broken down by macrophages and the debris is removed. Years later, all that is left is a cystic lesion in the brain with brown or orange staining in its walls. In some cases, aspiration of a recent haemotoma may bring dramatic relief to the patient. This applies particularly to those patients who show initial improvement followed by later deterioration. Spontaneous haemorrhage into the brain stem or pons is often a catastrophic event as there are vital neurological structures in these regions and the patient rarely survives. The haemorrhage which accompanies venous infarction in the compressed midbrain in patients with space-occupying lesions in the cerebral hemispheres, has already been mentioned and should not be confused with spontaneous brain-stem haemorrhage.

Haematomas in the cerebellum act as space-occupying lesions, but they may be amenable to surgery; removal of the haematoma can be a life-saving procedure.

Subarachnoid haemorrhage

Patients with subarachnoid haemorrhage usually present with sudden severe headache and transient or prolonged loss of consciousness. Lumbar puncture reveals fresh or altered blood in the cerebrospinal fluid. Since many of the abnormalities causing subarachnoid haemorrhage can be treated surgically, this condition is of considerable interest to the surgeon.

In many patients, investigation fails to reveal the origin of the subarachnoid haemorrhage, but when the cause is found it is most frequently a ruptured berry aneurysm of the circle of Willis. Less frequent causes are arteriovenous malformation, mycotic aneurysm, bleeding diatheses or tumour.

Berry aneurysm (saccular aneurysm)

The majority of berry aneurysms are found in patients over 40 years of age and these lesions are rare in childhood. Clinically, berry aneurysms may present when they rupture and bleed, or they may present before rupture, due to the local effects of the aneurysm on surrounding neurological tissue. For example, the third cranial nerve may be compressed by an aneurysm on the posterior communicating artery, or temporal lobe epilepsy may develop in association with an aneurysm on the middle cerebral artery.

Haemorrhage from an aneurysm may be immediately fatal; of the many patients who survive, 30–40 per cent will die in the next two months from recurrent haemorrhage. Investigation by cerebral angiography will localize an aneurysm in approximately 50 per cent of patients with subarachnoid haemorrhage, and surgical intervention with clipping of the neck of the aneurysm reduces the mortality rate.

Examination of the brains of patients who die following the rupture of a berry aneurysm usually reveals an extensive, and sometimes thick, coat of fresh blood over the surface of the brain trapped between the arachnoid and the cerebral cortex or front of the brain stem (Fig. 16.4). The blood in the subarachnoid space surrounds the large cerebral arteries supplying the brain; spasm of these arteries some three or four days after subarachnoid haemorrhage may result in extensive cerebral infarction. It is not entirely clear why spasm occurs, but it may be due to the release of vasoactive pharmacological agents from the blood clot surrounding the arteries and it is certainly a severe complication of subarachnoid haemorrhage. Further examination of the arteries of the circle of Willis may reveal the aneurysm. Most are found on the anterior part of the circle of Willis and particularly on the anterior communicating artery, on the internal carotid artery (Fig. 16.5) at the origin of the posterior communicating artery, and on the middle cerebral artery as it forms its three major terminal branches. A minority of aneurysms arise from arteries in the posterior part of the circle of Willis and on the basilar and vertebral arteries. If the aneurysm is projecting into the subarachnoid space then a massive subarachnoid haemorrhage will result from its rupture. In some cases, however, an aneurysm arising from the middle cerebral artery is buried deep within the lateral fissure and its rupture may result in a mas-

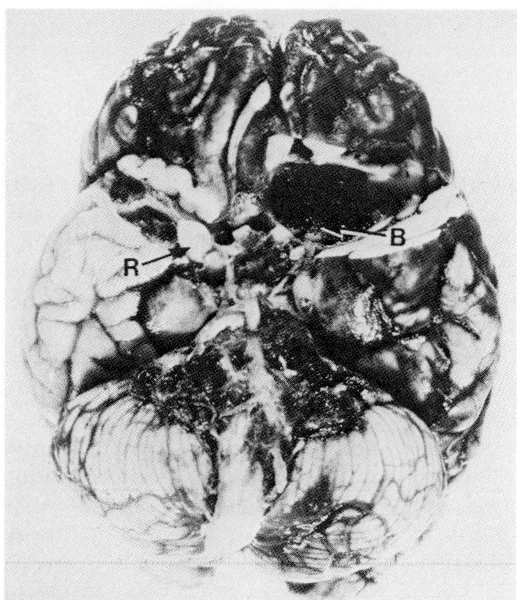

Fig. 16.4 Rupture of a berry aneurysm (B) on the left middle cerebral artery has resulted in a massive subarachnoid haemorrhage and intracerebral haemorrhage. Further berry aneurysms which have not ruptured are seen on the right (R). The temporal lobes have been resected to reveal the aneurysms and intracerebral haemorrhage.

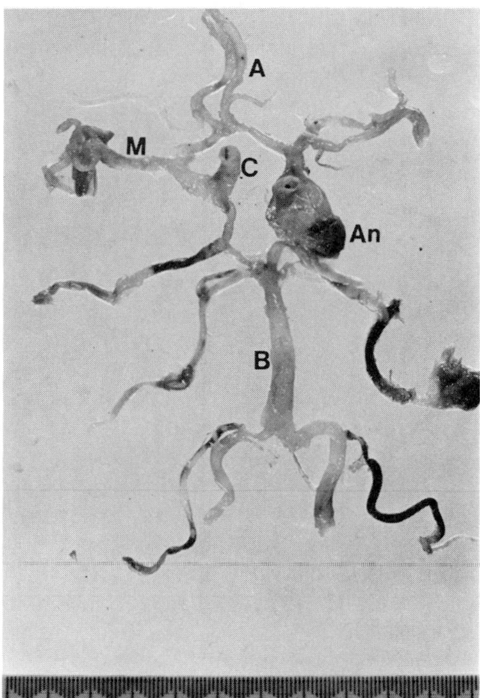

Fig. 16.5 Arteries of the circle of Willis dissected from the brain. A large (5 mm) aneurysm (An) is arising from the termination of the left carotid artery.
Labelled arteries: (A) anterior cerebral; (B) basilar; (C) right carotid; (M) right middle cerebral artery.

sive haemorrhage into the cerebral hemisphere and into the cerebral ventricles (Fig. 16.4).

Histological studies of berry aneurysms have shown that they arise as fibrous pouches from vessel bifurcations. The lack of smooth muscle and elastic tissue in the wall of an aneurysm allows it to enlarge. Aneurysms may form due to a combination of different factors. Haemodynamic stresses on the cerebral artery throughout life may well alter the shape and consistency of the arterial wall proximal to a bifurcation; aneurysms may form in those patients in whom the changes in the vessel wall enhance the haemodynamic stresses on the bifurcation itself. Hypertension does not appear to be a factor in the formation of aneurysms although it may be associated with their rupture.

Repeated haemorrhage from a berry aneurysm may be prevented by the application of a metal clip across the mouth of the aneurysmal sac. This requires meticulous dissection using an operating microscope.

A complete examination of the fixed postmortem brain will produce a record of the events that have followed rupture of the aneurysm and the subsequent distribution of the arterial haemorrhage throughout the subarachnoid space, cerebral ventricles or both. In a patient dying after clipping of an aneurysm, it is particularly important that the surgeon examine the site of operation and the position of the clip. Cerebral infarction is a complication of surgical intervention, mostly due to diffuse spasm of cerebral arteries.

Hydrocephalus may be a late complication of subarachnoid haemorrhage, probably because blood in the cerebrospinal fluid and in the arachnoid granulations result in eventual fibrosis and occlusion of the cerebrospinal fluid drainage pathways.

Arteriovenous malformations

Although less common than berry aneurysms, arteriovenous malformations may be the cause of subarachnoid or intracerebral haemorrhage. They may also present with epilepsy or with neurological deficit due to the arteriovenous malformations "stealing" blood from surrounding brain tissue. On cerebral angiography, the lesion may be visualized as a mass of abnormal blood vessels. The malformation may not be accessible to surgery if it is located deeply within a hemisphere; in such cases there is often local disruption to brain tissue, and several episodes of bleeding may result in severe disability, particularly if important neurological tracts, such as the internal capsule, are damaged. Arteriovenous malformations on the surface of a cerebral or cerebellar hemisphere may bleed and cause a subarachnoid haemorrhage, although the haemorrhage is not usually as severe as that from a berry aneurysm. At operation the malformation may be seen as a large number of interconnecting and entwined arteries and veins, extending as a wedge-shaped lesion into the white matter, and surrounding by gliotic discoloured brain showing evidence of previous haemorrhage. Veins draining the malformation may contain red, oxygenated blood confirming the presence of an arteriovenous shunt. Accessible lesions can be treated by surgical removal; the arteries supplying the abnormality are identified and ligated first, the lesion then collapses and the veins can be ligated as the malformation is removed. Deep lesions which are inaccessible to surgery have been treated by radiotherapy and embolization, but the results are uncertain.

Histological examination of an arteriovenous malformation reveals a tangled mass of vessels surrounded by scarred gliotic brain, usually containing brown haemosiderin pigment as evidence of previous haemorrhage. The scarring around an arteriovenous malformation is thought to be responsible for the associated epilepsy. Detailed examination of the vessels in the malformation reveals a mixture of large, poorly formed arteries and veins, often with fibrous walls and defective elastic laminae. Smaller vascular lesions, which may not be detected on angiography, are cavernous haemangiomas or capillary telangiectases which are structurally different from arteriovenous malformation.

Head injury

Although many patients present with minor injuries to the head and may be admitted to hospital, they present little problem to the surgeon. A far more important problem for the surgeon is serious head injury.

Broadly speaking, serious head injuries fall into two categories, depending upon how the energy of the blow has been applied to the head. Concentrated violence results in a penetrating injury which is at its most severe in the case of a high velocity missile wound to the head. If the blow is more diffuse, then the injury is described as a blunt head injury. As blunt injuries are the most common problem in civilian surgical practice, they will be considered first.

Blunt head injuries

Logical treatment of the wide variety of blunt head injuries that occur in road traffic accidents and in industry, is based upon the recognition that damage to the central nervous systems may occur in two stages: *primary brain damage* occurs at the time of the head injury and is already present by the time the surgeon first sees the patient, whereas *secondary brain damage* is the result of complications which occur following the head injury and are potentially treatable. A full understanding of the pathological mechanisms involved in primary and secondary brain damage are essential for the planning of appropriate management for each head injury patient.

Primary brain damage in blunt head injuries

Much of the energy expended upon the head during a blunt head injury results in bruising and laceration of the scalp tissues and in fracture of the underlying skull. The severity of skull fracture is often a good indication of the force applied to the head and the likely severity of the underlying, and usually much more important, brain damage.

The brain is attached to the dura, and thus to the skull, by the tenuous connection of cortical veins draining into the superior sagittal sinus, and by the carotid arteries and cranial nerves at the base of the brain. Under normal circumstances, the brain floats in its surrounding bath of cerebrospinal fluid and is buffered against injury during normal movements of the head. The sudden acceleration and deceleration of the brain incurred during blunt head injury has two main effects on the brain. Firstly, the brain is thrown against the skull and the sheets of dura forming the falx cerebri and tentorium cerebelli; this results in surface bruising and contusions with petechial haemorrhage or sometimes severe bleeding from brain tissue. Although bruising occurs on the surface of the brain at the site of injury, and thus usually under the site of fracture, the more severe contusion frequently occurs as a contrecoup lesion on the opposite side of the brain. For example, a severe blow on the occiput may cause minor contusions at the site of direct injury, but severe surface contusion of the frontal and temporal poles may result from 'cavitation' as the brain is separated from the skull on impact.

The second major type of primary brain damage which occurs in head injuries is shearing and disruption of nerve fibres and small blood vessels throughout the brain substance. A living brain is very soft and, during a head injury, swirling movements and eddies are set up, particularly within the white matter. During the very short time that the swirling movements are operating within the brain, many nerve fibres are torn, especially in the long tracts such as the corpus callosum (Fig. 16.6), cerebral peduncles and other pathways in the brain stem. In addition, small blood vessels may be torn and cause petechial haemorrhages at this time (Fig. 16.6) and blood vessels themselves may tear nerve fibre tracts; rather like pulling a piece of cotton through swirling blancmange.

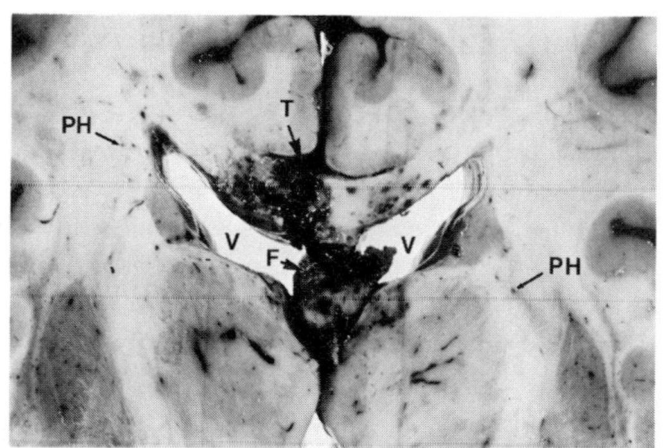

Fig. 16.6 Blunt head injury—shearing lesions occur as primary brain damage. Here the corpus callosum is torn (T); many petechial haemorrhages (PH) due to torn blood vessels are seen in the corpus callosum and in cerebral white matter. The fornix (F) is also damaged. Lateral ventricles (V).

Extensive primary brain damage occurring at the time of injury produces the familiar clinical picture of coma, fixed dilated pupils, and gross disturbance of muscle tone, power and reflex activity. Furthermore, such damage may account for much of the residual neurological deficit which follows severe head injury.

Clearly the degree of primary brain damage depends upon the severity of the injury but, as has been shown particularly in professional boxers, repeated minor head injuries may result in extensive brain damage and neurological deficit.

Secondary brain damage in blunt head injuries

The main importance of this category of damage is that the surgeon may have the opportunity to prevent or treat the lesion as all the pathological processes mentioned below develop after the primary injury. Such secondary effects of head injuries fall into two main categories: intracranial haemorrhage and brain swelling.

Intracranial haemorrhage Intracerebral haemorrhages may occur, following head injury, due to the tearing of blood vessels within the hemispheres. Only in a minority of patients are these haematomas of surgically significant size, but defects in blood clotting, as found in haemophiliacs and patients on anticoagulants, may predispose to the formation of large intracerebral haematomas. Subarachnoid haemorrhage may also result from trauma due to spread of blood from areas of contusion on the surface of the brain.

By far the most important types of intracranial haemorrhage, which follow head injuries, are subdural haematomas and extradural haematomas; these two lesions will be dealt with separately below.

Subdural haematoma By definition, a subdural haematoma is a collection of blood between the arachnoid, on the surface of the brain, and the dura mater.

Acute subdural haematomas may form soon after a head injury as bleeding occurs from contusions on the surface of the brain or from veins torn during the head injury. Blood clot forms a layer between the dura and the surface of the brain and is frequently found over the convexity of a cerebral hemisphere or under a temporal lobe. The layer of blood clot may be one or more centimetres in thickness and may reach three to four centimetres in elderly patients with atrophic brains. As the blood clot accumulates, there is a steady deterioration in the level of consciousness and the signs of brain displacement with transtentorial herniation develop. The pupil on the same side as the haematoma dilates and a hemiplegia develops on the contralateral side; these signs are due to compression of the oculomotor nerve and the cerebral peduncle as they pass through the tentorial opening on the same side as the subdural haematoma.

Surgical removal of an acute subdural haematoma at an early stage is certainly worthwhile, but the results of treatment are poor.

Chronic subdural haematomas may develop following only a minor injury, especially in older people who have some brain atrophy. The initial injury and bleeding often passes unnoticed, but a vein may be ruptured and blood slowly oozes into the subdural space. As the blood clot accumulates, it becomes adherent to the dura and starts to organize into a tough brown membrane of fibrous tissue and granulation tissue which may require stripping from the overlying dura; the membrane is usually not adherent to the underlying brain. Increase in size and thickness of the chronic subdural haematoma may occur due to repeated, minor bleeding, but absorption of fluid into the hypertonic blood clot may also result in gradual enlargement of the chronic haematoma. Clinically, the patient gradually deteriorates as the brain becomes compressed and distorted. There is a picture of headache, a varying level of consciousness and dementia. The haematoma is not uncommonly bilateral, and tends to occur in the elderly, the alcoholic and in early infancy. Aspiration of the fluid usually effects a cure.

Extradural haematoma This well known complication of head injury is the least common form of intracranial haematoma. Its importance lies in its readily recognized clinical onset and the excellent results of treatment, providing the haematoma is identified, evacuated and treated at an early stage. Since the primary brain damage is frequently not severe, there is a characteristic lucid interval between the head injury and the progressive loss of consciousness.

Extradural haematomas usually form in the temporal regions due to bleeding from a middle meningeal artery. More rarely, haematomas develop in the parietal or frontal regions or in the posterior fossa due to tearing of the walls of venous sinuses or from bleeding from diploic veins. Injury to arteries, veins or venous sinuses is usually a result of fracture of the skull bones. In the classical site of extradural haematoma in the temporal region, the middle meningeal artery and its major branches run between the dura and the bone. Following damage to the artery, the haematoma accumulates between the skull and dura probably at the time of injury or soon after. The underlying damaged brain, however, takes some hours to swell due to the accumulation of oedema fluid but with the combination of brain oedema and haematoma, the intracranial pressure rises and brain shift and distortion occurs. It is this combination of events which probably accounts for the lucid interval. Small chronic extradural haematomas may be associated with persistent focal neurological signs and epilepsy. An extradural haematoma may be readily seen on a CAT scan as a lentiform radiodense space-occupying lesion.

Brain swelling The normal weight of an adult brain is between 1200 and 1300 g but in some patients dying three to four days after a severe head injury the brain may weigh 1700 g. The extra 400 g is due to oedema fluid.

There are various causes of such massive cerebral oedema some of which are preventable; furthermore, if recognized, cerebral oedema can be treated.

Brain swelling may be a result of primary brain injury. Shearing lesions and tissue disruption result in an inflammatory reaction and oedema; fluid pours out into the damaged areas particularly during the first 24–48 hours and greatly increases the brain volume. There are also well recorded changes in the cerebral microcirculation at this time which may contribute to the brain swelling. A further cause of cerebral oedema is hypoxia and an increase in blood carbon dioxide levels due to respiratory depression, airway obstruction or chest injury. The increased capillary permeability to fluid resulting from these lesions may add significantly to the brain swelling.

As the brain increases in size, particularly around the major sites of injury, the intracranial pressure rises markedly and this may result in further brain distortion, brain stem compression and eventually a reduction of cerebral perfusion. Ultimately, the intracranial pressure may rise so high that effective blood flow to the brain ceases and the patient dies.

Penetrating head injuries

Many of the features of a blunt head injury may be present in penetrating head injuries. In addition, there is penetration of the skin, subcutaneous tissue and skull with the entry of foreign bodies, bone and possibly infection into the brain tissue. Of special importance are the high velocity missile injuries; as a bullet passes through the brain it leaves a track surrounded by a wide sleeve of necrotic and haemorrhagic brain tissue. Pressure waves within the brain may result in tissue damage even more remote from the missile track. In general, transverse injuries of the brain are more severe than longitudinal injuries. However, much depends upon the energy transferred from the missile to the brain. In high velocity injuries, the brain and skull may almost explode and little treatment is possible. Low velocity missiles, on the other hand, may ricochet off the skull and re-enter the brain and cause further damage.

The role of pathology in the management of head injuries

Much of the information available to the surgeon regarding brain damage in head injuries has come from careful clinicopathological documentation and from experimental studies. If a surgeon is to plan the appropriate management for head injury patients, there is no substitute for a direct visual appreciation of the types of brain damage which result from head injuries. Such observation will aid the understanding of the differences between primary brain damage and potentially treatable secondary brain damage. Furthermore, it may be realized that the same lesions that have had such a devastating effect in the brain of those who die as the result of a head injury, are frequently present, albeit to a lesser degree, in the brains of those patients who survive.

Disorders of the spinal cord

Disorders of the spinal cord which concern the surgeon usually present with varying degrees of paraplegia and tetraplegia; the onset of the neurological disability may be acute or slowly progressive. There are many similarities between the pathology of the brain and of the spinal cord and the major categories which will be considered here are those of trauma, neoplasia, and congenital disorders.

Spinal cord trauma

The spinal cord may be damaged in flexion, extension and rotational injuries to the vertebral column. This type of injury usually affects the cervical and thoracic spine, whereas compression injuries with crushing of vertebrae are usually seen in the lumbar region. As in the brain, there is primary damage to the spinal cord at the time of injury; it may be crushed or stretched and partial or complete transection of the cord may occur. Secondary damage to the cord may follow due to compression from an extradural haematoma or from bony fragments penetrating the cord from damaged vertebrae. Extensive swelling of the cord, due to the outflow of inflammatory oedema fluid into regions of contusion and laceration, may follow a spinal injury. Such swelling may impair the circulation of the cord and cause further haemorrhage and infarction, particularly in the central part of the cord. Penetrating injuries may introduce infection into the damaged area.

As in the brain, no effective regeneration of nerve fibres occurs in the spinal cord so that axons distal to the site of injury degenerate and as the damaged tissue is removed by macrophages, the injured region is transformed into a cyst and the distal part of the cord becomes atrophic.

Cervical spondylosis and intervertebral disc lesions

The spinal cord may be damaged by osteophytes and enlarged intervertebral joints in patients with cervical spondylosis. In addition, emerging nerve roots may be compressed. Similar problems arise, particularly in the lumbar region, following intervertebral disc protrusion. Surgical decompression or fusion of cervical intervertebral joints may arrest the neurological damage, and relieve symptoms, if the disase of the spine is localized.

Spinal tumours

Tumours affecting spinal cord function can be divided into different categories based on the anatomical site and the origin of the neoplasm.

Extradural tumours

Numerically, extradural tumours are the commonest forms of cancer which affect the spinal cord. Tumours may arise in the bone of the vertebral column or may grow in the extradural space. In both these cases the tumours are usually metastatic, spreading from breast, bronchus, prostate, kidney or thyroid. Frequently the patient has a history of a primary tumour and the pathology of specimens taken at laminectomy for decompression of the cord will confirm the presence of a known tumour. Occasionally, however, no primary site has been discovered and the spinal lesion may be of primary diagnostic importance. This is particularly so with lymphomas which may infiltrate extradural fat and cause paraplegia from cord compression in the absence of evidence of widespread disease. Characterization of lymphomas, for example myeloma, follicular lymphoma, etc., is essential if appropriate chemotherapy and irradiation treatment is to be given to the patient. Fresh tissue is required for this characterization so it is advisable to inform the pathologist prior to the operation on an unidentified extradural tumour.

Rarely, primary tumours such as osteoblastoma, giant cell tumours of bone, and chordoma, compress the spinal cord or cauda equina. Once the pathological character of the tumour is known, the appropriate treatment by surgical decompression, radiation, chemotherapy, or a combination of all of these methods, may be instituted.

Extramedullary intradural tumours

This group of tumours offers the most satisfactory

prospects for treatment by the surgeon. They are almost entirely benign tumours and include meningiomas and Schwannomas and surgical removal results in a cure. Occasionally, a lipoma, or dermoid cyst may present in the spinal canal and is often associated with a congenital abnormality of the spine.

Intramedullary tumours

Most tumours arising within the cord itself are gliomas, but intramedullary tumours form the rarest group of all tumours in the spine. Unlike those gliomas arising in the cranial cavity, well differentiated slowly growing gliomas are the commonest form of tumour in the spinal cord. Astrocytomas may cause significant enlargement of the spinal cord as may ependymomas which also spread within the subarachnoid space. Glioblastoma multiforme is a rare tumour in this site, and metastatic carcinoma is only occasionally found within the cord. Spread of medulloblastoma from the cerebellum, or diffuse involvement of the cord by carcinomatous meningitis may also occur. Specimens of cerebrospinal fluid may contain free-floating cells from metastatic carcinoma or medulloblastoma, but rarely can cells from the more benign tumours be detected in the cerebrospinal fluid. Myelography or whole body CAT scan may be used to investigate the extent of the intrinsic cord lesion, and although resection is usually not possible, small fragments of tissue may be obtained at laminectomy and must be treated with extreme care if a tissue diagnosis is to be obtained.

Occasionally, enterogenous cysts, lipomas and epidermoid cysts present as intrinsic tumours in the cord. Surgical removal of intrinsic cord tumours is difficult, but with microscope techniques, total removal of tumour may be achieved in a small proportion of cases.

Congenital disorders of the spinal cord

The central nervous system develops from ectoderm on the dorsal aspect of the embryo. By two weeks of gestation in the human embryo, the neural tube has become established and has closed by four weeks. The developing spinal cord is submerged within the embryo and surrounded by mesoderm which forms the bony structures of the spine and the muscles of the back. If the process of neural tube closure is arrested at an early stage of development, the vertebrae fail to develop properly and spina bifida results. This congenital lesion may occur throughout the spine but is most commonly found in the lumbar region. In its least severe form, spinal bifida occulta, the failure of fusion of the neutral arch may not be apparent externally. Underlying developmental abnormalities of the spinal cord are known by the general term of "spinal dysraphism" and are usually associated with progressive weakness and muscle wasting in the lower limbs and poor control of sphincter function. Surgical intervention with division of fibrous bands of adhesion at the lower end of the spinal cord may result in some improvement.

More serious abnormalities are present in spina bifida cystica, of which myelomeningocoele is the most common variety. Children presnt at birth with a cystic swelling, often confined to the lumbar region, and sometimes covered with skin. In its most severe form, the flattened spinal cord is exposed on the surface, whereas in those lesions covered by skin, the spinal cord tissue and nerve roots may be firmly bound to the deep aspects of the cyst wall. Tissue removed from the sac wall during surgical closure of the myelomeiningocoele defect, should be examined histologically for the presence of neural elements. Myelomeningocoeles are associated with a severe defect of motor function in the legs and approximately half the patients have an associated Arnold–Chiari malformation and hydrocephalus.

Meningocoeles are much less common and the covering of the lumbar sac contains no neural tissue; this type of cystic swelling may be associated with a lipoma of the cauda equina and filum terminale. There is usually little neurological defect with a meninogocoele and the lesion may be repaired with reconstruction of normal anatomical layers.

Diagnostic procedures in non-surgical disorders

The surgeon may be asked to perform a purely diagnostic biopsy, particularly in cases of peripheral neuropathy, muscle disease, and hereditary or dementing disorders of the central nervous system. As the whole purpose of removing the tissue is not therapeutic but diagnostic, the pathologist should play a major role in advising the surgeon on the nature of the tissue required and on the biopsy procedure.

Muscle biopsy

With modern histological and histochemical techniques, muscle biopsy has now become a valuable adjunct to the diagnosis of muscle disease. Biopsies can be taken under local anaesthesia as long as precautions are taken not to infiltrate the muscle with the local anaesthetic, or to use diathermy near the site of biopsy. As an irritable tissue, muscle tends to contract readily if traumatized; a suitable biopsy, therefore, is taken with as little injury to the muscle as possible. A piece of muscle for histochemistry and a futher piece for electron microscopy, usually taken in a clamp or attached to a piece of swab stick, are all that is usually required. On some occasions, however, specimens are taken and snap frozen for biochemical estimations. Muscle tissue for histochemistry is taken fresh to the laboratory, and frozen in liquid nitrogen; histochemical techniques applied to cryostat sections will aid the pathologist in classifying the type and severity of the muscle disease. Specimens for electron microscopy are fixed immediately in glutaraldehyde; they are attached to a clamp or a piece of swab stick prior to removal from the patient in order that the muscle fibres should not go into contracture as they come into contact with the fixative.

Peripheral nerve biopsy

Peripheral nerves are extremely delicate and can easily be damaged by inappropriate handling. Even touching the nerve with a swab may cause irreparable damage to the tissue and impede histological evaluation. Carefully taken lengths of nerve are fixed in glutaraldehyde and later prepared for teasing and for light and electron microscopy.

Cerebral biopsy

Although infrequently performed, cerebral biopsy may be the essential diagnostic procedure in a number of different neurological disorders. If a biopsy is performed, adequate specimens of cortex and white matter should be taken to allow for reasonable histological study.

Conclusion

The importance of pathology of the nervous system for the practising surgeon lies in three main areas. First, and most obvious, is the histopathological diagnosis of tumours and other lesions biopsied or removed at surgery. Second is attaining the full understanding of the range and anatomy of pathological lesions in the brain that is necessary for the interpretation of powerful new imaging techniques such as radiology, CAT scanning and nuclear magnetic resonance.

Third, and probably most important, is the part that pathology plays in demonstrating to the surgeon those changes that occur in diseased brain which are not visualized by imaging techniques. As already emphasized, the management of head injuries especially relies heavily upon a clear appreciation of the range of pathological damage in the patient's brain.

Further reading

Neuropathology and neurosurgery

Adams JH, Graham DI, Doyle D. *Brain Biopsy: The smear technique for neurosurgical biopsies*. London: Chapman and Hall, 1981.

Adams JH, Corsellis JAN, Duchen LW (eds). *Greenfield's Neuropathology*, 4th edn. London: Edward Arnold, 1984.

Jennet WB. *An Introduction to Neurosurgery*. London: Heinemann, 1975.

Northfield DWC. *Surgery of the Central Nervous System*. Oxford: Blackwell Scientific, 1973.

Russell DS, Rubinstein LJ. *Pathology of Tumours of the Nervous System*, 4th edn. London: Edward Arnold, 1977.

Weller RO. *A Color Atlas of Neuropathology*. Oxford: Harvey Miller and Oxford University Press, 1984.

Weller RO, Swash M, McLellan DL, Scholtz CL. *Clinical Neuropathology*. Berlin: Springer, 1983.

Muscle and nerve biopsy

Swash M, Schwartz MS. *Neuromuscular Diseases: A practical approach to diagnosis and management*. Berlin: Springer, 1981.

Weller RO, Cervos-Navarro J. *Pathology of Peripheral Nerves*. London: Butterworth, 1977.

17

The Skin

P S Boulter and N M Gibbs

Introduction

The skin is the largest organ of the human body. It is exposed to the stresses of normal life and subject to insult from physical and chemical trauma. A wealth of primary, degenerative, inflammatory and neoplastic conditions occur and it is a frequent site for secondary manifestations of disease. These, as will be seen, include metastases from distant primary tumours. Also the skin may present abnormalities which represent cutaneous markers of visceral disease. In the interpretation of skin disease there is need for very close collaboration between the surgeon, the dermatologist and the histopathologist. Since the skin is a frequent site for infection, there is also considerable microbiological and virological interest.

The majority of cutaneous irregularities are of little importance. Warts, most naevi in children and adults, and the seborrhoeic keratoses and other marks of ageing, are blemishes which need cause no alarm. Action is thus indicated only on cosmetic grounds. Amidst the multitude of unimportant lesions is a minority which are, or may become, malignant. The warning sign of danger is always alteration in appearance. Increase in area or thickness, change in pigmentation or the development of ulceration can never be ignored. If the patient thinks that something has changed he is usually right and clinical and histological assessment will be required.

Treatment is often dictated by histopathological findings. Wherever possible skin lesions should be excised rather than biopsied. Curettage should be avoided in lesions of uncertain origin. Vascular lesions may not be detected unless the whole thickness of the dermis, the epidermis, and sometimes subcutaneous tissue, is included in the biopsy.

The technique of biopsy

In order to give the histopathologist a chance of providing essential diagnostic information, tissue biopsy should be reasonably generous in size and should include a representative sample of the lesion if total excision is not possible. In the skin, the knife is the essential instrument for biopsy: diathermy excision can produce gross thermal distortion which can serve to confuse the histological appearance.

The successful histological interpretation of a skin biopsy depends firstly on the adequacy of tissue sampling and secondly on accurate clinical information relating to the size, distribution and multiplicity of lesions. Finally, the histopathologist may need to see the lesion for himself prior to biopsy or a good colour photograph.

Where disease is widespread, such as in bullous conditions, typical lesions should be sampled—preferably early rather than gross ones so that tissue relationships are preserved. In some dermatological conditions, immunofluorescent tests will be performed in addition to examination using traditional histological stains and it is particularly important for the surgeon to know how the pathologist wants the specimen to arrive. Formol fixation, admirable in some circumstances may be disastrous when immunochemical tests are being done. Before taking a specimen it is always advisable to ascertain whether fresh or formalin-fixed specimens are wanted and there may, of course, be indications for the use of special fixatives.

When the surgeon is carrying out a biopsy of a pigmented skin lesion, excision should include any flare when present.

Cutaneous manifestations of visceral disease

Metabolic diseases may present with skin manifestations. Jaundice is an obvious example and here pathological aid to diagnosis will be biochemical rather than histological. This applies also to the cutaneous manifestations of thyroid disease and xanthomata of long-standing diabetes and other rarer metabolic diseases. The clinical recognition of xanthomata may call for the service of a clinical biochemist and electrophoresis of blood lipids may enable abnormalities of lipid metabolism to be categorized.

Cutaneous manifestations of visceral neoplasms

Bowen's disease often occurs in skin of areas unexposed to sunlight and is occasionally associated with the presence of visceral carcinomata. Multiple sebaceous adenomas of the face and scalp may be associated with visceral carcinomas, particularly those of the colon. Telangiectasis of blood vessels of the skin occurs in carcinoma of the breast and certain sarcomata, and direct invasion of the skin by underlying cancers from any organs may occur. Carcinoma of the pancreas may produce subcuticular nodular necrosis.

Metastatic deposits in the skin may be the first indication of deeper malignancy. Tumours of the lung, breast, ovary and kidney may sometimes have very silent primary lesions and the clinical diagnosis may be facilitated by appropriate biopsy of a suspicious skin lesion. Acanthosis nigricans may be the first presentation of carcinoma of the stomach. In each of these situations, clinical recognition and pathological confirmation go hand in hand.

Purpura

Many systemic conditions are associated with purpura which of course may have very serious implications signifying systemic disease of the haemopoietic organs. Infection such as meningococcal septicaemia in children is associated with purpura and thrombocytopenia is an important cause with surgical significance. In elderly people, loss of skin elasticity may occur and purpura will be accompanied by skin haemorrhage. It can be found also in Cushing's syndrome and from excessive steroid administration. When ulceration is present in addition to purpura, an inflammatory vasculitis is likely and this may be due to infective processes or to the collagen diseases such as polyarteritis nodosa or systemic lupus erythematosis. Skin haemorrhages in bacterial endocarditis may be embolic, or the result of an inflammatory vasculitis. When there are no absolutely clear-cut diagnostic features, combined investigation by physician, haematologist and histopathologist may be indicated and here the surgeon may play a valuable part in procuring specimens for examination. These should be taken from areas where reasonably discrete lesions on the non-dependant areas of the body will give a better chance of making a diagnosis than in dependant areas which tend to have more complicated and confluent lesions and where healing of even a small biopsy wound may be impaired.

The surgeon's help is often required when bullous lesions occur. Typical areas should always be chosen and tissue fluid samples for immunological and virological tests should be taken.

Inflammatory skin diseases

The dermis and epidermis are continuous with the mucosal layers of the alimentary canal, and lesions present in the skin may mirror lesions occurring in the intestinal tract. Lichen planus and herpes simplex can involve the skin, the mouth and the genitalia. The cutaneous manifestation associated with ulcerative colitis and Crohn's disease are well known and here biopsy may be an essential part of the investigation. There is a very substantial grey area in inflammatory skin disease. Chronic processes with bullous formation may occur with epidermolysis—as in erythema multiforme and lupus erythematosis—but in some cases acantholysis will indicate pemphigus. Viral diseases such as herpes simplex or herpes zoster can be identified exactly by ctyological examination of blister fluid, together with indirect immunofluorescence tests. Sometimes, antibodies to plasma proteins may be noted and of course infection such as staphylococcal, streptococcal and fungal infections can be diagnosed by taking the right specimens under the correct conditions and seeing that they are comprehensively examined in the pathological laboratory.

Non-bullous inflammatory lesions have many aetiological factors and provide a large part of the work of the dermatologist. The distribution of the lesions and the history, together with exposure to chemical agents, will often facilitate the diagnosis. Examination of parings of nail and skin are often vital. Some diseases are great rarities in one country but common in others: anthrax is a good example of this, where occupational exposure to wool and similar substances may induce infection, which in the skin often has a very insidious course.

The surgeon may be called on to aid in the diagnosis of lesions which occur in special sites. Mucocutaneous junctions are often of great importance. Herpes simplex commonly involves the lips—the classical cold sore—but cracks at the angle of the mouth complicate bacterial infections at all ages and moniliasis in the debilitated and the elderly. Solar exposure, tobacco and alcohol may produce keratoses and these may progress to squamous carcinoma. Mucoceles and salivary adenoma occur on the lip and the pigmented spots of the Peutz–Jegher syndrome are well known. It may not be easy by inspection to determine the exact cause of a lesion on the lips and biopsy is required.

Genital herpes is an increasingly common condition with premalignant significance in the female. *In situ* squamous carcinoma of the glans penis and prepuce (Queyrat's erythroplasia) has a histological resemblence to Bowen's disease, but a marker of visceral cancer. The benign condition of hidradenoma papilliferum, a condition of the vulva, may be confused, both clinically and histologically, with a metastasis from endometrial carcinoma.

The perianal skin is accident-prone and Crohn's disease produces giant cell granulomas which may be the first sign of this disease, but similar lesions occur in erythema nodosum. Extramammary Paget's disease is a known producer of symptomless red, raised and rather moist patches, and only careful histological examination of skin biopsies will allow of diagnosis. Warts can occur anywhere, but the condylomata caused by the human papilloma virus occurs in homosexuals, who incidentally have an increased incidence of rectal cancer. This, of course, means that examination of the perianal skin is incomplete without rectal examination and proctosigmoidoscopy, with the taking of appropriate mucosal, as well as cutaneous, samples.

The hands and soles of the feet are not common places for tumours but keratoacanthoma, apocrine carcinoma and melanoma can all occur. Benign cellular naevi are much more frequent and usually show junctional change. The nail beds are a known site of melanoma, but commoner by far is the pigmentation associated with trauma and infection such as that by *Bacillus pyocyaneus* and certain fungi. The taking of an appropriate nail specimen under ring-block anaesthesia is sometimes needed and when a specimen is taken it should not be consigned into fixative for histological examination alone, the collaboration of the microbiologist should be sought so that valuable diagnostic material is not wasted.

Any area of the skin can produce epidermoid cysts containing the characteristic degenerate amorphous squames with a gruel-like consistency, often foul smelling, and prone to secondary infection. Pilar cysts are rather different. They are found mostly on the head and neck but have a solid content often rather brownish in colour, occasionally associated with calcification and with a much lower risk of infection which, when it occurs, is usually the result of trauma. Careful excision biopsy is both diagnostic and curative.

Scars

Multiple scars may be the result of previous infection and surgery but may arise as the result of steroid administration, Cushing's syndrome and the rarer congenital defects such as the Ehler's–Danlos syndrome. Depressed scars are often left by the self-limiting benign cutaneous tumour known as keratoacanthoma or molluscum sebaceum. Radiation in any part of the body will lead to cutaneous atrophy with alteration in skin pigmentation and may precede the development of radiation dermatitis and basal or squamous carcinomata. Pigmentation occurs in radiation scarring and may arouse the suspicion of melanoma. Lower dosage radiation tends to lead to basal cell carcinoma and higher dosage will produce more intense change and a greater incidence of squamous carcinoma with its attendant risk of distant lymphatic metastases. Endometriosis, implantation dermoids, keloids and granulomas occur in scars and may be delayed in their appearance. There is always an indication for biopsy in any skin lesion in which progression is observed.

Skin tumours

The surface of the body teems with excrescences. The overwhelming majority of these are entirely benign. There is, however, a second group which represent unstable lesions having a potential for malignant change and finally, of course, there is frank malignancy. Some of these lesions are very obvious. The common viral wart is frequent, especially in childhood, and often multiple. Diagnosis is seldom a problem and most are self-curing. There are naevi of all varieties: some smooth, some warty, many containing enlarged hair follicles and an appreciable number may be pigmented.

Some pigmented lesions have a halo and this does not by any means always indicate the presence or future risk of malignancy.

Pigmented lesions

The presence of black or brown pigmentation in lesions arouses more concern than is pathologically justified. Many epidermal naevi are pigmented and sometimes haemangiomata have pigmentation especially during their phase of regression. The raised blue naevus, a dermal lesion, grows during childhood and unless removed will stay unchanged through life.

The vascular lesion often incorrectly referred to as a 'juvenile melanoma' is a spindle cell self-limiting benign tumour. The main object in making an exact diagnosis in pigmented lesions is to identify and treat melanomata for reasons of safety and to remove unsightly but benign lesions for cosmetic reasons.

There should be some caution about the interpretation of pigmentation in a lesion. Hypertrophic sebaceous keratoses change from pink to a brown colour by ingraining with dirt.

Yellow lesions include spiroadenoma, xanthelasma and sebaceous adenoma. Histiocytomata are often rather yellow in their cut surface, but the external appearance is usually of white or dull red colour.

Calcification

This is seen in some skin lesions, such as scars, acne, pilar cysts and pilomatrixoma. This latter lesion is the commonest calcified skin lesion in children but it can occur anywhere on the body surface at any age. Gouty tophi are recognizable and biochemical investigation will confirm the nature of the lesion without recourse to histology.

Ulceration

This may be a worrying and unpleasant phenomenon and chronic gravitational ulcers and certain granulomata break down; lupus vulgaris and gumma are important in this connection, also the pseudocarcinomatous hyperplasia of epidermoid cysts.

Lesions which bleed also produce alarm and from more sinister ones must be separated pyogenic granuloma which is a very vascular papilloma usually associated with subpapillary staphylococcal infection. This lesion may last for many weeks and can enlarge spectacularly, simulating in its appearance that of some malignant tumours, though the rapid growth tempo and evil smell of a pyogenic granuloma are characteristic.

Most skin lesions are not painful, but when marked tenderness is a clinical feature, glomus tumours, pilar leiomyoma and eccrine spiroadenomas should be thought of.

It can be seen, therefore, that in many benign skin lesions, cosmetic reasons, discomfort, discharge or bleeding may be an indication for surgical excision.

Premalignant dermatoses

Solar keratosis

This is a consequence of ultraviolet damage to the skin with alteration of collagen formation with thickening. While most of these lesions do not undergo malignant change, basal cell and invasive squamous carcinoma may supervene occasionally.

Radiation dermatitis

Therapeutic and accidental exposure to ionizing radiation may lead to skin atrophy and telangiectasia. When radiation dosage has been low, basal cell carcinoma may arise, and when more excessive, squamous cell tumours occur and may go on doing so many years after the exposure. Chronic inflammatory ulcers may be premalignant. Tropical sores, lupus vulgaris and Marjolin's ulcer, together with the heat-induced lesions of Kangri cancer, are all examples of this.

Leukoplakia

This is a lesion characterized by a white thickening of the epidermis and is a precursor of squamous carcinoma in the lips and genital areas. Increase of thickness and fissuring are all warning signs in this condition. Not all lesions of white appearance are luekoplakic. Lichen planus and the cutaneous lesions of moniliasis may be confusing: biopsy, either by incision or the examination of surface scrapings, may be necessary.

Arsenical keratoses

These are often multiple, having a long-term tendency to undergo multifocal malignant change and are a dramatic example of chemically induced precancerous lesions which may also result from tar and other hydrocarbons.

Naevi

Some naevi are precancerous and these, together with Hutchinson's freckle, will be discussed separately.

Bowen's disease, Paget's disease, Queyrat's erythroplasia and the intradermal epithelioma of Jadassohn

These are all examples of very superficial tumours which strictly speaking are *in situ* malignancy rather than merely premalignant.

These conditions can only be properly managed if a biopsy is performed with interpretation of the histological appearance. Considerable surface extent may make excisional biopsy unnecessarily mutilating and incisional biopsy is both effective and safe. This is especially important as the proper treatment is often by radiation or the use of local chemotherapy.

Malignant skin tumours

Basal cell carcinoma (BCC) or 'rodent ulcer'

Rodent ulcer is a name which should be forgotten as this tumour does not necessarily ulcerate, though it is always locally invasive. Men are more often affected than women and the disease is uncommon under the age of 50. It is often very slow-growing and, unless bone or cartilage is involved, there is usually no pain. Only superficial discharge or disfigurement will make the patient seek medical attention. Metastases have been recorded but are exceptionally rare.

Site

Basal cell carcinomas can arise anywhere on the body especially in areas exposed to the sun such as the face, scalp and neck, with the inner canthus, the eyelids and the temple particularly common sites. The hands, forearm, back and upper chest are also affected. These areas are most often involved in white people in hot climates, such as Australians and South Africans. In Britain there is an occupational incidence in agricultural workers and fishermen. An exception to this generalization is that of the naevoid basal carcinoma syndrome (multiple BCC, jaw cysts and bifid ribs). Histologically, this form cannot be distinguished from the ordinary tumour.

Clinical features

In its earliest stage BCC usually presents as a firm papule which is little different from the surrounding healthy skin. Some lesions appear, however, as thinning of the skin with a pink atrophic area. Both of these types are followed by ulceration and extension both deeply and laterally when the characteristic rolled pearly edge become apparent. Pigmentation is not uncommon and the presence of haemosiderin and melanin in a lesion showing ulceration and crusting will mimic superficial spreading melanoma.

Histopathology

Basal cell carcinoma arises in the epidermis or the hair follicles and is composed of cells that resemble the basal cells of the epidermis. Histologically, there are three variants: the superficial multicentric type is slow-growing and often appears on the trunk; the morphoeic variety has strands of cells producing a desmoplastic reaction, and these tumours have a greater tendency to progress and to recur after treatment; the third or fibroepithelial type is characterized by an elevated tumour with stromal islands divided by cords of basal cells and is the least aggressive form. Recurrent BCC may show squamous characteristics and then have a higher invasive potential, and it is in these that metastases have been reported.

Diagnosis

The clinical diagnosis is often obvious and the histopathological confirmation in small lesions should be made by excisional biopsy with a lateral margin of 3 or 4 mm. The full thickness of the skin and the superficial part of the subcutaneous tissue should be taken. Excision satisfactorily combines investigation and treatment. When the tumour is in an awkward situation or is extensive in area or depth, then incisional biopsy is perfectly proper and has no danger. Paradoxically, the more extensive and advanced is the lesion, the easier it is to obtain a histological diagnosis on the first outpatient visit, as excisional procedures usually require both planning and refined technique.

Treatment

Small BCC should be excised as described above but larger lesions, and those in special sites such as the eyelid, will require the next stage of decision, that is between surgery and radiation therapy.

Surgery This is indicated when the tumour has extended down to cartilage or bone, and it is also desirable if a patient is to be exposed to very cold climates and if there is difficulty in follow-up. The problem of the larger lesion is reconstruction, which may be by free graft (with either split or full thickness skin) or by local flaps. Ideally, the choice of treatment should be by joint decision between surgeon, dermatologist and radiotherapist, each provided with a histological diagnosis. There is one absolute indication for surgery, and that is disease recurrent after irradiation.

Radiotherapy The majority of BCC are radiosensitive. With radiotherapy, hospital admission and general anaesthesia can be avoided in patients who are often elderly or infirm.

Other treatments In countries where BCC is common, other treatments have been tried. Some are outpatient procedures practised by dermatologists and include (a) curettage; (b) cryosurgery; (c) laser therapy; and (d) local chemotherapy using 5 Fluorouracil cream. Local recurrence is more common, but in very early disease and in those unfortunates who have multiple BCC, less radical therapies are justifiable, but careful follow-up is needed.

Basisquamous carcinoma

This entity is uncommon. It occasionally occurs *de novo*, but is more common when tumours have recurred after irradiation or superficial chemotherapy. The tumour grows more rapidly, ulcerates earlier and may metastasize.

Treatment, either by surgery or radiotherapy, should be to a wider area and follow-up should be even more careful.

Squamous cell carcinoma (SCC)

This is in a different category of danger. The SCC grows more rapidly, is liable to metastasize to the regional lymph nodes and shows considerable clinical and histological variation.

Aetiology

Squamous cell carcinoma seldom happens in previously normal and unirritated skin. There are a number of antecedent conditions. These include (a) tars and oils which lead to the development of a chemical dermatitis; (b) arsenic which may be followed after many years by keratoses which progress to cancer; (c) radiation of all sorts succeeded by dermatitis and keratotic change; and (d) chronic irritation which may be bizarre, such as the continued use of heat, for example the Kangri cancer found in people in Himalayan countries who use a portable warming pan under their clothes. This never-forgotten rarity is much less common than the SCC which arise following recurrent inflammatory change around scars and sinuses associated with tuberculosis and tropical ulcers. Irritation from tobacco, smoked or chewed, leads to lesions around the mouth and lips. Here, and in the genitalia, the condition of leucoplakia may be a precursor. Finally, most of the premalignant dermatoses described previously, such as Bowen's disease, may progress to SCC. It need hardly be emphasized that early recognition, histological diagnosis and treatment of predisposing lesions will prevent malignant transformers.

Site

Any area of the skin can be affected depending upon the site of action of carcinogens. The aggression manifested by this tumour varies somewhat with its aetiology and metastases are least common when ultraviolet radiation is the underlying cause and most frequent after chemical insult.

Diagnosis

Biopsy is essential in these lesions and may be achieved by limited incision, superficial curettage or cytological methods. Local factors and availability of resources will often dictate the choice between irradiation and surgical treatment, but therapy will require to be more radical than in BCC. Lymph nodes must be watched and treated when indicated.

Pathology

Squamous cell carcinoma arises from the squamous epithelium of the epidermis and forms a warty tumour sometimes with a central keratin plug. Keratinization is characterized histologically by the presence of epithelial pearls and intercellular bridges. In less differentiated forms, these characteristics become less obvious and more rapidly growing tumours will have a spindle-celled infiltrating form which may even resemble the cellular appearance of connective tissue sarcoma.

Treatment

A number of factors will effect the choice of treatment and many of these are common to those previously described in BCC. Whether surgery or radiotherapy is chosen will depend upon the same local factors as have been described above. Both methods have their advantages, though it is possible to be dogmatic about squamous carcinoma metastatic to regional lymph nodes where surgery should always be chosen.

Tumours and lesions of the melanogenic system

The commonest of all pigmented tumours is the pigmented naevus. While all pigmented lesions cause worry, the chance of malignancy is very small indeed except in the uncommon giant pigmented naevus which is followed by melanoma in a high proportion of patients.

Blue naevus

This is formed by collections of dendritic melanocytes in the dermis. It is usually small and most commonly occurs on the face, the forearms and hands. The cellular blue naevus is an uncommon tumour in which melanocytes are more numerous and extension into subcutaneous tissue is a feature.

Precancerous melanosis

This includes a group of pigmented skin disorders where dysplastic melanocytes recur in the basal and superficial layers of the epidermis. Hutchinson's melanotic freckle (lentigo maligna) is found characteristically in solar-damaged facial skin in the elderly. A similar condition—more dangerous and variable in site and occurring in younger patients—is known as Pagetoid melanoma. Both these precursor lesions should be regarded as melanoma *in situ*.

Melanoma

This disease is becoming universally more common. In the United Kingdom there has been a steep rise in registration of melanomas. There is increased exposure to ultraviolet light with modern clothing and sunbathing and tropical holidays are risk factors. It is not suprising that in Australia, South Africa and the USA, this disease is much more frequently found in white-skinned people. The closer to the equator, the greater is the chance of fair-skinned people developing the disease. Conversely, there is no such increase in incidence in dark-skinned residents. Ultraviolet radiation is thought to be becoming more intense over much of the world's surface because the ozone barrier which serves to protect us from ultraviolet radiation is believed to be damaged by chemical pollution at very high altitudes.

Pathology

Melanoma virtually always arises at the epidermodermal junction and is associated with pre-existing naevi in approximately 10 per cent of cases. Partial regression is not unusual, but complete regression is rare. This may be a demonstration of immunocompetence, as any degree of regression is characterized by heavy lymphocytic infiltrate and this may be seen in excised melanomata. Melanomata can occur at any age but are rare in childhood, seldom reported before puberty and become commoner with advancing age. They may be flat or raised, sessile or pedunculated and arise not only on the skin but on mucosal surfaces such as the vagina, anal canal, rectum and mouth.

They occur in the protected situation of the nail bed and, uncommonly, on the sole of the foot, though strangely this site is commoner in black races. Skin pigmentation provides protection, but incidence increases in albinism and strikingly so in xerodermia pigmentosum.

Melanoma may arise in previously normal skin, but may be preceded by Hutchinson's freckle or naevi.

Types of melanoma

Four distinct varieties are described.

Melanoma arising in lentigo maligna (LMM) This tumour has probably the best prognosis of all melanomas and is most common on the face of elderly people. It may be recognized by increase in area, but more often by change in the surface of a lentigo with ulceration or increase in thickness. Lentigo is never palpable. If the sensitive finger can detect alteration in thickness then invasive change is likely.

Superficial spreading melanoma (SSM) This is the commonest variety; in this condition change in previous junctional naevi may be noted—concern being aroused by increase in area, variation in pigmentation, crusting, discharge or bleeding. Superficial spreading melanoma is a condition more frequent in young and middle-aged adults. It lies intermediate in malignancy between SSM and those melanomata of greater thickness.

Nodular melanoma (NM) This is the most sinister melanoma. It grows more quickly, rises further above the surface and correspondingly invades deeper with a greater chance of metastasis. While most melanomata are pigmented, nodular tumours—possibly by virtue of more rapid growth with corresponding failure of melanin maturation—often have pale or totally amelanotic areas.

Melanomas of mucosal surfaces (MMS) These are singularly evil lesions by virtue of their rate of growth and also because their site of origin often precludes early recognition and their routes of metastasis make surgical inoperability likely. The mouth, vagina and rectum are the commonest sites.

Diagnosis

The diagnosis of melanoma is essentially a matter of clinical acumen, but must be confirmed histologically. Where a suspect lesion is small, excisional biopsy with a margin of 3 or 4 mm is atraumatic, and when excision is complete will provide specimen which can be assessed by the histopathologist. Most important of all is the assessment of depth and this, as will be seen later, is the most important index of prognosis. Frozen-section diagnosis can of course be used, but in a small lesion recognition of histological pattern may not be easy and the finer points of histopathological diagnosis, such as change at the edge of a naevus, may be difficult. A frozen-section specimen often prevents depth assessment and the whole of a limited lesion may be used up in this process. Excision biopsy with paraffin section is to be preferred.

In the past incisional biopsy has been condemned, but this is perfectly reasonable in thicker lesions. A locally removed specimen of the surface will confirm the diagnosis and justify radical treatment. Histological diagnosis is mandatory before embarking on extirpative surgery to rid the patient of melanoma.

Prognostic variables in cutaneous melanoma

These include clinical features such as rapidity of growth, the sex of a patient (the prognosis is poorer in males), the anatomical site of the lesion, whether ulceration has occurred and whether there are depigmented areas within the tumour. Clinical and histological type of tumour, the presence or absence of lymphocytic infiltration and the existence of satellites or distant metastases, are significant, as is the number of mitoses seen. The area of the tumour is less important than the depth.

Depth of melanoma Allen and Spitz recognized that dermal and subcutaneous invasion were related to prognosis. Clark divided the skin into a series of layers—the epidermis (level 1), dermal invasion into the papillary dermis (level 2) to junction of papillary and reticular dermis (level 3). Level 4 is invasion of the reticular dermis, and level 5 is subcutaneous infiltration. By this staging, prognosis can be predicted. Breslow has correlated risk with actual tumour thickness. Lesions under 0.75 mm have virtually no tendency to metastasis, while increasing thickness is matched by decreasing prognosis. Lesions over 3 mm in depth are overwhelmingly followed by metastatic disease. It is important, therefore, for the removed surgical specimen to be given to the histologist as soon as possible so that accurate depth measurements can be made. Depth is not only a prognostic index, but a guide to prophylactic block dissection and other adjuvant therapy.

Management of metastatic disease

If lymph-node invasion is noted at the time of diagnosis, then elective block dissection is indicated. Decisions about the extent of excision of a melanoma and the desirability of prophylactic block dissection are influenced by clinical and histological features. In general, shallower lesions have less chance of metastasis, longer survival and justify wider excision more than thicker lesions with their increased metastatic rate and poorer life expectancy. Tumours extending to Clark's level 4 or Breslow's 2 mm are those in which lymphatic metastasis is more likely to occur. Prophylactic block dissection in these deeper-extending melanomas becomes more logical, though with increasing lymphatic spread comes greater likelihood of haematogenous metastasis.

Metastatic patterns in melanoma There may be satellites in the skin and subcutaneous tissues, lympathic vessel and node involvement, and haematogenous spread to the brain, lung and abdominal organs. The liver is frequently involved and melanoma shows a particular affinity to the mucosa of the proximal small bowel.

Adjuvant therapy This is disappointing. Radiation may produce diminution in size of both primary and secondary melanomas, but is not reliable enough to commend it as a form of primary therapy. Drugs such as phenylalanine mustard and vindesine can be given either systemically or by isolated limb perfusion. Combination chemotherapy using the more drastic agents such as DTIC and BCNU has been disappointing and associated with unpleasant side effects.

Conclusion

There is no single skin condition in which the accurate collaboration of surgeon and pathologist is more essential than in melanoma. The interpretation of biopsies is a key to the nature of the lesion and augments clinical opinion. Histological assessment of the depth of the tumour has emerged as the most important prognostic parameter other than the observed presence of metastatic disease. It is the guide to choice of excisional area, the use of prophylactic lymph-node dissection and may in the future indicate a place for chemotherapy.

Rarer primary skin tumours

Basal cell carcinoma, squamous cell carcinoma and melanoma constitute the overwhelming majority of skin cancers. Nodular dermatofibrosarcoma is the most common connective tissue tumour. It may arise from pre-existing dermatofibroma or *de novo*. It seldom metastasizes and has a slow rate of growth. Excision biopsy is usually required to differentiate it from benign dermatofibroma. Malignant histiocytoma is rarer. It arises from the skin or subcutaneous tissue. Excisional biopsy followed by histological examination is important as this lesion has a tendency to metastasize both to lymph nodes and viscera.

Reticuloses affect the skin. Lymphosarcoma and reticulum-cell sarcoma being more frequent than Hodgkin's disease and the leukaemias. Occasionally the presenting lesion is in the skin, but systemic disease often produces skin manifestations. Mycosis fungoidies is a cutaneous disease from the start and systemic change a secondary phenomenon. Biopsy is usually invaluable in producing the diagnosis, though haematological studies may help.

Kaposi's sarcoma, a cutaneous malignancy affecting skin capillaries and perivascular tissues, produces multiple purple circumscribed lesions which may ulcerate. The course is variable, there is spontaneous disappearance of some of the patches and systemic involvement is common.

Metastatic disease

As many cancers progress, skin nodules may appear and their nature is often very obvious. Tumours of the breast, the thyroid, the kidney and some gastrointestinal lesions may produce skin metastases. Peri-umbilical skin infiltration is a late feature in cancer of the stomach and pancreas. Visceral malignancy, especially carcinoma of the bronchus, may make its first clinical appearance by skin nodules. Histological confirmation of the nature of an expanding bizarre skin lesion may initiate a search for primary tumour, though with the necessary proviso that early skin metastasis even from a small primary is of dire significance. After histological confirmation, systemic treatment by chemotherapy or local treatment by radiotherapy is the only way in which the patient may be helped.

Conclusion

As we stated at the beginning, the skin has a multitude of diseases of its own and acts as a surface indicator of many metabolic and visceral conditions. The surgeon will find that his closest ally is the histopathologist but biochemistry, microbiology, virology and immunology may help in diagnosis, management and assessment of prognosis.

Further reading

The literature on skin disease is extensive. The reader is directed to the following text books where reference is given to papers on special aspects of skin pathology.

Ariel IM. *Melanoma*. New York: Appleton-Centry-Crofts, 1981.

Hadfield GJ and Hobsley M. *Current Surgical Practice*, Vol I 1976. Chapter on 'Skin Tumours' by P. S. Boulter.

Levene, GM, and Calnan, CD. *Colour Atlas of Dermatology*. London: Wolfe Medical Publications, Ltd., 1973.

Lever, WF. *Histopathology of the Skin*. Pitmans Ltd., 1975.

Rooke A, Wilkinson DS, Ebling FJG. *Text Book of Dermatology*. Oxford: Blackwell Scientific Publications, 1979.

18

Soft Tissue Tumours

B T Jackson and J R Tighe

Introduction

Many benign soft tissue swellings, such as the ubiquitous lipoma or subcutaneous neurofibroma are common, present an easy clinical diagnosis, require little or no investigation and are simple to manage by either local surgical excision or mere reassurance to the patient. Other benign soft tissue swellings, however, such as nodular fasciitis, may be erroneously diagnosed and treated by the clinician as malignant, while true malignant soft tissue tumours are often badly managed due to a poor understanding by the surgeon of their pathology. It is therefore important for all surgeons to be aware of the many pitfalls in diagnosis and management of these tumours, just as all pathologists should be aware of the importance of close collaboration with the surgeon before offering a definitive opinion on the pathological specimens received.

Pathological classification

Unfortunately, the distinction between true soft tissue tumours and other tumour-like lesions, including hamartomas and reactive proliferation of connective tissues, cannot always be established clinically or by macroscopic examination of the excised specimen. Microscopic assessment is essential. Any useful classification should therefore cover both true tumours and tumour-like lesions.

Soft tissue tumours may be defined as those arising from non-epithelial extraskeletal connective tissue, excepting the lymphoreticular system and neuroglia. Most are mesodermal but some are neuroectodermal in origin. Their pathological classification is complex and controversial and, despite several revisions in recent years, there is still not universal agreement. Table 18.1 should therefore be regarded as a guide rather than a definitive statement. From the surgeons point of view, however, the importance is to distinguish tumour-like lesions from true tumours, and benign tumours from malignant. The minutiae of classification beyond this are relatively unimportant because the principles of diagnosis and treatment are similar within each group.

Clinical presentations

Depending on the anatomical site of origin, soft tissue tumours and tumour-like lesions usually present as a swelling which may be both easily observed and easily palpable. Tumours arising within body cavities may produce symptoms and signs of displacement, compression or obstruction of neighbouring viscera. Rarely, hypoglycaemia may be caused, especially by tumours of the retroperitoneum. The mechanism of this is unknown. The duration of history is sometimes surprisingly long even in the case of malignant tumours, for not all soft tissue sarcomas are fast-growing. In general, however, sarcomas are rapidly growing, in which case the history will be short and the swelling often painful. Palpation then may demonstrate an increase in overlying skin temperature cause, by vascularity of the tumour and, on occasion, pulsation may be felt. Inspection may show dilated veins overlying the swelling.

The criteria by which the clinical diagnosis of a soft tissue tumour is made is by the history of localized swelling of increasing size and by careful clinical examination which demonstrates that the swelling is solid and arising in mesenchymal tissue. By assessment of its relation to skin, muscle or bone, the anatomical plane from which the tumour arises may often be determined, although this is by no means always possible with certainty. Imaging techniques may be necessary to demonstrate this.

It is unusual for a patient to present with clinical symptoms or signs from metastatic spread of a soft

Table 18.1 Classification of soft tissue tumours.

Tumour-like lesions of fibrous tissue ('pseudotumours')		
Nodular fasciitis		
Keloid		
Elastofibroma		
Proliferative myositis		
Fibromatoses		
Palmar, plantar and penile fibromatoses		
Abdominal wall, extra-abdominal and intra-abdominal fibromatoses (desmoid tumours)		
Fibrous proliferations of infancy and childhood		
Tumours and tumour-like lesions of known histogenesis		
SITE	BENIGN	MALIGNANT
Adipose tissue	Lipoma	Liposarcoma
Fibrous tissue		Fibrosarcoma
Fibrous histiocytes	Fibrous histiocytoma Atypical fibroxanthoma Giant cell tumour of tendon sheath Juvenile xanthogranuloma	Malignant fibrous histiocytoma
Muscle	Leiomyoma Rhabdomyoma	Leiomyosarcoma Rhabdomyosarcoma
Blood vessels and lymphatics	Haemangioma Glomus tumour	Haemangiosarcoma
	Haemangiopericytoma	Haemangiopericytoma
	Lymphangioma	Lymphangiosarcoma
Synovial tissues		Synovial sarcoma
Mesothelium	Fibrous plaque Adenomatoid tumour	Mesothelioma
Neural origin	Neurofibroma Neurilemmoma Granular cell myoblastoma	Neurofibrosarcoma
	Ganglioneuroma Paraganglioma	Neuroblastoma Ganglioneuroblastoma
Tumours of uncertain histogenesis		
		Kaposi's sarcoma Clear cell sarcoma Epithelioid sarcoma Alveolar soft part sarcoma

tissue sarcoma. Such spread is typically blood-borne to the lungs and is normally asymptomatic until after the primary tumour has presented.

Pathology

Tumour-like lesions of fibrous tissue ("pseudotumours")

These lesions may be slow-growing but can increase rapidly in size. This feature, together with their capacity to infiltrate, may falsely give an impression of a malignant tumour. They may be safely treated by local excision, however, as they never metastasize and rarely recur. The two most important conditions in this category are nodular fasciitis and keloid. Less common than these are elastofibroma and proliferative myositis.

Nodular fasciitis

Nodular fasciitis is a lesion of uncertain aetiology which presents most often in the upper limbs and trunk of young adults. It can easily be mistaken for a sarcoma, as the history is normally short and the lesion fast-growing and often tender. It is sometimes called a pseudosarcoma. In published series, up to 36 per cent have been initially wrongly diagnosed as being a malignant tumour. In fact, the lesion is benign and may be treated by local excision. Histologically, it shows fibrous tissue often infiltrating muscle and containing chronic inflammatory cells.

Keloid

Keloid is a common proliferative lesion occurring in a previous scar. It is more common in black races and there appears to be a relationship between the development of keloid scars and uterine fibromyomata. The lesion affects the collagen in the dermis which forms thick hyaline bands. There is a tendency to recur after excision which may be reduced by cutaneous radiotherapy or intradermal steroids. Keloid should be distinguished from the more common hypertrophic scar which does not spread into surrounding tissues and regresses spontaneously over the course of several months.

Elastofibroma

This is a rare lesion that occurs most often in the scapular region of the middle-aged and elderly. It is usually firm and ill-defined with a slow rate of growth but may be bound down to surrounding structures. The lesion is benign and may be safely treated by local excision.

Proliferative myositis

Like nodular fasciitis, proliferative myositis is a rapidly growing lesion which can also be confused with a sarcoma. It involves skeletal muscle, especially of the upper limbs, and tends to occur in middle age. It is thought to be reactive to injury and is cured by local excision.

Fibromatoses

The term fibromatosis is applied to lesions which show fibroblastic proliferation with infiltration of surrounding tissues. These lesions differ from the previous fibrous proliferations because they are much more liable to recur after excision but they do not metastasize. In this respect they have a behaviour intermediate between that of a fibroma and a fibrosarcoma.

Palmar, plantar and penile fibromatoses

Palmar fibromatosis is well known as *Dupuytren's contracture*. There is an association with other diseases, particularly alcoholic cirrhosis, diabetes mellitus and epilepsy. The lesion usually starts as a firm nodule, but progresses to thickening of the palmar fascia with dimpling of the skin and eventual contractures. *Plantar fibromatosis* is a similar condition affecting the sole of the foot.

Penile fibromatosis (*Peyronie's disease*) may occur in association with palmar and plantar fibromatosis. It affects the dorso-lateral aspect of the penis involving particularly the corpus cavernosum. It leads to abnormal curvature of the penis and may cause pain on erection and intercourse.

Abdominal wall, extra-abdominal and intra-abdominal fibromatoses (desmoid tumours)

Although desmoid tumours are most commonly associated with the abdominal wall in women of child-bearing age, similar lesions may occur elsewhere in the body, particularly the chest wall, shoulder region and thigh. They present as a firm indurated mass of mature fibrous tissue which infiltrates and destroys skeletal muscle. These fibromatoses are notoriously difficult to excise and often show persistent local recurrence.

Although similar to the abdominal wall and extra-abdominal fibromatoses, *intra-abdominal fibromatosis* is worthy of special mention because it may be associated with sebaceous cysts, intestinal polyposis and osteomata in Gardner's syndrome, a condition which is inherited as an autosomal dominant trait with variable expression. Intra-abdominal fibromatoses may also occur after colonic resection and are found in the omentum, the mesentery or in the retro-peritoneal tissues. They are similar to other desmoid tumours in that local recurrence after excision is common.

Fibrous proliferations peculiar to infancy and childhood

Although children may be affected by fibrous proliferations similar to those found in adults, there are certain lesions which are found almost exclusively in childhood.

Fibrous hamartoma of infancy grows usually in the first year of life and is found most commonly in the axilla. The mass is usually superficial in the skin or immediate subcutaneous tissues and rarely involves neighbouring muscle. This lesion differs from other fibromatoses in that recurrence is unlikely to occur after surgical excision.

Infantile digital fibromatosis occurs on the fingers and toes and may be single or multiple. It is usually poorly circumscribed and extends from the skin into the underlying tissues. It frequently recurs after excision, but if left often undergoes spontaneous regression.

Fibromatosis colli is a lesion which develops in the sternocleidomastoid muscle in the early weeks of life and leads to wryneck. The aetiology is uncertain, although there is often a history of forceps delivery or breech delivery which must raise the possibility of a traumatic origin. The lower part of the muscle is replaced by fibrous tissue which continues to grow for up to two years and then undergoes spontaneous regression.

Infantile myofibromatosis may be single or multiple and occurs in the newborn. The nodules appear to consist of proliferating myofibroblasts and occur anywhere in the soft tissues or in the skeleton. When the lesions affect internal organs such as the lung, heart and intestine, there may be interference with vital function, but in other sites the prognosis is good as spontaneous regression occurs during ensuing months.

Tumours and tumour-like lesions of known histogenesis

These are more common and more easily recognized than the preceding fibrous proliferations. The distinction between benign tumours and hamartomas is not always satisfactory or useful and they are therefore best grouped together.

Tumours of adipose tissue

Lipomas are so common that they barely justify description. They may be single or multiple, small or large, situated in subcutaneous tissue or in deep tissues between fascial planes. Lipomas of the retroperitoneum are often very large while visceral lipomas may produce symptoms of obstruction, as with endobronchial or intestinal lipomas. They consist of mature adipose tissue which is usually soft and surrounded by a thin fibrous capsule. However, variants of this pattern are common. Some tumours are mixed with strands of collagen (*fibrolipomas*) and some have a mucoid consistency (*myxolipomas*). The latter must be distinguished from myxoid liposarcomas. *Angiolipomas* occur mainly in the subcutaneous tissues where they may present as painful tender masses. Other variants are the so-called *spindle cell lipomas* and the *pleomorphic lipoma*. In both of these tumours there is a danger of misdiagnosis of a liposarcoma, but the clinical history of a circumscribed tumour which has been present for several years, together with the histological features, should indicate the benign nature. Local excision is adequate for all types.

Angiomyolipomas are hamartomas which occur particularly in relationship with the kidney. The tumours may reach the size of a large grapefruit and can give rise to symptoms suggestive of a renal carcinoma. They tend to be found at a younger age, however, and the histological pattern of a mixture of smooth muscle, blood vessels and adipose tissue is characteristic. There is an association with tuberose sclerosis. In spite of its large size and sometimes worrying histological appearances, it is benign.

A benign tumour of brown fat is known as a *hibernoma*. These tumours, which occur particularly in adults, are usually found in the interscapular region. They are slow-growing, well defined and soft in consistency. The colour is usually light brown. Histologically, they have typical granular cells of brown fat.

Liposarcomas are the most common of the soft tissue sarcomas. They occur in adults with a peak incidence in the sixth decade and vary considerably in their degree of malignancy as well as in size. They are commonly sited in the limbs, especially the thigh, and the retroperitoneum. The behaviour of the tumour can be predicted from its histological appearances. The latter allows subdivision into four main types: well differentiated, myxoid, round cell and pleomorphic. All four types commonly recur locally after excision, but the myxoid and well differentiated types are less likely to metastasize than are the round cell and pleomorphic types. Over 50 per cent of patients with the round cell and pleomorphic type develop metastases within five years. Metastases are almost always haematogenous, principally to the lungs. The site of origin of the tumour also affects prognosis: those that arise in the retroperitoneal tissues have a worse prognosis than those that arise in the limbs.

Tumours of fibrous tissue

In recent years there has been an appreciable change in terminology of many soft tissue tumours and this applies particularly to those which are predominantly fibrous in nature. In the past these were loosely grouped together as fibroma and fibrosarcoma, but it is now appreciated that these terms have been used to cover a number of different tumours.

The term *fibroma* is now rarely used unless qualified, *viz.* neurofibroma, ovarian fibroma. Most lesions which in the past have been called fibromas are now recognized as being reactive fibrous proliferations and not true tumours. Likewise, the term *fibrosarcoma* is now used much more selectively. Conditions which in the past have been classified as fibrosarcoma have included leiomyosarcomas, malignant fibrous histiocytomas and malignant Schwannomas. True fibrosarcomas can occur at all ages and in all sites. They vary considerably in size. Although the tumour usually appears firm and well circumscribed it must never be merely enucleated for the histology shows that microscopically it infiltrates surrounding tissues. It consists of interlacing bands of spindle cells in a collagenous stroma with frequent mitoses. Pleomorphism is not a characteristic feature of these tumours. Because of infiltration, fibrosarcomas tend to recur after excision and when they metastasize they do so by the blood stream spreading principally to the lung but also to the skeleton. Because of the variety of lesions included under this heading, accurate figures for survival are not easily obtained. Recent figures suggest that a five-year survival of 50 per cent can be expected, provided the tumour is adequately treated, with longer survival for the well differentiated tumours and less for the highly cellular and mitotically active tumours.

Tumours of fibrous histiocytes

The diagnosis of *fibrous histiocytoma* has become fashionable in recent years, although their histogenesis remains in doubt. Some believe that they are facultative histiocytes with the ability to form collagen and others believe that they are mixed tumours of two cell patterns—histiocytic and fibroblastic. *Benign fibrous histiocytomas* occur most often in the skin and are more usually called *dermatofibromas*, *histiocytomas* or *sclerosing angiomas*. They present as cutaneous nodules, often on the extremities, are well circumscribed and easily excised. Similar tumours may occasionally occur in deep tissues. Pigmentation overlying the cutaneous lesions is common.

A second variant of fibrous histiocytoma is the *atypical fibroxanthoma* which occurs in the light-exposed skin of elderly patients. This tumour presents as a solitary nodule which may become ulcerated. Histologically, there is an alarming appearance with giant cells and frequent mitoses. In spite of their bizarre appearance they have a good prognosis if locally excised. Recurrence is unusual.

The *giant cell tumour of tendon sheath* is regarded by some as a fibrous histiocytoma of synovium. This benign tumour develops in tendon sheaths most often on the flexor surface of the fingers. They are usually small, firm and brown in colour. A similar lesion occurring as a diffuse change of large joints, especially the knee, is known as *pigmented villonodular synovitis*.

In infancy a variant of fibrous histiocytoma is the *juvenile xanthogranuloma*. These tumours present as red papules usually in the skin of the extremities. Histologically, they have a characteristic appearance with foamy histiocytes and multinucleated giant cells. If left they tend to undergo spontaneous regression.

Malignant fibrous histiocytomas occur most commonly in the deep tissues of the limbs of the elderly. Although they may appear well circumscribed they are not encapsulated and may infiltrate between muscles or along fascial planes. Grossly, they vary in appearance from firm fibrous cream-coloured swellings to soft mucoid tumours. They frequently recur after excision and approximately one-third metastasize, both by the blood stream and by lymphatics. A variant of malignant fibrous histiocytoma which occurs in the skin is *dermatofibrosarcoma protuberans*. This tumour differs from a benign dermatofibroma in its larger size and its infiltrative properties. Histologically, it may show mitotic activity but pleomorphism is not usually great. Dermatofibrosarcoma tends to recur locally but rarely metastasizes.

Tumours of muscle

Tumours of smooth muscle are most commonly sited in the uterus and the gastrointestinal tract, but they also occur in subcutaneous soft tissues. The commonest is the *vascular leiomyoma*, a tumour which usually presents as a tender, well circumscribed subcutaneous nodule, very often in the lower limb, arising from proliferating smooth muscle around blood vessels. Leiomyomas may also be found in the skin arising from the erector pilae muscle or from the smooth muscle found in scrotal and labial skin or around the nipple. These are benign tumours which may be easily excised without further recurrence.

Although *leiomyosarcomas* are found in the gastrointestinal tract and in the uterus, they are relatively uncommon in soft tissues. When they do arise in these tissues the commonest site is in the retroperitoneum where they usually present as large masses which have a fleshy or grey/white appearance. The histological assessment of malignancy is unreliable as most of the features of pleomorphism, hyperchromatic nuclei and tumour necrosis may be seen in smooth muscle tumours which behave in a benign fashion. The most reliable feature is the degree of mitotic activity. Those that do behave in a malignant fashion usually infiltrate locally and metastasize by the blood stream to the liver and lung.

Benign tumours of striated muscle, *rhabdomyomas*, are exceedingly rare. The malformation of the heart called a "rhabdomyoma of cardiac muscle" is now accepted as a hamartoma. This lesion is associated with tuberose sclerosis and occurs particularly in childhood.

Rhabdomyosarcomas are most common in childhood, usually occurring in children under the age of ten years. These are classified as either embryonal or alveolar depending on the microscopic appearances, and are most common in the head and neck and the genito-urinary tract including the spermatic cord and the urinary bladder. These childhood tumours characteristically appear as mucoid or grape-like growths, known as *sarcoma botryoides*, which are destructive of local tissues including bone. In adult life a third type may occur, the *pleomorphic rhabdomyosarcoma*, and these tumours are usually sited in the main muscle mass of the limbs. They infiltrate skeletal muscle and cannot be distinguished macroscopically from any other aggressive sarcoma. All these types infiltrate surrounding tissues and metastasize readily by the blood stream to the lungs and also to regional lymph nodes.

Tumours of blood vessels and lymphatics

Opinion varies as to whether haemangiomas are true neoplasms, hamartomas or reactive vascular proliferations. They may be subdivided into localized and diffuse forms, the latter if affecting a limb, sometimes leading to hypertrophy of the limb as in the Klippel–Trenaunay syndrome. Localized forms of haemangioma may affect either the skin or deep tissues, the two most common types being the capillary haemangioma and the cavernous haemangioma. The infantile form of capillary haemangioma often presents soon after birth in the region of the head and neck where it gives rise to the so-called "strawberry naevus". These lesions grow quite alarmingly, but the vast majority will undergo spontaneous regression with minimal scarring if left untreated. Ectate capilary haemangiomas form the so-called "port wine stain" of the skin.

Pyogenic granulomas are also vascular proliferations that frequently occur around the fingers. Similar lesions may occur on the gum margin, particularly during pregnancy. They may become ulcerated and secondarily inflamed. The term "pyogenic granuloma" is unfortunate for it is neither primarily pyogenic nor is it granulomatous.

Glomus tumours or *glomangiomas* occur in the skin of the limbs, especially in the subungual areas of the fingers, where the classical story is of severe pain often related to changes of temperature or to touch. They are said to arise from glomus cells in the dermis which are concerned with temperature regulation. Similar tumours may occur in deep tissues, but here they are usually symptomless. In the skin they appear as firm nodules which histologically consist of a haemangioma, the vessels cuffed by rows of orderly glomus cells. These are benign tumours cured by local excision.

Haemangiosarcomas arising from blood vessels are not always easy to distinguish from lymphangiosarcomas arising in lymphatics. Angiosarcomas may occur in the skin or in the deep tissues. Those that arise in the liver have an association with exposure to vinyl chloride monomer. Angiosarcomas may also occur in the breast where they are often deceptively benign in their appearance although their behaviour is that of a highly malignant tumour. In the skin, haemangiosarcomas tend to occur in the elderly and present with multiple red nodules often clustered together. As might be expected, haemangiosarcomas are usually haemorrhagic tumours and blood-borne metastases occur readily.

Lymphangiosarcomas are most frequently associated with chronic lymphoedema. Originally described in lymphoedematous arms developing after mastectomy postoperative radiotherapy, they have now been found in many other examples of chronic lymphoedema.

Haemangiopericytomas are tumours that arise from pericytes surrounding the endothelium of blood vessels. They may appear as vascular tumours or they may be more solid and fibrous in consistency. Their behaviour varies from benign to highly malignant.

Lymphangiomas may be of capillary type, but cavernous lymphangiomas made up of widely dilated lymphatic channels are much more common. Extreme forms of these comprise the so-called *cystic hygroma* which occur most commonly in the neck and axilla, although other sites are well recognized. These lesions cause difficulty in treatment because of their size and involvement of important structures. They extend through muscle and fibrous tissue and may be difficult to excise.

Tumours of synovial tissues

Synovial sarcomas occur throughout adult life. Despite their name they do not usually arise from synovial membranes of joints, but from the soft tissues surrounding tendons and aponeuroses. They are most common in the lower limb, but also occur in the trunk and neck. Radiologically, there may be evidence of calcification within them. Macroscopically, they may be solid or cystic, well circumscribed or infiltrating surrounding tissues. Histologically, they characteristically have a biphasic pattern with clefts lined by epithelioid cells and a spindle cell stroma. They are highly malignant.

Tumours of mesothelium

Mesothelioma is a tumour which has attracted attention in recent years because of its association with industrial exposure to asbestos, particularly crocidolite (blue asbestos). This exposure may result in pulmonary fibrosis and carcinoma of the lung in addition to mesothelioma. The latter tumour develops as firm or gelatinous nodules on the visceral and parietal layers of the pleura or peritoneum. These nodules fuse to form a diffuse mass of white tissue which encases the underlying viscera. In the peritoneum the pattern is more variable than in the pleura and it may appear to affect the omentum as a localized tumour. There is superficial invasion of the underlying tissues, but metastases to regional lymph nodes are relatively uncommon. Hypertrophic pulmonary osteoarthropathy is a well recognized association.

Distinct from this diffuse form of mesothelioma are fibrous plaques (localized fibrous mesothelioma) and adenomatoid tumour. *Fibrous plaques* occur more on the pleura than the peritoneum. They may rarely be associated with hypoglycaemia but are usually asymptomatic. The association with asbestos exposure is not established in most cases and they are almost always benign. *Adenomatoid tumours* occur most frequently in the uterus and adnexae or in the testis and spermatic cord. They may be found incidentally or they may present as a firm mass. The microscopic appearance of small mesothelial-lined spaces in a fibrous stroma has raised the possibility of lymphangioma, but these benign tumours are now regarded as being of mesothelial origin.

Tumours of neural origin

Both *neurofibromas* and *neurilemmomas* (Schwannomas) are common tumours. They may be single or multiple and both may be associated with von Recklinghausen's disease (neurofibromatosis). Neurilemmomas occur most frequently on cutaneous nerves and intracranial nerve roots. They are usually encapsulated and mobile and may undergo cystic change. Involvement of deep nerves is uncommon. Only very rarely does malignant change occur. In contrast, neurofibromas are not encapsulated although they may appear circumscribed. They may cause diffuse expansion of the nerve, the so-called "plexiform neuroma", and affect both cutaneous and deep nerves. When multiple, and particularly when involving deep nerves, malignant change to *neurofibrosarcoma* (malignant Schwannoma) may occur. The latter tumours are usually much larger than their benign variant. Because of their close connection with major nerves, resection of the tumour may necessitate amputation of the affected limb. The tumour can spread along the nerve for a considerable distance so that microscopic examination of the cut ends of the nerve should always be undertaken.

Of uncertain histogenesis, but now usually thought to be of nerve sheath origin, is the so-called *granular cell myoblastoma*. The term "myoblastoma" is inappropriate for there is little evidence to support a muscle origin. These tumours occur in the skin, deep tissues and in the viscera. They are usually small, asymptomatic and are found incidentally. Although they are benign they may induce hyperplastic change in the overlying epithelium, particularly of the tongue, which can mimic squamous carcinoma.

Ganglioneuroma, *ganglioneuroblastoma* and *neuroblastoma* are tumours that arise in the sympathetic nervous system. Neuroblastoma accounts for 10 per cent of childhood malignancies and most occur in the first five years of life. These tumours arise in the adrenal gland or sympathetic chain. They are soft, fleshy and often necrotic. The tumour consists of small primitive neural cells that may cluster to form rosettes. If differentiation of the neural cells to ganglion cells is apparent, the tumour is classified as a ganglioneuroblastoma. These are highly malignant tumours that metastasize to lymph nodes, bone and liver. Prognosis depends on age of presentation, site, stage and histological differentiation. Ganglioneuromas are fully differentiated tumours containing ganglion cells and Schwann cells. They are found usually in the mediastinum, retroperitoneum or adrenal in late childhood and adult life as encapsulated fibrous tumours. In contrast to neuroblastoma and ganglioneuroblastoma, these are benign tumours amenable to local resection.

Tumours of chemoreceptor cells in the carotid and aortic bodies and in the glomus jugulare are uncommon tumours. They are usually classified as *paragangliomas*, the commonest being the *carotid body tumour*. These are firm encapsulated tumours arising at the carotid bifurcation and may measure several centimetres in diameter. The tumour may rarely be bilateral and familial. They are usually benign although a few may recur and metastasize. Paragangliomas in other sites are more prone to infiltration (glomus jugular tumours) and to metastasize (aortic body tumours).

Tumours of uncertain histogenesis

Of the tumours of uncertain histogenesis, one, *Kaposi's sarcoma*, is of particular importance, not only because of its sex and geographical distribution, but also because of its association with immunocompromized patients. The tumour occurs most frequently in Africa, predominantly in males. More recently it has been found to be associated with the acquired immune deficiency syndrome (AIDS) caused by HTLV III virus infection most commonly in promiscuous male homosexuals but also in those receiving multiple blood transfusions or blood products, for example, haemophiliacs. The lesions usually develop in the skin of the lower limb as bluish-red nodules accompanied by oedema. With time, the lesions spread and coalesce and there may be visceral involvement. In children and in AIDS patients, lymph node spread is more common. Although the cell of origin of these tumours has not been identified, microscopically they appear vascular with red blood cells lying in clefts formed by the tumour spindle cells. Outside of Africa, development of Kaposi's sarcoma is frequently followed by a second malignancy, often malignant lymphoma.

Other tumours of uncertain histogenesis include *clear cell sarcomas*, *epithelioid sarcomas* and *alveolar soft part sarcomas*.

Management of soft tissue tumours

The management of a soft tissue swelling depends not only on the clinical diagnosis, but also on the size and site of the swelling. For example, a clinically obvious lipoma or a small mobile subcutaneous nodule of uncertain nature will normally be treated without investigation by simple excision and histological examination. A larger swelling, however, possibly malignant and sited deep within the tissue of a limb or in the retroperitoneum must be investigated before operation so as to answer three questions: (i) What is the diagnosis? (ii) What anatomical structures are involved? (iii) If a sarcoma, can it be resected? Without this knowledge, mistakes in treatment can easily occur due to the pathological behaviour of these tumours. Unlike epithelial tumours, fixity and infiltration are not pathognomic of malignancy as both the "pseudotumours" and the fibromatoses may infiltrate deeply and yet they do not metastasize. A soft tissue swelling must therefore not be judged "inoperable" without a tissue diagnosis. Conversely, mobility and encapsulation are no guarantee of benignity. Fibrosarcomas, especially, may appear encapsulated and therefore mistaken at operation for benign lesions. Inadequate excision will result in local recurrence. In no circumstances should a simple enucleation be performed however easy and tempting this may seem. The guiding principle is always to remove the tumour in total with a generous margin of surrounding normal tissue. In former times this often resulted in high amputation of a limb, sometimes even a hind-quarter or fore-quarter amputation. Today, major amputation is rarely indicated.

What is the diagnosis?

Although many different imaging techniques have been used to try and answer this question none have been found satisfactory and surgical biopsy is still essential. Plain radiographs show no more than a non-specific tissue mass, although occasionally erosion of adjacent bone may be observed. Focal calcification within the mass is non-specific. Arteriography will show a non-specific tumour circulation in approximately two-thirds of soft tissue sarcomas, while displacement of surrounding vessels may be observed if the tumour is hypovascular. Unfortunately, the appearances do not correlate with the histology. Ultrasound is unhelpful in diagnosis and while CT scanning may distinguish liposarcomas from other soft tissue tumours, in general the appearances are non-specific. In short, modern technology has not yet replaced the histopathologist in making an accurate diagnosis by histological examination of either an adequate biopsy or a totally excised neoplasm with a surrounding margin of normal tissue.

Surgical biopsy

In contrast to epithelial tumours where small amounts of tissue may be sufficient for the histopathologist to make a diagnosis, mesenchymal tumours require large and generous biopsies to ensure an accurate diagnosis. *Small biopsies are dangerous as they may be unrepresentative of the disease.* Sometimes the entire tumour is removed for analysis, but for larger tumours a generous incision biopsy is generally indicated. In the case of deep tumours, multiple Trucut needle biopsies may be performed through a single skin puncture which will subsequently be excised *en bloc* with the tumour, but this technique gives less material than ideal. Care must be taken to avoid the inadvertent biopsy of the periphery of the tumour where non-specific degenerative changes may be present and which can lead to a wrong diagnosis being made and the wrong operation performed.

In addition to the biopsy material itself, the pathologist requires clinical information which should be correlated with the histological appearances before a diagnosis is made. This information includes the length of history, the site and size of the swelling, details of previous treatment if any, the presence or absence of a family history of similar swellings and details of any trauma that the patient may have sustained.

Peroperative frozen tissue section analysis of soft tissue tumours is best avoided as it is fraught with difficulty of interpretation and may lead to wrong information being given to the surgeon.

What anatomical structures are involved?

Accurate localization of a tumour is necessary for deeply sited lesions when planning surgical operations or radiotherapy. If available, *xeroradiography* is preferable to plain radiography in defining the tumour margins, but both *ultrasound*, and especially *CT scanning*, are more accurate still and therefore to be preferred. Using these techniques it is possible to determine whether a lesion is contained within a particular muscle or fascial compartment or is extracompartmental or extending along fascial planes. Invasion of major blood vessels may also be shown using CT scanning, although this can also be demonstrated by *arteriography*.

Can it be resected?

The recurrence rate of an apparently localized sarcoma or fibromatosis is closely related to the adequacy of excision. It is therefore essential for the surgeon to have a maximum amount of information about the extent of the tumour before embarking on attempted removal. Infiltration of bone or large blood vessels may preclude immediate resection and indicate rather the need for radiotherapy, chemotherapy or arterial embolisation. Computerized axial tomographic scanning is the most effective investigation currently available to demonstrate infiltration and should ideally be performed in all cases.

The presence of lung metastases should routinely be excluded before radical excision is attempted. It is well established that CT scanning is a more sensitive technique in demonstrating small pulmonary metastases than either plain radiography or whole lung tomography. If clinically suspected, liver metastases may be shown by ultrasound or CT scanning and bone metastases by skeletal scintigraphy.

Treatment

Benign soft tissue tumours

Local excision with preservation of function and an acceptable cosmetic result is the appropriate treatment for most benign soft tissue tumours. Occasionally, this may not be possible as with large cavernous haemangiomas or with neurofibromas arising from major nerves.

"Pseudotumours" and fibromatoses

Local excision is also adequate for both "pseudotumours" and fibromatoses, but a wide margin of normal tissue is essential for the latter swellings or recurrence will almost certainly occur. Enucleation should never be performed.

Malignant soft tissue tumours

Complete surgical excision with a surrounding margin of normal tissue is the treatment of choice for malignant soft tissue tumours but this may not be feasible if there is widespread infiltration and fixity to surrounding tissues or metastatic spread. Some of these tumours are sensitive to high dose radiotherapy and a few are chemosensitive. This has resulted in much interest in combination treatment in recent years, although the exact place of these techniques in treatment is not yet agreed. Preoperative radiotherapy, possibly in association with chemotherapy, certainly may render an initially unresectable tumour amenable to surgical excision or allow a less mutilating operation to be performed. Tumours that have already metastasized may also be best treated by high dose radiotherapy and combination chemotherapy.

Because the characteristic local spread of these tumours is along fascial planes within a muscle compartment, and because they most often occur in the soft tissues of the limbs, it is usually possible to excise the tumour together with surrounding groups of muscle and fascia from origin to insertion *en bloc* with an ellipse of overlying skin containing the preoperative biopsy site. The surface of the tumour itself should ideally not be observed. This operation is known as a compartmentectomy. Spread across a major fascial septum into another compartment is unusual. Major nerves should where possible be preserved, but involved blood vessels can be sacrificed and, if appropriate, a graft used to bridge a major defect. A preserved but deformed limb, even with motor or sensory deficits, is almost always better than a high amputation and prosthesis. Grossly mutilating amputations are now rarely indicated.

Prognosis with soft tissue sarcomas

The results of treatment have very often been published in small retrospective series that are difficult to interpret due to the uncertainties of pathological classification as well as the wide range of treatments performed. It is therefore difficult to give an accurate prognosis for an individual patient with a soft tissue sarcoma. Using the surgical principles described in this chapter, the local recurrence rate for sarcomas of the limbs is in the order of 5 per cent, but is markedly greater if the excision is less than ideal or the tumour is sited in the trunk or retroperitoneum. Distant metastases developing after excision may occur in up to 50 per cent of patients although again there is wide variation depending on the site and nature of the tumour. In general, patients with limb sarcomas fare much better than patients with sarcomas of the trunk, limb girdle or retroperitoneum.

Further reading

Reviews

Aust JB. Soft tissue sarcomas. In *Clinical Oncology*, pp 645–63. Ed by J Horton, GJ Hill. Philadelphia: WB Saunders, 1977.

Gerner RE, Moore GE, Pickren JW. Soft tissue sarcomas. *Ann Surg* 1975; **181**:803–8.

Krementz, ET, Muchmore JH. Soft tissue sarcomas: behaviour and management. In: *Advances in surgery*, pp 147–96. Ed by LD MacLean. Chicago: Year Book Medical Publishers, 1983.

Mackenzie DH. *The Differential Diagnosis of Fibroblastic Disorders*. Oxford: Blackwells, 1970.

Mackenzie DH. Miscellaneous soft tissue sarcomas. In *Recent Advances in Pathology*, pp 183–216. Ed by CV Harrison and K Weinbren. Edinburgh: Churchill Livingstone, 1975.

Simon MA, Spanier SS, Enneking WF. Management of adult soft tissue sarcomas of the extremities. In *Surgery Annual*, pp 363–402. Ed by LM Nyhus. New York: Appleton-Century-Crofts, 1979.

Stower MJ, Hardcastle JD. Malignant retroperitoneal sarcoma: a review of 32 cases. *Clin Oncol* 1982; **8**:257–63.

Thomsen S, Morales AR. Soft tissue tumours. In *Principles and Practice of Surgical Pathology*, pp 205–44. Ed by SG Silverberg. New York: John Wiley, 1983.

Pathology

"Pseudotumours"

Enziger FM, Dulcey F. Proliferative myositis. *Cancer* 1967; **20**:2213–33.

Hutter RVP, Stewart FW, Foote FW. Fasciitis. A report of 70 cases. *Cancer* 1962; **15**:992–1003.

Mackenzie DH, Wilson JF, Cooke KB. Elastofibroma. *J Clin Path* 1968; **21**:470–75.

Price EB, Silliphant WM, Shuman R. Nodular fasciitis: a clinicopathological analysis of 65 cases. *Am J Clin Path* 1961; **35**:122–36.

Soule EH. Proliferative (nodular) fasciitis. *Arch Path* 1962; **73**:437–44.

Tighe JR, Clark AE, Turvey DJ. Elastofibroma dorsi. *J Clin Path* 1968; **21**:463–9.

Fibromatoses

Allen PW. The fibromatoses: a clinical classification based on 170 cases. *Am J Surg Path* 1977; **1**:255–70, 305–21.

Rosenberg HS, Stenback WA, Spjut HJ. The fibromatoses of infancy and childhood. *Perspectives in Pediatric Pathology* 1978; **4**:269–348.

Tumours of adipose tissue

Enterline HT, Culberson JD, Rochlin DB, Brady LW. Liposarcoma. A clinical and pathological study of 53 cases. *Cancer* 1960; **13**:932–50.
Enziger FM, Harvey DA. Spindle cell lipoma. *Cancer* 1975; **36**:1852–9.
Evans HL. Liposarcoma. A study of 55 cases with a reassessment of its classification. *Am J Surg Path* 1979; **3**:507–23.
Shmookler BM, Enziger FM. Pleomorphic lipoma: a benign tumour simulating liposarcoma. *Cancer* 1981; **47**:126–33.
Weinberg T, Feldman M. Lipomas of the gastro-intestinal tract. *Am J Clin Path* 1955;**25**:272–81.

Tumours of fibrous tissue

Pritchard, DJ, Soule EH, Taylor WT, Ivins JC. Fibrosarcoma—a clinicopathologic and statistical study of 199 tumours of the soft tissues of extremity and trunk. *Cancer* 1974; **33**:888–97.

Tumours of fibrous histioctyes

Kearney MM, Soule EH, Ivins JC. Malignant fibrous histiocytoma. A restrospective study of 167 cases. *Cancer* 1980;**45**:167–78.
Taylor HB, Helwig EB. Dermatofibrosarcoma protuberans. A study of 115 cases. *Cancer* 1962; **15**:717–25.
Weiss SW, Enziger FM. Malignant fibrous histiocytoma. An analysis of 200 cases. *Cancer* 1978; **41**:2250–66.

Tumours of muscle

Horn RC, Enterline HT. Rhabdomyosarcoma. A clinicopathological study and classification of 39 cases. *Cancer* 1958; **11**:181–99.
Phelan JT, Sherer W, Mesa P. Malignant smooth muscle tumours (leiomyosarcomas) of soft tissue origin. *New Engl J Med* 1962; **266**:1027–30.
Stout AP, Hill WT. Leiomyosarcoma of the superficial soft tissues. *Cancer* 1958; **11**:844–54.

Tumours of vessels

Danese CA, Grishman E, Oh C, Dreiling DA. Malignant vascular tumours of the lymphedematous extremity. *Ann Surg* 1967; **166**:245–53.
Enziger FM, Smith BH. Hemangiopericytoma. An analysis of 106 cases. *Human Pathol* 1976; **7**:61–82.
Mills SE, Cooper PH, Fechner RE. Lobular capillary hemangioma. The underlying lesion of pyogenic granuloma. *Am J Surg Path* 1980; **4**:471–9.
Rosai J, Sumner HW, Kostianovsky M, Perez-Mesa C. Angiosarcoma of the skin: a clinicopathologic and fine structural study. *Human Pathol* 1976; **7**:83–109.
Shugart RR, Soule EH, Johnson EW. Glomus tumor. *Surgery, Gynecology and Obstetrics* 1963; **117**:334–40.

Tumours of synovial tissues

Cadman NL, Soule EH, Kelly PJ. Synovial sarcoma. An analysis of 134 tumours. *Cancer* 1965; **18**:613–27.
Mackenzie DH. Synovial sarcoma. A review of 58 cases. *Cancer* 1966; **19**:169–80.

Tumours of mesothelium

Roberts GH. Diffuse pleural mesothelioma. A clinical and pathological study. *Br J Dis Chest* 1970; **64**:201–11.
Taxy JB, Battifora H, Oyasu R. Adenomatoid tumours: a light microscopic histochemical and ultrastructural study. *Cancer* 1974; **34**:306–16.

Tumours of neural origin

Lack EE, Cubilla AL, Woodruff JM. Paraganglionomas of the head and neck region. A pathologic study of tumours from 71 patients. *Human Pathol* 1979; **10**:191–218.
Lack EE, Worsham GF, Callihan MD, Crawford BE, Klappenbach S, Rowden G, Chun B. Granular cell tumour: a clinicopathologic study of 110 patients. *J Surg Oncol* 1980; **13**:301–16.
Russell DS, Rubinstein LJ. *Pathology of Tumours of the Nervous System*. pp 372–436. London: Edward Arnold, 1977.

Tumours of uncertain histogenesis

Ekfors TO, Kalimo H, Rantakokko V, Latvala M, Parvinen M. Alveolar soft part sarcoma. *Cancer* 1979; **43**:1672–7.
Enziger FM. Epithelioid sarcoma. *Cancer* 1970; **26**:1029–41.
Enziger FM. Clear-cell sarcoma of tendons and aponeuroses. An analysis of 21 cases. *Cancer* 1965; **18**:1163–74.
Templeton AC. Studies in Kaposi's sarcoma. *Cancer* 1972; **30**:854–67.

Investigation

Golding SJ, Husband JE. Radiology of soft tissue sarcoma: discussion paper. *J Roy Soc Med* 1982; **75**:729–35.

Surgical treatment

Abbas JS, Holyoke ED, Moore R, Karakousis CP. The surgical treatment and outcome of soft tissue sarcomas. *Arch Surg* 1981; **116**:765–9.
Bowden L, Booher RJ. The principles and technique of

resection of soft parts for sarcoma. *Surgery* 1958; **44**:963–77.

Shiu MH, Castro EB, Hajdu SI, Fortner JG. Surgical treatment of 297 soft tissue sarcomas of the lower extremity. *Ann Surg* 1975; **182**:597–602.

Radiotherapy

Coe MA, Madden FJ, Mould RF. The role of radiotherapy in the treatment of soft tissue sarcoma. *Clin Radiol* 1981; **32**:47–51.

Lindberg RD, Martin RG, Romsdahl MR, Barkley HT. Conservative surgery and postoperative radiotherapy in 300 adults with soft tissue sarcomas. *Cancer* 1981; **47**:2391–7.

Chemotherapy

Eilber FR, Mirra JJ, Grant TT, Weisenburger T, Morton DL. Is amputation necessary for sarcomas? A seven year experience with limb salvage. *Ann Surg* 1980; **192**:431–7.

Rosenberg SA, Tepper J. Glatstein E, Costa J, Young R, Seipp C, Wesley R. Adjuvant chemotherapy for patients with soft tissue sarcoma. *Surg Clin Nth Am* 1981; **61**:1415–23.

19

Arteries

R M Greenhalgh and N Woolf

Introduction

Diseases of the arteries express themselves clinically for the most part in the form of *underperfusion* of one or more tissue beds. The logical correlate of this is that any process, which encroaches significantly on the integrity of the arterial lumen, must be of concern to the vascular surgeon. A second important group comprises those conditions in which the integrity of the *wall* is lost and this will naturally lead to haemorrhage in the affected area. The final group of conditions to be considered is that in which the normal *architecture* of the vascular system is disturbed, either because of arteriovenous malformations (congenital or acquired) or, more rarely, by neoplasm.

In this group of disorders, the morphological changes found in tissue removed at operation rarely influence the management of the case, except in the fields of neoplasia and the arteritides. However, an understanding of the natural history and mechanical effects of the spectrum of processes seen in this field of surgery is essential and for this reason this chapter is organized by initially describing the various pathological lesions encountered and then discussing how this information affects the handling of the different clinical syndromes.

Disorders causing arterial obstruction

If one disregards for the moment the nosologic entities which are subsumed under this heading and considers instead arterial stenosis and obstruction in terms of *process*, the pathogenetic factors which are of most importance are occlusive and mural thrombosis and hyperplasia of the modified smooth muscle cells of the arterial intima. These versatile cells express not only some of the characteristics normally expected in muscle cells, but also the ability to synthesize and secrete a number of the extracellular components of the arterial intima including collagen, the microfibrillar elements of elastin and the glycosoaminoglycans of the intercellular and interfibrillar ground substance. Intimal smooth muscle cells can be induced to proliferate in any situation where endothelium is damaged and mural thrombosis occurs; the trigger for proliferation in this situation probably being the release of a factor stored in the alpha granules of the platelet which is mitogenic for arterial smooth muscle. Other cell-derived "growth factors" which are relevant to the artery wall almost certainly exist, among them molecules secreted by endothelial cells and macrophages.

Atherosclerosis

Of all the disorders causing arterial narrowing or occlusion, atherosclerosis is by far the most important. Our understanding of many of the elements in its genesis and natural history is still inchoate, and this forces us to define atherosclerosis in terms which are predominantly morphological. It is a widely prevalent disorder affecting chiefly large elastic and muscular arteries and characterized by the presence of focal intimal thickening; these intimal elevations being made up of a mixture of proliferated connective tissue, necrotic tissue debris and accumulations of lipid, much of the last-named being derived from the plasma.

Morphology of mature atherosclerotic lesions

It would seem logical to approach the question of the morphology of atherosclerotic lesions by describing first the earliest structural manifestations of the disorder and then the sequence of changes leading to mature clinically significant plaques. This we cannot do since there is controversy as to what constitutes the precursor lesion of the mature plaque, no certainty that the common morphological endpoint cannot be reached from different beginnings, and no agreement that what many workers have termed "early" atherosclerotic lesions develop inevitably into characteristic fibro-lipid lesions. For these reasons we shall concentrate only on the morphological features of the mature fibro-lipid plaque or *raised lesion*.

This is the archetypal lesion of atherosclerosis and appears to function well as a predictor for the amount of clinical arterial disease within a given population group. Its basic constituents are uniform, but within these limits many morphological variants exist. Essentially the lesion consists of a lipid-rich basal pool of "atheromatous" debris which is covered on its luminal aspect by a "cap" of connective tissue which varies in thickness from lesion to lesion. In some, the proliferated connective tissue is the predominant element and this gives the luminal aspect of the plaque an opaque, white "pearly" appearance. When such a lesion is bisected the yellow, lipid-rich base may be inconspicuous or even absent. In other lesions, the basal accumulation of lipid and tissue debris may be of massive proportions, separated from the vessel lumen only by a thin, easily ruptured sheet of connective tissue and hence very likely to be the site of a complicating thrombus.

Complications

From the clinical point of view the most important event in the natural history of the plaque is thrombosis which may lead to crippling or life-threatening events. In the coronary tree, and probably in other parts of the arterial system, the key event preceding occlusive thrombosis is splitting of the intimal connective tissue cap with exposure of the subendothelial elements of the vessel wall to the passing stream of blood. In such circumstances massive thrombi can form very rapidly indeed; the platelet aggregation possibly being related to sharp rises in the local concentrations of adenosine diphosphate (ADP) as a consequence of distortion of red blood cells occurring as blood flows rapidly into the substance of the plaque. It is not without interest that masses of aggregated platelets are frequently seen within the depths of the plaque as well as in the lumen. Whether these represent the end results of haemorrhage from the arterial lumen into the plaque, as described above, or represent the remains of mural thrombi which have become incorporated into the vessel wall, is uncertain.

Distribution of lesions

Even the most inexperienced cannot fail to be aware of the different degrees to which different arteries and different areas within the same artery are affected by atherosclerosis. Since the chemical composition of the boundary layer of the blood in contact with the lining endothelium is unlikely to differ significantly from one segment of an artery to another, it seems reasonable to attribute the localization of atherosclerotic lesions and, to some extent, their severity, to the interaction between variations in the fluid mechanics of blood flow on the one hand, and variations in the reactivity of arterial tissues in different parts of the vascular tree on the other.

In the *aorta*, the distribution of mature raised lesions differs markedly from that which obtains in the case of the fatty streak, a lesion found in all population groups and apparently with little predictive value for significant atherosclerosis in the future. The lesions occur in greater numbers in the abdominal than in the thoracic portion of the aorta, a fact which is probably significant in relation to the distribution of atherosclerotic aortic aneurysm. Unlike fatty streaks, which often spare the intima immediately around the ostia of the intercostal vessels, the mouths of these vessels are often involved by raised lesions. In the case of renal and mesenteric arteries, a relative degree of sparing is usually present. Atherosclerosis of these vessels does not occur in the absence of significant aortic disease. If a significant degree of atherosclerosis is present in the mesenteric and renal arteries, one can predict with confidence that the coronary arteries will be severely affected, but the reverse does not hold true.

In the *carotid arteries*, the *carotid sinus* is by far the most severely affected site and the predilection for serious disease, characterized by ulceration and mural thrombosis, to occur here is in sharp contrast with the relative freedom from raised lesions enjoyed both by the common carotid and by the cervical segment of the internal carotid adjoining the sinus. The petrous segment of the internal carotid is usually only minimally affected, but the terminal portion of the artery, which is often very tortuous, shows the presence of severe atherosclerosis almost as often as the carotid sinus region itself. In the *vertebal arteries*, the extent of intimal surface involvement by atherosclerotic plaques is low, but the prevalence of severe stenosis is high.

As in the carotid and vertebral systems, the

distribution of atherosclerotic lesions within the *iliac arteries* varies quite markedly from one segment to another. Severe disease is more common in the right common iliac artery than in the left, and this tendency is more marked in women. As compared with the common and internal iliac arteries, the external iliacs are relatively free from disease.

Risk factors and atherosclerosis

Many variables have been implicated as "risk factors" for the development of clinically significant arterial disease and hence, by implication, as factors which might promote the development of atherosclerotic lesions. The risk factor concept is important and should be examined critically since significant progress in controlling atherosclerosis-related clinical disease is likely to be made only if severe atherosclerosis can be prevented—so called *primary prevention*. For primary prevention to succeed it is clearly of the first importance that potentially reversible "risk factors" be identified. However, it may well be that some of the factors that have been found to be related to the prevalence of arterial disease may have a relationship that is not a direct causal one and removal or reversal of such a factor would not materially affect the prevalence or severity of atherosclerosis.

Age Of all the factors canvassed, age has the strongest and most consistent association with atherosclerotic lesions. The different arterial beds are affected at different rates. Lesions appear in the aorta in the first decade of life, in the coronary arteries in the second and in the cerebral arteries in the third. It would be useful to know whether the fact that atherosclerosis is so closely age-related is due to some intrinsic ageing process or whether it is simply an expression of the time required for other factors to exert their effect. In this connexion there are certainly some population groups that have a life span not significantly different from the human species in general in whom ageing is not accompanied by the *clinical* manifestations of atherosclerosis.

Sex In so far as the coronary arteries are concerned, there is no doubt that the clinical expressions of atherothrombosis in the middle decades of life are far commoner in males than in females, though with increasing age this difference decreases but never disappears. These clinical data are, at least in part, mirrored by studies of the prevalence and severity of atherosclerosis in autopsy populations. It is obviously tempting to try to ascribe these sex-determined differences in terms of a putative role for sex hormones. Many experimental data exist on the effect of oestrogens on the induction of experimental atherosclerosis in a variety of animal species. However, many of the results are contradictory and, since they have been obtained for the most part in small animals not known for their propensity to develop atherosclerosis spontaneously, it is difficult to know how much significance to attach to them. In humans, the use of oestrogens in a large-scale secondary prevention study has not proved encouraging. One should not, in our view, adopt too nihilistic a stance in relation to applying the results of this "experiment of nature". If we have not so far obtained the "right answer" to the problem of sex-determined differences in extent and severity of atherosclerosis, it is likely that the "right questions" have not been asked. Some differences between the sexes certainly seem to exist in the field of lipid metabolism and perhaps these should be more extensively explored. In females taking contraceptive compounds the effect, in terms of lipid concentrations in the plasma, depends on the type of compound administered. In general, High Density Lipoprotein (HDL) concentrations increase with increasing doses of oestrogen and the reverse is seen with progesterone.

Race There are striking geographical differences in the prevalence of atherosclerosis-related clinical disease. These differences correspond roughly to the distribution of various racial groups and they are, by and large, mirrored in the data obtained in the course of necropsy studies related to the extent and severity of atherosclerosis. Within individual racial groups quite steep gradients exist insofar as extent and severity of lesions in the coronary artery tree is concerned and these large intra-group variations suggest that membership of one or other racial group does not *per se* confer either relative immunity from, or increased susceptibility to, atherosclerosis. This view is strengthened by a consideration of epidemiological data relating to immigrant populations who seem to acquire a risk for the development of atherosclerosis-related clinical disease closer to that of the host population than to that of the population from which they have stemmed.

Lipid metabolism A vast literature exists which relates to the association between lipid metabolism, atherosclerosis and clinically significant arterial disease. Despite the complexity of this subject, which it is impossible to review adequately here, this association can be expressed in a series of simple propositions each of which deserves critical examination.

1. Atherosclerotic lesions contain far more lipid than adjacent areas of normal intima.

2. The production of increased plasma concentrations of certain lipid classes in a variety of animal species by dietary and/or pharmacological means is followed by the appearance of intimal lesions which have at least some features in common with human atherosclerosis.

3. An association exists between populations in which the prevalence of atherosclerosis-related disease and of raised lesions is high, and high plasma concentrations of certain lipid classes (notably low density lipoproteins). The converse applies in those groups in which the prevalence both of clinically manifest arterial disease and of raised intimal lesions is low. Such associations are particularly strongly expressed in the case of certain genetically determined hyperlipidaemic states as, for example, familial hyperlipidaemia Type IIa. One lipid class of particular interest in recent years is high density lipoprotein, in relation to which epidemiological data suggest an inverse risk relationship between plasma concentrations of HDL and coronary heart disease. The question which arises from these data is whether high plasma concentrations of HDL merely constitute a predictor of ischaemic heart disease or whether the HDL in some away acts as a *protector* against it. A recent angiographic study suggests a strong inverse relationship between coronary artery narrowing and the HDL_2 subfraction concentration in the plasma, and there are many experimental data suggesting that HDL may actually remove free cholesterol from the artery wall.

Diabetes mellitus In rather overprivileged Western communities there is no doubt that diabetes constitutes a potent additional risk factor for atherosclerosis-related clinical disease. For diabetes to operate in this way a certain "background" level of atherosclerosis appears to be necessary, since in populations in whom atherosclerosis is not a serious problem, diabetes does not produce any significant effect on the frequency of the major clinical syndromes associated with atherosclerosis. The question of whether diabetes increases the severity of artery wall disease is not easy to answer, since ideally one would need to compare two groups alike in every way except in respect of the presence or absence of diabetes. However, from a study of such data as exist it seems that there is a real difference between diabetics and non-diabetics insofar as raised atherosclerotic plaques in both the aorta and the coronary arteries are concerned. Whether the increment in extent and severity of the artery wall lesions is sufficient to account for the increase in *risk*, is a legitimate question, but one which is impossible to answer in the present state of our knowledge. Certainly it would be unwise totally to disregard the possibility that the diabetic state might affect other factors which might be implicated in the genesis of atherosclerosis-related disease, such as platelet function, microangiopathic changes affecting the arteriolar and capillary beds of key target areas, and changes in the susceptibility of underperfused tissues.

Hypertension Several studies have shown quite clearly that elevation of blood pressure is associated with an increased risk of death from coronary and cerebral artery disease. This increased risk is accompanied by an increase in extent and severity of atherosclerosis, at least in respect of the epidemiologically significant raised lesion, where there is a statistically significant difference between hypotensive and normotensive cases at all ages, in both sexes and both in the aorta and in the coronary arteries. It is impossible here to consider in any detail the manner in which raised blood pressure produces an incremental effect on the process of atherogenesis, but the evidence that it is the *mechanical* effect of the elevated pressure which is the dominant element is, in our view, compelling.

Cigarette smoking Strongly positive epidemiological correlations exist between heavy smoking (of cigarettes) and a high risk of Ischaemic Heart Disease (IHD) and/or peripheral vascular disease. Data gathered in Britain show that smoking more than 15 cigarettes a day trebles the risk of dying from ischaemic heart disease in men aged 45–54 and similar results have been obtained in the long-running Framingham study in the USA. In the latter, the degree of risk appeared to be related to the *number* of cigarettes smoked each day rather than to the duration of the habit and this, coupled with the observation that the risk of IHD decreases quite rapidly in people who stop smoking, suggests that the major effect of smoking may lie outwith a simple increase in the severity and extent of artery wall disease.

However it is unwise to conclude from these data that cigarette smoking is without any effect on the artery wall itself. Retrospective necropsy studies show that atherosclerosis is greatest in heavy smokers and least in non-smokers and a prospective study in Hawaii has shown that on multivariate analysis there is a statistically independent association between aortic and coronary artery atherosclerosis and daily consumption of cigarettes. To date, the evidence that smoking is associated with structural changes in the artery wall remains fairly scanty. Changes quite obvious on ultrastructural examination, have been observed in relation to the endothelial cells of the umbilical arteries of infants born to smoking mothers, and the exposure of small mammals such as rats and rabbits to graded doses of fresh cigarettes regularly produces similar endothelial cell changes (contraction of the cells and the formation of numerous blebs and complex plasma membrane processes on the luminal aspect of the cell). In addition, the experiments alluded to here also show the occurrence, in the vast majority of animals exposed to smoke, of small platelet thrombi which form in relation to the low wall shear areas of arterial branches. Whether this reflects a change in platelet function or some change in the underlying endothelial cells is not yet known.

Many possibilities have been canvassed in the search for *mechanisms* by which cigarette smoking may affect the artery wall and the interaction between this wall and circulating elements of the blood. These include a possible direct effect of nicotine, a possible effect of carbon monoxide and a possible hypersensitivity to certain antigens in tobacco. At present the Scottish verdict of "not proven" is the only appropriate one, but this is an area of very considerable interest in which progress can be expected with a reasonable degree of confidence.

The natural history of atherosclerosis

From the clinical point of view, the importance of atherosclerosis lies in its ability to compromise the integrity of an arterial lumen. This is accomplished, in part, by the increase in plaque bulk inherent in the process of atherogenesis and, more importantly, by the occurrence of occlusive thromobosis in relation to underlying atherosclerotic lesions. In the majority of cases where thrombosis is rapid and the residual lumen becomes occluded, the "trigger" for platelet adhesion and aggregation appears to be cracking or fissuring of the connective tissue "cap" of the plaque with loss of covering endothelial cells and exposure of the passing stream of blood to the subendothelial elements of the arterial intima. Whether the change in platelet behaviour is mediated by exposure of the platelets to collagen or whether, as some have suggested, the distortion of red blood cells consequent on rapid flow of blood into the plaque substance leads to a steep increase in the local concentration of ADP, causing aggregation of platelets, need not concern us here, Let it suffice that, under these circumstances, bulky thrombi form very quickly, much of the mass of aggregated platelets lying within the substance of the atherosclerotic plaque and continuous with the intraluminal portion of the thrombus. If the plaque shows the presence of a large basal pool, the flowing blood from the artery lumen tracks within the soft, "atheromatous" debris leading to some very complicated morphological patterns and, sometimes, pushing the intima inwards towards the lumen, thus causing a still greater degree of narrowing. Post-mortem studies on segments of thrombosed arteries derived from patients injected with radioactive fibrinogen prior to death, suggest that propagation or extension of such thrombi frequently takes place in both cephalad and caudad directions. If the degree of tissue underperfusion is not so severe as to lead to death, changes in the mass of thrombus take place quite rapidly, the nature of these depending very largely on whether the thrombus is *occlusive* or whether it is *mural*. (It is worth bearing in mind that a marked degree of retraction of an occlusive thrombus can take place, thus re-establishing some degree of blood flow across the thrombosed segment.) In occlusive arterial thrombi, the normal processes of tissue repair by granulation tissue appear to be triggered and the mass of platelets and fibrin become converted into a plug of granulation tissue with an abundant microvasculature and later into a fibrous tissue core within the lumen of the artery. Superimposed on this is *recanalization*, in the process of which cracks appear in the thrombus, these being aligned in the long axis of the vessel. Within a few days these clefts become lined by flattened cells and in due time by fully differentiated endothelium. In some instances, new smooth muscle cells become arranged in layers round the new small lumina passing through the occluded segment.

Where mural thrombus is present, the most striking reaction in the underlying vessel wall is smooth muscle cell proliferation, this presumably being triggered by the release from platelet alpha-granules of platelet-derived growth factor (PDGF). This is a fairly low-molecular weight basic protein which remains stable after exposure to urea, an acid environment and after heating to 100°C. This growth factor is not merely a mitogen; it increases endocytosis by smooth muscle cells, stimulates the synthesis of cholesterol by these cells and also enhances protein synthesis, particularly that of collagen. Other growth factors derived most notably from endothelial cells have also been identified and it is not without interest that in arteries which have been injured experimentally by means of a balloon catheter, the greatest degree of smooth muscle proliferation occurs in those areas covered by regenerating endothelium.

The clinical presentation of stenosing atherosclerotic disease depends on the arteries involved. Examples given here include coronary, renal and peripheral arterial disease.

Coronary artery disease

The mildest symptom of coronary artery disease is angina pectoris of effort. The patient experiences a cramp-like pain in the middle of the chest which sometimes passes down the left arm or up the neck. This comes on with severe exercise at first, but later occurs with milder exercise. If angina becomes more severe it can occur at rest. Excitement or worry can also bring it on. When the patient rests the symptoms go away and on clinical examination no abnormality can be detected. In many ways this is very similar to cerebral transient ischaemic attacks. Without warning one day a patient can have a more severe attack of chest pain which does not go away. Once again the pain may go down the left arm or up the neck. Frequently the patient has been a very heavy cigarette smoker. On examination, the patient may have signs of cardiogenic shock associated with a poor cardiac output state. The jugular venous pressure would be raised. The patient may be cold and clammy and have a fast pulse. The respirations are frequently shallow and rapid. An electrocardiogram may show Q waves, raised ST segments or inverted T waves suggesting that a myocardial infarction has taken place.

Renal artery stenosis

Whenever a patient is being investigated for hypertension the clinician listens over the renal artery for a systolic bruit. This might imply that a renal artery stenosis is causing the hypertension. It is important to discover this because renal artery stenosis is one of the few correctable causes of hypertension. In such a patient, the renin levels are raised and an aortogram with selective renal artery views is performed to demonstrate the stenosis.

Peripheral arterial disease

The commonest symptom of peripherial arterial disease is intermittent claudication, so named after the emperor Claudius, who limped. The patient, who is five times more likely to be male, and is usually aged between 40 and 70 years, experiences a cramp-like pain in the calf or buttock muscles on exercise. The pain always comes on after the same degree of exercise and goes away when he stops walking. If the common iliac arteries are involved, then the patient experiences calf and buttock claudication on one side only. If the aorta is involved in the male, bilateral calf and buttock claudication is associated with impotence (the Leriche syndrome). In the female, bilateral calf and buttock claudication is sometimes found in short-statured "little women" with blocked aortas. In these ladies the arterial disease is confined to the bifurcation of the abdominal aorta; in other parts of the arterial tree the vessel are curiously spared from disease.

On examination, the clinician feels carefully for the femoral, popliteal, dorsalis pedis and posterior tibial pulses which helps him to decide which artery is involved. In addition, patients frequently have arcus senilis and xanthelasmata.

If the arterial disease is more severe, ischaemic rest pain can follow. The patient experiences severe pain in the toes at first which keeps him awake at night. The pain is relieved by hanging the foot out of bed and made worse by raising it. This is an intolerable pain which requires urgent intervention. If disease progresses further, gangrene occurs, first at the more distal part usually in the hallux.

Some other conditions leading to luminal stenosis or occlusion

Arterial embolism

Ninety per cent of major arterial emboli originate within the chambers of the left side of the heart and 5 per cent from the aorta itself, these latter being associated with ulcerated atherosclerotic plaques. However, the most important form of embolism from the clinical point of view is from the extracranial arteries, principally in the neck, whence small athero-embolic particles usually from the carotid bifurcation pass up to the brain and cause symptoms of stroke. Those conditions within the heart most likely to be complicated by systemic embolic phenomena are myocardial infarction, post-ischaemic ventricular aneurysm, the presence of prosthetic valves, congestive cardiomyopathy and atrial fibrillation from any cause. Less frequent causes are left atrial myxoma and the various forms of infective endocarditis. Somewhere between 10 and 25 per cent of such emboli involve the aortic bifurcation.

The fate of venous and prosthetic grafts when placed in the arterial stream

When autologous vein is used for arterial bypass, it is either in-situ or reversed. When the vein is reversed it is completely taken out of its normal bed and thus loses any blood supply from the surrounding tissues which would normally supply the adventitia and more outer aspects of the vein. A vein normally derives most of its blood supply from the lumen, but in a reversed vein bypass the whole of the blood supply is supplied from the lumen. For in-situ bypass the valves are divided and the vein is left lying in its usual bed and it is thought that less disturbance of blood supply occurs. It is imagined that this enables the vein to stay more elastic and for the bypass to work for longer periods. Whether reverse or in-situ, when used as an arterial bypass, the vein is suddenly subjected to a much higher pressure. This distends the vein and at re-operation the vein bypass is invariably thicker and whiter macroscopically than at the time of implantation. In many respects it comes to resemble an artery after some months, very much more than at the time of implantation.

Prosthetic graft materials are said to "heal". They do not have a normal intima, but an intima grows along the prosthetic graft quite rapidly after implantation. The "healing process" also continues through the meshes of the Dacron and velour surfaces are said to facilitate this process. The continued patency of all graft material depends upon a maintenance of elasticity, lack of thrombosis and absence of significant progression of arterial disease above and below the bypass.

Atheromatous emboli

These emboli, consisting of a mixture of cholesterol-rich plaque debris and aggregated platelets are usually very small (150–600 μm) and are released in showers. The commonest anetecedent event is said to be surgery involving manipulation of an atherosclerotic aorta. In most instances, the release of such emboli does not produce significant clinical effects, but acute renal failure, acute pancreatitis and segmental ischaemia within the gastro-intestinal tract have been recorded and rarely, quite large arteries may be occluded.

Athero-embolic stroke

Presently, the vast majority of patients with symptoms of cerebral ischaemia have evidence of athero-embolism from an extracranial vessel. Amaurosis fugax is a symptom of transient blindness in which the patient describes loss of vision as if a blanket is being placed over his eye. The blanket then slowly passes away and he can see again. This symptom implies that embolization has taken place through the ipsilateral internal carotid artery and its branch the ophthalmic artery. Another patient would complain of transient weakness of the hand such as dropping a cup or saucer. Sometimes the leg is also involved and if it is the dominant limb, then the patient may well notice difficulty in finding the words or speaking them—expressive and motor dysphasia. If such an attack passes off within 24 hours, it is described as a transient ischaemic attack. On clinical examination during an attack, the clinician detects motor and sensory loss, brisk reflexes in the affected limbs and an up-going plantar response. If a neurological deficit is detected after three days, it is said that a completed stroke has occurred. A CAT scan in such a patient shows a poorly attenuated area corresponding to a cerebral infarct.

Thrombo-angiitis obliterans (Buerger's disease)

In 1908 Leo Buerger described a disorder occurring, for the most part in young men, which was characterized by segmental obliteration of the lumina of both arteries and veins associated with local manifestations of an inflammatory reaction. This clinical and pathological picture occurred almost exclusively in cigarette smokers. They may present with symptoms of Raynaud's phenomenon or ischaemic rest pain of the fingers or toes. In addition, they may have attacks of superficial thrombophlebitis causing an inflamed hard lump to be noticed under the skin. On examination the proximal pulses such as the femoral or sub-clavian are always present. There is an absence of pulses in the distal part of the limbs such as the radial, ulnar, dorsalis pedis and posterior tibial. The patient curiously has no symptoms of intermittent claudication, but the degree of ischaemia in the distal portion of the limb is severe. If he stops smoking cigarettes the progression of the disease can be halted, but if he continues to smoke there is nothing more sure than that amputation will follow.

In the early 1960s some doubts were expressed

as to whether the disease described by Buerger was indeed a distinct entity, the view being put forward that thrombo-angiitis obliterans was simply a variant of arteriosclerosis and not a specific disease with a specific histological pattern. It may well be that some of the cases diagnosed as thromboangiitis obliterans are examples of other types of thrombotic arterial occlusion, but the combination of features said to be characteristic of Buerger's disease is so striking as to enable a clinician to recognize the syndrome described.

Histological appearances

The lesions have a definite segmental distribution and usually start in small or medium-sized arteries most frequently in the lower limb, though the upper limb may also be affected as also vessels in the heart, lung, brain, gastro-intestinal tract etc. Obviously, the vast majority of the lesions which have been studied histologically are derived from amputation specimens, surgery having been resorted to only after a prolonged clinical course. In the few early lesions described, the presence of an acute inflammatory reaction characterized by neutrophile infiltration is a striking feature and the association of micro-abscess formation within occlusive thrombi in small vessels is a striking feature not found in atherosclerosis-related thrombotic occlusion.

Aetiology and pathogenesis

The basic aetiology is still unknown, though the influence of a genetic factor is suggested by the high prevalence of HLA-A9 and HLA-B5 in sufferers from this disease. The association with cigarette smoking is a constant one and the possibility has been raised that allergy to one of the constituents of cigarette smoke might play a role. A glycoprotein with a molecular weight of 180 000 has been extracted both from tobacco leaf and from condensates of smoke, and about one-third of the population, whether smokers or non-smokers, exhibit immediate-type cutaneous hypersensitivity to this compound. This apparently paradoxical finding may be due to cross-reactions with antigens of other members of the Solanaceae family (e.g. tomatoes and potatoes) to which tobacco belongs. When the tobacco glycoprotein is added to human plasma, there is shortening of the partial thromboplastin time, activation of plasminogen and generation of bradykinin. These effects are all mediated by the activation of Hageman factor by the tobacco glycoprotein and, on the basis of these findings, it has been suggested that smoking might be related to the initiation of an inflammatory reaction either through IgE-mediated release of vasoactive amines or through the activation of Hageman factor-dependent pathways.

Takayasu's arteritis

This disorder was described 75 years ago by a Japanese ophthalmologist in a young female who had cataracts associated with an unusual wreath-like pattern of arteriovenous anastamoses surrounding the optic papilla. Later, these eye changes were found to be associated in a number of patients with absent radial pulses and it is, of course, with this latter finding that we are primarily concerned. The majority of case reports have emanated from Asia and Africa and there is a marked predilection for females (female : male ratio—8.5 : 1).

The basic pathological picture is of a marked degree of intimal proliferation associated with scarring of the media and patchy loss of medial elastic fibres. A degree of lymphocytic infiltration is usually present, but is overshadowed by the fibrosis. The adventitia becomes considerably thickened and vasa vasorum appear to be destroyed. The macroscopic appearances in the advanced stages of this condition bear a striking resemblance to the "tree-bark"-like intima seen in luetic aortitis. The proliferative process leads ultimately to stenosis or even obliteration of the lumen of the aorta or its major branches. Aneurysm formation, post-stenotic dilatations and calcification in the arterial wall are among the late complications that have been recorded. The parts of the vascular tree most often involved are the aortic arch and its major branches, the changes frequently being most severe at the origins of the branch vessels. Takayasu's arteritis may present as a multisegment aortic disorder with intervening segments of apparently normal aorta, a diffuse involvement of the aorta, or as an isolated lesion involving one of the aortic branches. Three varieties have been described, the classification depending on the location of the lesions. Type I involves the aortic arch and its branches. In Type II the arch is spared and the main sites are the descending thoracic aorta and the abdominal aorta. Type III combines the features of both Types I and II and is, by far, the most common.

The aetiology remains unknown but, as so often in the arteritides, an auto-immune origin has been canvassed. It is not without interest that some investigators have reported a higher frequency of positive skin reactions to tuberculin in patients than in controls. The retinopathy originally described by Takayasu is only seen in approximately 25 per cent of the patients.

The *clinical features* of this condition depend upon the extent and severity of the arterial lesions, usually worst in the aortic arch. Stroke symptoms, blindness, paralysis and poor mentation may present, or on other occasions the patient may complain of intermittent claudication of the arm. Major arterial reconstruction is often required.

Giant cell arteritis (temporal arteritis)

This is a disorder found chiefly in the elderly and typically it involves medium-sized vessels such as the temporal arteries, though the aorta or its branches are affected in about 15 per cent of the patients. In its fully developed state, the characteristic pathological picture is that of focal medial necrosis with patchy loss of elastic fibres, the latter feature being associated with the presence of a few lymphocytes and occasional multinucleate giant cells. The changes are often segmental and there is a considerable degree of sampling error involved in obtaining a biopsy from an affected vessel. A negative report from the pathologist therefore, should not be regarded as ruling out the diagnosis if the clinical grounds for suspicion are strong, and blocks of tissue sent for histological examination should be sectioned at many levels. Sometimes the whole thickness of the vessel wall is infiltrated by acute inflammatory cells, and granulomatous features as described above are completely absent. Thrombosis very often complicates the inflammatory process and the arterial lumen eventually becomes occluded by fibromuscular connective tissue by the ordinary processes of organization of occlusive thrombus. The great fear of this condition is irreversible blindness. The patient may have pain in the temporal distribution and the visual fields become reduced. The erythrocyte sedimentation rate (ESR) is always high. Diagnosis is by temporal artery biopsy and steroids are commenced at once when the diagnosis is made.

Fibromuscular dysplasia

Fibromuscular dysplasia was originally described in the renal artery and there is a mistaken tendency to regard this lesion as being confined to the renal arterial system. In fact it can occur in many large muscular vessels, though the renal artery is most commonly affected. The peak incidence is in the third and fourth decades, but cases occurring in childhood have also been reported. The most common variety is *medial fibroplasia* which is found predominantly in young women and chiefly affects the distal two-thirds of the main renal artery. There may be many segmental stenoses in any affected vessel, the stenoses consisting of disorderly masses of fibromuscular medial tissue interspersed with segments which are relatively thinned. This gives rise to the characteristic "string of beads" deformity seen on aortography. The second most common variant is what has been termed *perimedial fibroplasia*. Here there is replacement of the outer portion of the media by scar tissue. *Primary intimal fibroplasia* is among the least common varieties and, as the name implies, is expressed in the form of a markedly thickened intima, the new connective tissue appearing rather loose and oedematous on light microscopy. There is no obvious inflammatory component and, in adults, the internal elastic lamina is for the most part intact. In cases occurring during childhood, however, there may be some fragmentation or reduplication of the internal elastic lamina.

The recent importance of this condition is that it can so easily be managed by dilatation. It is extremely suitable to manage renal arteries so diseased by transluminal angioplasty. This method involves the percutaneous passage of an intraluminal balloon catheter which dilates the lesion.

Arterial disorders leading to haemorrhage

Aortic dissection

This is a relatively common condition; one publication states that some 60 000 cases occur annually in the USA. Though the term "dissecting aneurysm" is often used, there is no dilatation of the aorta and the condition is best regarded as a dissecting haematoma which tracks along planes in the region of the middle and outer one-third of the media of the aorta and (sometimes) of its major branches. In most cases this haematoma is accompanied by a sharply demarcated transverse tear in the aortic intima through which blood from the lumen presumably tracks both proximally and distally. In a small proportion of the cases of fatal aortic dissection (some 5 per cent), no trace of such an intimal tear has been recorded and this has given rise to the hypothesis that some cases of dissection owe their origin to intramedial haemorrhage. De Bakey has devised a classification of aortic dissection based on the distribution of the lesion. In Type I, the dissection starts in the ascending aorta and extends past the subclavian vessels into the descending aorta along which it may continue to track. Type II dissections are confined to the ascending aorta and the arch and do not extend past the subclavian vessels, and Type III dissections begin distal to the subclavian vessels. More recently there has been a move to simplify this classification slightly by grouping Types I and II together to form a Type A, and redesignating Type III as Type B.

The pathogenesis of aortic dissection is still poorly understood and there is little agreement on the relative importance of intimal tears and intrinsic medial weakness in this condition. A majority of aortic dissections show histological abnormalities in the media which consist essentially of the accumulation of connective tissue mucins, this being so marked on some occasions, as to give an impression of mucin-filled cystic cavities. There is loss of medial cells (hence the term *cystic medial necrosis*), but no evidence of this loss being associated with an inflammatory response. Elastic tissue fragmentation may be seen, but does not appear to be an essential element in the morphological picture. Such changes may be found in the aortae of aged persons and in association with a long-standing history of hypertension without any evidence of dissection, and some writers have cast doubt on the relevance of cystic medial change to aortic dissection. On the other hand, it is quite clear that certain disorders of connective tissue (chiefly genetically determined) such as Marfan's syndrome and the various Ehlers–Danlos syndromes, carry with them a greatly enhanced risk of aortic dissection. In the former, such dissections account for 30–45 per cent of the fatalities. In all but a few, the biochemical defects responsible for the medial changes are not known, though it seems likely that collagen synthesis and polymerization are affected. In this connexion it is not without interest that feeding beta-amino propronitrile (derived from the sweet pea *Lathyrus odoratus*) to small laboratory animals leads to impairment of normal collagen synthesis and such animals develop medial necrosis and may die of aortic dissection. Similarly, the administration of oestrogen to turkeys leads to a similar set of circumstances and aortic dissection appears to be related to pregnancy. Despite all this evidence, the most appropriate verdict at present on the role of medial weakness in the genesis of aortic dissection is probably the Scottish one of "not proven". A role for hypertension (perhaps mediated via increased shearing stresses on the intima) in relation to intimal tears, appears very likely indeed and in some instances the extent of dissection may be limited by the institution of vigorous antihypertensive treatment.

This condition clinically presents with pain in the chest which radiates around along the course of the aorta. Occasionally re-entry of the lumen by the dissection occurs which is ideal. If not, urgent surgery is required which either provides re-entry or replaces the diseased aorta.

Aneurysms

Aneurysms—localized abnormal dilatations of vessels—may occur in any vessel, but are most commonly found in the aorta. They may be classified on the basis of their location, their shape (either saccular or fusiform) or their aetiology. With the dramatic decline in the prevalence of syphilis, the vast majority of aneurysms encountered in large musculo-elastic arteries arise on a basis of atherosclerosis. They are found, for the most part, in the abdominal aorta usually distal to the origins of the renal arteries and, not surprisingly, there is a marked male preponderance. Unlike what occurs in syphilitic mes-aortitis, where there is fragmentation and loss of elastic laminae, the deficient element in atherosclerotic aneuryms is the medial smooth muscle cell. If one examines any large atherosclerotic plaque histologically, there is obvious medial thinning immediately beneath the thickened intima, and, in appropriately stained sections, this can be seen to be associated with a closer than normal apposition of the elastic laminae and loss of smooth muscle. In experimental situations where comparatively thick mural thrombi form, such smooth muscle cell loss can take place with great speed and shallow aneurysms appear within two to three weeks. Presumably such changes are due to changes in the depth reached by nutrients and oxygen diffusing from the arterial lumen across the intima and a similar mechanism may well operate in the human situation. Once there is some degree of dilatation of the arterial lumen, the lateral pressure on the wall increases markedly and a vicious cycle of ever-increasing dilatation and ever increasing pressure on the wall operates. The aneurysms usually contain large amounts of laminated thrombus which, however, exhibits a striking lack of organization by granulation tissue. This mass of thrombus and clot appears as laminated and gelatinous material and, since there is no firm anchorage between the undersurface of the thrombus and the aortic wall, blood can track behind the thrombus. The mass of thrombus therefore provides little or no protection against haemorrhage in the event of rupture of the wall of the aneurysm.

Aortic aneurysm

Aortic aneurysm can occur anywhere from the ascending aorta along the thoracic aorta or abdominal aorta. Patients with an aneurysm of the ascending aorta frequently present with symptoms of cardiac failure from aortic valve incompetence. Such a patient is dyspnoeic, has orthopnoea, paroxysmal nocturnal dyspnoea cough and all the symptoms of left-sided heart failure from a raised left atrial pressure. On examination there is usually an aortic systolic and early diastolic murmur heard loudest in the aortic area over the heart. Occasionally a patient with an aneurysm of the ascending aorta may present with difficulty in swallowing as a result of pressure on the oesophagus. An aneurysm of the descending thoracic or abdominal aorta can frequently remain asymptomatic for years and is a common cause of sudden death. The warning symptoms, if any, are of backache related to the site of the aneurysm. Abdominal aortic aneurysms can sometimes produce the symptoms of diarrhoea associated with occlusion of the inferior mesenteric artery causing mesenteric ischaemia. On examination it is difficult to detect a thoracic aneurysm, but an abdominal aortic aneurysm is felt in the epigastrium slightly to the left as a pulsatile and expansile lump which may be tender. The clinician frequently finds that arteries in other parts of the body, such as the popliteal arteries, are enlarged in patients with aortic aneurysm. Surgery is frequently required for aneurysms. Usually they are replaced by a section of Dacron tubing.

Neoplasms and malformations of blood vessels

The distinction between benign neoplasms of the vascular system and malformations and hamartomas is, conceptually, not an easy one. In practice the word *haemangioma* may be broadly defined as a benign but non-reactive process in which there is an increase in the number of blood vessels, these being either normal or abnormal in appearance. These lesions may be localized or may, more rarely, involve large areas such as an entire limb. Angiomatous lesions may be classified as:

A. Benign vascular tumours

1. Localized
   (a) Capillary haemangiomas (including the juvenile type)
   (b) Cavernous haemangioma
   (c) Venous haemangioma
   (d) Arteriovenous haemangioma
   (e) Epithelioid haemangioma
   (f) Haemangioma of granulation tissue type pyogenic granuloma
   (g) Miscellaneous haemangiomas of soft tissue (e.g. intramuscular)
2. Diffuse angioma

B. Vascular tumours of intermediate or borderline malignancy

C. Malignant tumours

(a) Angiosarcoma
(b) Kaposi's sarcoma
(c) Malignant endovascular papillary angioendothelioma
(d) Proliferating angioendotheliomatosis

In a chapter of this length it is impossible to consider other than very few of these and the reader is advised to refer to other sources for more adequate coverage of this topic.

Capillary haemangioma

This is the most common of vascular tumours and tumour-like malformations. It usually appears during infancy or early childhood and is located in the skin or subcutaneous tissue. Many variants have been described. One of the commonest of these is the *juvenile haemangioma* which is an immature form of capillary haemangioma. It occurs in about 1 of every 200 live births and is not uncommonly multiple. In the early stages of their natural history they resemble common birth marks in that they are flat red lesions which darken when the baby cries. With the passage of time they grow into elevated protruding masses and it is this feature that has earned them the name *strawberry naevus*. This enlargement occurs rapidly, usually over a period of a few months. However, the period of growth is almost always followed by a period of regression and by the age of seven years between 75 and 90 per cent will have involuted leaving a small pigmented scar.

The tumours are often multinodular, but despite

this can be shown to be fed by a single arteriole. In the early stages the lumina of the capillaries are slit-like and inconspicuous, the endothelial cells that line them are plump and hyperplastic and mitoses are by no means rare. At this stage the vascular nature of the lesion may not be apparent unless appropriate staining methods (such as the reticulin stain) are used. As the lesions mature so does the luminal pattern become more obvious and the endothelial cells flatten giving the whole lesion an appearance more akin to that seen in adult capillary haemangioma.

Epithelioid haemangioma

This is an unusual but distinctive lesion which occurs most frequently between the ages of 20 and 40 years and is more common in women. Most are located in the head and neck region with a particular concentration round the ear. The lesions often start as small, itchy nodules which later coalesce and ulceration and crusting are not infrequent. The abnormal vessels which make up the lesion are lined by plump endothelial cells which have scalloped luminal surfaces which project into the lumina. A mixture of inflammatory cells surrounds the vessels and eosinophils are especially prominent though lymphocytes, plasma cells and mast cells are also seen. Lymphoid aggregates with germinal centres are seen occasionally. Large lesions persist and there are occasional reports of local recurrence after excision. The most distinctive feature of this lesion is the plump, so-called "epithelioid endothelial cell" and many workers believe that this appearance is related to a functional change in the neoplastic endothelium which may be the assumption of some histiocyte functions.

Angiosarcoma

These are frankly malignant tumours the cells of which exhibit functional and morphological characteristics of endothelium. There is a wide spectrum of differentiation and the more poorly differentiated examples may present very difficult diagnostic problems, though in some instances it is possible to identify the histogenesis of the tumours by means of immunocytochemical techniques in cases where the tumour cells are synthesizing Factor VIII associated antigen. Angiosarcomas constitute only a small proportion of all sarcomas and, unlike most malignant connective tissue tumours, have a distinct predilection for the skin. Chronic lymphoedema is a recognized association and some 200 cases of malignant vascular tumours have been described under these circumstances, the majority following on mastectomy. It is not without interest, however, that no case has been reported in patients with filariasis.

Kaposi's sarcoma

Kaposi's sarcoma is a neoplasm in which there is a spectrum of histological appearances dictated, in part at least, by time. In some cases the appearance of these tumours appears to be related to the immunological competence of the host. It has long been recognized to have a distinct regional bias in its distribution and while rather rare in Europe and America, Kaposi's sarcoma may account for up to 9 per cent of all reported malignancies in Central Africa. There have been suggestions that viral infections may be implicated and the DNA of cytomegalovirus has been identified in the cells of some of these tumours. The high incidence among certain sub-populations, notably homosexuals in whom the helper/suppressor T cell ration is reversed, adds strength to this view of the origin of the tumour.

Arteriovenous fistulae

A fistula is an abnormal communication between two epithelial surfaces and in this case the epithelial surfaces apply to an artery and a vein. Broadly speaking these fall into two separate categories, traumatic and congenital.

The traumatic arteriovenous fistula usually results from deep injury in which a solid object, such as a knife or blunt object is forced into the body, usually a limb. This injury disrupts the normal relationship of the arteries and the veins and leads to the abnormal communication. From the clinical point of view a very careful history is vital in making this diagnosis.

The congenital variety presents in a number of ways, usually in the teens. Frequently one limb is longer than another and this is because of increased blood flow associated with a congenital arteriovenous malformation. The increased blood flow past the epiphysis leads to the lengthening. On other occasions prominent veins can be noted over a rather swollen limb. Sometimes these can be mistaken for varicose veins. In the worst variety the prominent veins become arterialized and are sometimes pulsatile.

When an arteriovenous fistula, of whatever

cause, is large enough, high output cardiac failure can occur. In this situation, Branham's sign is positive and on occlusion of the arterial blood supply to the fistula, pulse pressure and heart rate reduce.

Further reading

Bergan JJ(Ed), *Arterial Surgery*. Churchill Livingstone, 1984.

Bernard Victor M, Towne Jonathan B (Eds), *Complications in Vascular Surgery*. Grune and Stratton, 1981.

Dard H, Cockett FB (Eds), *The Pathology and Surgery of the Veins of the Lower Limb*. Churchill Livingstone, 1976.

Eastcott HHG (Ed), *Arterial Surgery*. Pitman, 1973.

Greenhalgh RM (Ed), *Smoking and Arterial Disease*. Pitman Medical, 1979.

Greenhalgh RM (Ed), *Hormones and Vascular Disease*. Pitman Medical, 1980.

Greenhalgh RM (Ed), *Femero-distal Bypass*. Pitman Medical, 1981.

Greenhalgh RM (Ed), *Extra-anatomic and Secondary Arterial Reconstruction*. Pitman Medical, 1982.

Greenhalgh RM, Clifford-Rose F (Eds), *Progress in Stroke Research 2*. Pitman Medical, 1983.

Miller NE (Ed), *Atherosclerosis; Mechanisms and Approaches to Therapy*. New York: Raven Press, 1983.

Nicolaides AN, Yao JST (Eds), *Investigation of Vascular Disorders*. Churchill Livingstone, 1981.

Woolf N, *Pathology of Atherosclerosis*. London: Butterworth Scientific, 1982.

Woolf N (Ed), *The Biology and Pathology of the Vessel Wall*. A Symposium of the Royal College of Pathologists, Praeger, 1983.

20

Veins and Lymphatics

D Negus and S J Machin

Introduction

As in all other surgical conditions, the surgeon and pathologist must work together for the effective diagnosis and management of venous and lymphatic disorders. However, their relationship differs in some respects from that required for the management of tumours, bacterial infections and other surgical diseases. Diagnosis and treatment of disorders of the veins and lymphatics is usually made without direct help from the histopathologist. At the same time, it must be appreciated that effective diagnosis and management depends on a thorough knowledge of the underlying pathology. The pathology of venous thrombosis and its sequela is dependant on a detailed knowledge of the coagulation system which comes within the interest of the specialist haematologist. Also the prophylaxis and management of thrombotic disorders is dependant on the laboratory tests and advice from a specialized coagulation unit.

Certain fundamental anatomical features are important in considering the pathology and clinical management of venous and lymphatic disorders. In the upper limb, there is no distinct division of superficial and deep veins; in the lower limb this division is functionally very important. The deep veins of the calf, which are the venae comitantes of the main limb arteries and the high capacitant soleal sinusoids, lie within muscles which are themselves enclosed in a tight investing deep fascia. Contraction of these muscles creates high intravenous pressures, of the order of 140 mm/Hg, which forces blood proximally to the popliteal, femoral and iliac veins. Reflux during muscle relaxation is prevented by bicuspid valves, which are most numerous in the distal veins. Valves also prevent reflux to the superficial, long and short saphenous, veins and into the direct calf and ankle perforating veins, which receive the supramalleolar venules. This network of small veins is exposed to the greatest pressures in direct perforating vein incompetence, and this produces the sequence of events which results in venous ulceration. Numerous smaller, indirect, perforating veins penetrate the deep fascia more proximally in the leg, to join intramuscular veins. These are of little functional significance.

The main lymphatic trunks lie in the superficial fascia and follow the course of the saphenous veins. Deep lymphatics are few and are functionally less important. A few lymph trunks terminate in the popliteal lymph nodes, but most end in the superficial and deep inguinal nodes which communicate with the iliac and lumbar nodes, and then with the cisterna chylae and thoracic duct. Like veins, lymphatics are profusely valved, and occasionally valvular incompetence results in dilated and "varicose" megalymphatics.

We will first discuss problems relevant to superficial veins and lymphatics. Our consideration of the lymphatics will be confined to their function in draining tissue fluid from the limb and to their role in acute infections. Acute inflammatory disorders affecting these structures are superficial thrombophlebitis and acute lymphangitis. The aetiology, pathology and management of varicose veins completes this section, as inadequacies of lymphatic drainage are more appropriately discussed with other causes of peripheral oedema in the subsequent section. This is followed by consideration of the aetiology, diagnosis, prevention and treatment of deep vein thrombosis and then by its sequel, the post-thrombotic syndrome. Finally, we will discuss the rare venous and lymphatic abnormalities of arteriovenous fistula, haemangiomas and lymphangiomas.

Superficial veins and lymphatics

Acute inflammatory disorders

Acute lymphangitis presents as a series of fine, red, tender lines along the length of the limb.

Infected lymph from an acute infection causes bacterial invasion of the lymphatic trunks. The infection stops at the regional lymph-nodes and if antibiotic therapy is delayed or inappropriate, this will result in an acutely inflamed, tender lymph-node, acute lymphadenitis and possibly abscess formation. The surgeon and microbiologist must therefore cooperate to minimize the course of the disease.

For example, as soon as the paronychia, whitlow or abscess is drained, a sample of pus is sent to the laboratory where Gram staining is performed. The appearance of many white blood cells associated with Gram-positive cocci in clusters suggests *Staphlococcus aureus*, the most common responsible organism. The presence of Gram-positive cocci in chains suggests beta-haemolytic streptococcus, Lancefield Group A, C, or G. However, the latter organisms are more commonly associated with cellulitis. Gram-negative rods are less commonly seen and their significance should be discussed with the microbiologist. Culture of the pus, aerobically (and anaerobically if required) is performed on blood agar.

Following drainage, appropriate antibiotic therapy is commenced. A useful regime would be flucloxacillin, (to cover *Staphlococcus aureus*) and ampicillin (to cover beta-haemolytic streptococci and many "coliforms"). This may be modified when the causative organism and its sensitivities are known. It is often forgotten that, in the pre-antibiotic era, these conditions were very serious and indeed life-threatening. The easy availability of antibiotics today should not make the approach to their management any less serious.

Once an inguinal or axillary abscess is diagnosed, it must be drained. Prolonged use of antibiotics without prior surgical drainage may encourage the abscess to develop a thick-walled cavity.

Superficial thrombophlebitis is most commonly a complication of an intravenous infusion. The inflammatory process, with invasion of the vein wall by macrophages, mast cells and leucocytes, may follow thrombus formation in the infusion cannula. It is important, therefore, to use non-irritant cannulae, and to change these at regular intervals. A little heparin, (2000 units per 24 hours) minimizes thrombus formation in the cannula. Care should also be taken to avoid irritant solutions, particularly concentrated dextrose. Where these have to be given, the cannula should be inserted into a large vein, such as the superior vena cava. All clotted infusion cannulae should be sent directly to the microbiology laboratory for culture. Hence the results of culture and sensitivity will be available if the patient subsequently develops septicaemia or bacteraemia. It must never be forgotten that though modern management of seriously ill patients depends very much on intravenous infusions and their monitoring by a central venous pressure line, these lines and cannulae provide a portal of entry for opportunistic pathogens.

Spontaneous superficial thrombophlebitis is an uncommon complication of varicose veins. Thrombophlebitis ascending along the course of the long saphenous vein is an indication for emergency sapheno-femoral ligation to prevent propagation of the thrombus into the common femoral vein. Small thrombosed varices do not require the use of anticoagulants. Crepe bandages, elevation and local applications such as Hirudoid ointment are usually sufficient treatment.

Painful spontaneous superficial thrombophlebitis in previously normal veins, which resolves in one vein only to reappear in another, is known as *thrombophlebitis migrans*. Unlike the thrombophlebitis of varicose veins, this often affects the arm veins. This condition may be the first evidence of *thrombangitis obliterans* (*Buerger's disease*), particularly if the patient is a cigarette-smoker. It is also said to be evidence of occult carcinoma, though spontaneous deep vein thrombosis is more usual in this context. A final diagnosis of this condition depends on biopsy when the affected segment of vessel often contains an organized recanalized thrombus.

It is appropriate to pause here to consider the words: "thrombophlebitis" and "phlebothrombosis". It was originally taught that superficial venous thrombophlebitis was predominantly inflammatory; while deep vein thrombosis had little inflammatory reaction, and was therefore termed "phlebothrombosis". It is now recognized that thrombosis and an inflammatory reaction of the adjacent vein wall normally co-exist to a greater or lesser degree. Superficial thrombophlebitis may either follow thrombus formation in a cannula, or infection around such thrombus formation. In either case, thrombosis and vein wall inflammation "phlebitis" co-exist. In the deep veins the vein wall reaction is less in evidence in the early stages, thrombus formation normally starting as a result of stasis and the accumulation of activated clotting factors. In most cases, this then sets up a vein wall reaction, which in turn fixes the thrombus and initiates the process which leads to re-canalization. The dangerous situation is when this reaction fails to take place and the thrombus remains lying loose in the venous stream, propagating proximally and then detaching to embolize to the pulmonary circulation. The pathology, diagnosis and management of deep vein thrombosis will be considered in more detail later.

Varicose veins

Varicose veins are defined as distended, elongated, tortuous, superficial veins with incompetent valves. Obvious superficial veins in a thin leg can be mistaken for varices, but mistakes will not be made if this definition is remembered. It has been suggested that varicose veins are the penalty that man pays for assuming the upright posture; that they are the result of pressure from the gravid uterus; or even that they result from pressure produced by the constipated sigmoid colon. It takes little thought to explode the fallacy of such explanations. Gravity is hardly a likely explanation since much taller animals than man have no varicose veins; and there is no demonstrable relationship with constipation. Certainly many women develop varicose veins during pregnancy, usually the second pregnancy, but a careful history will reveal that over 90 per cent of these women have a strong family history of varicose veins.

It has been postulated that varicose veins are the result of rupture of the upper valve at the saphenofemoral junction, perhaps following straining at stool. A little experience in a vein clinic will show that many patients present with distal varices, the saphenous vein becoming dilated and varicose later. It has also been demonstrated that the valve leaflets themselves are by far the strongest part of the vein, the vein wall, in particular that adjacent to the valves, being much weaker.

A more convincing explanation, based on recent studies, is that varicose veins are a congenital disorder which results from inherited weakness of the vein wall. This weakness is histologically demonstrable as a defect in collagen crossbanding with an increase in local collagenase and also an increase in circulating collagen-splitting enzymes. The collagen abnormality in the walls of varicose veins has also been demonstrated in the undilated arm veins of the same patients.

This increased distensibility is exacerbated in pregnancy, when collagen tissue and smooth muscle become softer and more distensible, and when there is also a 30 per cent increase in blood volume, the greater proportion being in the venous circulation.

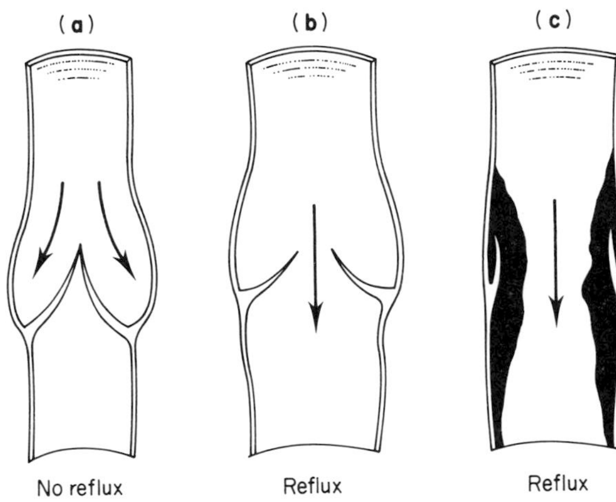

Fig. 20.1 Normal and abnormal veins. A—normal valve with no reflux. B—primary familial varicose vein with a dilated vein and a distended weak vein wall. C—secondary varices following venous thrombosis with a retracted and recanalised thrombus, causing valvular damage and subsequent reflux.

It is important to realize that this theory of aetiology applies only to primary varicose veins. Secondary varices resulting from venous thrombosis, and its subsequent recanalization, results in damage to the valve cusps themselves, which become either destroyed or firmly adherent to the vein wall, with resultant venous incompetence. This subject is considered further below. Normal and abnormal venous valves are shown in Fig. 20.1. Small varicose veins can be treated by injection scleropathy. This treatment consists of injecting a sclerosant, usually sodium tetradecyl sulphate, which produces a sterile inflammatory reaction of the vein wall. Subsequent compression by elastic bandages causes these walls to adhere. This is followed by permanent replacement of the lumen by a thin fibrous cord. Inadequate compression leads to lumpy thrombus formation, rather than the sclerosis which is the aim of this form of treatment. Injection sclerotherapy is satisfactory for small isolated varices of the lower leg. If the long or short saphenous veins are incompetent, the long-term effects of injection sclerotherapy are poor, due to the persistent high venous pressure exerted on the smaller veins. Ligation of the responsible saphenous vein is then necessary with avulsion of varices through small stab incisions. A grossly incompetent, dilated saphenous vein is stripped at the same time.

Primary familial varicose veins may include the perforating veins which join the superficial venular network to the deep veins. However, these are less common than following deep vein thrombosis, and venous ulceration is very much more likely to be associated with a past history of venous thrombosis than by simple primary varices.

The swollen limb

The diagnosis of limbswelling includes both general and local causes. It can be clarified by a simple classification of the responsible pathological and physiological factors (Fig. 20.2).

Oedema of the upper limb is not common. The arms, as well as the legs, may become swollen in acute anaphylaxis or severe nephritis; but acute swelling of one arm usually results from axillary vein thrombosis, with obstruction of venous return. Distal veins are distended and the arm is cyanosed and painful. Treatment is by elevation and anticoagulants. Chronic swelling of the upper limb is sometimes seen following axillary block dissection and deep X-ray therapy for carcinoma of the breast. Most of these patients have a scarred and narrowed axillary vein as well as absent lymphatic pathways.

The general causes of lower limb oedema are congestive cardiac failure, renal failure and hypoproteinaemia. Venous congestion, an increase in tissue fluid, and a reduction in plasma osmolarity, are the prime causes in each case. All must be excluded in investigating any patient with bilateral lower limb oedema of unknown cause by examination of the cardiovascular system and jugular venous pressure; examination of the urine for protein; and measurement of the total plasma protein and albumen levels.

Local causes include acute deep vein thrombosis, its sequel the post-thrombotic

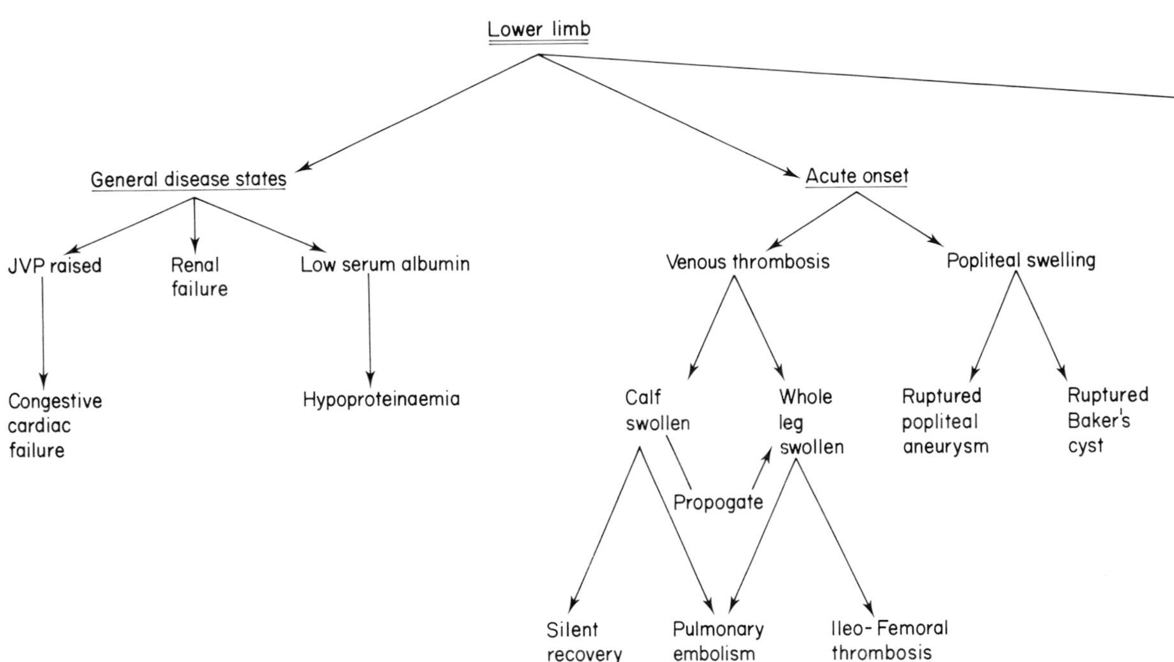

Fig. 20.2 The swollen limb.

syndrome, lymphoedema (which may be either primary or secondary) and obstruction or damage to both iliac veins and lymphatics by malignant disease following surgical block dissection or radiotherapy.

Deep vein thrombosis

Thrombosis of the deep veins is the most common cause of the acutely swollen lower limb. The calf is most frequently affected, and the swelling is usually accompanied by pain, tenderness on palpation and an increase in local skin temperature. At the same time, it must be realized that many deep vein thromboses give rise to no symptoms or physical signs whatsoever, and these are often the cause of "silent" pulmonary embolism, which may be fatal. An understanding of the pathology of this common complication of major illness and surgery is essential to its prevention, diagnosis and management.

Pathology of venous thrombosis

Venous thrombi are intravascular deposits, composed mainly of fibrin and red cells. In this they differ from arterial thrombi, which are initially largely composed of platelets.

Venous thrombi form in regions of slow flow, beginning as small deposits in valve cusp pockets in the deep calf or thigh veins, in large calf venous sinuses, or in venous segments exposed to local trauma. Initial deposits consist of masses of platelet aggregates or of fibrin and trapped red cells. The initial composition may vary according to the predominating thrombogenic stimulus; fibrin and red cell thrombi form in areas of stasis, while platelet thrombi form at sites of endothelial cell damage.

The nidus of the thrombus grows out of the valve cusp, being composed of successive layers of aggregated platelets and fibrin (Fig. 20.3). The

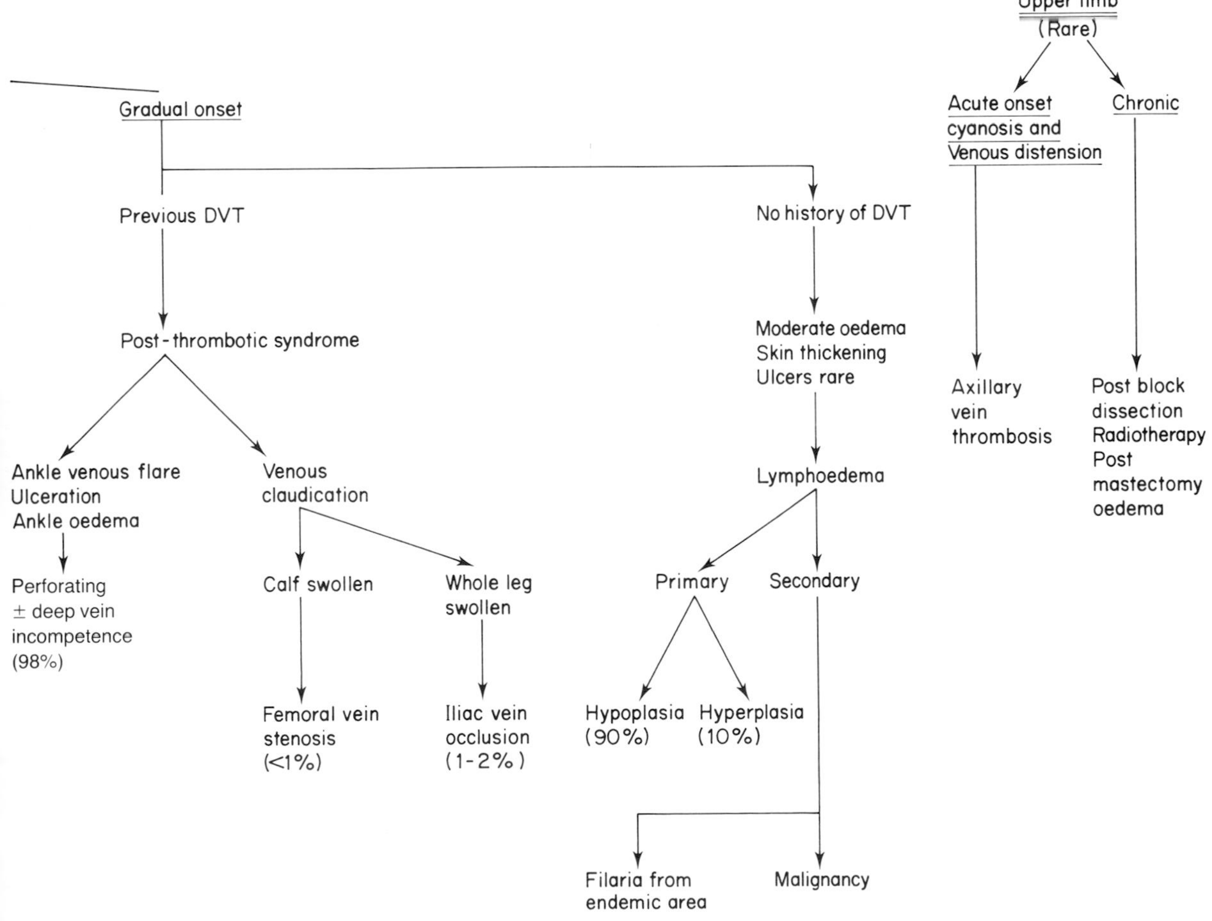

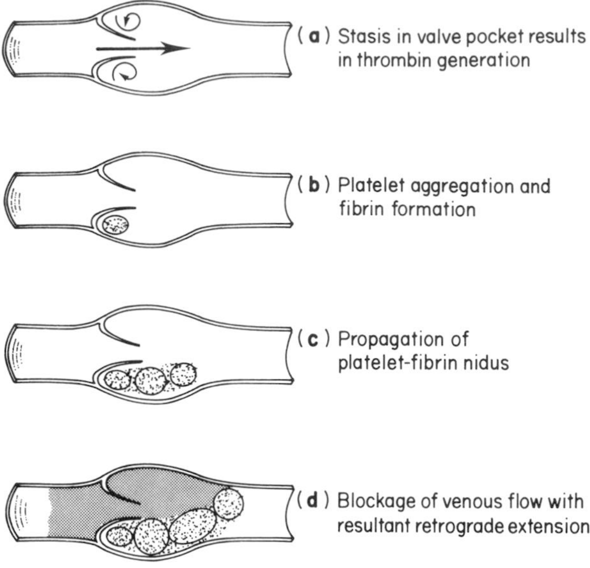

Fig. 20.3 The development of venous thrombosis.

propagating thrombus gradually occludes the vein, flow is slowed and the thrombus extends mainly proximally in the direction of flow. When the lumen is totally occluded, a red coagulation thrombus spreads distally. Propagation continues until the next tributary is reached, when it extends into the lumen of the flowing vessel as a mixed thrombus.

Varying degrees of inflammatory change occur in the underlying vein wall. Local inflammation, the venous distension and raised venous pressure which occur because of the obstruction, explain the pain, tenderness and swelling that occur in acute deep vein thrombosis. Lack of inflammation results in loose propagating thrombus, with a higher risk of embolization. A simple scheme representing the pathological events in deep vein thrombosis is shown in Fig. 20.4.

Natural history of venous thrombosis

Once a thrombus has formed, it may extend, undergo lysis, become organized or embolize. If the initial thrombogenic stimulus persists, extension is likely to occur. Complete lysis rarely occurs depending on fibrinolytic activity and digestion of fibrin by leucocytes. Pulmonary embolism is frequently associated with venous thrombosis, but if the embolus arises from a calf vein thrombus it is usually small and asymptomatic. Most large pulmonary emboli originate from thrombi in the proximal veins of the leg.

Thrombi which do not completely embolize or undergo dissolution, slowly organize and become recanalized. Destruction of the venous valves during recanalization raises the venous pressure in the affected leg. This predisposes patients to the post-thrombotic syndrome and to recurrent acute venous thrombosis.

The pathogenesis and subsequent outcome of venous thrombosis is shown diagramatically in Fig. 20.4.

Thrombosis initiation is the result of a combination of activation of blood coagulation, vascular damage, and local stasis. These important factors in the aetiology of deep vein thrombosis are still the same as those summarized by Virchow's triad in 1864. These predisposing factors overcome the natural protecting mechanisms such as inactivation by circulating inhibitors of activated coagulation factors, clearance of these activated products by the liver and reticuloendothelial cells, and dissolution of fibrin clots by the fibrinolytic system.

Activation of coagulation The coagulation proteins circulate as inactive proenzymes, which are sequentially activated to serine proteases leading to the generation of thrombin. Thrombin interacts with fibrinogen and converts it into fibrin monomer. These fragments copolymerize to form a precipitate of insoluble fibrin, which is further stabilized with covalent bands by activated Factor XIII. This is shown schematically in Fig. 20.5. The coagulation system is activated in vivo by tissue thromboplastin at the level of Factor VII (the extrinsic pathway) or by contact activation of Factor XII (the intrinsic pathway). Tissue thromboplastin is made available by vascular cells at sites of damage, and by migrating activated leucocytes, and is released into the bloodstream during surgery and following tissue injury. Vascular injury exposes subendothelial tissues which contact activate Factor XII in the circulating blood.

Vessel damage The normal intact endothelial surface is non-thrombogenic. This non-reactivity is due to several factors, which include electrostatic repulsion by the negative charge on the cell surfaces, and the synthesis and secretion by the endothelial cells of fibronectin, prostacyclin (which inhibits platelet aggregation) and a heparin-like anticoagulant, heparan sulphate.

It used to be thought that pressure on the calf veins during operation was an important cause of vessel damage, and much care is still taken to protect the calf muscles. While such care is certainly

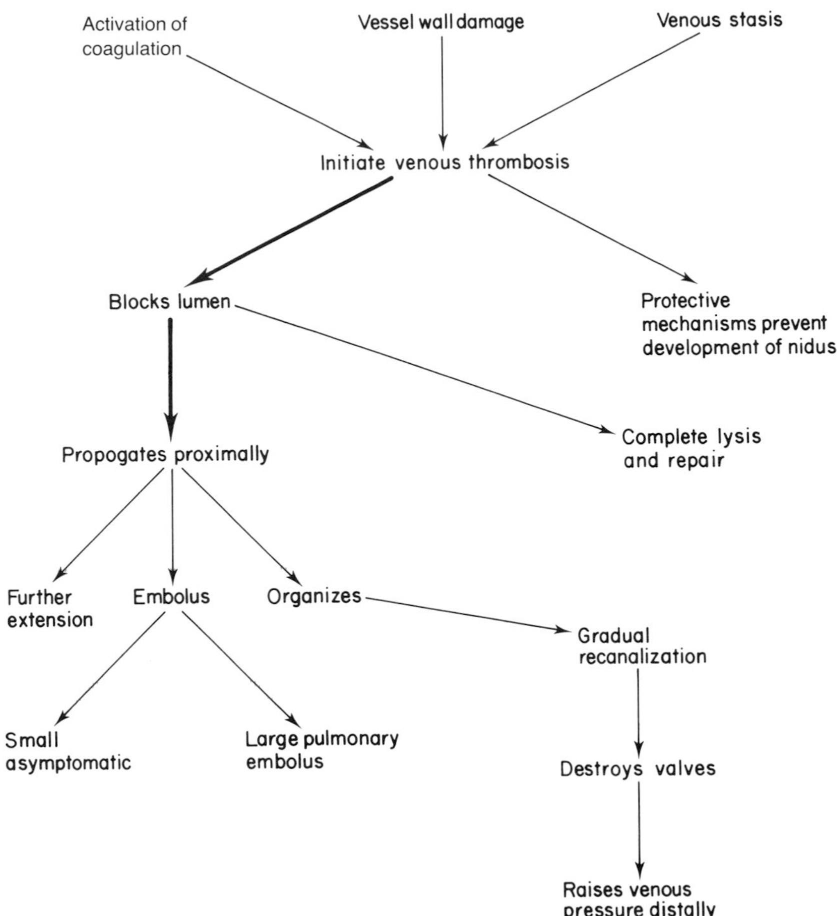

Fig. 20.4 Pathology of venous thrombosis.

sensible, there is no real evidence that simple compression of the calf muscles causes any damage to the deep veins at all. It is traditional to elevate the heels of an anaesthetized patient on rubber pads in order to stop the calf muscles lying in firm contact with the table and this in itself may contribute to venous stasis. It is also sensible to protect the calves by elastic stockings or bandages. These confer some degree of protection and also counteract stasis. By contrast, trauma to the lower limb, whether accidental or surgical, can produce severe venous damage and many patients with fractures of the lower limb subsequently develop deep vein thrombosis.

Following vascular damage and exposure of the subendothelium, platelets adhere and then aggregate to the damaged surface, releasing adenosine diphosphate (ADP) and thromboxane A_2 (TXA_2) and then they undergo a change in the external platelet membrane, which further accelerates thrombin generation. Leucocytes also migrate to the damaged area, releasing tissue thromboplastins, and contact of Factor XII with exposed collagen and other subendothelial tissues activates the coagulation pathway.

Venous stasis Venous return from the legs is considerably aided by contraction of calf muscles. Immobilized patients lose this action, with resultant pooling of blood in the calf sinusoids. Impaired venous return and stasis can result from cardiac failure, venous obstruction (external compression such as a pelvic mass, or internal obstruction relating to a previous thrombosis) or excessive venous dilatation, which may occur with varicose veins or as a direct effect of oestrogens on smooth muscle tone. Venous stasis is most marked during general anaesthesia, with a low cardiac output, particularly if intra-operative blood-loss results in temporary hypotension.

It should be remembered that muscle relaxants

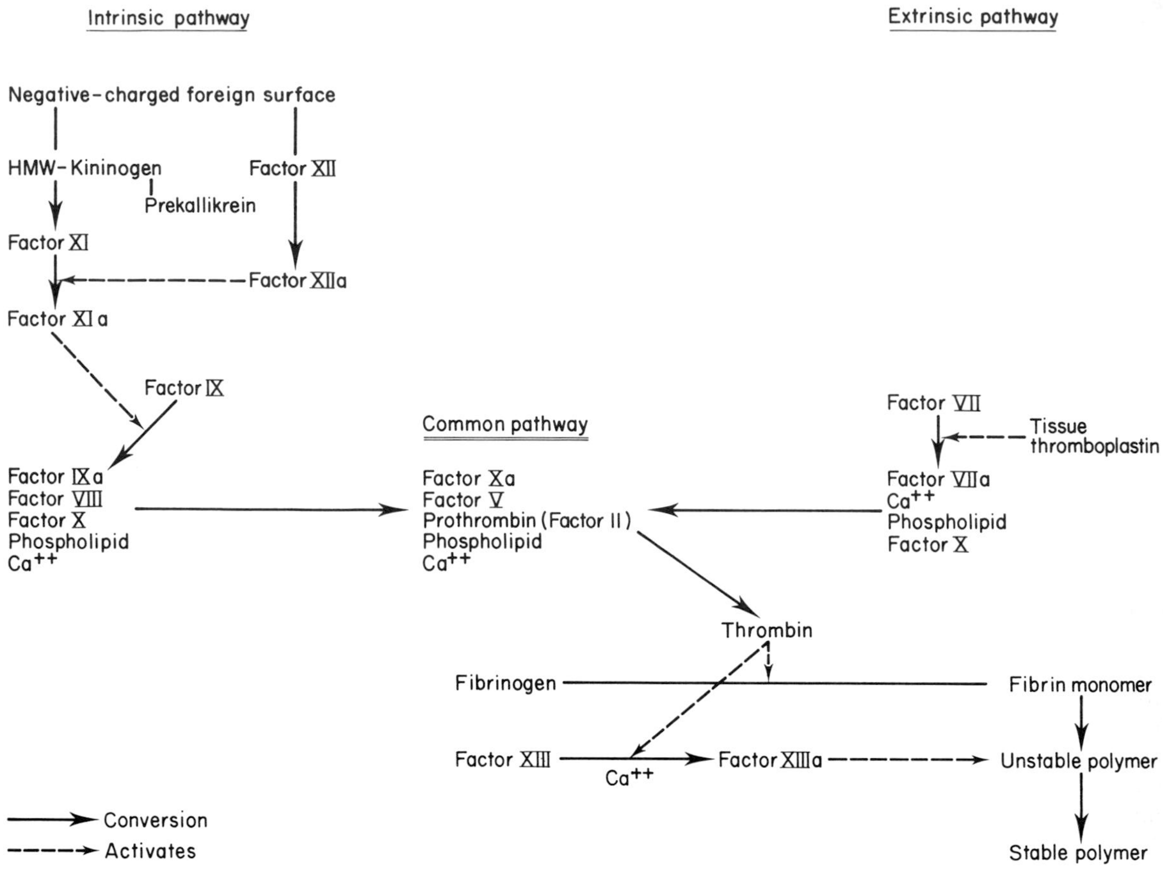

Fig. 20.5 Blood coagulation process.

not only relax the abdominal muscles, in order to make the surgeon's work possible, but also relax all other striated muscle, and this of course includes the calf muscles. Blood will then tend to pool in the dependent soleal venous sinusoids and valve pockets in the calf veins. Activated clotting factors, particularly Factor Xa, accumulate in such areas of relative stagnation, with resulting initiation of thrombosis. Surgical operations in which no muscle relaxants are used, such as repair of inguinal herniae, have a much lower incidence of postoperative thrombosis than laparotomy, where relaxant drugs are mandatory.

Clinical risk factors and incidence of venous thrombosis

A number of clinical conditions and laboratory abnormalities predispose to venous thrombosis. The clinically recognized high risk states are listed in Table 20.1, along with some less common dis-

Table 20.1 Clinical risk factors associated with a high incidence of venous thrombosis.

High risk factors	*Uncommon diseases with a high incidence*
Surgical and non-surgical trauma	Homocystinuria
Age	Myeloproliferative disorders
Malignancy	Polycythaemia
Immobilization	Systemic lupus erythematosus
Heart Failure	Behçet's disease
Previous venous thrombosis	Paraproteinaemias
Myocardial infarction	Nephrotic syndrome
Paralysis of lower limbs	
Varicose veins	
Obesity	
Oestrogen therapy	
Pregnancy and puerperium	
Diabetes Mellitus	

Table 20.2 Classification of venous thromboembolism according to type of major operation

Thromboembolic event	*Abdominal and thoracic surgery in patients under 40. No risk factors*	*Abdominal surgery in patients over 40 plus previous DVT, or malignancy*	*Elective hip and knee surgery*
Calf vein thrombosis (%)	2	40	50–60
Proximal vein thrombosis (%)	0.4	10	20
Clinical pulmonary embolism (%)	0.2	5	5–10
Fatal pulmonary embolism (%)	<0.02	1	1–3

orders which are frequently complicated by venous thrombosis.

The incidence of venous thrombosis following surgery is related to the severity, site, extent and duration of the procedure and the length of time of postoperative immobilization. The approximate incidence of venous thrombosis and pulmonary embolism for major surgical procedures are summarized in Table 20.2.

Patients undergoing elective hip surgery differ from other surgical patients developing venous thrombosis in several respects. These patients have a high incidence of isolated femoral vein thrombi. This probably results from local damage due to operative manipulation and excessive intra-operative venous stasis. Venographic studies have demonstrated stretching and distortion of the femoral vein during disarticulation of the hip, which is an essential part of hip replacement surgery. Secondly, the relative failure of prophylactic heparin in these patients may represent the inability of heparin to prevent an injury-based thrombus related primarily to intimal and endothelial cell damage.

The association between venous thrombosis and malignancy may be related to the fact that procoagulant material, which has both tissue thromboplastin-like and Factor X activating activity, has been isolated from malignant tissue. Secondly, malignant patients in general have reduced vascular fibrinolytic activity and tumours may readily compress or infiltrate veins.

A number of potential thrombogenic factors operate during pregnancy. These include a decrease in vascular fibrinolytic activity, the release of tissue thromboplastins into the circulation during delivery and venous stasis due to pressure from the uterus and venous dilatation. There is also an increased level of fibrinogen and the coagulation Factors II, VII, VIII and I. Although the risk of fatal pulmonary embolism during pregnancy is low (approximately 1–2 deaths per 100 000 deliveries in England), it remains the commonest cause of maternal death. These patients often have other high risk factors such as age over 30, obesity, previous venous thrombosis, prolonged bed rest or an operative delivery. Oestrogen therapy also has a reported increased risk of venous thrombosis related to a decrease in functional antithrombin III (AT III) activity, decreased vascular fibrinolytic activity, venous dilatation and an increased level of a number of coagulation factors.

Laboratory risk factors and the hypercoaguable state

Several laboratory abnormalities are associated with venous thrombosis. These may be long-standing hereditary or acquired defects, or transient acute phase reactions which have arisen in response to recent tissue injury.

Chronic defects Predisposition to venous thrombosis has been reported in several families now with congenital deficiency of AT III. Patients with levels of functional AT III activity below 60 per cent of normal, seem to be at risk. Antithrombin III is an important physiological regulator of inappropriate activation of the coagulation pathway by its ability to complex and inactivate thrombin, Xa and other activated coagulation factors including IXa and XIa. Heparin exerts its catalytic action of inactivating clotting enzymes by binding to AT III. This binding induces a conformational change which facilitates thrombin inactivation. Heparin then dissociates from the AT III-thrombin complex and may interact again with other available AT III molecules.

Acquired deficiency of AT III may be found in liver cirrhosis, the nephrotic syndrome, disseminated intravascular coagulation and after prolonged intravenous heparin infusions. In all these conditions, a significant clinical venous thrombotic event may occur. However, a reduced function level of AT III below 70 per cent of normal only occurs in a small proportion of patients with venous thrombosis. This usually represents greatly increased AT III consumption or a latent depression of synthesis.

Antithrombin III accounts for about 70 per cent of the natural inhibitors of activated coagulation proteins. Deficiency of the other inhibitors—α_1-anti-trypsin and α_2-macroglobulin—does not seem to predispose to thrombosis; although the vitamin-K dependent factor protein C, which has recently been described, inhibits the pro-enzymatic action of Factors V and VIII and its deficiency may be associated with venous thrombosis.

There are several inherited defects of the fibrinogen molecule, known as dyfibrinogenaemia, which have been associated with recurrent thrombosis. These are detected by a prolonged thrombin and reptilase time and defective absorption of thrombin may account for a thrombotic tendency.

The main protective mechanism following thrombus formation involves activation of the fibrinolytic enzyme system. Plasminogen is converted to the active proteolytic enzyme plasmin by the release into the circulation of plasminogen activators from vascular endothelial cells and other tissues. Plasmin hydrolyses fibrin and various coagulation proteins including fibrinogen. Abnormal plasminogen and decreased vessel wall synthesis and release of plasminogen activator have occasionally been reported in patients with recurrent venous thrombosis, especially in those with lesions involving the superficial veins.

Polycythaemia, increased blood viscosity, and thrombocytosis over prolonged periods, contribute towards a thrombotic tendency.

Acute phase reactions Following any form of tissue injury, including surgical procedures, there is a systemic acute phase reaction caused by activation of blood coagulation. This non-specific reaction causes an elevation of several plasma proteins (fibrinogen, Factor VIII and the anti-plasmins), the platelet count and white count, and also causes a fever. These changes cause increased thrombin generation and platelet reactivity, which may be exacerbated locally by vascular damage and stasis.

Thrombin generation cleaves fibrinopeptides A and B from fibrinogen and converts it into fibrin monomer. These monomers co-polymerize with each other and large polymers are precipitated intravascularly as fibrin. These deposits are usually small asymptomatic microvascular events which are subsequently digested by fibrinolytic activity, but they may be large enough to form the nidus of a thrombus in larger veins at susceptible sites.

The effect of these interactions can be monitored by a series of sensitive blood tests. These include radio-immunoassay of fibrinopeptide A, para-coagulation tests for co-polymerizing fibrin monomers (protamine sulphate or ethanol gelation tests) and assays of fibrinogen and fibrin degradation products. Similarly platelet activation may be assessed by radio-immunoassay of thromboxane B_2 (TXB_2) or products of platelet α-granule release (β-thromboglobulin and platelet Factor 4).

Blood tests to predict and diagnose venous thrombosis

The predictive values of numerous blood tests have been evaluated in many clinical trials involving surgical patients. Of these tests, only two have shown any consistent predictive value. They are decreased fibrinolytic activity by the euglobin clot lysis time and increased platelet coagulant activity.

Similarly, many tests have been evaluated for their ability to confirm or exclude a diagnosis of venous thrombosis. Although many of the tests employed have been highly sensitive to intravascular fibrin formation and platelet activation, they all suffer from lack of clinical specificity, and false positive or negative results are still in the order of 10 per cent.

Prevention of deep vein thrombosis

Although deep vein thrombosis may occur in any patient undergoing a surgical procedure, it is the high risk groups of patients which have been outlined above, whom it is most important to protect. The last decade has seen an energetic search in many centres for suitable methods of prevention. These must be reliable, safe and preferably simple and inexpensive. As in considering the natural history of venous thrombosis, one can approach the problem of prophylaxis in terms of Virchow's triad—vascular damage, venous stasis and hypercoagulability.

It is obviously impossible to prevent vascular damage in major limb trauma, but care should be taken in operative technique and in particular the orthopaedic surgeon can modify his approach to the hip joint so as to minimize distortion of the femoral vein.

Venous stasis can be reduced, either passively or actively. Passive elevation of the legs during and after surgery may have some effect, but this has not been proved by clinical trials. Compression stockings, on the other hand, have been shown to effect a 50 per cent reduction in isotope-detected small deep vein thrombi. Active mechanical methods include intermittent galvanic stimulation of the calf muscles to produce regular small contractions, or intermittent compression of these muscles by an air-inflated bag. Both methods have been demonstrated to reduce the incidence of isotopically detected thrombi but, to date, no major study of their effect on pulmonary embolism has been carried out. In addition, early ambulation remains an important preventive measure. All these methods are quite simple, extremely cheap and free of complications, and may be used in combination with other forms of prophylaxis in high risk patients.

The hypercoagulability of the acute phase reaction which follows surgical operations can be counteracted in a number of ways. Low dose subcutaneous heparin given in a dose of 5000 units 2 hours preoperatively and then every 8 or 12 hours postoperatively is now the most widely adopted form of prophylactic therapy. Low-dose heparin has been shown by Kakkar and his colleagues to significantly reduce the frequency of ^{125}I-fibrinogen detectable thrombosis and major pulmonary embolis. However, there have been several reports of increased episodes of wound haematomas and bleeding, especially in the high risk patients receiving the eight-hourly regime. The routine use of laboratory control is probably unnecessary, although some workers have claimed to reduce haemorrhagic complications by maintaining the peak heparin level below 0.05 U/ml. To reduce the bleeding complications associated with low-dose heparin prophylaxis, several new approaches including the combined use of only 2500 units of heparin with the venoconstrictor dihydroergotamine, the use of a semi-synthetic heparin analogue and the use of low-molecular-weight heparin, are all at present being assessed in clinical trials.

As an alternative to the subcutaneous route, it has been suggested that intravenous heparin prophylaxis might be used in patients who already require intravenous therapy. It has been shown by Negus that only a very small dose of heparin is required, 1 unit per kilogram body-weight per hour. In a 70 kilogram man, the 24-hour dosage is less than 1700 units. This method has been shown to be effective in two studies using ^{125}I-fibrinogen detected venous thrombosis, but larger-scale studies are required for confirmation. Heparin is unstable in dextrose or dextrose saline, and must be given in normal saline, which is then 'piggybacked' into the main infusion line. It appears to be free of complications, in particular there is no increased risk of haemorrhage.

Other proven effective prophylactic approaches include oral anticoagulation with warfarin starting one day preoperatively or immediately postoperatively or the infusion of 500 ml of low-molecular-weight dextran 40 over a 4–6 hour period starting during the operation and repeated daily for up to 5 days later. Although warfarin is effective, it is unpopular with surgeons because of the considerable incidence of increased bleeding episodes and the stringent laboratory control that is required postoperatively. Dextran 40 also carries a slight increased risk of bleeding, may produce circulatory overload and, rarely, anaphylactic shock.

Diagnosis of deep vein thrombosis

As we have seen, the pain, tenderness and swelling that usually occur in deep vein thrombosis can be explained by local inflammation, venous distension and raised venous pressure. This is most marked in iliofemoral thrombosis, when the whole limb is swollen and pale—the latter due to a decrease in arteriolar perfusion. This painful "white leg" (phlegmasia alba dolens) may proceed to even more severe venous occlusion with a cyanosed "blue leg" (Phlegmasia cerulia dolens) and digital gangrene. The latter is more common in patients with underlying arterial insufficiency.

There is little difficulty in diagnosing such florid presentations of venous thrombosis. However, only too often deep vein thrombosis is 'silent' and this, because the thrombus is non-adherent, is the most likely to embolize to the pulmonary circulation, and therefore the most dangerous.

Several methods of diagnosis have therefore been introduced in recent years. These include examination of the patency of the deep veins by Doppler ultrasound. Firm compression of the calf vein, with the ultrasonic probe placed over the groin, will normally result in a transmission of an audible pulse wave. This is reduced or abolished by thrombotic venous obstruction. A more sensitive method, which is more used in research than in clinical situations, is the ^{125}I-fibrinogen uptake technique. This depends on the fact that human fibrinogen, obtained from hepatitis-free donors and labelled with radioactive iodine, is incorporated into forming thrombus following its intravenous injection. The consequent rise in radioactivity can be detected by a scintillation counter.

Deep vein thrombosis results in a local increase in temperature, and this can be detected by infra red thermography. The only bar to the more widespread use of this method is its considerable expense. In addition to Doppler ultrasound, venous occlusion can be detected by various plethysmographic methods. Venous occlusion is produced by inflation of the thigh cuff. Following its release, with the leg elevated, there should be a rapid fall in calf volume. Occlusion or partial occlusion of the venous drainage will slow down this reduction in calf volume; and these changes in volume can be detected by either strain-gauge, air, or impedance plethysmography.

Phlebography is the most accurate and widely used method of detecting deep vein thrombosis, by injecting contrast medium into a dorsal foot vein. Until recently these media were irritant and could produce pain and further thrombosis. Modern, non-irritant media, have very much reduced the discomfort and risk associated with this technique.

Treatment

Diagnosis of deep vein thrombosis must be followed by its effective treatment. The aims of treatment are to prevent extension of venous thrombosis and the development of pulmonary embolism, to prevent the post-thrombotic syndrome and to relieve the acute local symptoms. Very small thrombi below the knee can be treated by simple compression and elevation, but if there is the slightest risk of propagation, or if even a small embolic episode has already taken place, treatment by anticoagulants is mandatory.

Anticoagulant therapy is usually initiated by a continuous intravenous infusion of full-dose heparin, preferably by means of a syringe pump. An initial bolus injection of 5000 units of heparin should be followed by a continuous infusion of between 20 000–30 000 units every 24 hours. A number of laboratory tests are available to monitor the anticoagulant effect of heparin, one of which should be performed approximately 6 hours after starting the infusion and then repeated daily. Ideally the heparin dosage should be maintained between 0.3–0.4 U/ml. Of the most frequently available tests, the whole blood clotting time (Lee and White method) should be maintained between 2 and 3 times control level, the activated partial thromboplastin time (APTT) between $1\frac{1}{2}$ and 2 times control level or the calcium thrombin time (TT) between 2 and 4 times control level. At this heparin concentration, thrombus extension is prevented without exposing the patient to the risk of excessive bleeding.

Heparin therapy should be continued for 7–10 days and then replaced by oral anticoagulant treatment. This should be started 4–5 days before the heparin infusion is discontinued, so as to maintain an adequate anti-thrombotic effect. The oral anticoagulants are vitamin K antagonists. Vitamin K acts at a post-ribosomal site in the hepatic synthesis of the coagulation Factors II, VII, IX and X by promoting γ carboxylation of glutamic acid residues at the amino terminal end of these molecules. This enables these coagulation factors to participate in the coagulation cascade by binding to phospholipids on the platelet membrane by ionic calcium bridges. During oral anticoagulant therepy, biologically inactive proteins are formed and the coagulation process of thrombin generation retarded. However, the full anticoagulant effect of these drugs is delayed until the normal clotting factors are cleared from the circulation. When oral anticoagulants are administered, the biological activity of the vitamin K dependent factors decrease according to their circulating half life (Factor VII—2–4 hours, Factor IX—25 hours, Factor X—40 hours and Factor II—60 hours).

Warfarin sodium is the oral anticoagulant of choice and therapy should be started with 10 mg on two successive days. If a large loading dose such as 20 mg or even higher is given on the first day, the patient is at risk from severe bleeding due to rapid disappearance of active Factor VII, which has the shortest half-life, and the full anticoagulant effect is still not achieved for 4–5 days. On the third day no therapy should be given but, on the fourth day, the prothrombin time should be measured and maintenance warfarin therapy started. The therapeutic range for the prothrombin time is $2\frac{1}{2}$–4 times the control value, but this may vary in different laboratories according to the source of tissue thromboplastin used for the test. Only when the prothrombin time is in the therapeutic range should the heparin infusion be discontinued. Maintenance warfarin therapy should be continued and the dosage regularly monitored by prothrombin time estimations by attending an anticoagulant clinic. Many patients on long-term anticoagulants are taking various other drugs, some of which may potentiate or antagonize the effects of warfarin.

The mechanisms of drug interactions with warfarin are numerous, but include the following basic principles:

1. Reducing absorption of vitamin K (i.e. cholestyramine)
2. Reducing or increasing warfarin absorption.
3. Reducing warfarin binding to albumin so resulting in an increased level of free, unbound warfarin (i.e. phenylbutazone, sulphonamides).
4. Altering the rate of hepatic inactivation of warfarin (i.e. barbiturates).
5. Increasing the rate of hepatic synthesis of the vitamin K_I dependent proteins, so producing a relative resistance to warfarin therapy (i.e. oestrogens, oral contraceptives).
6. Increasing the breakdown of the vitamin K_I dependent proteins (i.e. thyroxine).
7. Any other drug which affects the haemostatic mechanism will potentiate the action of oral anticoagulants (i.e. aspirin).
8. Changes in the dietary sources of vitamin K_I (i.e. patients receiving long-term intravenous nutrition).

Patients receiving oral anticoagulants should avoid other drugs, especially those compounds known to increase or decrease the anticoagulant effect. Commonly used drugs reported to interfere with oral anticoagulation are listed in Table 20.3. Obviously, when a change in a patient's medication is made, the prothrombin time should be regularly monitored and the daily dose of warfarin therapy appropriately adjusted.

In most patients, oral anticoagulants should be continued for 3–6 months. There is approximately a 10 per cent recurrence rate of thrombosis after stopping oral anticoagulants, but this is usually in patients with continuing risk factors. Such patients should be maintained on permanent warfarin anticoagulation.

If the prothrombin time becomes grossly prolonged and spontaneous bleeding develops, the warfarin effect must be temporarily reversed. An intravenous dose of vitamin K_I takes 6 hours before any synthesis of biologically active factors occurs and then subsequently the prothrombin time will shorten. Complete correction is not obtained until 24 hours later. So to control acute bleeding an infusion of fresh frozen plasma or prothrombin complex concentrate is required. If an intravenous dose of 10 mg of vitamin K_I is given, effective warfarin anticoagulation cannot be restarted for another 2 weeks, whereas 1 mg of vitamin K_I allows immediate redosage with warfarin after the bleeding episode has been controlled. Obviously, patients receiving oral anticoagulants who require surgical procedures or dental extractions, must have their prolonged prothrombin time corrected before the procedure and for several days postoperatively. The regular warfarin dosage should be stopped 3 days preoperatively and if the prothrombin time is greater than 6 seconds longer than the control value immediately prior to the operation, an infusion of fresh frozen plasma should be given to further correct the prothrombin time. Twenty-hour hours postoperatively, the regular dosage of warfarin should be restarted, so allowing full anticoagulation to be achieved again 2 days later.

Table 20.3 Commonly used drugs which interfere with oral anticoagulant control

Drugs which increase the effect of oral anticoagulants	*Drugs which decrease the effect of oral anticoagulants*
Acetylsalicyclic acid	Barbiturates
Allopurinol	Cholestyramine
Ampicillin	Diuretics
Anabolic steroids	Oestrogens
Chloramphenicol	Oral contraceptives
Clofibrate	Phenytoin
Neomycin	Rifampicin
Phenylbutazone	
Sulphonamides	
Thyroxine	
Tricyclic antidepressants	

Surgery has only a small place to play in the management of deep vein thrombosis. A few years ago, the operation of thrombectomy was popular, but re-thrombosis was only too common, and the operation is now reserved for patients who can be demonstrated to have very small, loose thrombi and in those with massive ilio-femoral thrombosis which threatens limb viability.

Interruption of veins to prevent embolism is also not often indicated, though it may be in cases of recurrent pulmonary embolism, or when anticoagulants are contraindicated by peptic ulceration or some other potentially haemorrhagic lesion. Ligation or plication of the inferior vena cava has now largely been superceded by the introduction of metal "sieves" such as the Kimray Greenfield filter. This is passed into the inferior vena cava by way of an incision in the jugular vein, under image intensifier control.

The post-thrombotic syndrome

The post-thrombotic syndrome is characterized by valve incompetence in the deep and perforating veins of the leg which follows thrombus recanalization and retraction. Following their infiltration by phagocytes, macrophages and mast cells, most thrombi retract and recanalize sufficiently to restore an adequate lumen. However, in this process, the valves are damaged. These may either be destroyed completely, or else rendered so firmly adherent to the adjacent vein wall as to make them functionally useless. In addition, post-inflammatory fibrosis in the vein wall makes it stiff and inelastic, and this also predisposes to venous reflux.

Incompetence of the valves in the perforating veins of the lower calf and ankle results in the high venous pressures of the deep veins being transmitted directly into the subcutaneous ankle venules. Muscle contraction creates an intramuscular pressure of up to 250 mm/Hg. This high pressure is normally necessary to expel blood from the deep calf veins and the soleal sinusoids proximally to the femoral vein and so to the heart. If the lower deep calf veins and their associated perforating veins are incompetent, the high pressure (approximately 100 mm/Hg) is transmitted directly to the supramalleolar veins with which the perforating veins connect. These dilate to form an "ankle venous flare" and this in turn leads to capillary dilatation and leakage of fibrinogen through the capillary endothelium, to form per-capillary fibrin cuffs. These inhibit the transfer of metabolites from blood to the skin and subcutaneous tissues so that skin necrosis eventually follows. Haemosiderin also leaks from these dilated capillaries, resulting in brown pigmentation of the skin. The subcutaneous fibrin results in induration or lipodermatosclerosis. This process is more severe if, in addition to incompetence of perforating and the lower calf veins, the more proximal femoral and popliteal vein valves are also incompetent. The resulting high pressure in the deep veins makes these ulcers very difficult to treat.

Many ulcerated legs follow a definite history of deep vein thrombosis; and, although this cannot be absolutely proved in all cases, it is sufficiently likely that the name "post-thrombotic syndrome" has been applied to all such patients. It must be emphasized that venous ulceration is a most uncommon complication of primary familial varicose veins.

Thrombus recanalization takes place in over 90 per cent of all cases. Occasionally, the superficial femoral vein or iliac vein may fail to canalize, and the resulting stenosis gives rise to a painful swollen lower leg. Most commonly, the left common iliac vein may fail to recanalize. This is related to the pre-existing stenosis which occurs in many patients where the vein passes between the body of the lower lumbar vertebrae and the overlying right common iliac artery, to join the inferior vena cava. Often a sufficient collateral circulation develops to overcome such stenosis, but sometimes a vein bypass operation may be necessary to relieve the symptoms of venous hypertension.

Apart from those few patients with venous stenosis, leg swelling is not a prominent feature of the post-thrombotic syndrome; indeed, fibrosis and cicatrization from recurrent ulceration often leads to narrowing of the gaiter area of the leg. Treatment is aimed at interrupting incompetent perforating veins by injection sclerotherapy or ligation. At present this must be followed by strong elastic graduated stocking support with a pressure of 25–35 mm/Hg at the ankle in patients with deep vein incompetence. Valve replacement in the deep veins has been attempted, but results are disappointing.

The pathology of the ulcer itself can usually be appreciated by simple observation and biopsy is not normally necessary. The floor of the ulcer consists of granulation tissue. This represents the surface of the dilated capillary loops which result from venous hypertension. This granulation tissue is usually covered by debris or slough consisting of coagulated lymph and it is very often secondarily infected, usually by staphylococci. The edges of the ulcer consist of sloping endothelial cells. There is no undercutting, as is seen in tuberculous ulcers. Should the edges appear at all everted or elevated, or should the ulcer not respond to simple cleaning with mild antiseptics and antibiotics combined with compression, then the possibility of squamous carcinoma change (Marjolin's ulcer) must be seriously considered, and biopsy performed without delay.

Like other skin tumours, this may metastasize to the inguinal lymph-nodes and these must be carefully examined, both clinically and preferably also by either lymphography or CT scanning. Treatment is by wide excision and skin grafting for a small carcinoma, but a larger one may need a combination of amputation and radiotherapy.

Lymphoedema

The prime function of the lymphatic trunks is to drain protein-rich tissue fluid. The abnormal physiological effect of absence of lymphatic drainage is therefore a high concentration of pro-

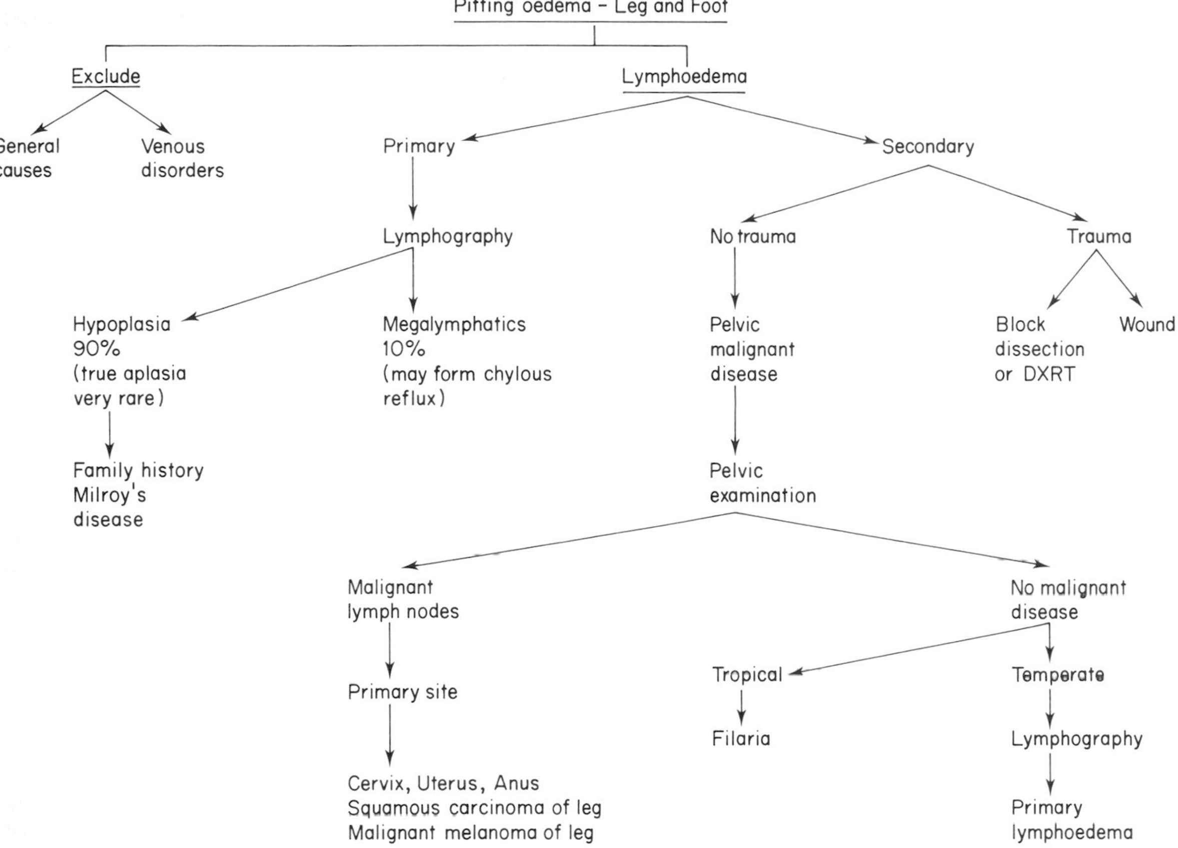

Fig. 20.6 Lymphoedema.

tein in the tissues, which are waterlogged and under tension. These factors are probably responsible for the changes which gradually take place in cases of long-standing lymphatic oedema. The skin becomes thickened and horny, and warts may form giving rise to the name 'elephantiasis'. Lymphoedema may be the result of a primary disorder of the lymph trunks or secondary to disease or trauma to the lymph-nodes. An approach to the classification of lymphoedema is shown in Fig. 20.6. Primary lymphoedema is the result of congenital hypoplasia of the superficial lymphatics. Milroy's disease is both familial and congenital. In about 10 per cent of patients with lymphoedema, the lymphatics are dilated and varicose (megalymphatics) and vesicles on the ankle and foot may discharge milky lymph, the rare condition of chylous reflux. It has not proved possible to establish pathological differences among the primary lymphoedemas by histology. Node biopsy has been performed, but histological examination shows only fibrosis or sometimes atrophy, and is of little help. In cases of underdeveloped lymphatics and lymph-nodes, destruction of some of the few remaining nodes by biopsying them may worsen the condition. The diagnosis, therefore, rests on lymphography. Lymphatic trunks can be demonstrated by insertion of a very fine needle into a dorsal foot lymphatic after visualization by the injection of 2 per cent patent blue violet into the web spaces of the foot. Ultrafluid lipiodol is injected slowly by means of a constant infusion pump, and the lymph trunks and nodes can be demonstrated by serial radiographs.

As well as lower limb chylous reflux, chylous ascites may occur, caused by intraperitoneal leakage from abnormal megalymphatics.

Secondary lymphoedema in the United Kingdom most commonly results from malignant invasion of lymph-nodes, or following their block dissection and radiotherapy for malignant disease. Lymph-node biopsy is important to obtain histological material and to confirm the diagnosis. Lymphography should also be performed to assess the extent of metastatic lymph-node involvement. This can now be supplemented or replaced by CT scanning. These investigations form the basis for rational treatment of metastatic disease.

In tropical countries, particularly South India, Guyana and parts of West Africa, secondary lymphoedema due to infection by the microfilaria *Wuchereria bancrofti* is common. The progressive oedema is accompanied by gross thickening of the skin, giving the appearance known as 'tropical elephantiasis'. The condition is due to scarring and obstruction of lymphnodes invaded by the microfilaria. Lymph-node biopsy is not usually necessary, as a diagnosis can be made by examination of a blood film which will show the organism often accompanied by a marked eosinophilia. Filarial infection may also give rise to chyluria, due to abnormal communications between dilated lumbar lymphatics and the renal pelvis. Filaria is treated by Banocide, 3 mg/kg given three times daily after meals for 6 weeks.

Mild to moderate swelling can be kept under control by elastic compression stockings and elevation of the leg which oppose the high colloid osmotic pressure of the tissue fluid. More advanced cases require excision of the oedematous subcutaneous tissue, with replacement of the superficial layers of the skin onto the deep fascia.

Rare venous and lymphatic abnormalities

Congenital arteriovenous fistula formation may produce large pulsatile varices. Generalized enlargement of the limb is often present. Intra-arterial embolization, using X-ray control, can now be performed and is the treatment of choice.

The Klippel–Trenaunay syndrome consists of port-wine staining (diffuse capillary haemangioma formation) of the limb, associated with enlargement of the underlying superficial veins, arteriovenous fistula formation and sometimes limb enlargement.

Benign tumours of lymph vessels, lymphangiomas, are often found to be mixed with blood vascular elements and should usually therefore be termed "haemo-lymphangiomas". These do not usually become malignant, and surgical excision is the treatment of choice, and this also applies to benign venous haemangiomas. Cystic hygromas are congenital lymph cysts which require surgical excision. Angiosarcomas, called "Kaposi sarcoma" are malignant tumours which arise in oedematous limbs.

Further reading

Bloom AL, Thomas DP (eds). *Haemostasis and Thrombosis*. Edinburgh: Churchill Livingstone, 1981.

Dodd H, Cockett FB. The Pathology and Surgery of the Veins of the Lower Limb, 2nd Ed. Edinburgh: Churchill Livingstone, 1986.

Hirsh J, Genton E, Hull R. *Venous Thromboembolism*. New York: Grune and Stratton, 1981.

Hume M, Sevitt S, Thomas DP. *Venous Thrombosis and Pulmonary Embolism*. Cambridge, Mass.: Harvard University Press, 1970.

Kinmonth JB. *The Lymphatics; Diseases, Lymphography and Surgery*, 2nd Ed. London: Edward Arnold, 1982.

Kwaan HC, Bowie EJW (eds). *Thrombosis*. Philadelphia: WB Saunders, 1982.

Negus D. The Peripheral Venous System: In *Operative Surgery and Management*. Ed G Keen. Bristol: Wright, 1981.

Strandness DE, Tuiele BL. *Selected Topics in Venous Disorders*. New York: Futura, 1981.

Verstraete M, Machin SJ (eds). Clinical Usage of Heparin, Present and Future Trends. *Scand J of Haem* 1980; **25**: Suppl 36.

21

Heart and Great Vessels

M F Sturridge and N Woolf

Introduction

There are few instances in the practice of surgery to the heart and great vessels when recourse can be made to the services of the histopathologist during the conduct of an operation. There are many occasions, however, when the safety of surgery is dependent upon suspicion or recognition of tissue pathology by the surgeon. Subsequent histological examination of specimens taken during surgery will reinforce the diagnosis and may considerably affect the prognosis that is given to the patient. The surgeon needs to anticipate, so far as possible, or at least appreciate at the time, pathological changes in tissues that can make standard techniques unsafe and in some cases render surgery extremely hazardous.

During an operation, the surgeon is concerned with cutting, dissecting and re-apposing tissues with or without the interposition of prosthetic materials. In each of these fields of activity, the accuracy and effectiveness of his work is influenced by the state of the tissue he is dealing with. Surgery has developed only because the body is constructed of materials that lend themselves to this sort of treatment. Experience tells that the tissues of children are infinitely stronger that those of adults and that this fact permits the intricate procedures that can be performed on tiny organs. The tissues of the elderly are by comparison flimsy, even though the correlation with chronological age is poor. At whatever age, the influence of inflammation, degeneration or congenital deficiencies on these tissues calls for the use of special techniques to achieve successful treatment.

For the purposes of this chapter, it is proposed to consider the tissues encountered during cardiac surgery and indicate the affect that certain disease processes have on them and how the surgeon may overcome the problems created.

The pericardium

The pericardium is encountered during the approach to all operations on the heart. It consists of a fibrous sac lined by a serous membrane which continues over the great vessels as the visceral pericardium and over the heart as the epicardium.

Many cardiac surgeons retract the cut edges of the pericardium with stay sutures to facilitate exposure of the heart and in the elderly patient these stitches may cut out, giving the first clue that the tissues are friable and that extra care will be required both when retracting and suturing.

As with any other tissue, the pericardial response to any injury is an acute inflammatory reaction of widely differing degrees of severity. Pericarditis is seldom encountered by the surgeon during its acute phase but its effects, mediated by the production of adhesions, are seen in many cases. Pericardial adhesions, basically the expression of repair by granulation tissue of unresolved inflammatory reactions, may follow a wide range of conditions but, in British practice, the. most commonly encountered causes are previous cardiac surgery and previous rheumatic heart disease, though the latter is ever less frequent. In developing countries, tuberculosis is still an important cause of adhesive fibrous pericarditis and may, not infrequently, be followed by constrictive pericarditis.

The adhesions which follow previous cardiac surgery should not be regarded as inevitable. Experience in dealing with "second operations" indicates that some surgeons produce dense and extensive adhesions whilst others produce hardly any. In addition, there is also a variation from patient to patient treated in the same way by the same surgeon, but this is less noticeable. Reduced handling and abrasion of the surfaces seem to be important and, of course, the deposition of glove powder within the pericardial sac must be avoided. Since increasing numbers of patients can expect to return for re-operation, the avoidance of pericardial adhesions is not a trivial matter.

Constrictive pericarditis

The one result of pericarditis, which *per se* may require surgical intervention, is constrictive pericarditis. The term is a complete misnomer, since the heart is usually enlarged and, at the time of presentation, there is usually no evidence of active inflammation of the pericardium. The clinical manifestations of the disease arise from the gross reduction of the effective compliance of the two ventricles which results in a heart of fixed stroke volume.

Many aetiologies have been described, but the commonest worldwide are tuberculosis and suppurative (probably staphylococcal) pericarditis. In Britain, viral infections and connective tissue disorders are the predominant causes of an infrequently encountered condition. The importance of these less obviously associated diseases is to remember that the heart may appear *enlarged* radiographically and a presumptive diagnosis should always lead to an exploratory operation.

At operation, the two layers of the pericardium may not be adherent all over the heart and some fluid may be present. When the sac is opened, if it is restrictive, the heart will be seen to try to "herniate" through the opening. Both the parietal and visceral pericardium are affected and segments of epicardium should be removed to see, in the same way, whether it too is restrictive. The original infection must also affect the myocardium as the freed heart is always dilated and, in many cases, never returns to normal size. Particular surgical hazards attend dissection over the coronary vessels, where the disease seems more aggressive perhaps because of the related course of the lymphatic channels, and over the right atrium, which is characteristically thin-walled and tense in this condition. It is necessary to try to remove all the pericardium anterior to the two phrenic nerves, but small islands left behind are inconsequential and, if the disease extends into the myocardium, it should be left. The posterior pericardium is freed from the heart but not removed.

The atria

The atria can be looked upon as dilatations with muscular walls at the confluence of their tributary veins. Their size is dependent upon the flow of blood which they each receive; thus if there is a congenital misconnection of veins—as in hemi-anomalous pulmonary venous connection, where the right pulmonary veins drain to the right atrium—the right atrium will be of larger volume than the left. In Fallot's tetralogy, pulmonary blood flow is reduced and the left atrium is small. Neither of these changes alters the substance of the atrial wall, but the small volume of a chamber may be significant when surgical correction suddenly increases the atrial inflow. It is with this consideration in mind that some surgeons prefer a palliating procedure as a preliminary to one stage total correction in some severe congenital defects.

Septal defects in the atrium are associated with a deficiency of septal tissue. Provided that the atrial pressure is normal, defects in the soft tissues, septum secundum and sinus venosus defects, can usually be repaired by simple suture. Septum primum defects, however, have semi-rigid margins anteriorly and inferiorly formed by the atrial wall overlying the ascending aorta and the ventricular septum between the two atrio-ventricular valves. To repair this, a patch is always required, partly because of the extent of tissue loss and partly because of the inability to place deep sutures which would compromise the conducting tissues in the ventricular septum.

The right atrial wall, anteriorly and into the appendage, is thin between the musculi pectinati whereas posterior to the sulcus terminalis it has a more consistent thickness similar to that of the left atrium. Incisions between the cavae are thus more easily closed than those made anteriorly.

Hypertrophy occurs when there is obstruction to outflow from the atria due to atrio-ventricular valve stenosis or atresia, or to ventricular hypertrophy causing reduced compliance during diastole. Atrial incisions are more easily closed in the presence of hypertrophy, but since the blood supply of hypertrophied muscle is often increased, bleeding from small arteries in the wall may be troublesome.

Left atrial volume in mitral stenosis is variable. Normal sized chambers, with no thrombi in the appendages, may be seen and a complete spectrum up to massive dilatation exists.

Atrial fibrillation is a well recognized complication of rheumatic carditis and, once established, is a stable rhythm. When it is associated with mitral valve disease, the increased pressure, caused by the increased atrial transit time, produces progressive dilatation of the left atrium. The really large atria have very little muscle left in their wall, although whether this is due to direct muscle damage in the course of rheumatic carditis is not known. The typical marker of rheumatic fever, the Aschoff body, may be found in biopsies of the atrial appendix at operation. This finding, by itself, is not, however, an indication of active disease and should not affect clinical policies regarding penicillin prophylaxis against streptococcal infections. The large chamber and the slow-moving blood with abnormal eddies induced by the arrhythmia, predispose to thrombus formation, such thrombus being an important potential source of systemic embolization. Radiographically, thrombus which is old may be visible due to calcification which can occur in the deepest layers. Old thrombus is seldom a danger as long as it remains undisturbed, but its surface acts as a nidus for further platelet deposition and this recent thrombus may embolize. Systemic emboli from atrial thrombi are common in mitral stenosis occurring in up to 30 per cent of patients and is one of the main reasons for recommending surgical treatment.

Atrial tumours

Primary tumours of the heart are uncommon. Of these, myxoma is the commonest. They usually arise from the atrial septum (about three-quarters occur in the left atrium) near the lower margin of the fossa ovalis and grow into the left atrium as a pedunculated, frond-like lesion often presenting with systemic embolization, the emboli being either portions of tumour or thrombus formed on the surface of the tumour. The risk of embolism is very high and, once diagnosed, surgical treatment should not be delayed. If the lesions grow sufficiently large, they may eventually cause obstruction of the mitral valve, this obstruction being typically intermittent and, sometimes, posturally dependent. Less commonly, they may arise from the right side of the septum and may nearly fill the right ventricle before they give rise to symptoms. With right-sided tumours, embolization occurs to the lungs. The base of the stalk arises from the endocardium of the atrium and is very seldom invasive so that the tumour can usually be shaved off together with a disk of normal endocardium without perforating the septum. If the procedure is inadequately performed, recurrence has been reported, so the limit of resection must be carefully examined. It should be remembered that large arteries and veins are frequently found at the tumour base. These communicate with subendocardial vessels but do not cause trouble at operation. There has been considerable controversy as to the true nature of these lesions. Most would accept that they are indeed true benign neoplasms consisting of multipotential mesenchymal cells. Factor VIII related antigen has been found within the cells of 18 cardiac myxomas, which suggests an origin from endothelial cells.

The ventricles

The ventricles consist of the branching myocardial cells arranged on the left in a spiral fashion around a cone-like cavity. The base of the cone provides the entrance and exit of an extremely powerful muscular chamber. The spiral formation causes the apex of the cone to twist during ventricular contraction to produce the characteristic left ventricular impulse as it strikes the chest wall at the "apex beat". The right ventricular muscle is arranged in a more orderly manner at right angles to the direction of flow through it. This ventricle is tubular in shape with inlet and outlet ends. Its posterior wall is formed by the interventricular septum.

All muscle presents a problem for the surgeon, particularly in relation to suturing. The left ventricular muscle is even more troublesome because of its thickness, low collagen content and the condensed formation of its cells. Added to these is the continuing forceful contraction of the muscle and the necessity for the surgeon to reconstitute the integrity of the ventricular cavity against the systolic force of the blood within it. As with all muscle suturing, success is dependent upon the collagen in the investing layers being incorporated in the sutures. In the case of the ventricles, these layers are the epi- and endocardium and every effort should be made to preserve the integrity of these when operating on the heart.

Stab wounds of the heart are an increasingly frequent problem of the present day and are probably the commonest occasion on which the problems of cardiac surgery are landed in the hands of the general surgeon who may have little or no experience of dealing with this organ. There is seldom an opportunity to acquire advice at the time, as the patient will either be losing blood profusely from the wound, or blood, collecting within the pericardium, compromises the heart action to the point of death. Normal heart muscle is in fact more difficult to manage than the diseased muscle with which the cardiac surgeon more often deals, since the latter usually contains more fibrous tissue. Steps should immediately be taken to reduce the blood pressure using vasodilator drugs, whilst the blood volume is being replaced and the heart exposed through a left anterior thoracotomy. The pericardium is widely opened anteriorly to the phrenic nerve and, if the right ventricle is involved, a transverse extension in "T" fashion across to the right will permit the right ventricle to be brought into view. Bleeding from the ventricle must be controlled immediately if the situation is to be rectified and the flat of the thumb over the hole, if it is near the base of the heart, or a firm grip between fingers and thumb if the more common apical wound is found, should enable some effective fluid replacement to be achieved before further action is taken. Taking advantage of induced hypotension or, if necessary, temporarily cross-clamping the inferior vena cava for one or two minutes, will enable deep nonabsorbable sutures to be placed. These should be tied gently with the primary intention of reducing the size of the hole and the consequent blood loss, rather than aiming for perfect apposition initially. More sutures can be added as required as the situation is brought under control. Particularly if the epicardium has been damaged around the vicinity of the wound, teflon buttresses should be used as an artificial epicardium to support the sutures. In almost every case, internal damage to the heart can be dealt with electively after the initial repair to the surface of the heart.

Elective operations on the ventricules are performed for aneurysms, septal defects and muscular outflow tract obstruction. More rarely, operations are performed for fibroelastosis or for aberrant conduction pathways causing dysrythnmias.

Aneurysms

Aneurysms of the ventricles occur only in scar tissue. On the right side, they may form in relation to surgical scars following inadequate relief of outflow tract obstruction. Such aneurysms are easily excised when corrective surgery is undertaken. Left ventricular aneurysms result from transmural ischaemic damage consequent on occlusion of a major branch of a coronary artery and anterior aneurysms are about ten times as common as posterior ones.

Anterior aneurysms of the left ventricle follow occlusion of the anterior descending branch of the left coronary artery and the anterior part of the interventricular septum is usually also involved in the ischaemic process. Initially the scar is quite narrow but, as fibrous replacement of the necrotic muscle takes place, the full thickness scar stretches to produce a thin-walled sac which, moving paradoxically with the phases of the cardiac cycle, limits the output of the left side of the heart and causes pulmonary congestion.

Large aneurysms can reach the size of a grapefruit. Such aneurysms may develop from two weeks to two years after the acute ischaemic episode. Mural thrombus lines the cavity in approximately 70 per cent of cases and this causes death by systemic embolization in about 15 per cent. Anterior aneurysms are usually adherent to the overlying pericardium and seldom rupture spontaneously, but the risk of systemic embolism justifies early surgical treatment.

Excellent results can be achieved by excising the aneurysm to improve left ventricular function, but a rim of scar tissue should be preserved to facilitate sound closure of the defect. In practice, this is done by opening into the centre of the aneurysm and removing any mural thrombus present. The interior of the sac is free from trabeculae which characterize the inside of the normal ventricle and the rim of the aneurysm can be identified both by sight and by feeling the thickness of the wall. Any extension to the septum or, more rarely, to the anterior wall of the right ventricle should be left untouched. Anterior aneurysms are elliptical in shape and are repaired by a suture line which follows the course of the anterior descending artery. Inferior aneurysms, caused by infarction of the posterior wall of the left ventricle by occlusion of the right coronary or distal circumflex branch of the left coronary, differ in several ways from anterior aneurysms. Many are small and not full thickness and require no treatment.

Full thickness inferior infarcts seem to result in a spreading intramural haematoma which ruptures sooner or later into the pericardium. Death will follow very soon unless pericardial adhesions have formed, in which case a false aneurysm is produced. Because of the proximity of the papillary muscles, or perhaps because the infarct may extend to the atrio-ventricular groove, mitral valve regurgitation is not uncommon. There appears to be a high incidence of important ventricular dysrythmias associated with posterior aneurysms and this may be the main indication for surgery, to which they are amenable, although mitral valve replacement may also be required.

Septal defects

Ventricular septal defects occur as congenital lesions or as a result of transmural infarction of the septum. All such defects reflect loss of tissue and, because of the resistance of the thick left ventricular wall, all but the smallest require the use of some form of either natural or artificial patch.

Congenital defects are most commonly related to the membranous septum at the root of the aorta and it must be remembered that the conducting tissue runs along the posterior and inferior borders of these defects. Complete right bundle branch block and left anterior hemi-block may complicate repair of the defects in as many as 17 per cent of patients and some may exhibit complete heart block. The strength of the endocardium is a critical factor which allows the patch to be held in position by multiple, shallow, fine sutures.

Ischaemic septal defects may occur anywhere in the septum, but are found most commonly towards the apex of the septum in association with anterior or antero-lateral infarction. They constitute a major surgical problem complicating the early stages of recovery from a serious myocardial infarction. Such ruptures occur approximately four times as frequently in women as in men and hypertension is a significant risk factor. Early operation is often indicated, but the results of such intervention have been most unrewarding. The undefined margins of the infarct make the placement of secure sutures unreliable and the ragged tear in the septum is difficult to close even with a patch. In some cases, however, time is bought by reducing the size of the defect and reclosure is possible. If the patient can be brought out of the acute phase, the margin between the necrotic and viable myocardium becomes defined and fibrous and, 4–6 weeks from onset, the defect can be closed relatively easily.

Outflow tract obstruction

Outflow tract obstruction can affect the right or the left ventricle.

Right ventricular outflow tract obstruction is most commonly found in Fallot's tetralogy. The condition is brought about by an abnormality of the embryonic spiral valve such that the division of the primitive aorta and bulbus cordis is unequal. The resulting large aorta overrides the ventricular septum, the bulbar septum does not meet the ventricular septum leaving a defect, and the right ventricular outflow tract is comensurately reduced in calibre. As the right ventricular cavity is normally trabeculated, resection of muscle bundles will often clear the approach to the pulmonary valve. In other cases, the associated right ventricular hypertrophy can be thinned by internal resection of muscle from the anterior wall of the outflow tract but, if there is hypoplasia, a gusset may also be required to increase the lumen. In all such cases, it is the epicardium which allows easy withdrawal from the right ventricle and which predominantly holds sutures or a patch securely.

Left ventricular outflow tract obstruction may be muscular or fibrous in hypertrophic obstructive cardiomyopathy. The latter may be associated with a normal or abnormal aortic valve and surgical treatment is seldom undertaken other than as an extension of aortic valve surgery. The procedure is then carried out through the aortic incision, thus avoiding left ventriculotomy. The condition is best appreciated if the operation on the valve is performed with coronary perfusion at near normal body temperature and with a beating heart. Viewed from the aorta, the outflow tract can be seen to narrow as the septum approximates the inferior surface of the anterior cusp of the mitral valve during systole. A finger passed retrogradely through the valve can appreciate the force of the constriction.

The presence of the conducting tissue in the superficial layers of the ventricular septum precludes muscular resection in this area. A wedge of tissue can be cut from the angle where the septum meets the mitral valve annulus anteriorly. The wedge is cut sufficiently deeply to divide the transverse fibres and this process can be completed by careful finger pressure until relief of the constriction is appreciated by digital examination. The obstructing bands may extend well down into the cavity of the ventricle requiring a long incision in the axis of the tract.

Excised muscle should always be sent for histological examination when the myofibrillar disarray characteristic of hypertrophic cardiomyopathy should be identified.

Fibrous subvalvar stenosis is also approached through an aortic incision. The valve cusps are gently retracted and the stenosis can then be seen as a crescentic shelf of tissue attached around the septal wall of the outflow tract and posteriorly to the mitral valve cusp. It is removed by careful sharp or blunt dissection from the surface of the septum so as to avoid the conducting tissue deep to it.

The heart valves

The valves of the heart are treated surgically by valvotomy, annuloplasty or replacement.

Valvotomy is the operation of choice for stenotic lesions of the pulmonary or mitral valves when long-term relief of obstruction can be obtained in suitable cases. It has seldom been effective in tricuspid stenosis, which is almost invariably associated with post-rheumatic deformity and significant regurgitation. The aortic valve is particularly unsuited to valvotomy except as a temporizing measure in infancy and young children.

Annuloplasty entails a procedure which reduces the diameter of a valve and thereby restores the ratio of cusp area to orifice area. Its use is restricted to regurgitant lesions of the mitral or tricuspid valves.

Replacement is reserved for any valve which is so diseased that restoration of effective function is impossible or unlikely to last.

Congenital stenosis

Congenital lesions of the valves usually result from malformation. In the most severe forms, there is atresia of the valve and if life is sustainable, there must be other abnormalities present to allow alternative pathways for the blood. Cases of severe stenosis die in infancy, though a few now survive through surgical valvotomy and other palliative procedures. Less severe cases that survive infancy, tend to present during their growth spurts at five years and at adolescence or later in life when the myocardium shows signs of strain.

All stenotic lesions represent obstruction to the circulation and are therefore serious and potentially fatal conditions. Stenosis of an inlet valve produces symptoms as the back pressure is transmitted to the venous end of the capillaries in the systemic or pulmonary circulations with resulting oedema. Stenosis of an outlet valve will be compensated by hypertrophy of the ventricle, the hypertrophy being of the high pressure, overload type with a normal or small ventricular cavity, and may remain unnoticed for a long time. However, the effect of this hypertrophy is to reduce the compliance of the ventricle and, thus, its end-diastolic volume. The cardiac output can then only be increased by increasing the heart rate, but as this shortens filling time it is self-limiting. During exercise, there is reduced perfusion either of the brain, causing syncope, or the coronary circulation, causing ventricular arrhythmias or angina.

The aim of surgery is always to relieve obstruction without replacing a valve. Complicated plastic procedures may be required in individual cases. The abnormal aortic valve alone always requires replacement sooner or later whether it is either congenitally stenotic or bicuspid. The normal left ventricle of a child or adolescent will sustain a tremendous work load for years before it shows electrocardiographic evidence of strain. As valve replacement can never be an elective procedure, with the prosthetic materials, man-made or tissue, that are yet available, replacement is certainly undesirable before growth is complete. Congenital aortic stenosis is usually treated by replacement between the age of 20 and 40 years. By this time, the valve has undergone degenerative changes with thickening and calcification of the cusp tissue, perhaps as a result of the stress and vibration caused by turbulent blood flow.

True bicuspid aortic valves are very rare. More commonly the valve is bicuspidized by fusion of the commissure between two smaller than normal cusps which appose a larger, free cusp. The rudimentary commissure is then always apparent. The valve initially provides no significant obstruction to blood flow and maintains its function for much longer than the congenitally stenotic valve. However, the bicuspid valve is subject to severe dystrophic calcification and then is the commonest indication for aortic valve replacement after the age of 60 years. In the majority of cases, the calcification is confined to the valve cusps, but sometimes nodular calcium extends superficially down the inferior surface of the anterior cusp of the mitral valve and deeply into the interventricular septum, sometimes affecting the conduction tissue to produce heart block. Except in the septum, the calcium can be peeled off the surfaces like candle wax, but care must be taken not to leave loose particles which would embolize when the circulation is re-established.

Rheumatic heart disease

Rheumatic heart disease is believed to result from a hypersensitivity reaction to antigens in the cell wall components of the beta-haemolytic streptococcus, Lancefield Group A. The antigens, which are thought to be implicated, are closely related to the bacterial M protein and to the Group A polysaccharide. The immune response which follows absorption of the antigens leads to damage of tissue elements in the host which share antigenic components with the streptococcus. These cross-reacting antigens are found in the myocardium (sarcolemma and subsarcolemmal cytoplasm), heart valves, thymus, skeletal muscle, human glomerular basement membrane, neuronal cytoplasms of the human subthalamic and caudate nuclei, skin and human lymphocytes. Acute rheumatic fever is characterized by both exudative and proliferative inflammatory reactions in connective tissue with particular emphasis on the heart, large joints and skin. The acute inflammatory phase is self-limiting, but recurrent attacks not infrequently occur. In pathological terms, the inflammation is a pancarditis affecting the epicardium, myocardium and the endocardium.

The valves exhibit a typical tissue response to inflammation including vascularization and infiltration by pleomorphic cells. Pain only occurs if there is pericardial involvement, but the inflammed, thickened and stiffened valve draws attention to itself clinically through the medium of loss of function, which is easily understood when comparison is made between such a valve and normal delicate, avascular and thin cusp tissues. Small sessile thrombi (vegetations) may be present along the line of contact of the cusps, reflecting damaged valve collagen.

Following clinical control of the acute phase of the disease, a slow but progressive change takes place in the valves resulting in thickening, shrinkage and some degree of fusion at the commissures. This commisural fusion is the diagnostic marker for post-inflammatory aortic valve stenosis. Progression towards chronic rheumatic valve disease may be explained by recurrent attacks of valvulitis and secondary alterations in haemodynamics likely to favour deposition of mural thrombi, the organization of which would lead to fibrosis of the underlying valve substance. Typically, the mitral valve alone is affected, but isolated aortic valve disease also occurs. In more severe cases, the mitral and the aortic or tricuspid valve, and less commonly all three valves, are diseased.

The discovery and common use of antibiotics in childhood illness has enormously reduced the incidence of rheumatic fever in the Western world, but the disease has not been abolished and rheumatic heart disease remains a common condition requiring cardiac surgery. In this country most cases of mitral stenosis present for treatment between the ages of 30 and 60 years, but on the Asian continent a much younger age group is severely affected, needing surgery from the age of seven years onwards. In these young subjects, treatment is particularly dangerous because the acute rheumatic process is still active in the myocardium.

Surgically, stenotic rheumatic valves that have to be replaced, provide good anchorage for sutures, except when extensive calcification is present. Calcification of the mitral valve frequently extends into the annulus and sometimes into the posterior wall of the left ventricle. Deep sutures in this area run the risk of interrupting the posterior end of the atrio-ventricular course of the circumflex coronary artery. To avoid this, carefully placed sutures passing not too deeply through the calcified tissue are tied with only sufficient tension to secure the valve without cutting through the tissue.

Valvar regurgitation

Regurgitation through a cardiac valve may result from shrinkage of the cusp tissue, destruction of cusp tissue or weakness of the supporting tissues leading to dilatation of the valve ring.

Tissue shrinkage

Shrinkage of cusp tissue occurs in rheumatic aortic and tricuspid valve disease so that such lesions always present with a clinical picture of mixed stenosis and regurgitation. Shrinkage much less commonly affects the mitral valve cusps, although the chordae below the valve are often markedly shortened as well as thickened and fused together.

Tissue destruction

Destruction of cusp tissue results from infection in subacute bacterial endocarditis. The infection, which occurs as a metastatic lesion from focal infection elsewhere in the body, but most often from dental sepsis and its treatment, has a predilection for congenial or acquired cardiac lesions. Of those sites that can be securely identified, the aortic and mitral valves are most frequently affected, but ventricular septal defect and persistent ductus arteriosus are other lesions at risk. Currently, tricuspid valve endocarditis is seen in addicts who take their drugs intravenously using unsterile materials.

The infections may arise as a result of deposition of small infected emboli or by the settling out of bacteria from a bacteriaemia onto susceptible tissue. A classical inflammatory response ensues which proceeds to the formation of an abscess with a central zone of necrosis. Because the valve cusps are so thin, rupture of such an abscess results in perforation of the cusp and a regurgitant murmur may become audible.

Surgical treatment may be called for during the acute phase of the disease if the infection is life-threatening and cannot be controlled by medical treatment, if there is electrocardiographic evidence of disease extending to involve the conducting tissue, or if destruction of valves produces a severe haemodynamic strain on the heart which is already overworked to support the increased metabolic demands brought about by the infection. Valve replacement under strict and overwhelming antibiotic control is required and can be life-saving, although the operative mortality is high. Mortality stems from extensive destruction of tissue which may be present around the affected valve and the occasional coincidence of diffuse intravascular coagulopathy. The presence of the latter should always be looked for before proceeding to operation and is an absolute contra-indication to immediate surgery.

Other surgical considerations in this disease are the clearing out of abscess cavities, their separation from the circulation by oversewing the mouth of the cavity and the difficulty of suturing a prosthetic valve to inflamed tissues. Fewer sutures should be used and these should be deeply set. Tying the sutures requires careful judgement—if they are too tight they cut through the tissues and if too loose the prosthetics becomes unstable when the inflammatory oedema has resolved.

Because of the difficulty not infrequently experienced in identifying the organisms responsible for this disease and the possibility that bacterial re-colonization may have occurred before operation, the excised valve should be placed immediately into warmed culture medium for immediate transport to the laboratory where it can be homogenized before culturing it under appropriate circumstances.

Replacement of valves after full and effective treatment of the infection presents no special problems.

Tissue weakness

Weakness of supporting structures is a factor in some cases of mitral or aortic valve regurgitation. The mitral valve is regurgitant during the acute phase of rheumatic fever due to dilatation of the mitral valve annulus and, probably, impairment of ventricular support. Surgical treatment should be avoided because of the high mortality associated with operations during this phase and because successful medical treatment is often associated with restored valve function.

Mitral regurgitation also occurs following myocardial infarction affecting the papillary muscles and chordae of the valve. Rupture of a papillary muscle can occur producing an acute surgical emergency in a patient in the first few days of recovery from a myocardial infarction. Rupture of an isolated chorda or the base of several chordae may occur, producing a less dramatic effect treatable at a more propitious occasion. Infarction can also lead to fibrous replacement of a papillary muscle which later stretches and allows the cusps to prolapse into the atrium in systole permitting regurgitation. Valve replacement in all these circumstances is made more difficult by the thin texture of the normal valve tissue. Multiple small sutures to distribute the strain of the systolic force against the valve are required.

Increasingly these days, patients are presenting with a condition called (in the UK) ‘floppy’ mitral valve. In this condition the valve cusps increase in area while the chordae become elongated and attenuated and may rupture. The essential lesion which produces floppy valve is disintegration of the valve fibrosa. The collagen bundles in the central portion of the cusp appear fragmented and this is associated with an accumulation of acid mucopolysaccharide. Similar changes are also seen in the chordae. These changes cause the valve apparatus to become weaker and the effect of the normal systolic forces on the valve is to stretch the cusps and elongate the chordae. The condition may be distinguished from other causes of mitral regurgitation by echocardiographic and angiographic appearances. At operation, the valve appears slightly thickened and may be yellowish in colour. There is a considerable amount of apparently redundant tissue. The chordae are long and thin often have a waisted appearance in their centre and allow prolapse of the valve into the atrium. The condition is attributed to an abnormality of the collagen in the valve substance. Surgical treatment involves valve replacement and is made difficult by the friable nature of the tissues. Teflon buttressed sutures are not only helpful during the operation, but may prevent late disruption of the prosthesis.

Weakness of the supporting structure of the aortic valve is encountered chiefly in two conditions: syphilis and Marfan’s disease.

Syphilis

Syphilis affecting the aorta is now an uncommon problem in this country. A patient presenting with aortic regurgitition and found on angiography to have an aneurysmal dilatation of the ascending aorta should, however, be suspected of the disease. Destruction of the elastic fibres in the tunica media of the aorta leads to progressive dilatation, in spite of considerable thickening and sometimes calcification of the aortic wall. The pathological changes extend to involve the aortic root which dilates so that the cusps become separated in the commissural regions and produce a large triangular orifice in diastole. The cusp edges become secondarily thickened which gives the cusp a "tadpole" shape on cross-section. Following a course of antibiotic therapy, if appropriate, the valve is replaced using a mechanical prosthesis to which the dilated annulus is secured with multiple sutures. It may be deemed necessary to replace the ascending aorta using graft material from the prosthesis to the origin of the innominate artery and implanting the origins of the coronary arteries into the sides of the graft.

Marfan's disease

Marfan's disease is associated with cystic medial necrosis in the ascending aorta and may be a purely localized lesion or may be part of the full manifestation of Marfan's syndrome. The aorta is typically very thin and the lack of elastic tissue makes suturing extremely difficult with a tendency for leakage to occur around each stitch. In contrast to syphilitic aortic valve disease, the cusp tissue is thin and glistening with slightly rolled edges, but regurgitation is brought about in the same way by stretching of the cusps between the three commissures. As with syphilis, the valve and usually the ascending aorta have to be replaced. The use of teflon buttresses for the sutures makes surgery easier and safer. The long-term prognosis is good only if the diesase is localized to the ascending aorta.

Aortic root dilatation is also seen after the age of 40 and extends well into the geriatric age group, but seldom comes to surgical treatment. Some association with floppy mitral valve has been noted and some cases have shown a familial trend.

Prosthetic valves

There are three basic differences in the prostheses used to replace diseased valves in man. There are valves derived from human or animal tissue which are attached in direct continuity to the host tissues, similar valves mounted on a frame which separates the two tissues, and valves made entirely from synthetic materials.

A wide variety of tissues have been used in the search for the ideal prosthesis, which is characterized by requiring a minimal opening force and having a central flow pathway permitting non-turbulent flow without a pressure gradient. It should be flexible, to move with the heart action, have a low susceptibility to infection and be non-thrombogenic. These properties should be retained throughout the normal life expectation of the patient. In practical terms it is also desirable to have valves in a selection of sizes, readily available, with a long shelf-life and economical to produce.

Needless to say such a valve has not been found, but many of those currently used fall into two categories: tissue valves that fulfil most criteria well, but progressively degenerate, and mechanical valves which are thrombogenic and necessitate the use of anticoagulants.

The human homograft aortic valve, obtained from cadavers, was the first tissue valve to be used in large numbers and was inserted with a cylinder of donor aortic root into the subcoronary position in the host. It satisfied all criteria except availability and durability. Variations in the preparation of the grafts, including early salvage and sterilization, increases their longevity, but inevitably the gradual degeneration of the dead collagen structure leads to their eventual attrition. The problems associated with collection of grafts, the technical skill needed to insert them accurately and the availability of adequate substitutes has diminished their use.

Porcine xenografts mounted on flexible metal or plastic frames covered with a synthetic material sewing ring are the most common tissue valves used today. The valves are processed with glutaraldehyde to preserve the collagen, but there is no evidence to suggest that their active function will exceed a mean of about 10 years. Because these valves are non-viable, they do not initiate an immune response. High calcium metabolism in the young, however, has predisposed to rapid heavy deposits in these valves. Their use in patients below the age of 35 years who have the greatest need for such a non-thrombogenic valve, has had to be discontinued.

Mechanical valves are either of caged-ball or tilting disc type and have the advantage of being theoretically indestructable. The ball valves have so far proved satisfactory in this regard over the longest period of time, but all of these valves have a greater or lesser tendency to thrombosis and thrombo-embolism and anticoagulant drugs, with their inherent risks of further complications, are normally employed.

Whenever valves are inserted in the circulation, non-absorbable sutures have to be used to retain the anchorage of the valve as tissue ingrowth is minimal and mostly the valves remain uncovered or develop a thin neointima which is poorly attached and contributes to the embolic risk.

Haemolysis is seldom a problem with mechanical valves unless there is a paraprosthetic leak. It may then be severe enough to need re-operation to correct it.

The thoracic aorta

Apart from those diseases which affect the aortic valve as well as the aorta and which have already been described above, the aorta is affected by true aneurysms, dissecting aneurysms and by coarctation.

True aneurysms

True aneurysms of the aorta were at one time common due to syphilis, but today they are uncommon. Atherosclerotic Marfan's disease and traumatic aneurysm occur, but syphilitic aneurysms are very rare in the Western world.

Arteriosclerotic aneurysms

These may affect any part of the thoracic aorta, but are found usually in the descending aorta just above the diaphragm in elderly patients and are often asymptomatic. They are discovered by radiographic demonstration during the course of investigation of possible chest disease. It is doubtful whether these will ever give rise to trouble and the elderly state of the patient often precludes surgical intervention.

The deficient element in arteriosclerotic aneurysms is the smooth muscle cell. If a large atheromatous plaque is examined histologically, there is obvious thinning of the media beneath the thickened intima and, in appropriately stained sections, this can be seen to be associated with a closer than normal apposition of the elastic laminae and loss of muscle. Once dilatation occurs, laminar flow is lost and the lateral forces of turbulent flow acting on the thinned wall leads to rupture. The aneurysms usually contains a large amount of laminated thrombus which exhibits a remarkable lack of organization to granulation tissue. Since there is no firm anchorage to the aortic wall, blood tracks between the layers. The mass of thrombus thus forms little or no protection against haemorrhage through the ruptured wall. Usually saccular in formation, the treatment consists of excision of the sac with repair of the aorta. The surrounding aortic wall may be diseased and require buttressed sutures but the main complication of such operations is the morbidity associated with surgery in arteriosclerotic patients.

Marfan's disease

Marfan's disease, or cystic medial necrosis of the ascending aorta, usually progresses to involve the aortic valve and the surgical treatment has been described. In Marfan's syndrome, there may be dilatation of all the proximal arterial tree with aneurysm formation. The problems of surgical treatment due to the thin friable tissues usually leads to surgery being deferred except to control threatened or actual rupture. In this case, a fabric graft is required to replace the most severely affected segment of the aorta. Between 30 and 45 per cent of patients die from rupture of a dissecting aneurysm.

Traumatic aneurysms

Traumatic aneurysms occur following deceleration injuries in which the mobile arch of the aorta hinges on the origin of the descending aorta which is splinted by its intercostal arterial branches. If the injury is severe, the aortic wall fractures posterolaterally and death is immediate. In a few, a false aneurysm forms in the scar. Chest radiographs taken 6–8 weeks after the injury, and sometimes years later, may show a shadow protruding from the aortic border in the left upper lung field.

Surgical treatment requires excision of the aneurysm with end-to-end anastomosis of the normal aortic wall proximal and distal to the scar. This is achieved through a left thoracotomy with the patient heparinized and perfusion of the descending aorta with an empirical 500 ml per minute of blood taken from the left atrium to maintain the blood supply to the spinal cord and kidneys.

Dissecting aneurysms

Dissecting aneurysm is probably the commonest condition of the aorta encountered surgically today. One publication states that some 60 000 cases occur annually in the USA. The patient may be known to have hypertension before the onset of symptoms of dissection, but this is not invariable. The cause is a tear through the intima of the aorta which permits blood to enter the media which is abnormal and separates between its middle and outer thirds to produce a false channel. The lesion then extends proximally and distally and can involve the branches of the aorta. The inelastic adventitia produces a sharp change of the pulse contour with a high pulse pressure and this in turn tends to extend the dissection and stretch the adventitia producing the wide aortic shadow typically seen radiographically. The dangers of the condition arise from rupture of the adventitia into the pericardium or pleura and from external pressure on the intima causing occlusion of major branches of the aorta and disruption of the aortic valve.

The condition has been divided into two types from the point of view of treatment. *Type A* includes the common dissection starting in the ascending aorta and confined to it or extending any distance beyond. *Type B* describes dissection starting at the end of the aortic arch or beyond it and extending predominently distally. *Type A* is now treated surgically in most centres because of the very poor prognosis with medical management, whereas the surgical treatment of *Type B* dissections is not significantly better than medical management.

The principle of surgical management is to transect the dissected segment of the ascending aorta and to suture the intima circumferentially to the adventitia to occlude the false channel proximal and distal to the site of the initial tear which is usually 2–3 cm above the aortic valve. A graft is interposed.

Type A dissections may extend to the root of the aortic valve cusps detaching the support of the commissures of the valve and allowing them to prolapse causing aortic regurgitation. This is normally corrected at operation by replacing the valve with a prosthesis either separately or as a composite valved-conduit graft. The origins of the coronary arteries are joined to the graft.

The surgical problems associated with dissecting aneurysms stem from the disproportion between the stretched adventitia and the normal diameter intima and the loss of substance of the media, which usually contributes to successful aortic surgery. The pathogenesis of dissecting aneurysm is still poorly understood. In a majority of cases there is histological abnormality of the media consisting of accumulation of connective tissue mucins, this being so marked on some occasions, as to give the impression of mucin-filled cavities (hence the term "cystic medial necrosis"). There is, however, no evidence of this loss being accompanied by an inflammatory response. Elastic tissue fragmentation may be seen, but does not appear to be an essential feature.

If the aneurysm leaks into surrounding tissues, the problems are accentuated by disruption of the tissues and haematoma formation which makes surgical dissection and tissue recognition more difficult.

Coarctation of the aorta

Coarctation of the aorta (the word is derived from Coarctare: to press together) is classically a localized stricture of the proximal descending aorta just distal to the ligamentum arteriosum. The obstruction is severe and blood reaches the lower half of the body by anastomotic channels between the subclavian arteries and the chest wall, thence retrogradely along the upper intercostal arteries to the descending aorta.

The effect of coarctation is to produce hypertension proximal to the obstruction and an inflexible flow to the descending aorta at a low pulse pressure. This in turn may lead to renal hypertension and in some cases produces claudication of the lower limbs during exercise.

As with all congenital lesions, there is considerable scope for variation in the site and severity of the lesion. There may be additional hypoplasia of the adjacent aorta proximal to the obstruction or variation of the disposition of the origins of the arch branches, but the classical form is commoner than all its variants.

All cases are treated surgically except in the rare elderly patient where it can be surmised that the particular circumstances are such that surgical treatment is not required. Excision of the narrowed segment, one of the earliest "cardiac" operations performed, remains the operation of choice, but numerous variants of gusset procedures have been tried. Generally, the surrounding tissues are good and the operation, carried out with elective hypotension, is both safe and effective in restoring pulsatile flow to the kidneys and lower limbs.

Surgical considerations in the treatment of coarctation include the approach via the left chest wall containing large tortuous and thin-walled anastomotic arteries, particularly in the substance of the latissimus dorsi muscle: the changes probably due to the abnormally high flow and high transmitted pressure within them. Apart from dealing with these in the approach to the chest, severe wound haematomas will develop if they are damaged by sutures when closing the wound.

At the aortic end of the upper intercostals, particularly in adult patients, there may be thin-walled aneurysms. These should be looked for in the preoperative angiogram, especially at the origin of the right highest intercostal which is not normally seen at operation. If they are present, the feeding intercostal should be ligated and the aortic wall repaired, as the subsequent exaggerated pulse pressure may cause them to rupture postoperatively.

A few cases are seen where the obstruction is less severe or where re-operation is required. In both circumstances, the anastomotic channels may be inadequate to protect the kidneys during the operation and in such cases a left atrio-descending aorta bypass should be used.

Persistent ductus arteriosus

The ductus arteriosus connects the left pulmonary artery to the junction of the arch and descending aorta. In intra-uterine life, it conducts reduced blood, which enters the right side of the heart from the superior vena cava, into the descending aorta whence it passes to the umbilical arteries. At birth, expansion of the lungs opens up the pulmonary vascular bed and blood-flow through the duct ceases. Under the influence of high arterial oxygen solutions and reduced levels of prostaglandins, the duct closes and becomes the ligamentum arteriosum. In a small proportion of normal infants (0.045 per cent) and in a higher proportion of premature infants (15–20 per cent), the ductus does not close at birth and may persist into childhood and adult life. A persistent ductus allows blood to shunt from the aorta into the pulmonary circulation causing a degree of cardiorespiratory embarassment related to the size of the shunt. All cases run the risk of bacterial endocarditis.

Ligation of the persistent ductus was the first elective surgical procedure related to the heart to become accepted and led to the development of cardiac surgery in the 1930s. Today, the operation is still recommended in all cases and the operative mortality for uncomplicated cases should approach zero, but inevitably is higher when it is associated with other congenital cardiac defects and in older patients.

Treatment is by ligation in most cases, but division with suture of the two ends may be required if the duct is short or very wide. The wall of the duct is thin and the intima cuts through easily when ligated. The operation, which is performed through a left thoracotomy incision, exemplifies techniques which should always be employed when dealing surgically with large vessels. It is first essential to gain control of the pressure within the duct by mobilizing the aorta sufficiently to enable it to be cross-clamped above and below the ductus using hypotensive anaesthesia and arterial pressure monitoring. With the pressure relieved, it is easier to gauge the tension applied to the wall of the vessel by the ligature. To avoid cutting through the duct, thick ligatures have been advocated, but these are very difficult to draw up into a tight snare around the vessel and are probably the cause of most cases of "recanalized" ductus. The thickness of a ligature should be related to the cross-sectional area of the obliterated vessel and then no undue tension is required. It is customary to ligate both ends of the ductus if its length permits but ligatures are foreign material and will harbour infection, so the least amount left behind the better.

A ductus is divided if ligation might result in shearing it from its attachment at either end. With the aorta clamped above and below the duct and with a narrow vascular clamp across the pulmonary end of the duct, division is performed and the aortic defect closed with interrupted sutures to give a circumferentially disposed suture line. After removing the aortic clamps and ensuring haemostasis, the pulmonary end of the duct is closed with a fine continuous suture.

Coronary artery disease

The effects of coronary arterial disease on the myocardium and the mitral valve have already been described and, historically, their surgical management preceded treatment of the underlying pathology.

Surgical treatment

Coronary artery surgery, as now practised, stems from the accurate delineation of disease in the coronary vessels by angiography, and it is both surprising and a matter for conjecture that cardiac imaging should have developed to such a high degree before coronary angiography was first attempted in 1962.

The principles behind modern surgical treatment are direct myocardial revascularization by bypassing localized obstructions in the proximal segments of coronary arteries. The primary objective is the relief of angina, but subsequent analysis of the results of surgery has demonstrated prolongation of life in the majority of patients that are treated; that is those with left mainstem stenosis or severe triple vessel disease. As the operative mortality has fallen towards 1 per cent with the expertise developed by the commonness of this procedure, it is likely that less severe cases will also be found statistically to benefit in this way, although advances in medical therapy make this less certain. It should be noted that although the disease is ten times as common in men than in women, the surgical risk in women is significantly higher for no defined reason.

Perhaps the unexpected finding from angiography was the predilection for atheroma to form in the larger coronary arteries rather than in the smaller branches and proximally rather than distally.

Surgically, the coronaries are defined as the anterior descending, the circumflex and the right as separate vessels with the left mainstem considered, again, separately.

At operation, it is usual to fashion the bypass graft from autologous saphenous vein which is joined proximally to the ascending aorta and distally to the affected artery end-to-side beyond an obstruction and preferably at a site where the vessel wall is normal. The internal mammary artery is sometimes used, freeing it from the chest wall, but preserving its origin from the subclavian artery. The patency of this vessel is high after successful anastomosis, but the inherent narrowness of the vessel, the tediousness of the dissection and the constraints it makes on the operation by tethering the heart, make its surgical popularity low.

Particularly the right coronary artery is often severely diseased throughout its length to its distal branches and in these cases endarterectomy may be performed, stripping the diseased intima and media out and forming the anastomosis to the remaining adventitia. The success of coronary arterial surgery, with a postoperative patency rate in excess of 90 per cent, is perhaps surprising in the light of experience with peripheral vascular surgery, but it is possibly attributable to the very high flows normally required by the beating heart which can enjoy no rest during the recovery period.

There remains an initial graft failure rate of 5 per cent and a perioperative infarction rate between 5 and 15 per cent to detract from the results. Progression of the disease in the native coronaries and a continuing attrition rate in the grafts due to thrombosis with or without atheroma formation in the arterialized veins, leads to a continuing failure rate currently estimated at about 10 per cent annum.

So far, the indications for treatment have tended to be confined to the treatment of stable angina in patients under the age of 50 years, angina poorly controlled by medical therapy beyond this age, unstable angina and the presence of left mainstem stenosis. Younger patients with a history of myocardial infarction, but without angina, may be recommended for surgical treatment if the disease is significant, but treatment of acute myocardial infarction has been associated with a higher operative mortality. Although it may be possible to reduce the extent of an infarct by emergency revascularization, so far it is not technically possible, in most instances, to intervene before cell death has occurred.

Further reading

Crawford T. *Pathology of Ischaemic Heart Disease.* London: Butterworth Scientific, 1977.

Davies MJ. *Pathology of Cardiac Valves.* London: Butterworth Scientific, 1980.

Jackson JW (ed). *Cardiothoracic Surgery.* In: Rob C, Smith R (series eds). *Operative Surgery.* London: Butterworths, 1978.

Sabiston DC, Spencer FC (eds). *Gibbon's Surgery of the Chest, 4th edn.* Philadelphia: W.B. Saunders.

Silver MD (ed). *Cardiovascular Pathology.* Edinburgh and London: Churchill Livingstone, 1983.

22

Upper Urinary Tract

C P Chilton, K M Cameron, W J Highman and M C Parkinson

Introduction

The aim of this chapter is to demonstrate the value of histopathology and cytology in the diagnosis and management of the commoner surgical problems of the adult upper urinary tract. It must be emphasized that the view presented is necessarily a restricted one as the other branches of pathology—biochemistry, microbiology and haematology—which also play an important part in clinical investigation and diagnosis, are only given brief mention.

As the problems to be described are those that are referred to the urologist by the general practitioner, diagnostic selection may already have occurred and the possible medical causes of the symptomatology discussed will not be enlarged upon.

It is essential to emphasize the importance of the preservation of functioning renal tissue in the planning of surgical and urological procedures. Normal intravenous urography (IVU), urea and electrolytes may be considered in the majority of patients to demonstrate normal kidneys. A more complete assessment of overall and individual renal function and anatomy can be achieved by the estimation of creatinine clearance, chromium labelled ethylene-diamine-tetra-acetate (EDTA) glomerular filtration rates, and by diethylene-triamine-penta-acetic acid (DTPA) and dimercaptosuccinic acid (DMSA) renal scans.

Before embarking on any major surgical procedure, an estimation of renal function should be performed. These investigations are particularly important where the pathology may have caused functional renal impairment, which may then be further compromised by surgery. Table 22.1 indicates the problems that can overtly or covertly cause such renal impairment: the patient undergoing vascular surgery or the individual with a pelvic or colonic condition which may be associated with obstructive uropathy, are important in this context.

Table 22.1 Causes of renal functional impairment.

Renal	*Post-renal*
Glomerulonephritis	Renal calculi
Chronic pyelonephritis	Pelvi-ureteric junction obstruction
Dysplasias	Retroperitoneal fibrosis
Polycystic kidneys	Vesico-ureteric reflux
Multicystic kidney	Neuropathic bladder
Analgesic nephropathy	Bladder outflow obstruction
Diabetes mellitus	Urethral stricture & valves
Hypertension	Phimosis
Interstitital nephritis	
Renovascular disease	

This anticipation and planning is one facet of the preservation of renal function. Maintenance of vital signs, adequate fluid and blood replacement, and the appropriate use of prophylactic and therapeutic antibiotics, are just a few examples of the general measures to prevent postoperative renal failure. Table 22.2 shows the common causes of renal failure in which attention to detail in pre and postoperative management can prevent many catastrophes.

Normal kidneys have the capacity to withstand considerable stresses such that one kidney can be removed without affecting the patient's well-

Table 22.2 Common causes of acute renal failure.

Hypotension
Myocardial infarction
Haemorrhage
Fluid loss
Septicaemia
Drugs
Toxins
Burns

being. When necessary, up to one half of a solitary kidney can be removed and the remaining half can maintain normal life.

Histopathology has a role to play in preoperative diagnosis, during the course of surgery and postoperatively. The preoperative role in renal surgical practice—apart from providing a background knowledge of possibilities and probabilities—is mainly cytological, though the advent of the nephroscope and ureteroscope has made possible endoscopic biopsy of the urothelium of the upper urinary tract. Peroperatively, a frozen section diagnosis may be requested as a guide to the extent of surgical resection or for an urgent report on any unexpected finding. Postoperatively the final diagnosis, though often merely confirmatory, is histopathological. Additional information of value in the context of prognosis and further therapy will be dealt with in the relevant sections of the chapter.

Renal problems present to the urologist in a number of well defined though sometimes overlapping ways. For each of the main clinical presentations—haematuria, renal mass, pain and obstruction—a plan of investigation and management designed as a flow chart has been devised (Figures 22.1–4). These are complex and independent of the text. It must, however, be stressed that the presentations are invariably not clear cut and that the patient may have any combination of the above. In addition to symptoms relating directly to the kidney or urogenital tract, renal problems may present with more non-specific symptoms such as weight loss, general malaise, fever, uraemia and anaemia. Thus, the importance of a carefully taken history and full physical examination as the basis on which further investigations are founded is emphasized.

Haematuria

The main causes of macroscopic haematuria are shown in Table 22.3.

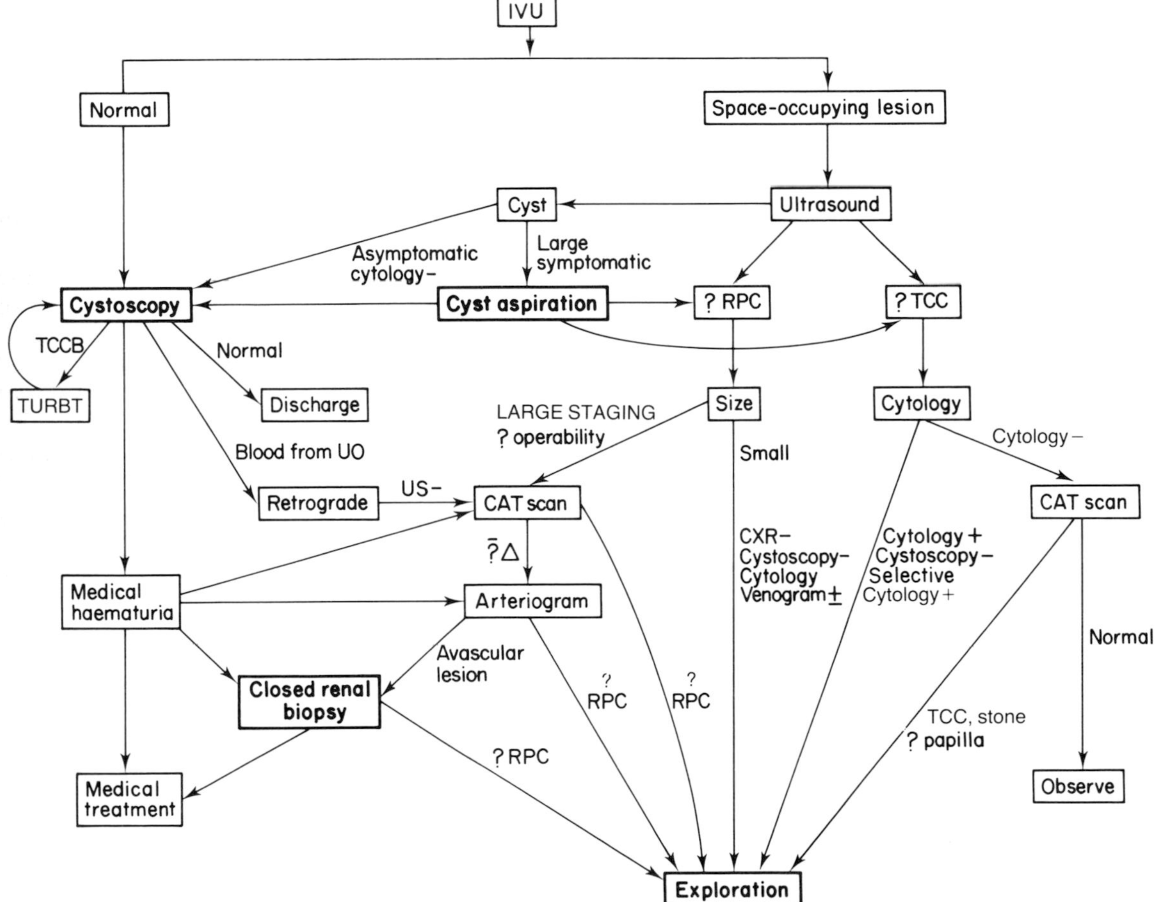

Fig. 22.1 Flow diagram demonstrating the diagnostic steps in a patient presenting with painless haematuria.

Table 22.3 Main causes of macroscopic haematuria.

<40 years	*>40 years*
Infection	Tumour
Stone	Infection
Tumour	Stone
Trauma	Trauma
Miscellaneous	Miscellaneous

Investigation of patients with haematuria

Virtually all patients who present in this way require full investigation of the urinary tract. Only occasional exceptions may be made, as in the case of the young woman of reproductive age in whom this symptom is part of a proved isolated episode of cystitis. Commonly, the bleeding may be caused by lesions which do not involve the histopathologist, for example calculi and infections. In these two conditions the value of biochemistry and bacteriology in investigation and treatment are found in specialized texts and will not be considered here.

An aggressive policy of investigation, including cytology, IVU and cystoscopy, is dictated by the knowledge that malignant tumour is a probable cause for which early diagnosis and treatment are essential. If these investigations are all normal and the bleeding does not recur, the patient may be reassured and discharged.

The intravenous urogram remains the mainstay in the diagnosis of surgical renal pathology in adults and of major concern is the demonstration of a space-occupying lesion in either the kidney or the ureter. The diagnostic possibilities in the former site include cysts and neoplasms (urothelial or renal parenchymal in origin) and in the latter, stones and transitional cell carcinoma. A urothelial neoplasm causing a filling defect has to be differentiated most commonly from radiolucent

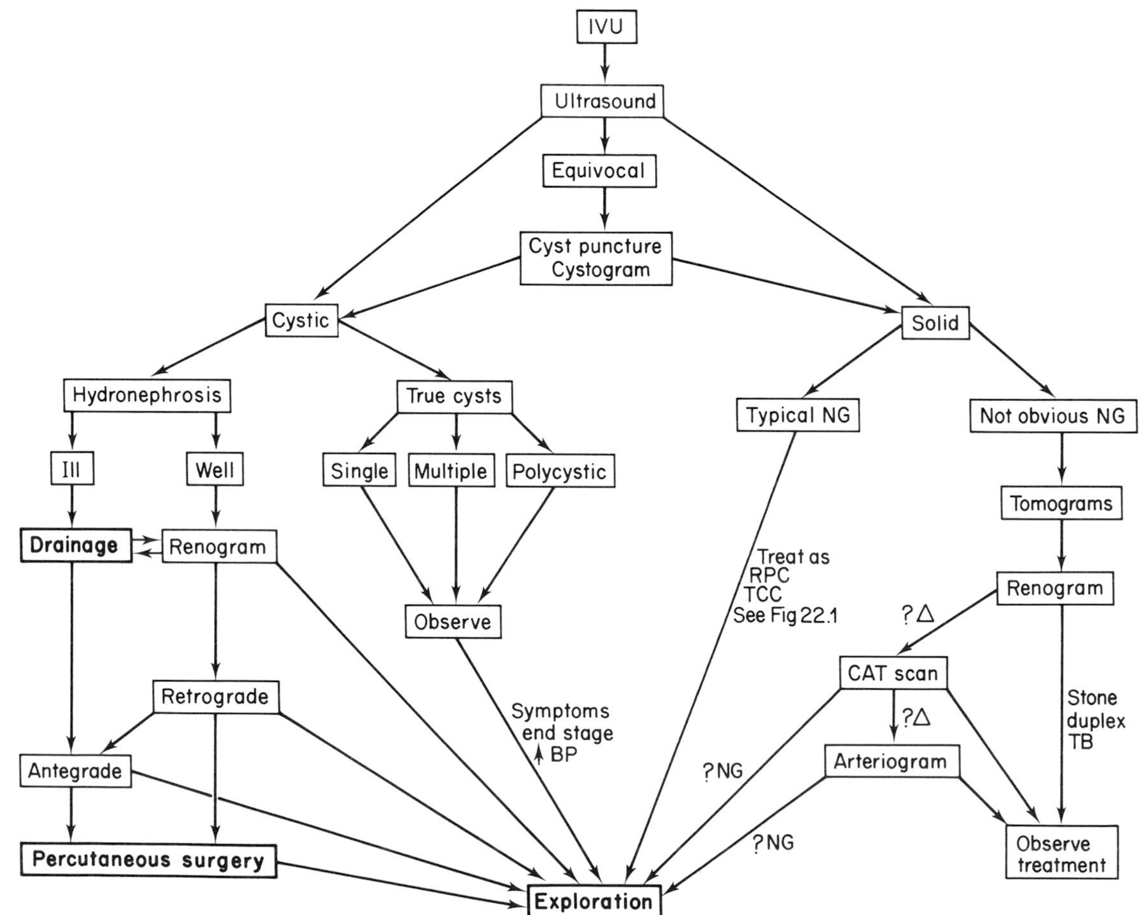

Fig. 22.2 Flow diagram demonstrating the diagnostic steps in a patient presenting with a renal mass.

stones (usually urate in type), blood clot and sloughed renal papillae. Other rare causes of luminal distortion as a result of intramural or extrinsic pathology will be found under the heading "Obstruction". Further discussion at this point will be limited to urothelial tumours, and information on cysts and renal parenchymal carcinoma will be found in the section concerned with those patients who present with a renal mass. Transitional cell carcinoma of the upper tracts is normally found in patients in their seventh decade, although the age range is wide, and occurs two to three times more commonly in men than in women.

Most diagnoses will be made by urine cytology, cystoscopy and retrograde imaging. At cystoscopy, urethral and intravesical causes of bleeding will be excluded (see Chapter 23). Upper urinary tract lesions may be confirmed if blood is seen issuing from a ureteric orifice and retrograde catheter studies may be performed at this stage. Whilst the popularity of retrograde pyelography has waned recently, bulb ureterograms and catheterized pyelograms do help to delineate filling defects which are not clear or have not been apparent on the intravenous urogram. Retrograde catheterization also allows specimens to be collected selectively for cytological examination.

Cytology

Cytology in experienced hands plays a useful role in the diagnosis of transitional cell carcinoma in the renal pelves and ureters, in addition to those arising in the bladder and urethra. This is especially so in patients with filling defects or other radiological abnormalities of the upper urinary tract. Cytological examination of voided urine taken prior to instrumentation from a well-hydrated patient forms an essential baseline. An aliquot of 50–100 ml of the entire specimen is required, with 20 ml of 95 per cent ethyl alcohol added as a preservative. Millepore filter preparations are superior to smears, both in the quantity of diagnostic material and in the morphological detail. A minimum of three specimens should be examined when investigating abnormalities in the upper urinary tract. Negative cystoscopy and bladder biopsy in these cases exclude carcinoma of the bladder as a source of malignant cells in the urine.

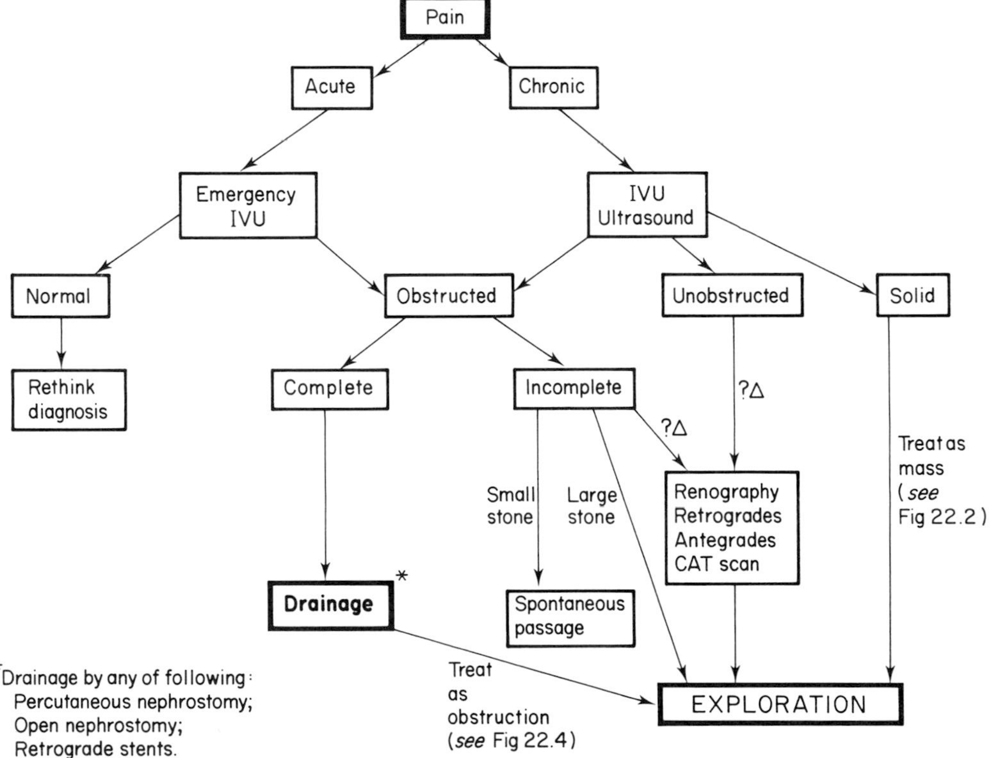

Fig. 22.3 Flow diagram demonstrating the diagnostic steps in a patient presenting with renal or ureteric pain.

Examination of ureteric urine followed by brushings from the suspicious area during retrograde pyelography with screening facilities may provide valuable diagnostic specimens. Saline irrigation after the brushing may yield more material. Brushings are made with a fine nylon bristle brush which is then cut off and immersed in 95 per cent ethyl alcohol. Cells and tissue fragments are detached by hard shaking and filter preparations made from the fluid. All solid material is fixed in 10 per cent formalin and sectioned. Serious complications following brush cytology have not been authenticated. Examination of antegrade aspirates of fluid from the renal pelvis may be useful in patients with obstruction at the pelvi-ureteric junction (PUJ). It must be stressed that the cytological diagnosis of malignancy in all material obtained by instrumentation should be made with caution because of the difficulty in distinguishing sheets of traumatically detached hyperplastic and atypical epithelium from differentiated transitional cell carcinoma.

In a personal series (WJH) of 45 patients with carcinoma of the renal pelvis, 62 per cent of tumours were detected by urine cytology. This is less than that for urothelial tumours arising in the bladder, for which experienced centres record a figure in the region of 80 per cent. This may be partly explained by the effects of peripheral location and inadequate urine flow past the tumour. False positive reports in experienced centres are uncommon and are more likely to represent early tumours initially undetected radiologically, rather than laboratory error. The presence of calculi may, however, cause problems in cytological interpretation. In a series of 135 patients with calculi, 7.2 per cent showed cytological features suspicious of well differentiated transitional cell carcinoma, but tumours were not detected on further investigation. However, careful follow-up of these

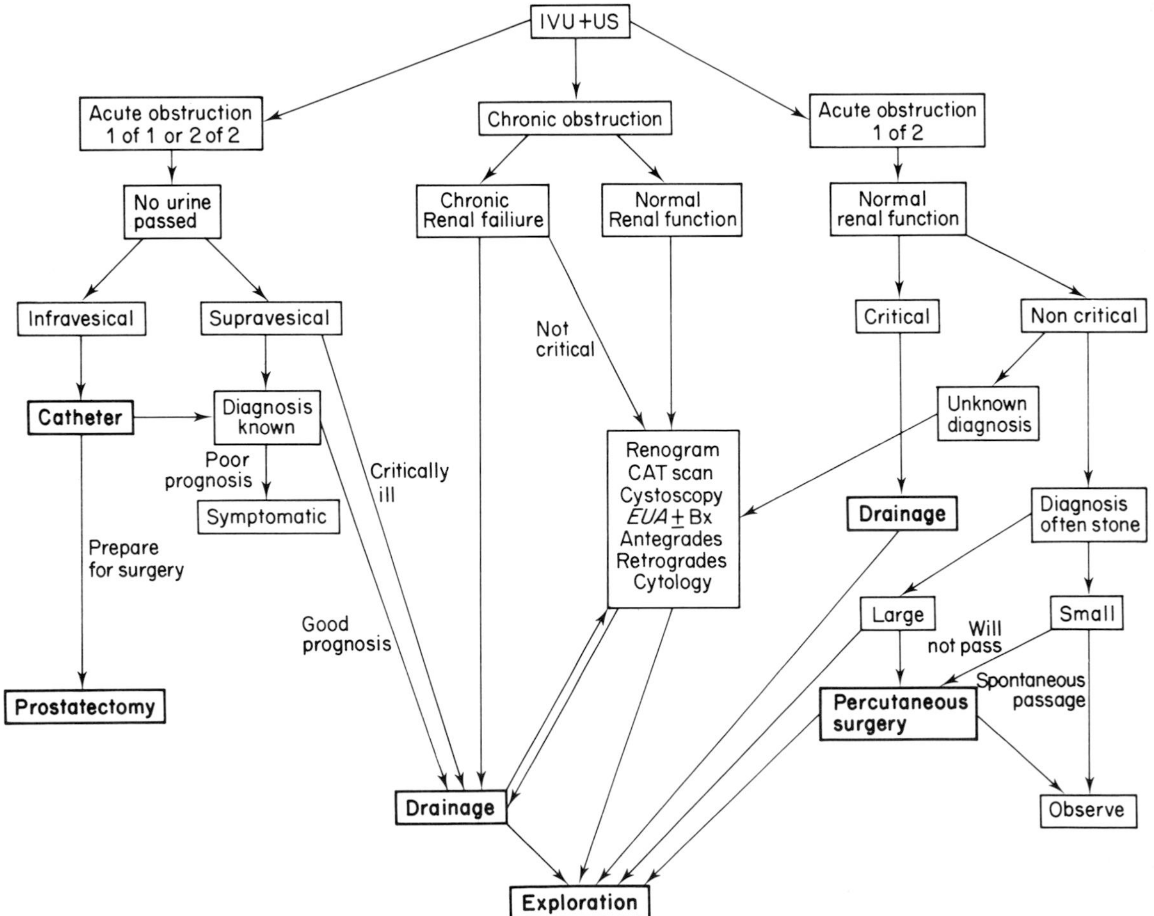

Fig. 22.4 Flow diagram demonstrating the diagnostic steps in a patient presenting with obstructive uropathy.

patients is important as tumours and calculi may co-exist.

Urine cytology is occasionally of value in diagnosing nonurothelial disease in patients with haematuria. If the pelvicalycine system is penetrated by a renal parenchymal carcinoma, tumour cells may be exfoliated and detected in the urine. Unrecognized medical renal pathology may be suggested by the presence of renal tubular cell casts, lumps of protein and degenerate renal tubular cells.

Tumours of the urothelium

Attitudes towards management of patients with pelvic and ureteric transitional cell carcinomas vary. A knowledge of the natural history and pathology of transitional cell carcinoma is essential to the understanding of this problem. Transitional cell carcinoma is not an isolated tumour but part of a field change involving the whole urinary tract. Radical surgery, in the form of nephroureterectomy with a cuff of bladder, has been the traditional approach and has the advantage that it removes the overt neoplasm, the surrounding area of pre-malignant change and the distal ureter. The latter has the proclivity for producing neoplasms and, on review of several series in which incomplete or partial nephroureterectomy has been performed, "stump" tumours were found in 20–58 per cent. Such tumours are difficult both to diagnose and treat. A criticism of nephroureterectomy is the fact that future treatment options will be severely depleted, notably in patients who have, or will develop, bilateral pelvic or ureteric disease—estimated at 1–2 per cent in large series, but found to be 8.9 per cent in 22 patients working in the dye industry and 9 per cent in 45 patients with Balkan nephropathy. The alternative is to treat pelvic and ureteric urothelial tumours by local resection and reconstruction of the urinary tract or, with advances in percutaneous surgery and transurethral ureteroscopy, by resection and diathermy. The conservative approach will be more acceptable when transurethral ureteroscopic follow-up becomes routine. Until this occurs, the overall survival figures do not fully support local resection.

Recently, it has been emphasized that both surgical approaches have a place dictated by the grade of the tumour. Thus, in low-grade tumours segmental resection is advocated as ipsilateral recurrence in this group is rare. In contrast, patients with neoplasms of intermediate grade benefit from nephroureterectomy as the incidence of ipsilateral recurrence in this grade is high (28 per cent). In patients with high-grade tumours, the prognosis is poor whatever the treatment and radical surgery may not therefore be justified.

In a proportion of cases tumour grading should be available preoperatively, based on the cytological appearances in the urine and in brush preparations. If this important information is not available, a frozen section at the time of surgery should be considered to establish the level of differentiation and to see whether the macroscopically normal urothelium adjacent to the overt neoplasm is the site of pre-malignant change. If a local resection is contemplated, a frozen section may also confirm that tumour excision is complete, but the pathologist and surgeon must realize that the statement "normal urothelium" is limited to the area of urothelium examined in this multifocal disease.

All these theoretical considerations and surgical procedures have to be tailored to the prevailing clinical situation. The surgical approach may be drastically altered in the presence of metastases; thus, chest X-ray and computerized axial tomography (CAT) scans should be performed to ensure accurate clinical staging and the management adjusted accordingly.

Pathology

The tissues received by the histopathologist include segments of ureter, nephroureterectomy specimens and, more recently, biopsies. The aim in all instances is the same, that of obtaining maximum information regarding grade and stage of the neoplasm and extent of the pre-malignant change in the surrounding urothelium—"field change". In the individual case this allows prognosis to be assessed and followup to be planned. In retrospective and prospective studies these facts are essential in order that tumours with a similar natural history can be compared. In addition, any differences between large series may reflect important epidemiological factors.

Fixation is best achieved in nephroureterectomy specimens (especially those that have been dilated) by redistending the ureter and pelvis with fixative and tying-off the ureter before putting the specimen into 10 per cent formalin. In the case of ureteric segments it is important to identify the proximal or distal limit—by a marker stitch for example—so that clinical impressions of tumour extent may be correlated with pathological findings. For research investigations involving tissue culture and ultrastructural and cytochemical studies of either tumour or attached normal tissue, the fresh specimen is taken rapidly to the laboratory. There, the pathologist responsible for the tissue diagnosis can select specimens for special fixation without prejudice to his/her reports.

Macroscopically, urothelial malignancies resemble those seen in the bladder (see Chapter 23). They may appear papillary with or without evidence of invasion, form an ulcer associated with invasion, or, in the case of carcinoma-in-situ, either produce a red granular mucosa or no abnormality. The appearances of the renal parenchyma is noted with special reference to papillary necrosis which may be found in association with pelvic carcinomas in analgesic abuse. Photographs of the outer and cut surfaces of the specimen provide a valuable record for surgeon and pathologist.

Blocks are selected to sample the neoplasms, adjacent tissue for evidence of pre-malignant change and the ureteric limits. Renal parenchyma is sampled to establish the extent of tumour spread or *in-situ* change within collecting tubules and to assess the possibility of papillary damage. When dealing with short segments of ureter, a section may be taken of the full length of the specimen and, for teaching purposes, when projected as a whole mount, provides an excellent demonstration of the microanatomy of the lesion.

The majority of epithelial pelvi-ureteric tumours are transitional in type and although true squamous and glandular carcinomas do occur (as opposed to squamous and glandular metaplasia within a transitional cell carcinoma), they are uncommon; therefore, discussion will be confined to the former group. The methods and prognostic value of grading and assessing the pathological stage of urothelial tumours of the pelvis and ureter in Britain are similar to those used for the morphologically identical carcinomas of the bladder (see Chapter 23). Although various systems are described in the literature, there is widespread agreement that tumour grade and stage are directly related and that both are indicators of disease behaviour. For example, in a recent series of 203 patients treated at the St Peter's Hospitals, the corrected five-year survival for those with grade I, II and III disease was 73.1, 46 and 33.3 per cent respectively. Patients whose neoplasms were not invasive, or only infiltrating into superficial muscle, had a corrected five-year survival of 72.5 per cent, whereas in those with deep muscle invasion or spread beyond the wall, the survival figure fell to 31 per cent. As most well differentiated tumours prove to be non-invasive, whereas those of high-grade malignancy are found to extend deeply into or through the muscle coat, for prognostic purposes subdividing tumour grades according to stage is most useful in those of intermediate grade.

Valuable prognostic information can also be derived from the histological assessment of "field change". Thus, flat carcinoma-in-situ in apparently "normal" urothelium adjacent to an overt tumour, indicates that bladder recurrences may be anticipated. Similarly, multiple tumours are associated with a worse prognosis than solitary neoplasms. For example, the corrected five-year survival for patients with solitary well differentiated papillary transitional cell carcinoma of ureter was 80.5 per cent, but only 50 per cent for those whose well differentiated carcinomas involved both pelvis and ureter (St Peter's study).

In series of upper tract neoplasms from the USA and Sweden, the well differentiated tumours are found to be the least common urothelial malignancies (1–22 per cent). In contrast are the findings in London where 64 per cent of upper tract urothelial neoplasms were well differentiated. This is unlikely to be the result of differences in grading methods as the survival rate for patients with low-grade neoplasms is similar in the different publications, but it may indicate an epidemiological difference. For example, in the Swedish series of 102 patients, phenacetin abuse, known to be associated with the development of high-grade renal pelvic carcinoma, was confirmed in nine patients and suspected in a further 16. The existence of such differences in the proportion of tumours in different grades underlines the importance of histological assessment for surgeons planning therapeutic trials.

Subsequent management of patients with urothelial tumours

Following surgery for transitional cell carcinoma of the upper tracts, patients require regular follow-up examination including cystoscopy, urine cytology and IVU. Cytological follow-up of the upper tracts, by examining freshly passed ileal conduit urine, is also essential in patients who have had a cystectomy for transitional cell carcinoma of the bladder and are candidates for further neoplasms in their remaining urothelium. Experience is needed to diagnose reliably malignant cells in conduit urine with its background of degenerate ileal cells. In such specimens additional information may be derived from the presence of abundant polymorphonuclear leucocytes and bacteria, from which upper tract inflammation may be inferred.

Other causes of haematuria

If urine cytology, IVU, ultrasound, CAT scan, cystoscopy and retrograde studies fail to demonstrate the source of bleeding, arteriography will be necessary in an attempt to make the diagnosis. This may show an arteriovenous malformation or angioma which can be embolized at the time of the arteriogram, ligated at open operation or necessitate a partial or total nephrectomy. Many of these vascular lesions are, however, small and difficult to demonstrate. Thus, it is not uncommon for nephrectomy to be performed because of severe prolonged haematuria and the diagnosis made postoperatively. Even at this stage the histopathologist may fail to sample such lesions initially because they are not apparent macroscopically or obscured by peripelvic haemorrhage. Arteriography may also demonstrate the typical tumour circulation of the small renal cell neoplasm which will be discussed under the heading "Renal mass".

Finally, although this chapter is only concerned with surgical conditions, it must be remembered that in the population as a whole glomerulonephritis is the most frequent cause of asymptomatic haematuria. In this context, the value of examination of the urine is stressed as the presence of red cell casts and dysmorphic red cells on phase contrast microscopy correlates closely with glomerular disease.

Renal mass

The commoner causes of a renal mass are shown in Table 22.4.

Table 22.4 Common causes of renal mass.

Cyst
Hydronephrosis
Tumour
Infection
Congenital lesions

Investigation of patients with renal mass

The mass may be clinically apparent on careful inspection of the abdominal and loin contours and on thorough bimanual palpation. A useful manoeuvre is to lie the patient on his asymptomatic side, when the abdominal contents and apron of subcutaneous fat will fall away and the lump become more easily felt.

More commonly a renal mass will present on IVU as a space-occupying lesion, the nature of which can usually then be ascertained by ultrasound examination. Basically, solid lesions are malignant and cystic ones benign until proved otherwise. True cysts may be single or multiple or the kidney may be polycystic. The so-called "false cyst" or hydronephrosis, most commonly caused by an obstructive lesion between the pelvi-ureteric and vesico-ureteric junctions, will be considered later. If the result of ultrasound examination is equivocal, aspiration cytology and cystography may resolve the problem.

Aspiration cytology

Cytology is of value in the diagnosis of cystic or solid masses in and around the kidney when imaging results are equivocal and when there is evidence of bilateral or disseminated disease. Aspiration is performed by the radiologist guided by a CAT scan or ultrasound. When cysts are aspirated, all the fluid should be sent for examination without the addition of fixative which precipitates the protein. A sample should be sent for culture if infection is suspected. Cysts producing clear, colourless or straw-coloured fluid are almost invariably benign. The presence of altered blood or necrotic debris is suspicious of renal parenchymal carcinoma. Cyst fluids are usually acellular, but occasionally benign cysts may contain many single degenerate cells. Inflammatory cells, haemosiderin-laden histiocytes and glomeruli are occasionally present. Benign transitional cells suggest that the fluid is urine and has been aspirated from a hydrocalyx. Malignant cells in clear cyst fluid may represent a tumour in the cyst wall, which is rare, or a separate tumour.

When aspirating solid masses adequate sampling is all important. The needle is moved back and forth in the mass as negative pressure is applied and aspirations from several sites may be required. The assistance of a cytotechnician is advisable in order to ensure good quality preparations. Smears made from aspirates of solid lesions are fixed immediately before drying in 95 per cent ethyl alcohol. An airdried smear for Romanowski staining is made if lymphoma is suspected. Blood clot and any solid material is fixed in 10 per cent formalin for surgical sections. Filter preparations of saline washings from the syringe and needle may contain useful diagnostic material. Morphological features in well prepared aspirates are sufficiently clearcut for reliable diagnosis of renal parenchymal carcinomas, including oncocytic forms. Transitional carcinomas can usually be distinguished morphologically, which is helpful in the differential diagnosis of masses in and around the kidney in patients with a history of urothelial carcinoma. Angiomyolipomas are recognized by the admixture of connective tissue and fat cells and small fragments of the tumour with abnormal blood vessels may be seen in sectioned blood clots.

The most significant theoretical complication of needle aspiration in the diagnosis of malignancy is needle-track seeding of tumour cells. Von Schreeb and his colleagues (1967) found no significant differences in the five-year survival rates between 77 patients with renal carcinoma operated on after diagnostic puncture with injection of contrast medium, and 73 matched controls. Haematomas were found in the renal region in ten cases and one developed acute pyelonephritis. One case of tumour developing along an 18-gauge needle track after aspiration of a grade II renal cell carcinoma has been reported and one retroperitoneal liposarcoma appeared in the needle track five years after aspiration with a 23-gauge needle. No evidence of seeding was found in 2500 trans-thoracic and trans-abdominal fine needle aspirations using 20–23 gauge needles. Small haematomas were the only complications reported in trans-abdominal aspiration of lymph nodes.

Further investigation and treatment

If the final diagnosis is that of a simple cyst, no further treatment, apart from observation, will be required. Should doubt still exist, further diagnostic steps will be similar to those taken in the case of a solid space-occupying lesion, which most commonly indicates a renal parenchymal carcinoma, and are performed with surgical exploration in mind. Small lesions may require no other special investigation apart from a chest X-ray to look for lung metastases. In modern practice, most lesions, and especially the larger masses, need further tests to assess local invasion and lymphatic spread—features which may influence the extent and even the practicability of radical surgery. Venography with ultrasound and CAT scanning will demonstrate vena caval involvement and its extent, and may indicate a thoraco-abdominal approach in order to remove tumour thrombus from the intra-thoracic vena cava. Selective coeliac and renal arteriography may suggest contiguous hepato-renal blood supply which would render the tumour inoperable.

The surgery for renal parenchymal carcinoma is radical nephrectomy removing the kidney, with its perirenal fat and fascia intact, the adrenal gland and para-aortic nodes. The need for open renal biopsy is very uncommon. Occasionally, however, renal parenchymal carcinomas occur in solitary kidneys or bilaterally and in these circumstances, if technically feasible, a lumpectomy or partial nephrectomy may be the only therapeutic option. In this situation, a frozen section may be required to confirm the diagnosis or to check the margins of excision.

Pathology

Postoperatively, the handling of the gross specimen in theatre is very important. Incisions made in the kidney prior to sending it to the pathology department may considerably reduce the value of the specimen for teaching purposes and can, on occasion, limit the amount of information that the pathologist can extract from it. Depending on the practice of the hospital, the uncut specimen should be placed immediately in fixative or delivered unfixed to the laboratory. The latter course should obviously be followed if fresh tissue is required for microbiology or other purposes. In the laboratory, following gross description and after examination of the hilar vessels, the kidney is bisected and photographed before blocks are removed for histological examination.

Renal cysts

All cystic kidneys sent for pathological examination require careful examination for the presence of co-existent tumour. This is particularly true in the case of the acquired renal cystic disease of long-term intermittent haemodialysis, in which tumours have been reported in up to 45 per cent of patients though their malignant potential is uncertain, and also of adult polycystic disease. It should be remembered that the latter is a familial condition transmitted as an autosomal dominant, which presents usually in adult life with chronic renal failure, hypertension, loin pain and haematuria. Other organs, especially the liver, may also be affected. Mention should also be made of medullary sponge kidney—an anomaly, generally considered to be congenital, in which there is cystic dilatation of the collecting ducts in the renal papillae of one or both kidneys or segments of kidneys, resulting in a characteristic radiological appearance. The lesion predisposes to both stone formation and infection which cause the symptomatology. In a proportion of cases there is associated hemihypertrophy of the body.

Renal neoplasms

Primary tumours of the kidney, excluding transitional cell carcinoma, which is urothelial rather than renal, can be classified simply as follows:

Epithelial	adenoma carcinoma
Mesenchymal	benign malignant (sarcoma)
Embryonal	congenital mesoblastic nephroma nephroblastoma (Wilms' tumour)
Miscellaneous	malignant lymphoma tumour of the juxta-glomerular apparatus

The type of neoplasm present will obviously influence both further therapy and prognosis. Epithelial tumours are by far the commonest, except in young children where the embryonal ones predominate. Of the malignant tumours, carcinomas account for about 89 per cent, sarcomas for 2–3 per cent and the embryonal tumours for 8 or 9 per cent.

Adenomas Adenomas, the incidence of which increases with age, are usually incidental findings. They are small, yellow or grey nodules situated in the cortex, commonly near the surface, in any part of the kidney—in contrast to adrenal cortical rests with which they may be confused grossly and which are confined to the upper pole. They arise from the renal tubules, as do the parenchymal carcinomas, and there are no histological, ultrastructural, immunofluorescent or other features which will distinguish an adenoma from a carcinoma.

It is usual, therefore, to accept the findings of Bell (1938) that tumours less than 3 cm in diameter seldom metastasize and to accept lesions over this size as carcinomas. Nevertheless, as smaller tumours occasionally do behave in a malignant fashion, it is safest to treat them as malignant if they show histological evidence of pleomorphism or mitotic activity. By and large, there is a linear relationship between size and the likelihood of metastases. One exception to this is the oncocytoma—a tumour composed entirely of altered epithelial cells which have abundant, granular, eosinophilic cytoplasm due to the presence of large numbers of mitochondria. Such tumours also have distinctive gross features, being well circumscribed, often large, and tan in colour, usually with a central area of scarring. Characteristic angiographic features have been described but their specificity has been challenged. Even when large these tumours tend to behave in a benign fashion.

Renal parenchymal carcinoma (*synonyms*: hypernephroma, Grawitz tumour, renal cell carcinoma, renal adenocarcinoma) is more common in the male (ratio 3:1) with a maximum incidence in the sixth decade, though rare cases do occur in childhood. It accounts for 2 per cent of all male and 1 per cent of all female malignancies and has a link with certain hereditary conditions, being common in von Hippel–Lindau disease. Although considered here under "renal mass" it should be remembered that its presentation is very variable and local, toxic and endocrine effects may all be present.

Grossly, the tumour characteristically forms a lobulated mass protruding from the surface of the kidney. The cut surface is commonly variegated with yellow areas, areas of haemorrhage and cyst formation, though the more anaplastic varieties tend to be white and solid with areas of necrosis. Gross invasion of the renal vein is common, being present in about 30 per cent of operation specimens, and should be looked for before the kidney is sectioned. (Retrograde venous spread to the genital organs occurs via the spermatic or ovarian vein and is therefore more common on the left side.)

Microscopically, there are two main cell types—clear and granular—and a variety of patterns including tubular, alveolar and papillary. The pathologist's job is not ended when a diagnosis of renal parenchymal carcinoma has been made. Certain features which may be of prognostic significance must be included in the report. Apart from neoplasms composed entirely of oncocytes, which have an excellent outlook, and those with spindle cell areas (see below) which do badly, cell type is no longer considered to be important in prognosis. Three histological grades are usually described, grade I being the best differentiated, and correlate well with both stage and prognosis. Although grading is a subjective exercise there is, in general, agreement about the poorly differentiated tumours which have the worst prognosis. Some such tumours develop a spindle cell appearance and are especially malignant in behaviour. Distinguishing them from sarcomas and Wilms' tumours may be difficult and transition forms between spindle and obviously epithelial cells must be looked for. Immunocytochemistry is likely to become of increasing value in this situation.

The most significant factor affecting prognosis is the presence of metastases and the majority of patients with metastases at presentation are dead within two years. The lung is the commonest site, being involved in 76 per cent of autopsy cases in a recent large series. The next commonest sites were lymph nodes (66 per cent), bones (42 per cent) and liver (41 per cent). Metastasis to one organ only was found in 8 per cent of the patients in this series and it should be remembered that surgical removal of a solitary metastasis in renal parenchymal carcinoma may be curative.

In the non-metastatic case, the local extent of tumour at the time of surgery is usually considered to be the most important single variable in determining survival. Suggested staging schemes, however, reflect the varying emphasis placed by authors on the invasion of different structures. Perhaps the two best known are those of Robson and of the Union Internationale Contre le Cancer (UICC). (See Table 22.5.)

Five-year survival figures for patients treated by nephrectomy vary considerably in reported series, with ranges for Robson's stages I–IV of 56–82 per cent, 43–100 per cent, 8–51 per cent and 0–13 per cent respectively.

Table 22.5 Staging schemes

Extent of tumour		*Robson (1969)*	*UICC (1978)*
Confined to the kidney	small	I	pT1
	large	I	pT2
Perinephric or peripelvic fat involved		II	pT3
Main renal vein invaded		III	pT3 V1
Regional lymph nodes invaded		III	N+
Extension to neighbouring organs		IV	pT4
Distant metastases		IV	M+

Invasion of the renal pelvis is of little prognostic importance and metastasis to the lower urinary tract extremely rare. The significance of renal capsular penetration is controversial and there may be a pathological explanation for this. The enlarging tumour may erode the renal capsule on a broad front—forming a false capsule as it spreads outwards in the perinephric fat. This is an entirely different matter from invasion of the perinephric fat by small tongues of tumour cells and is much less likely to have an adverse affect on prognosis. The two are not distinguished in currently used staging schemes. Invasion of the hilar vein, seen in one-third of operation specimens, is generally accepted to be a bad prognostic sign, though in one computer analysis its presence was found to be of no predictive value.

Mesenchymal tumours The benign mesenchymal tumours are usually considered to be hamartomatous rather than neoplastic. The majority are small, incidental findings and need no further consideration. Two are of interest—the haemangioma in the pericalyceal region (see under "haematuria") and the *angiomyolipoma* which occurs in two forms. When small, multifocal and often bilateral, they are usually associated with the familial condition of tuberous sclerosis and frequently lead to renal failure. Because of the associated severe problems, surgery is rarely indicated. When single, they tend to be large and to have no association with tuberous sclerosis. Angiomyolipomas occur over the age of 40 and are more common in women (ratio 4.5:1), presenting as space-occupying lesions which account for less than 1 per cent of renal neoplasms found at surgical exploration. Presenting symptoms, which result from haemorrhage into and around the tumour, include flank pain and shock. Hypertension is occasionally a feature.

Grossly, the cut surface is yellow-grey, depending on the relative proportions of fat and smooth muscle, and microscopically they are composed of fat, smooth muscle and tortuous blood vessels. Malignant transformation is extremely rare and the pathologist must not be misled by apparently disquieting histological features; the smooth muscle element is often pleomorphic and this does not imply malignant change. The finding of similar tissue in a regional lymph node or even in the spleen does not seem to affect the excellent prognosis and may represent multifocal development rather than metastasis.

Sarcomas of the kidney are rare, accounting for only 2–3 per cent of malignant renal tumours. Fibrosarcomas were once considered to be most common but, with more careful study, including the use of electron microscopy, most of the spindle-celled tumours have proved to be carcinomas or of smooth muscle origin. They are usually locally invasive before surgery and the prognosis is poor.

Embryonal tumours The embryonal tumours, which predominate in children, are dealt with in Chapter 29. A rare case of nephroblastoma (Wilms' tumour) does, however, occur in the adult. The incidence is uncertain as some of the tumours so designated in the past are now thought to have been "sarcomatoid" parenchymal carcinomas. The prognosis in the adult is also uncertain, but it is suggested that therapy should be aggressive and multimodal as in childhood, and long-term survival has been reported.

Malignant lymphoma Infiltration of the kidneys, either nodular or diffuse, is found at autopsy in approximately one-third of patients with malignant lymphoma and may rarely lead to acute renal insufficiency. This condition may also present as an apparently primary renal tumour, though the majority of the patients die of disseminated disease.

Juxta-glomerular-tumour The rare juxta-glomerular tumour, which is included here for completeness, does not present as a mass. It produces renin, leading to a secondary form of aldosteronism and hypertension, and occurs in a younger age group than carcinoma with a range of 2–37 years. Its behaviour is benign. Grossly, it is small and well circumscribed and situated in the renal cortex. Microscopically, it is composed of small uniform cells in compact clusters separated by thin-walled blood vessels. The cells contain cytoplasmic granules which give a positive immunofluorescence with anti-human renin antibodies and are ultrastructurally identical with the secretion granules of the normal juxta-glomerular cell.

Inflammatory lesions

Some inflammatory conditions may present as space-occupying lesions and mimic tumours on ultrasound examination. They include the tumefactive form of xanthogranulomatous pyelonephritis, malakoplakia, renal carbuncle and some fungus diseases. The clinical presentation and findings are likely to be of help in the diagnosis and, with the exception of xanthogranulomatous pyelonephritis, the conditions mentioned tend to occur in the severely debilitated patient.

Xanthogranulomatous pyelonephritis This is a non-specific chronic inflammatory condition which is usually associated with a non-functioning kidney, stones and urinary infection—especially with Proteus species. It may occur as an expansile yellow mass resembling renal parenchymal carcinoma, but more commonly it is seen in the form of a calculus pyonephrosis, in which the dilated pelvi-calycine system is surrounded by shaggy yellow tissue. The yellow colouration is due to the presence of large numbers of foamy macrophages, laden with intracytoplasmic fat, which are thought to result from suppuration and bear some resemblance to the clear cells of a parenchymal carcinoma. Bilateral involvement is extremely rare. The affected kidney tends to adhere to adjacent organs and to form fistulae—features which, in association with the yellow colour of the inflammatory tissue, have sometimes led to a diagnosis of inoperable carcinoma or to the performing of, in retrospect, unnecessarily radical surgery.

Malakoplakia A rare chronic inflammatory condition, malakoplakia was first described in the bladder, where it is most common and usually self-limiting. It has since been reported in other parts of the genito-urinary tract and also other systems. Involvement of the renal parenchyma is rare, but may be bilateral and progressive leading to renal failure. In 75 per cent of cases it is associated with an *Escherichia coli* urinary infection, and ultrastructural studies on such a lesion in the colon have demonstrated bacteria in various stages of degradation within the phagocytic vacuoles of macrophages. This defective digestion of coliform bacteria has been attributed to an intracellular abnormality of the macrophages, and defects of blood monocytes have also been demonstrated in one case. Malakoplakia has been reported in a renal transplant and in a patient with lymphoma.

Grossly, in the bladder, ureter and renal pelvis, the lesions of malakoplakia consist of soft yellowish plaques, while in the renal parenchyma they are described as yellowish nodules—mainly within the medulla. Unlike xanthogranulomatous pyelonephritis, obstruction does not appear to be a feature and IVU shows only intrarenal calyceal compression. Ureteric obstruction, due to a plaque of malakoplakia has, however, been recorded.

Microscopically, the condition is characterized by the presence of eosinophilic macrophages with round intracellular inclusions, resulting from the metamorphosis of phagolysosomes, which are often laminated and contain calcium (Michaelis–Gutmann bodies).

Renal carbuncle, which is a rare lesion, is essentially a confluent collection of abscesses in the renal parenchyma which does not communicate with the renal pelvis. It appears to be confined to debilitated or diabetic subjects—especially drug addicts using dirty needles for intravenous injections. The IVU may show a soft tissue mass compressing the calyces, but evidence of severe infection and renal pain should help in the diagnosis.

Fungus diseases, such as primary renal aspergillosis or candidiasis, may present as large inflammatory masses and fungus balls and inflammatory debris can obstruct the collecting system.

Pain

Any of the previously described conditions can present with pain. Renal tumours in an advanced state may cause a dull loin ache which is rarely severe unless associated with infection, clot colic or spontaneous haemorrhage. Renal cysts are rarely painful unless there is intracystic haemorrhage, often caused by trauma. Congenital lesions such as polycystic disease or horseshoe kidneys may also present as painful abdominal masses. Horseshoe kidneys are often associated with other congenital abnormalities, and an accompanying hydronephrosis may be due to congenital narrowing of the PUJ rather than to the abnormal course of the ureters over the anterior aspect of the renal isthmus, as is often suggested. The main causes of renal pain are shown in Table 22.6.

Table 22.6 Main causes of renal pain.

Infection
Stone
Hydronephrosis
Tumour
Trauma
Congenital lesions

The commonest cause, infection, occurs in the form of pyelonephritis, abscesses or pyonephrosis. Specific infections and infestations such as tuberculosis, schistosomiasis and hydatid disease may also present in this way.

Surgical intervention, however, is most often required for renal/ureteric colic due to an obstructing lesion of the ureter or renal pelvis. Urinary calculus disease is the most frequent cause and suitable cases may be treated percutaneously. Kidneys removed because of staghorn calculi show varying degrees of parenchymal destruction with associated pyelonephritic changes. The distended pelvicalycine system has a congested granular lining which on microscopic examination usually contains areas of ulceration and foci of urothelial atypia and/or metaplasia of squamous, adenomatous or, rarely, glandular type. Any stone received in a surgical specimen should be sent for analysis.

Obstruction

The commonest causes of renal obstruction are shown in Table 22.7.

Table 22.7 Commonest causes of renal obstruction.

Bilateral	*Unilateral*
Infravesical pathology	Stones
Pelvic/retroperitoneal neoplasia	Pelvic/retroperitoneal neoplasia
Idiopathic retroperitoneal fibrosis	Idiopathic retroperitoneal fibrosis
Stones	Ureteric neoplasia
PUJ abnormalities	PUJ abnormalities
Miscellaneous	Infection
	Miscellaneous

The obstruction may be at supravesical, vesical or infravesical level; only the first will be discussed in this chapter. Patients present typically with renal pain or ureteric colic, often complicated by infection causing fever, malaise and rigors and not uncommonly associated with lower tract symptoms of frequency and dysuria. Bilateral obstruction or obstruction of a solitary kidney may lead to acute renal failure.

Investigation and early management

Intravenous urography and abdominal ultrasound will confirm the obstruction and often, in conjunction with the history, will indicate its site and cause. In the acute situation, where there is severe renal damage or the patient's condition is critical, emergency relief of the obstruction is vital and further diagnostic tests must be deferred.

The kidney can be drained and the urine diverted in a number of ways. Open nephrostomy or ureterostomy, retrograde intubated ureterostomy and percutaneous nephrostomy are examples. Which method is employed will depend on the clinical circumstances and the facilities available. Once the acute situation is resolved, further investigations may proceed at a more leisurely pace—as in the non-acute case. Much more information regarding the site, cause and effect of the obstruction can be obtained from DTPA renography with lasix provocation, and ascending and descending pyeloureterograms will give confimatory evidence.

Pathology

When considering the pathology of obstruction only three major causes of importance to the surgeon and histopathologist will be discussed, as stones are not within the scope of this chapter and urothelial tumours are described above.

Lesions in the retroperitoneal space and pelvis commonly produce bilateral obstruction in contrast with those discussed below. Thus, patients have an insidious onset of ill health secondary to chronic obstructive uropathy and renal failure. The underlying pathology is usually that of an infiltrating pelvic tumour, idiopathic retroperitoneal fibrosis (RPF) or a neoplasm in the retroperitoneal space, as inflammatory processes, haemorrhage and cysts are rare. If neurological changes are present, a malignant aetiology is almost certain. The most common pelvic neoplasms include those extending from the cervix, prostate, bladder or intestine. Neoplasms found in the retroperitoneum include primary or secondary germ cell tumours, metastases, neoplasms of soft tissue or peripheral nerve origin and lymphomas but, of these, obstructive uropathy is most often associated with secondary deposits. The common primary sites are those listed under pelvic neoplasms and may have been established prior to the development of obstruction. On the other hand, the latter may be the presenting symptom necessitating investigation of the possible primary sites. Fine-needle aspiration of peri-ureteric masses and lymph nodes under fluoroscopic control may be valuable as false positives are rare, and a laparotomy to establish the diagnosis may thus be avoided. Negative cytological results do not, of course, exclude tumour.

If laparotomy is performed, the common primary sites may be examined and the distribution of the fibrosis noted. Pelvic fibrosis commonly has a malignant basis, whereas idiopathic RPF is usually centred on the lumbar aorta. Frozen sections may be considered, but are only of value when a positive diagnosis of tumour can be made. The histology is often difficult to interpret as carcinomas frequently invade in a single-celled manner evoking a dense fibrosis which may be difficult to distinguish from idiopathic RPF or a lymphomatous infiltrate. Therefore, in practice, the definitive diagnosis is commonly made on paraffin sections taken from the retroperitoneal tissue during ureterolysis.

Further management

The aim of exploration is to free the ureters from the dense fibrous tissue, wrap them in omentum and place them intra-peritoneally to prevent further obstruction. Postoperatively, if a diagnosis of idiopathic RPF has been made, the patient may respond to treatment with steroids, while some malignant retroperitoneal lesions may respond to therapy suited to the nature of the primary tumour, for example stilboestrol for carcinoma of the prostate.

Idiopathic pelvi-ureteric junction (PUJ) "obstruction"

This typically presents with loin pain, often exacerbated by a high fluid intake, recurrent urinary tract infection and a palpable renal mass. Once diagnosed, the treatment is to re-establish a freely draining pelvis which is most commonly achieved by removal of the abnormal junction and reconstructive pyeloplasty. The specimen should not be incised prior to fixation as orientation to display a longitudinal section of the junction may be relevant to diagnosis. As indicated in the nomenclature, the cause of this condition is not definitely known. The abnormalities seen in idiopathic PUJ obstruction have been variously described as an increase in fibrous tissue in the lamina propria and muscle in the dilated segment, a deficiency of the spiral muscle at the PUJ, adhesions and obstructing polar vessels. In addition to an assessment of fibrosis and of the disposition of the muscle fibres, the pathologist will be able to exclude some of the other causes of obstruction discussed in this chapter.

Amongst post-inflammatory strictures, tuberculosis is implicated with increasing frequency. As renal tuberculosis results from haematogenous spread from a primary site elsewhere, usually in the lungs, the initial lesions are in the cortex from which spread occurs to the medulla leading to ulcerative lesions of characteristic appearance on renal papillae. Involvement of the pelvicalycine system, ureter and bladder follows and a positive microbiological diagnosis should be obtainable. Healing of the lesions is accompanied by fibrosis and the resultant strictures of individual calyces and ureter lead to stasis and hydronephrosis. The patients may present with symptoms of chronic urinary infection and obstruction. Quite often the obstructive uropathy occurs whilst the patient is on active anti-tuberculous chemotherapy. It is during the rapid healing phase that intense fibrosis occurs and the ensuing stricture can quickly cause irreparable renal damage. The possibility of stricture formation must be considered both during and after treatment and looked for by serial IVU. When they do occur, partial upper polar nephrectomy may be needed or local ureteric excision with reconstruction or reimplantation depending on the site.

Many other causes of ureteric obstruction, all of which are rare in urological practice in Britain, are listed for completeness: sloughed renal papillae, schistosomiasis, endometriosis, fibroepithelial polyps, inverted papillomas, metastatic tumours, amyloid, and "urinoma" (extravasated urine).

The main aim of the urologist in dealing with obstruction is the preservation of renal function. "End-stage kidneys" are the hallmarks of missed diagnoses and opportunities to reverse what, initially, were reversible conditions. Such kidneys may be the shrunken scarred organs resulting from reflux nephropathy or the large dilated shells following renal destruction by staghorn calculi or other obstructive lesions, and are treated by simple nephrectomy.

Further reading

Bell ET. A classification of renal tumors with observations on the frequency of the various types. *J Urol* 1938; **39**: 238–44.

Booth CM, Cameron KM, Pugh RCB. Urothelial carcinoma of the kidney and ureter. *Br J Urol* 1980; **52**: 430–35.

Chisholm GD, Williams DI. Ed. *Scientific Foundations of Urology* Second Edition. London: William Heinemann Medical Books Ltd, 1982.

Harmer MH. Ed. *T.N.M. Classification of malignant tumours (UICC)* Third Edition. pp. 109–112. Geneva: International Union Against Cancer, 1978.

Heney NM, Szyfelbein WM, Daly JJ, Prout GR, Bredin HC. Positive urinary cytology in patients without evident tumour. *J Urol* 1977; **117**: 223–4.

Johansson S, Angervall L, Bengtsson U, Wahlqvist L. A clinicopathologic and prognostic study of epithelial tumours of the renal pelvis. *Cancer* 1976; **37**: 1376–83.

Maskell R. *Urinary Tract Infection*. London: Edward Arnold, 1982.

Milroy EJG, O'Riordan JLH. Investigation and Management of Urinary Calculi of Metabolic Origin. In *Current Surgical Practice* Volume III, London: Edward Arnold, 1981 pp. 80–94.

Murphy DM, Zincke H, Furlow WL. Primary grade 1 transitional cell carcinoma of the renal pelvis and ureter. *J Urol* 1980; **123**: 629–31.

Murphy DM, Zincke H, Furlow WL. Management of high grade transitional cell carcinoma of the upper urinary tract. *J Urol* 1981; **125**: 25–9.

Nelson RP. New concepts on staging and follow-up of bladder carcinoma. *Urology* 1983; **XXI**: No. 2, 105–12.

Robson CJ, Churchill BM, Anderson W. The results of radical nephrectomy for renal cell carcinoma. *J Urol* 1969; **101**: 297–301.

Rose GA. *Urinary Stones: Clinical and Laboratory Aspects*. Lancaster, England: M.T.P. Press Ltd, 1982.

von Schreeb T, Arner O, Skovsted G, Wikstad N. Renal Adenoma—Is there a risk of spreading tumour cells in diagnostic puncture? *Scand J Urol Nephrourol* 1967; **1**: 270–76.

23

Lower Urinary Tract

P B Clark and C K Anderson

Introduction

There used to be a myth amongst urologists that they could always tell as much about a tumour by looking at it down a cystoscope as a pathologist could tell about it by looking at it down a microscope. Although this may be true with many vesical tumours, in a significant proportion a competent pathologist will be able to warn the urologist that the tumour is more aggressive than he thought, or on rare occasions he will tell him the lesion he had confidently diagnosed as a tumour is not a tumour at all. Similarly, with prostatic lesions, what appears to be benign may be malignant and what appears to be malignant may be benign. Without histological guidance, therefore, a urologist may often make a mistake; on rarer occasions, without clinical guidance a pathologist may also make a mistake; to avoid any mistake there should be close collaboration between them.

Clinical presentations

An abnormality is seen in the bladder on cystoscopy – is it malignant or benign?

It cannot be stressed too strongly that if anything suspicious is seen in the bladder on cystoscopy it should be biopsied. Only in this way can tragic errors be avoided.

The most serious error is to imagine a localized area of reddening or oedema is simply an area of inflammation, when in fact it is an area of anaplastic carcinoma, perhaps extending into perivesical fat. More extensive patches of reddening may be caused by carcinoma-in-situ. Biopsy will prove the diagnosis.

Conversely, what appears to be a tumour may be benign. The common "catheter reaction" may worry the uninitiated, but its characteristic situation in the fundus of the bladder and its appearance, perhaps with an ulcer where the tip of the catheter lay, will differentiate it so reliably from tumour that biopsy is not usually indicated. After radiotherapy a papillary lesion, thought to be a recurrence, may prove on histological examination to be no more than heaped-up mucosa. Sometimes chronic inflammation outside the bladder, for example associated with diverticulitis of the colon or a tubo-ovarian abscess, may produce a raised area in the bladder covered with inflammatory polypi which looks exactly like a sessile papillary tumour. The rare condition of primary amyloidosis of the bladder produces a raised reddened lesion looking for all the world like an aggressive carcinoma. In these conditions believe the histological and not the cystoscopic appearances.

A tumour has been found in the bladder – how can the pathological assessment affect management?

The most important prognostic factor about a tumour of the bladder is its clinical stage, and especially whether it has invaded muscle. Histological examination of an ordinary biopsy will show whether the tumour is entirely non-invasive or shows the earliest sign of invasion, namely of the basement membrane of the fronds. If a deep biopsy has been taken including muscle or the tumour has been resected, histological examination will show whether there is invasion of the submucosa, muscle or lymphatics. Invasion of muscle or lymphatics is usually an indication for radical treatment, for example radiotherapy or cystectomy.

Histological examination of an ordinary biopsy will show whether the tumour is well differentiated, poorly differentiated or anaplastic. The worse the grade, the worse the prognosis. If a deep biopsy has been taken or the tumour resected, histological examination will show whether the grade is uniform throughout the tumour or if its base is less well differentiated than the surface, indicating a worse prognosis. Sometimes certain areas of a tumour will show focal de-differentiation.

In addition to resecting or taking a biopsy of the original tumour, many urologists routinely take a biopsy of normal mucosa to detect unsuspected dysplasia or carcinoma-in-situ, which might affect management (Wallace *et al.*, 1979).

Tumours of the bladder are a continuing disease. Even after the original tumour has been treated successfully, recurrences are common and they too should be assessed histologically. Most are identical to the original tumour, but about 20 per cent are less well differentiated and more invasive.

A tumour has been found in the prostatic urethra – what is its clinical significance?

Tumours of the prostatic urethra have a sinister reputation. They may be superficial, relatively benign and respond to simple diathermy, they may grow down the lumen of the prostatic ducts and need deep resection or they may invade the protatic stroma and kill the patient within one or two years in spite of radiotherapy or cystectomy. Only careful histological examination will differentiate between these extremes of behaviour. Histological examination after frozen section may be needed to decide how deeply to resect a tumour growing down the ducts.

A solid tumour is present in the base of the bladder – is it vesical or prostatic in origin?

A solid tumour arising from the bladder will usually need to be treated by cystectomy or radiotherapy; radiotherapy may also be needed if it is arising from the prostate, but in this instance hormonal treatment, for example subcapsular orchidectomy, may also be beneficial. It is important, therefore, to differentiate between the two, if this is possible. The clinical history and cystoscopic appearances often suggest which it is, but careful histological assessment, for example by immunocytochemistry (see page 296), may be needed to make the final decision.

The patient has severe urinary symptoms and the vesical mucosa looks unstable – is this carcinoma-in-situ?

Carcinoma-in-situ means different things to different pathologists; the precise histological criteria by which it should be diagnosed will be described later (see page 299). In a group of 18 patients studied in Leeds, 15 died within two years of the initial diagnosis. Because of this, for the last ten years cystectomy has been performed on patients with carcinoma-in-situ and severe urinary symptoms, usually severe frequency and pain on micturition; examination of the cystectomy specimens showed that the majority had co-existing poorly differentiated, superficially invasive tumours of the bladder and that associated tumours of the ureter, prostate and urethra were also common. Carcinoma-in-situ, therefore, is a very serious condition and accurate histological assessment is essential.

Methods of obtaining material for examination

Urine for cytology

To be of value, the sample of urine must be freshly voided and examined as soon afterwards as possible by a cytologist, preferably one who is examining large numbers of urine samples each week. Cells die quickly after being exfoliated, so that a random specimen is preferable to an early morning specimen and tumours of the bladder can be diagnosed more easily than those of the upper urinary tract; poorly differentiated tumours and carcinoma-in-situ can be diagnosed more easily than well differentiated tumours because there is a greater difference between the cells exfoliated from them than those from normal urothelium.

Biopsy of the bladder

Cup biopsy forceps may be used to pinch off samples of normal-looking mucosa in a patient with a bladder tumour, or when taking random biopsies in a patient with positive urine cytology in whom no tumour can be found; however, use a resectoscope to biopsy the tumour itself or whenever there is doubt as to the diagnosis, in order to give the pathologist an adequately large piece to tissue.

Resect a small lesion in its entirety, digging the loop of the resectoscope into the tissues behind it, cutting underneath it and bringing the loop out again on its near side. Limit the depth of the cut to half the depth of the loop to avoid perforating the bladder. A circular or oval piece of tissue will be cut with the lesion near its centre. Remove it from the bladder with an Ellik evacuator.

Resection of bladder tumours

Much more will be learnt about a tumour of the bladder by resecting it transurethrally than by taking a cup biopsy from its surface. The pathologist will obtain the whole tumour and will be able to tell whether it is uniformly differentiated throughout and whether muscle or lymphatics are invaded. If the tumour has not spread beyond the submucosa, complete transurethral resection will cure that particular tumour, although recurrences may develop elsewhere in the bladder later.

If possible, therefore, resect the tumour until its base is flat, evacuate all the fragments from the bladder and send them as the "superficial specimen" to the pathologist. Resect the base of the tumour including samples of muscle and send these fragments separately as the "deep specimen". Remember to perform bimanual examination afterwards to find out whether any residual tumour is palpable.

If the tumour is large, solid and obviously invading widely, make no attempt to resect it completely, but instead take adequate samples from it with the resectoscope, if possible including the edge of the tumour and underlying muscle by cutting consecutive slices in the same furrow until muscle appears.

Perineal needle biopsy of the prostate

There are many different methods of obtaining material from the prostate for the pathologist to study. Cells may be aspirated from it through a Franzen needle introduced through the rectum (Williams *et al.*, 1967); cylinders may be cut from it with a biopsy needle introduced through the rectum or perineum; slices may be resected from it transurethrally. A needle biopsy is usually more accurate in diagnosing carcinoma of the prostate than a transurethral resection (Purser *et al.*, 1967); this is because a tumour often originates in the outer zone of the prostate and a needle guided by a finger in the rectum can be thrust accurately through the suspicious nodule. Perineal needle biopsy is preferable to rectal needle biopsy because the latter is associated with an unacceptably high incidence of infection (Fawcett *et al.*, 1975; Sharpe *et al.*, 1982). Transrectal Franzen needle aspiration probably has a lower infection rate, but most pathologists will prefer to receive a histological rather than a cytological specimen.

Many different biopsy needles have been designed. The Tru-cut needle (Travenol Laboratories) is disposable and can be relied on to obtain satisfactory specimens (Mellinger and Blackard, 1968). To take a perineal biopsy of the prostate with it, lubricate the left index finger if right-handed, introduce it into the rectum and locate the nodule to be biopsied. Make a tiny stab incision about 2.5 cm (1 inch) in front of the anus, push the tip of the biopsy needle through it and guide the biopsy needle with the left index finger up in front of the rectum to the prostate and to the nodule. Thrust the inner stilette of the Tru-cut needle through the nodule and then steady it with the right hand while the free fingers of the left advance the outer sheath over the stilette to cut a cylinder of tissue out of the prostate.

Withdraw the biopsy needle. The biopsy will lie in its notched stilette. Transfer it to fixative and cut further cylinders from the prostate until a sufficient number have been obtained. Then, and only then, remove the left index finger from the rectum and apply some plastic spray dressing to the perineal incision.

Fixation and handling of specimens

Fixation of the specimen

Buffered formol saline is the fixative of choice, but some laboratories may have special requirements and it is essential to check these. Specimens requiring electron microscopy are best fixed in 4 per cent glutaraldehyde, which is a toxic fixative and must be kept away from mucous surfaces, especially the eyes. If it is not possible to transfer the specimen to the laboratory within an hour, the samples—which should be finely minced to no larger than pin-head size—are best fixed in formol saline.

Partial and total cystectomy specimens require special treatment and are best sent to the laboratory fresh and unfixed. Failing this, a partial cystectomy may be pinned to cork and a total cystectomy inflated with formol saline through a urethral catheter; after this both should be suspended in a large volume of fixative, normally ten times that of the specimen.

Handling of specimens in the laboratory

Small biopsies should be described as to their gross appearance. Larger specimens should be spread out, examined, described and representative pieces taken for histological section. It cannot be too strongly emphasized that all specimens comprising more than a few tissue fragments must be weighed; this is very important as it is a useful guide to the surgeon of how much tissue has been removed.

Partial cystectomy specimens must be fixed pinned to cork. The lesion present should be fully described and the degree of involvement of the bladder wall and adventitial tissues carefully noted. Ideally the specimen should be photographed and a diagram made showing the lesion, the state of the surrounding mucosa and bladder wall and indicating where blocks of tissue have been taken for histological section.

Total cystectomy specimens should be opened by cutting with scissors up the urethra, around the right lateral margin and over the vault to the upper left lateral wall and fixed pinned to cork. Such specimens should be photographed and a diagram made showing the location, size and appearance of any tumour, or tumours, and any changes in the remainder of the bladder mucosa. The ureteric orifices and the lower ends of the ureters should be identified and sampled and the urethra carefully examined for the presence of tumour.

The proximal cut ends of the ureters, the prostate and the distal urethra must be sampled histologically for mucosal changes and a reasonable number of blocks taken from the apparently uninvolved bladder mucosa to detect carcinoma-in-situ, noting their position on the diagram. When the prostate is included this must be carefully examined as though it were an open prostatectomy specimen (see below); the prostate can be invaded by carcinoma of the bladder and this carries a very poor prognosis. A significant proportion of patients with bladder tumours also have small "intra-adenomatous" foci of prostatic carcinoma. The extent of invasion of all tumours must be carefully investigated by appropriate tissue blocks and the perivesical tissues thoroughly explored. Radical total cystectomy specimens have associated lymph node chains and these must be dissected out and the individual nodes identified, recorded on the diagram and taken from histological section. It is usually impossible to examine a total cystectomy specimen adequately with less than 15 tissue blocks, while "mapping" the overall mucosal changes may take many times that number.

Urethrectomy specimens should be opened on receipt using round-pointed scissors to avoid stripping the mucosa. The specimen is then fixed pinned out and is examined for the presence of tumour and is also sampled histologically along its entire length, including proximal and distal margins, for mucosal changes.

Transvesical or retropublic prostatectomy specimens are weighed and the number and size of the lobes recorded. The specimen is then examined by a series of 2 mm slices. The slices are laid out and examined individually; representative histological blocks are taken along with any hard, solid, yellow or unusual areas.

Tissue sectioning and staining

For large blocks, which are well orientated, a single carefully cut section stained by haematoxylin and eosin is usually all that is required. For small specimens, a series of three to six sections cut at multiple levels may show a lesion at one level which is missing from the others; the laboratory should keep unstained spare sections from the various levels.

Special stains are generally of little help in most lesions of the lower urinary tract. Only in the case of the rare connective tissue tumours may special stains, such as trichrome and reticulin methods and phosphotungstic acid-haematoxylin for cross striations, be of help in reaching a correct histological diagnosis. Other obvious exceptions are stains for tubercle bacilli, amyloid and mucin.

Immunocytochemistry

In appropriate cases this can be of great help and the methods may be successfully applied to paraffin-wax-embedded tissues. The epithelial membrane antigen will enable a precise separation of anaplastic carcinomas from sarcomas and the prostate-specific antigen will allow discrimination between undifferentiated carcinoma of the bladder and the prostate (see page 294). Monoclonal antibodies against intermediate filaments may help in precise histological diagnosis; for instance, desmin and vimentin are only found in tumours of muscle.

Other immunocytochemical techniques, such as those for blood group isoantigens, are currently only of research interest.

Electron microscopy

Generally, electron microscopy of lesions of the lower urinary tract is a research tool only. An obvious exception is in connective tissue tumours where the ultrastructural appearances may well be diagnostic; this is the case in embryonal rhabdomyosarcoma.

Semi-thin sections

Large semi-thin sections using resin-embedded tissues cut on such instruments as the "Ultracut" are generally of research interest only. Their value lies in the clarity with which such structures as the basement membrane and individual cells in inflammatory cell infiltrates may be seen and identified.

Flow cytometry

This promises to be of great value in demonstrating some of the changes which take place with cellular de-differentiation and in subsequent generations of bladder tumours. The transfer of cellular material from the operating theatre to the cytometer is best effected if the specimen is sent fresh and unfixed to the pathology laboratory.

Histopathology of the bladder

Inflammatory lesions

These may produce a diagnostic problem at cystoscopy; many inflammatory lesions are seen histologically to have a variable inflammatory cell infiltrate in the submucosa with vascularity associated with combinations of hyperplasia, cellular atypia and ulceration of the overlying epithelium. Such appearances may be described by the histopathologist as "non-specific cystitis" with the additional qualification "acute", "chronic" or even "acute-on-chronic". It is important for the pathologist to be aware that tuberculosis may frequently have an atypical appearance in the bladder without classical ulceration or tubercle formation. Multiple sections may assist in the diagnosis, but tubercle bacilli are often very scanty in such lesions. Nevertheless, one section in every series of multiple slides should be stained by the Ziehl–Neelsen method; the fluorescent stain for tubercle bacilli using the auramine-rhodamine B technique may be helpful in identifying scanty organisms. Positive histological diagnosis will, almost invariably, be an indication for treatment with anti-tuberculous drugs. Similarly, a biopsy from a "sandy patch" in the bladder may show typical ova, making a positive diagnosis of schistosomiasis and leading to appropriate and specific treatment. If all the ova appear calcified, systemic treatment may not be necessary.

The phenomenon of denuding cystitis appears to be a real entity (Elliott *et al.*, 1973). Here the surface epithelium, probably because of imperfect cellular formation, desquamates readily into the urine, or is easily abraded by endoscopic manoeuvres and tissue handling. Histologically the epithelium is completely shed, or is limited to one or two layers of small, dark-staining cells. The submucosa is oedematous and usually shows a remarkable lack of inflammatory cell infiltration, in contrast to true inflammatory ulceration. It is important to recognize the condition which may well be associated with epithelial dysplasia, and even carcinoma-in-situ and tumour formation.

Reactive lesions

This group of lesions, characterized histologically by the accumulation of massed inflammatory cells or of material, such as amyloid, in the submucosa, may mimic a flat tumour on cystoscopic examination.

Follicular cystititis is a common condition; histologically there are aggregates of lymphocytes and lymphoid follicles in the submucosa; the overlying epithelium is usually normal; the cause is unknown. Eosinophilic cystitis is diagnosed histologically by the finding of submucosal accumulations of eosinophils; it occurs in children as well as adults (Littleton *et al.*, 1982). Malakoplakia, which often follows a urinary tract infection, is a quite specific entity; densely packed transformed macrophages (Hansemann cells) are present beneath the epithelium which is elevated into flat, yellowish plaques; small, intracellular calcospherites, called Michaelis–Guttmann bodies may be seen within the macrophages (Stanton and Maxted, 1981).

Amyloidosis of the bladder is usually primary, the material being deposited beneath the mucosa, throughout the submucosa and in vessel walls. The lesion may produce the appearance of a flat vascular tumour and the deposits may be associated with severe epithelial dysplasia and hyperplasia, which can easily be mistaken histologically for shallow, invasive carcinoma. Vesical amyloid usually stains positively with methyl violet producing a pink colour, or with Congo red producing an orange/red colour; it also shows green optical activity under polarized light. Thioflavine-T causes yellow fluorescence under ultraviolet light and this test may be positive when others are negative.

Proliferative lesions and metaplasia

Epithelial proliferation (hyperplasia), which may take either a flat or papillary form, is seen with obstructive lesions of the bladder as well as with inflammation, infection, irritation and the presence in the urine of drugs and chemical derivatives. Histologically, the lesion appears as an area of thickened epithelium with an increase in cell layers, which may be regular (simple hyperplasia) or may show varying degrees of dysplasia so that the lesion comes to resemble that of carcinoma-in-situ (see page 299).

Similarly, epithelial downgrowths may occur (von Brunn's nests) which may become detached from the surface and undergo central cyst formation (cystitis cystica) or clefts may be formed lined by columnar cells which can undergo mucinous metaplasia (cystitis glandularis). While the cause of cystitis cystica and glandularis may be apparent, the lesions are often idiopathic and simply associated with the process of ageing. The conditions do, however, indicate a degree of mucosal instability and they are often seen in association with tumours.

Polypoid cystitis is a florid form of papillary hyperplasia which is seen in association with tumours or around an inflammatory focus in the bladder, particularly a vesico-intestinal fistula. The lesion consists of finger-like papillary projections clad in hyperplastic urothelium; these are broader at the base than at the tip. The conical outline usually serves to differentiate the lesion from a papillary carcinoma, but sometimes this differentiation is impossible.

"Nephrogenic" adenoma is regarded as an example of adenomatous hyperplasia of the bladder mucosa (Molland *et al.*, 1976). Occasionally the condition may be mimicked by a focus of flat adenocarcinoma and such lesions must be carefully examined histologically for areas of cellular de-differentiation, mitotic activity and microinvasion.

Squamous and glandular metaplasia occur in the bladder mucosa as a result of infection, irritation and chemical activity. Both conditions occur in extrophy of the bladder and squamous metaplasia frequently accompanies vesical bilharziasis. Squamous metaplasia may be of clear cell, "vaginal" type, seen chiefly in female patients with the urethral syndrome, or it may show maturation to form a keratin band on the surface (leukoplakia). The first form appears entirely benign but the second form often undergoes malignant transformation to squamous carcinoma and this may be suspected whenever there is a significant element of cellular dysplasia. Irregular squamous metaplasia is seen in infected diverticula and in severe cystitis, particularly when a foreign body is present. It also occurs in patients with urethral stricture and sinus formation.

Glandular metaplasia, which is very rare as a spontaneous occurrence, may be strikingly regular in histological appearance, but, nevertheless, it appears to carry a high risk of the development of adenocarcinoma. The degree of mitotic activity may act as a guide to the likely malignant potential.

It is important when metaplastic lesions are diagnosed histologically that an assessment of cellular differentiation and mitotic activity be made and evidence of microinvasion carefully looked for.

Tumours

For the full histological assessment of a bladder tumour four features must be examined: the cell type involved in the tumour, the growth pattern, the degree of histological differentiation (grade) and the extent of invasion and spread (pathological stage).

Cell type

The commonest type of bladder tumour is the transitional cell growth, which accounts for over 90 per cent of all tumours. Pure squamous and glandular tumours account for 1–2 per cent each of the total. Such tumours should exhibit a uniform cellular type, even if poorly differentiated, and should, ideally, show comparable metaplasia in the epithelium adjacent to the tumour. Focal squamous and occasionally glandular metaplasia is seen in many poorly differentiated tumours and, while this should be recorded, such growths should not be classified as pure, squamous or glandular carcinomas. Adenocarcinoma occurs in the vault of the bladder, where it may originate from the urachus and also in the base where it arises from areas of intestinal-like glandular metaplasia having the same mucin histochemical pattern as the large bowel. Such tumours can be differentiated by this means from urachal carcinomas.

The remainder of the total of bladder tumours is made up of connective tissue tumours, carcinosarcomas and secondary tumours. Connective tissue tumours may be classified using electron microscopy for ultrastructure and immunocytochemistry to detect cellular intermediate filaments. It is particularly important to perform these investigations in embryonal rhabdomyosarcomas of children where the lesion may at first be mistaken for an oedematous polyp.

"Undifferentiated sarcoma of the bladder" should be diagnosed with extreme caution as most of such pleomorphic, spindle cell tumours are in fact anaplastic carcinomas and the cells will react, even if poorly, with a common epithelial membrane antigen.

Growth pattern

In bladder tumours, four types of growth pattern may be recognized: papillary, papillary and solid, solid and *in situ* (Fig. 23.1).

The majority of tumours are of papillary pattern, the stroma cores being covered by epithelium of varying cellular thickness. Invasion into the stromal cores and the base may be present. Some tumours have both papillary processes and a substantial solid component where invasion of the underlying lamina propria and muscle has occurred and such tumours should be classed as papillary and solid. This subdivision is helpful to the surgeon as these tumours carry a poor prognosis. Solid tumours are entirely invasive and lack any papillary component although the lumenal surface may be heaped up and elevated.

The term "papilloma" should be applied with extreme caution and only to tumours having a delicate, papillary configuration, showing flawless differentiation and maturation, and having large surface cells at right angles to the lower layers. The fronds of the tumour must at no point be more than five cell layers thick and there must be no invasion in sections cut at levels.

Carcinoma-in-situ is a localized, or generalized, epithelial change characterized by extreme cellular de-differentiation, similar to that seen in anaplastic carcinoma with marked nuclear pleomorphism and frequent mitoses, but showing no invasion. The term is best restricted to this type of lesion while lesser degrees of disorder are described as moderate or severe dysplasia.

The "inverted" papilloma, is a highly distinctive lesion marked by the presence of thin ribbons of well differentiated transitional cells growing downwards into the lamina propria from the surface epithelium. The tumour is usually completely benign, but where cellular atypicism and marginal invasion are present the behaviour will be that of an equivalent carcinoma (Cameron and Lupton, 1976).

Grading

The grading of bladder tumours is a most important function of the histopathologist and the results, despite intellectual objections to the procedure, usually correlate well with survival, although the tumour grade is not an infallible guide to prognosis in individual cases. Well differentiated carcinomas are of low invasiveness; undifferentiated tumours on the other hand are usually highly invasive and, even after successful local treatment, are often followed by equally malignant recurrences. The bladder mucosa in such patients is generally unstable and dysplastic. It is in the middle grade where the difficulty lies; many such tumours will prove relatively indolent while

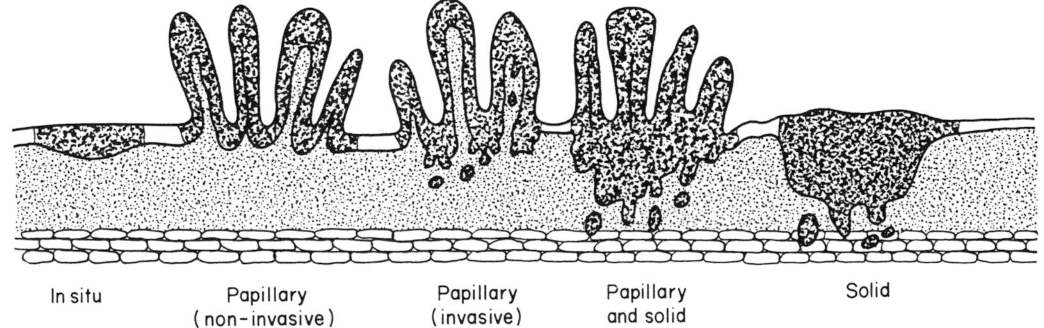

Fig. 23.1 Growth form of bladder tumours.

others will be aggressive and difficult to treat. It is in this subgroup that additional prognostic indicators are urgently needed and, in the future, they may be supplied by immunocytochemistry and flow cytometry.

In everyday practice it should be possible for the pathologist to grade tumours into Grade 1 (G1), which are low grade neoplasms demonstrating the minimal degree of cellular anaplasia consistent with a diagnosis of carcinoma and Grade 3 (G3), which are high grade tumours showing marked anaplasia. The remainder fall into Grade 2 (G2) and are assessed as medium grade. Because in many hospitals the histological examinations will be performed by only a small number of pathologists, or by a single pathologist, the accuracy of grading should be reasonably high. This accuracy can be improved by good communication between pathologist and surgeon.

Table 23.1 Histopathological staging of bladder tumours (TNM system).

Stage	*Urinary bladder*
pTis	Pre-invasive carcinoma (carcinoma-in-situ)
pTa	Papillary non-invasive carcinoma
pT0	No evidence of tumour found on histological examination of specimen
pT1	Tumour not extending beyond the lamina propria
pT2	Tumour with invasion of superficial muscle (not more than half-way through muscle coat)
pT3	Tumour with invasion of deep muscle (more than half-way through muscle coat) or with invasion of perivesical tissue
pT4	Tumour with invasion of prostate or other extravesical structures
pTX	The extent of invasion can not be assessed

Pathological staging

The assessment of the pathological stage is probably the most important single contribution the pathologist can make to the management of bladder tumours and with care and attention to detail it can be a very accurate investigation which correlates well with survival.

Transitional cell tumours of the bladder exhibit a well known propensity for invasion, so superficial invasion of the stromal cores of the fronds and of the base must be looked for carefully using sections cut at levels. When the base of the tumour has not been sent in a separate container it is important for the pathologist to try to identify it in the resected chips and with a little experience this can often be done.

The easiest way for the pathologist to record the extent of invasion is to use the TNM Classification of the International Union against Cancer (UICC, 1978) (Table 23.1).

The Institute of Urology, London, has a similar staging classification but subdivides stage pT1 into pT1a, invasion limited to the core of a papilla and pT1b, invasion of the true lamina propria of the bladder. Stage pT4a, invasion of the prostate, is further, and very sensibly, subdivided into pT4aa, invasion limited to the prostatic ducts and/or acini only and pT4ab, infiltration of the fibromuscular interstitial tissues of the prostate. These subdivisions are most useful.

Pathologists sometimes confuse densely cellular papillary tumours with compacted fronds for solid growth. Such tumours are often of low malignancy and while they may appear "solid" are certainly not infiltrating in that no true invasion is present. Again, the lamina propria, particularly in previously treated patients, may contain bars of collagen and these should not be confused with muscle.

In biopsies and transurethral resections it is obviously impossible to stage beyond pT2 (invasion of muscle). Where the tumour invades the lamina propria or muscle to the limits of the resection then this should be correctly recorded as pTX, but it will be helpful to the surgeon to add in brackets (pT1 minimum), or where muscle is involved, (pT2 minimum). It is important to look for superficial lymphatic invasion (L1) and in cystectomy specimens, deep lymphatic invasion (L2). The need to delineate fully the extent of extravesical spread and lymph node involvement has already been stressed. The stages of invasion by bladder tumours is set out in Fig. 23.2. Invasion of blood vessels, where seen, must be reported, although there is no section in the UICC rubric for recording this information.

Histopathology of the prostate and urethra

Prostatic hyperplasia

Prostatic hyperplasia commences in the region of the periurethral glands and involves both epithelium and stroma. Sometimes the material submitted for histology will comprise a large quantity of tissue chips or an enucleation of the en-

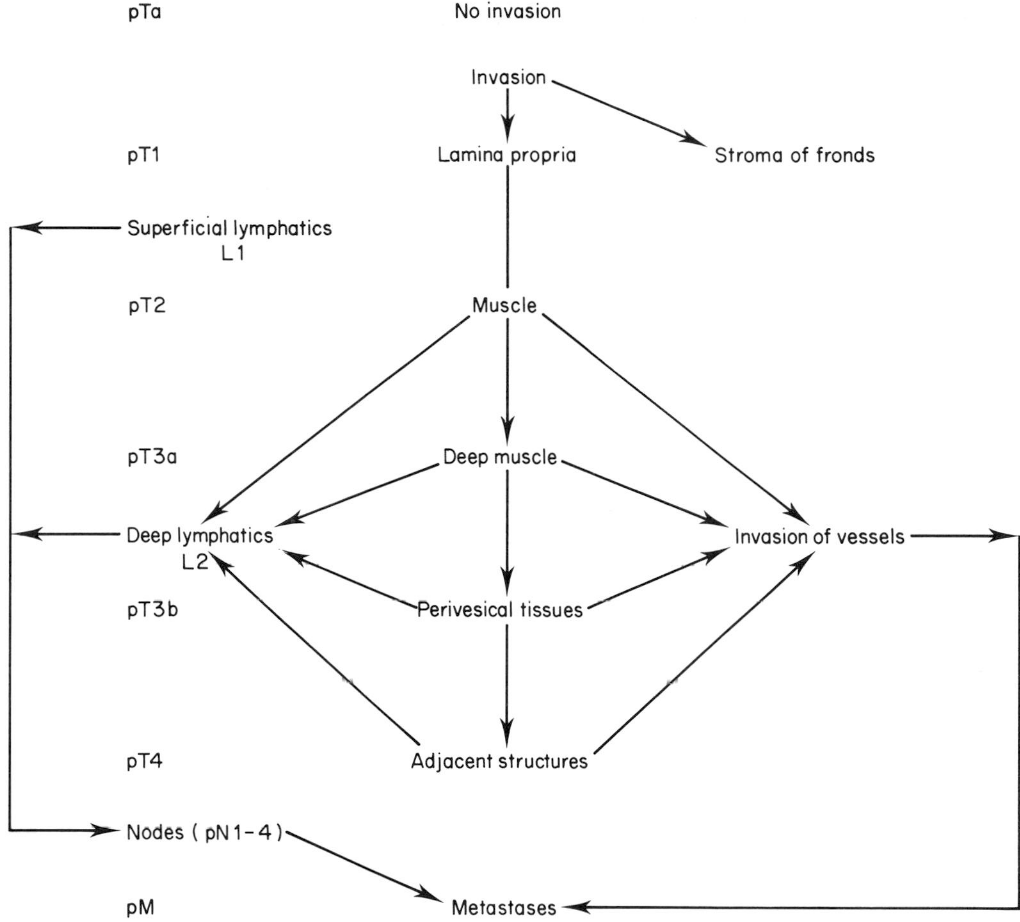

Fig. 23.2 Pathological staging of bladder tumours.

larged inner prostate as several large lobes with or without small accessory adenomas. Sometimes all that is needed to relieve bladder neck obstruction is a small resection of a few tissue chips, or even a simple incision and the pathologist should understand the differences in appearance of the various types of specimen. The importance of weighing the tissue and of taking adequate samples has been emphasized.

Histologically, the early stage of hyperplasia is marked by proliferation of the stroma, so that small bladder neck resections may consist exclusively of smooth muscle and no acini may be seen, even in multiple sections. In the established disease, hyperplastic acini lined by tall columnar cells are present. The acini frequently contain small papillary ingrowths of epithelium and stroma and, while acini are generally lined by a single layer of epithelium, cellular layering and heaping often occur and cribriform epithelial nests are formed. The stroma is prominent between the acini and contains a substantial amount of smooth muscle, the combined tissues forming the adenomatous nodules. Secretion occurs into the acini and is retained there while small concentric concretions, corpora amylacea, are formed which frequently calcify. Small calculi are sometimes present.

As the process continues cystic dilatation of acini occurs with focal loss of epithelium and infiltration by chronic inflammatory cells. Acinar atrophy occurs and the epithelium often has an hydropic appearance with small clusters of cells appearing to infiltrate the stoma; such appearances should not be mistaken for focal prostatic carcinoma. Larger foci of ischaemic necrosis are often seen and these destroyed acini are replaced by fibrovascular tissue to form the frequently seen fibrovascular nodule. Large nodules composed of fibrous tissue, fibromuscular tissue and pure smooth muscle are seen and may sometimes comprise virtually the whole of a large resection or enucleation (Franks, 1969).

Sudden, extensive areas of necrosis may occur in a hyperplastic prostate producing frank infarction. As organization occurs, the adjacent epithelium undergoes squamous metaplasia. This process may appear so florid and bizarre as to suggest squamous carcinoma, but the phenomenon is entirely benign. Pathologists should also learn to recognize the appearance of the ejaculatory ducts in resections and enucleations as this infolded, double-layered epithelium may be confused with carcinoma.

Prostatitis

The changes of hyperplasia are frequently accompanied by inflammatory cell infiltration which may impart the appearance of active inflammation. Such changes should be recorded in the report, but they may well not accord with a clinical history of prostatitis.

Eosinophilic prostatitis, however, is a real entity generally seen only in association with allergic states and where large areas of prostatic tissue are blanketed with a dense infiltrate of eosinophils. In granulomatous prostatitis, there is focal or generalized destruction of prostatic tissue and replacement by granulomas containing epithelioid cells, giant cells and mixed inflammatory cells.

Prostatic carcinoma

Clinical prostatic carcinoma often arises in a segment of the prostate (McNeal, 1969) which is why it may be evident on rectal examination when histological examination of resected juxtaurethral prostate shows no tumour. As the disease progresses the entire gland becomes involved.

Intra-adenomatous prostatic cancer also occurs and is usually small, focal and unsuspected clinically, being revealed only on histology. These incidental cancers are of little clinical importance as the patient with the condition seldom develops metastatic carcinoma. Nevertheless, the pathologist must record the presence of any such foci in prostatic material and try to determine whether the foci are small or large, discrete or infiltrating and their number few or many. In an open prostatectomy it is desirable to state where in the lobe the focus was found as peripheral nodules which are cut across are more sinister than central ones.

Clinically apparent prostatic carcinoma will present to the pathologist usually as a transurethral resection, which is often of modest size, or as a needle biopsy, or as both. The first duty is to confirm the diagnosis and it is important not to confuse atrophic acini merging with the stroma for invasive carcinoma, or regenerative squamous metaplasia for squamous carcinoma—a growth form which is practically unknown in the prostate. On occasions it is impossible to confirm the clinical diagnosis histologically and then it is important for the pathologist to look for features such as stromal nodules, calcified corpora amylacea, calculi and foci of granulomatous prostatitis which may impart a spurious impression of malignancy to the gland on clinical examination.

The grading of prostatic carcinoma is of dubious validity because well differentiated and anaplastic areas are frequently seen in the same tumour and the amount of material sampled is usually, and for good clinical reasons, small. Well differentiated tumours resemble normal prostatic epithelium except that the cells are large and frequently show nuclei containing large nucleoli. The normal acinar pattern is lost, at least in part, and back-to-back acini are seen; tumour cells frequently invade perineural spaces. In less well differentiated tumours there is increasing loss of acinar formation with the development of cribriform lobules (Ansell, 1982). The clear cell growth pattern, however, carries a good prognosis. Undifferentiated prostatic carcinoma resembles any other anaplastic carcinoma, but will usually stain positively, if only focally, with prostate-specific antigen. The pathological staging of prostatic carcinoma is not usually carried out in the United Kingdom as radical prostatectomy is seldom performed. The routine proposed by the International Union against Cancer (UICC, 1978) would appear to cover the requirements for staging adequately when this is called for.

While the majority of prostatic carcinomas arise from acini, very occasional tumours originate from ducts. Such tumours have usually an elaborately papillary pattern although this may be compressed in the smaller ducts. Ductal carcinoma does not appear to be attended by elevation of the serum acid phosphatase or to respond to oestrogen therapy so it is important to recognize the entity and its degree of invasiveness, as this has important clinical consequences. At present it is not known whether the tumour reacts with prostate-specific antigen. It is probable that the so-called "endometrioid" carcinoma is an example of a ductal tumour.

When prostatic carcinoma is treated by oestrogen therapy the cells first undergo hydropic degeneration and then condense with marked nuclear pyknosis. There is usually simple squamous metaplasia of the prostatic ducts and the urethra and it is important to recognize these changes in histological sections.

Other tumours of the prostate

Transitional cell tumours of the prostatic urethra are rare but important. Apart from direct invasion of the prostate by a tumour arising in the bladder, transitional cell carcinomas of the prostate may arise in three ways:

First, a transitional cell carcinoma may implant from the bladder onto the prostatic urethra. This is most likely to occur when the prostate has been resected in the presence of a bladder tumour, but may arise after any trauma to the urethra. Such tumours will have a similar structure and invasion potential to the tumour in the bladder.

Secondly, a transitional cell carcinoma may arise spontaneously from the transitional cell lining of the urethra, which may first have passed through a stage of carcinoma-in-situ. The same carcinogens initiating and promoting tumours in the bladder will act on the identical urethral epithelium to produce neoplasia.

Thirdly, the tumour may arise from the transitional cell lining of the terminal prostatic ducts; this being the urothelial analogue of the ductal adenocarcinomas already referred to. This tumour may be mistaken for a carcinoma of the prostate, particularly in the absence of any tumour in the bladder, but it will not respond to oestrogen therapy. Such transitional cell carcinomas tend to be restrained by the basement membrane of the ducts in which they form, or by the upper lamina propria of the urethra, and can be managed for long periods by endoscopic resection. Consequently it is necessary to detect invasion in biopsy material and any evidence of extensive infiltration and lymphatic permeation so that appropriate radical therapy can be undertaken.

Connective tissue tumours of the prostate are rare. Rhabdomyosarcomas are rapidly growing, leiomyosarcomas and fibrosarcomas less so. Infiltration by malignant lymphoma may also take place. Most "sarcomatoid" prostatic neoplasms are in reality undifferentiated carcinomas and should react with epithelial membrane antigen and prostate-specific antigen, if of prostatic origin. True sarcomas may be precisely identified by electron microscopy and immunocytochemistry as with sarcomas arising in the bladder.

So-called tumours of the seminal vesicles usually turn out to be examples of epithelial atypia due to involutional changes in the vesicular epithelium. When a true tumour involves the vesicles it is most likely to be of prostatic origin.

Urethral tumours

Simple fibrous and inflammatory polyps and adenomatous polyps may be encountered. It is important for the surgeon to attempt careful, complete excision biopsy so that the pathologist may see the entire lesion and its base. Transitional cell tumours may rarely be of primary occurrence or be associated with a history of bladder tumour. Such tumours have a structure identical to transitional cell tumours of the bladder and should be similarly assessed and reported as to growth pattern, grade and extent of invasion, if any. Squamous cell carcinomas may arise from areas of squamous metaplasia or from the terminal urethra. Squamous cell carcinomas appear to be more invasive than pure transitional cell growths.

Not infrequently when the urethra has been removed following previous cystectomy no tumour is seen in the main lumen but carcinoma-in-situ is present in the periurethral ducts and glands, a phenomenon also seen in frank urethral carcinoma. Very rarely adenocarcinoma may arise in the acini of periurethral glands or from Cowper's gland (Lieber *et al.*, 1983).

Summary

In the lower urinary tract there are many pitfalls to trap the unwary urologist as he looks through his cystoscope, or the inexperienced pathologist as he peers down his microscope. Most of these pitfalls can be avoided by close collaboration and communication between urologist and pathologist. Of the two, the pathologist is the more likely to make the correct diagnosis, and to give him the best chance the urologist should tell him all the relevant clinical facts, obtain an adequate specimen for him and make sure it is fixed properly.

References

Cameron KM, Lupton CH. Inverted papilloma of the lower urinary tract. *Br J Urol* 1976; **48**: 567–78.

Elliott GB, Moloney PJ. "Denuding cystitis" and in situ urothelial carcinoma. *Arch Pathol* 1973; **96**: 91–4.

Fawcett DP, Eykyn S, Bultitude MI. Urinary tract infection following trans-rectal biopsy of the prostate. *Br J Urol* 1975; **47**: 679–81.

Franks LM. The pathology of prostatic tumours. *Br J Hosp Med* 1969; **2**: 575–82.

Lieber MM, Malek RS, Farrow GM, McMurtry J. Villous adenocarcinoma of the male urethra. *J Urol* 1983; **130**: 1191–3.

Littleton RH, Farah RN, Cerny JC. Eosinophilic cystitis: an uncommon form of cystitis. *J Urol* 1982; **127**: 132–3.

McNeal JE. Origin and development of carcinoma of the prostate. *Cancer* 1969: **23:** 24–34.

Mellinger GT, Blackard CE. A new instrument for needle biopsy of the prostate. *J Urol* 1968; **99**: 228–9.

Molland EA, Trott PA, Paris AMI, Blandy JP. Nephrogenic adenoma: a form of adenomatous metaplasia of the bladder. A clinical and electron microscopical study. *Br J Urol* 1976; **48**: 453–62.

Purser BN, Robinson BC, Mostofi FK. Comparison of needle biopsy and transurethral resection biopsy in the diagnosis of carcinoma of the prostate. *J Urol* 1967; **98**: 224–8.

Sharpe JR, Sadlowski RW, Finney RP., Branch WT, Hanna JE. Urinary tract infection after transrectal needle biopsy of the prostate. *J Urol* 1982; **127**: 255–6.

Stanton MJ, Maxted W. Malakoplakia: a study of the literature and current concepts of pathogenesis, diagnosis and treatment. *J Urol* 1981; **125**: 139–46.

UICC. TNM Classification of Malignant Tumours, 3rd edn. (Harmer M. H. ed.). Geneva: International Union Against Cancer, 1978.

Wallace DMA, Hindmarsh JR, Webb JN, Busuttil A, Hargreave TB, Newsam JE, Chisholm GD. The role of multiple mucosal biopsies in the management of patients with bladder cancer. *Br J Urol* 1979; **51**: 535–40.

Williams JP, Still BM, Pugh RCB. The diagnosis of prostatic cancer: cytological and biochemical studies using the Franzen biopsy needle. *Br J Urol* 1967; **39**: 549–54.

Further reading

Urothelium

Koss LG. Tumours of the Urinary Bladder. Fascicle 11 of the Second Series of Atlas of Tumour Pathology. Washington DC: Armed Forces Institute of Pathology, 1974.

Mostofi FK, Sobin LH, Torloni H. WHO International Histological Classification of Tumours No. 10 – Histological Typing of Urinary Bladder Tumours. Geneva: World Health Organisation, 1977.

Pugh RCB. Urothelium: Histopathology. In: *Scientific Foundations of Urology*, Chapter 84 (Chisholm GD, Williams DI, eds). London: William Heinemann, 1982.

Prostate

Ansell ID. Histopathology of Prostatic Cancer. In: *Scientific Foundations of Urology*, Chapter 89 (Chisholm GD, Williams DI, eds). London: William Heinemann, 1982.

Mostofi FK, Price ED. Tumours of the Male Genital System. Fascicle 8 of the Second Series of Atlas of Tumour Pathology. Washington DC: Armed Forces Institute of Pathology, 1973.

Mostofi FK, Sesterhenn I, Sobin LH. WHO International Histological Classification of Tumours No. 22 – Histological Typing of Prostate Tumours. Geneva: World Health Organisation, 1980.

24

Testis

J P Williams and R C B Pugh

Introduction

This chapter is concerned with the investigation and management of three groups of patients—the boy or man with a scrotal swelling, the cryptorchid patient, and the male partner of an infertile couple. The differential diagnosis and treatment differ from group to group and it is therefore logical to consider them separately though many of the investigations that are essential for a correct diagnosis are common to more than one category of patient.

The patient presenting with a scrotal swelling

Clinical history

As will be discussed later, the age of the patient will often give some indication of a likely or possible diagnosis. The patient's ethnic group is also important as testicular tumour formation is more common in Caucasians, whereas parasitic infestation is more likely to be found in patients indigenous to, or recently resident in, certain tropical or subtropical regions. Filariasis in its acute form causes lymphangitis, epididymitis (often recurrent) and orchitis, and microfilariae and/or an eosinophilia may be found in the blood. Lymph varices and scrotal elephantiasis are late manifestations. In schistosomal infestation orchitis is rarely seen, but granulomatous nodules may occur in the cord or epididymis, sometimes with a hydrocele or scrotal sinus. The increased incidence of tuberculosis of all forms within recent years in the United Kingdom, especially amongst the immigrant population, must always be borne in mind.

Though it is generally accepted that trauma does not predispose to or cause tumour formation, it may nevertheless be responsible for a variety of benign swellings such as hydrocele, haematoma or, in severe injury, actual destruction of the testis. Testicular trauma without the usual accompanying sickening pain is, however, sometimes noted in patients with a tumour, so that all episodes of injury merit careful investigation and documentation. Evidence of extragenital disease, with or without constitutional upset, must be sought both in the history and in the full clinical examination that is mandatory in all patients. The commonest presentation of a patient with a primary tumour is a testicular swelling (usually, but by no means invariably, painless), whereas with a similar type of swelling and an accompanying lymphadenopathy there is more likely to be a leukaemic infiltration of the testis and/or cord. A history of preceding or concomitant urinary frequency, or overt urinary tract infection, points to epididymo-orchitis or granulomatous orchitis rather than to a neoplasm. A general constitutional upset may accompany orchitis or epididymitis due to a wide variety of bacterial, rickettsial or viral infections, such as brucellosis, Q-fever and mumps.

Clinical examination of the scrotum

At all ages, examination of scrotal contents can be difficult because of fear, pain and embarrassment on the part of the patient. Preliminary inspection is of critical importance, to note any inflammatory signs in the scrotal skin and to see the contour and position of the underlying swelling, as well as the lie of the testicle. Normally the testes hang vertically, but a lax mesorchium—which predisposes to torsion—causes the testis to lie transversely.

Palpation must be extremely gentle, noticing the relative position and consistency of the scrotal contents as well as the site of maximum tenderness.

A hydrocele can increase the difficulty of diagnosis and should be tapped before palpation (the fluid being sent to the laboratory for bacteriological and cytological analysis).

In inflammatory disease affecting the scrotal skin, inguinal nodes may be enlarged and tender. In cases of advanced testicular neoplasm, retroperitoneal abdominal nodes may be palpated. They are at the level of the first lumbar vertebra and therefore deep palpation is required high in the abdomen.

The first step in the diagnosis of scrotal swellings is to define the anatomy. Of paramount importance is the relation of any swelling to the testis itself. If anterior and transilluminable, it must be a hydrocele. If light is not transmitted, then the tunical sac probably contains blood. A large hydrocele may extend well up the cord and it may then be confused with a scrotal hernia. A swelling behind the body of the testis must be in the epididymis. A lesion above the body of the testis must be in the cord. Thickening or discrete tumour in the cord may be due to fatty deposition, infection or malignant infiltration. In all scrotal swellings, a hernia must be excluded.

Basic investigations

Although, as will be discussed later, immediate operation is indicated in a few patients, in the majority of cases there is less urgency and surgery should be deferred until certain investigations have been carried out or set in train. Microscopic examination of the urine in the clinic may indicate infection: a midstream specimen of urine should be sent to the laboratory as a routine. Any clinical suspicion of tuberculosis demands the collection of appropriate early-morning urine specimens. A blood count should always be requested and may provide confirmatory evidence of infection or may enable the diagnosis of blood disorder to be made. If there is any suspicion of tumour, it is absolutely essential that blood samples be taken for the estimation of beta human chorionic gonadotrophin (βHCG) and alpha fetaprotein (αFP) levels. In centres with a special interest in testicular tumour research, protocols will include the preservation of a separate deep frozen serum sample so that the value of new markers may be assessed in retrospective series. A serological test for syphilis is indicated if there is any evidence of urethritis or epididymo-orchitis or if there is firm testicular enlargement in an adult. A chest radiograph is necessary if there is suspicion of tuberculosis or malignant disease.

Differential diagnosis

At all ages a number of conditions other than tumour enter the differential diagnosis. From the clinical viewpoint, it is helpful to discuss the various conditions which may arise as age advances.

Infants and young children

The commonest scrotal swelling in the infant is usually diagnosed as a hydrocele, but exploration almost invariably reveals it to be a congenital (indirect) inguinal hernia. Several types of testicular *tumour* occur in young patients. Except when there is leukaemic infiltration (when there is often evidence of disease elsewhere or of constitutional upset), the only physical sign of yolk sac tumour, Sertoli cell/mesenchyme tumour and differentiated teratoma, is painless, moderate, usually smooth, enlargement of the body of the testis. The distinction between these different entities cannot usually be made until after orchidectomy. Mature teratomas have an excellent prognosis in childhood, whereas only two-thirds of the yolk sac tumour cases are cured by orchidectomy alone (Pugh, 1976).

Paratesticular embryonic sarcomas ("rhabdomyosarcomas") are relatively common, rapidly growing and potentially highly malignant tumours with their maximum incidence in childhood. These tumours have a soft, rather gelatinous, creamy-white appearance. In most cases it is impossible to determine their precise point or tissue of origin, but the maximal involvement is of cord and/or epididymal structures.

Pre-puberty and puberty

In the pre-pubertal and pubertal age group by far the most important and urgent condition to be dealt with is *torsion* of the testis, and time is of the essence if testicular function is to be preserved. Torsion is a relatively common condition which, sadly, is too often missed, the alternative diagnosis of epididymitis being made.

It cannot be overemphasized that *a painful swollen testis in a boy or young man is torsion until exploration has proved otherwise. Epididymitis in this age group is extremely rare.* If this condition is in fact present, a useful confirmatory sign is that supporting the scrotum tends to relieve the pain, whereas this manoeuvre will not bring relief in a case of torsion. In cases of torsion, an attempt to rotate the organ in the wrong direction will increase the pain. It is said that rotating the testis the other way will relieve the condition, but in our experience it has not proved effective. It is probable that the normal testis is incapable of rotation upon the cord to an extent to impair its blood supply, but a testis which has a long mesorchium may do so. These organs tend to lie transversely in the scrotum—a useful confirmatory sign if noted on the other side. The patient complains of pain and is found to have a tense, swollen testicle—often extremely tender to palpation, and the overlying scrotal skin is red and glazed. Fever is often present leading the unwary to assume that the process is infective. Once these signs are present, operation should be undertaken with the utmost speed. All too often schoolboys or young men are seen in whom the diagnosis has been mistaken and who betray the inevitable sequel of an atrophic testis on one side with a transversely lying, but otherwise normal, testis on the other side.

Recurrent subacute torsion can occur.

Rarely, a hydatid of Morgani can undergo torsion and similarly present with severe scrotal pain. Gentle examination may reveal a point of exquisite tenderness in the upper pole of the testis which may suggest this rare condition. Strangulated inguinal hernia can also cause difficulty in diagnosis.

The commonest *tumour* in this age group is the teratoma, though the other types seen in infants—the yolk sac tumour, Sertoli cell/mesenchyme tumour and malignant lymphoma—also occur. An occasional seminoma has been recorded. The teratomas are an interesting group and, though many have an incompletely differentiated histological appearance, this is often a measure of tissue immaturity rather than of malignant potential as metastasis rarely, if ever, occurs before the age of puberty.

Young adult

In the young adult, malignant teratomas are the most common tumours, followed by seminomas and combined tumours: all produce moderate (smooth or nodular) enlargement, which sometimes spreads into the lower end of the cord or into the epididymis, occasionally mimicking a primary lesion there. Gynaecomastia may occur as a manifestation of interstitial cell tumour or of Sertoli cell/mesenchyme tumour—only a minority (10 per cent) of which are malignant—but is more usually a portent of metastatic disease of a trophoblastic type.

Early middle age

In early middle age seminoma is commoner than teratoma. Paratesticular tumours also occur, but the embryonic type seen in young children is extremely uncommon—all varieties of smooth muscle, fibrous tissue and fatty tumour are found; these have a tendency to local recurrence rather than metastasis, but the overall prognosis is not good.

Late middle and old age

Malignant lymphoma is seen at all ages and is the commonest tumour to be found in late middle age and in the elderly, in whom it has a poor prognosis.

Testicular involvement sometimes occurs months or years after an apparently localized lymphomatous lesion, usually in the nasopharynx, has been successfully treated. In other patients, lymphomatous deposits, often in the skin, are found contemporaneously and in most cases the testicular lesions precede widespread dissemination.

Granulomatous orchitis is another lesion of the late middle-aged or elderly patient which may be confused clinically with malignancy, as it produces moderate rather firm enlargement of the body of the testis; the epididymis may also be thickened. There is often a history of preceding or concomitant urinary tract infection. In the very rare case there is suppuration and sinus formation.

Metastatic tumour deposits in the testis and lower cord may be mistaken for primary tumour. The list of tumours which have produced testicular secondaries is a long one, but the prostate has pride of place. Although *varicoceles* may appear earlier, it is in the young adult that they most commonly present. Often they are symptomless and noted for the first time when a patient is examined for infertility (see below).

Varicocele consists of tortuous varicosity of the pampiniform venous plexus and is much commoner on the left side. When one examines the patient in the erect posture, a "bag of worms" is seen and felt in the lower end of the cord above the testis and there may be dilated veins beneath the scrotal skin from cremasteric vein involvement. A cough impulse is present. The swelling diminishes when the patient lies down.

Epididymitis may be acute, subacute and relapsing, or chronic. The first two groups may be associated with a cystoprostatitis, the commonest organisms being *Neisseria*, coliforms and *Klebsiella*. The patient complains of pain and swelling on the affected side and fever may be present. Examination reveals redness and oedema of the overlying scrotal skin and a reactionary hydrocele may be present. Careful palpation reveals a tender and enlarged epididymis. In early cases, the testis is uninvolved and will not be tender. If due to the gonoccocus, a urethral discharge will have been noted two or three weeks previously, but not invariably so. Cases of so-called non-specific urethritis are frequently complicated by epididymitis. The relevant laboratory tests have already been described.

Occasionally in men of this age one sees what is clinically an acute epididymitis. Careful questioning reveals that a day or two before, the patient has been lifting heavy weights with a full bladder and it is likely that the condition is due to the forcing of urine up the vas. The condition settles down without treatment.

Recurrent or relapsing epididymitis should always lead to a search for tuberculosis, but characteristically tuberculous epididymitis presents as a chronic condition with the patient becoming aware of a thickening behind the testis and examination reveals a hard craggy epididymis. In late cases a sinus is present. Examination frequently reveals induration of the prostatic lobe on the affected side, and similarly the ipsilateral vesicle may be palpable. Sometimes only the cord is affected. A hydrocele may be present.

Treatment

Some conditions, such as varicocele in its early stages, require no active treatment, although the patient is usually in need of firm reassurance that no serious disease exists.

Urethritis, acute epididymitis and any accompanying cystoprostatitis require appropriate antibiotic therapy. It should be remembered that it is sometimes impossible to distinguish between inflammation and neoplasm on clinical grounds alone and it is therefore imperative that all patients treated for suspected inflammatory conditions should be re-examined carefully one or two weeks after commencing drug treatment.

The testes of patients in whom a confident diagnosis of haematocele or hydrocele has been made, require a firm scrotal support after tapping the fluid. Such patients need to be reviewed because reaccumulation is common, demanding curative surgery.

Operative treatment is essential if there is any suspicion of a strangulated hernia or torsion, if tumour is suspected, or if a lesion thought to be inflammatory has not responded to a course of drug therapy (in which case there is now suspicion of other underlying disease). *Urgent exploration is essential in all cases of torsion*. A scrotal incision is made. On opening the tunica vaginalis the surface of the testis will be seen to have lost its natural sheen and in cases where the torsion has been present for more than a few hours, untwisting the organ will not bring about relief of the purple congestion and restoration of the normal colour. The testis must then be removed *and the occasion taken to fix the remaining testis*. If intrascrotal neoplasm is suspected, the skin incision must be made in the groin with extension into the scrotum *only* if the mass is so large that it cannot otherwise be delivered into the wound. On no account should exploration be carried out through a scrotal incision, as there is a significant risk of tumour recurrence in the wound if this is done. The groin incision is made in a skin crease over the deep inguinal ring and the cord exposed after dividing the external oblique aponeurosis in the line of its fibres down to the external ring. Finger dissection permits the cord to be mobilized as it leaves the deep inguinal ring and a soft intestinal clamp is then applied across it at this point. Only then is the testis handled. Finger dissection alongside the cord at the neck of the scrotum will permit the testicle to be dislocated up into the wound. Handling of the testis itself should be kept to a minimum, though the clamp should prevent embolization of tumour cells. A hydrocele, characteristically small and only very rarely large, sometimes occurs with malignant disease, though tumour cells are seldom found in the fluid. Incising the external tunica allows inspection of the testis, epididymis and cord. Adhesions between the two layers of the tunica suggests inflammatory disease. Large ribbon-like vessels deep to the tunica albuginea, running at right angles to the long axis of the testis, may be found overlying a tumour and contrast with the fine ramifying vessels on the surface of the inflamed testis. Smooth generalized enlargement of the body of the testis is seen in both orchitis and neoplasm, especially malignant lymphoma and seminoma. In seminoma, too, there may be a discrete mass in one or other pole which deforms the testicular outline. The teratomatous testis may be smooth or nodular and is often smaller than the seminomatous. Gross enlargement favours tumour rather than orchitis.

Enlargement of the epididymis alone indicates non-specific inflammation or tuberculosis, or occasionally filarial infestation, but sometimes extension of an intratesticular tumour into the epididymis may be mistaken for primary disease there. Uniform thickening of the cord suggests lymphomatous infiltration and contrasts with the nodularity sometimes encountered with tuberculosis.

If there is any doubt as to the underlying pathology, orchidectomy should be performed, the cord being divided as high as possible at the deep inguinal ring and its proximal stump secured by transfixation ligature. There is no place for pre-orchidectomy biopsy when tumour is suspected and the patient has two scrotal testes, though a case could be made if the patient is cryptorchid. Biopsy carries the relatively small risk of disseminating intrascrotal malignancy, but its main drawback is that the information likely to be obtained may very well be misleading due, in the main, to the heterogeneous structure of many tumours, particularly the teratomas. The finding, for example, of differentiated somatic elements gives no indication of the potential behaviour of a tumour.

In centres with a research interest in testicular tumours, cord blood may be taken for estimation of βHCG and αFP before the testis is removed, as these substances are present in higher concentration in testicular than peripheral veins. Thus, an indication of which markers the tumour produces may be obtained in those instances where the quantity produced is too small to elevate the peripheral blood level. When there is obvious inflammatory disease, swabs should be taken from any exudate within the tunica, and after suitable surface searing from the testis and epididymis, sent to the bacteriology laboratory.

Examination of specimen, fixation, etc.

Once the special procedures that are recommended for the immediate handling of tissues in which there is obvious tumour or infection have been completed, the entire specimen should be placed in an adequate volume (ten times the specimen volume) of 10 per cent formol saline and left for several hours (for example, overnight). External examination will then give much useful information as to the likely diagnosis. Slicing the entire specimen in its long axis is usually all that is required to demonstrate non-neoplastic conditions, but should tumour be present or suspected, multiple slicings in several planes in the long axis should be the routine. In tumour cases, representative blocks for sectioning must be taken from the tumour itself, from the non-neoplastic parts of the testis, from the rete testis, epididymis, lower end of the cord and from the upper cord at the level of surgical section. This enables the pathologist to determine the pathological stage of the tumour which will be of assistance to the clinician in assessing the overall potential of the tumour. If tumour has been found, it is imperative that the entire surgical specimen be kept in the laboratory until such time as the clinicians are satisfied that the patient's post-orchidectomy course is as expected and is in keeping with the histological report and with any changes that occur in the postoperative serum marker levels. Any discordance demands re-examination of the specimen, and further sectioning may reveal additional features which would require amendment of the original histological diagnosis. Ideally, of course, there should be no need for such a "second look", but the extreme variation in the histological appearances in many teratomas makes accurate sampling extremely difficult: the only sure way to avoid the need for re-examination is to take a large number of tissue sections the first time round.

Histopathology

Testicular tumours

The tumours to be found in the testis and cord are listed in Table 24.1.

Table 24.1 Histological classification of tumours.

Tumours of the testis	*Paratesticular tumours*
Germ cell origin	Soft tissue tumours (embryonic sarcoma)
Seminoma	Adenomatoid
Teratoma	Metastases
Combined tumours	
Others	Mesothelioma
Malignant lymphoma	Cystadenoma of epididymis
Interstitial (Leydig cell) tumour	
Sertoli cell/mesenchyme tumour	
Miscellaneous (e.g. carcinoid, carcinoma of rete)	
Metastases	

Eighty-five per cent of adult testicular tumours are of germ cell origin and their histopathological classification is therefore important. The aim of classification may be to group together tumours expected to behave in a similar manner, and such a system will be prognostically valuable. Alternatively, neoplasms may be grouped according to morphological identity alone, thus enabling the development of a descriptive nomenclature which facilitates communication and epidemiological studies. The two classifications widely used in diagnostic pathology are examples of these differing approaches.

The classification applied in the United Kingdom is that associated with the British Testicular Tumour Panel and Registry. Neoplasms of germ cell origin are divided into seminoma, teratoma and combined tumours, the latter being a composite of both the former groups.

Seminomas are sub-divided into classical and spermatocytic types. The classical seminoma is radio-sensitive and therefore has a good prognosis. The spermatocytic seminoma constitutes only three per cent of seminomas, occurs in older men and has never been proven to cause metastatic disease.

Teratomas comprise—teratoma differentiated (TD), malignant teratoma intermediate (MTI), malignant teratoma undifferentiated (MTU), and malignant teratoma trophoblastic (MTT). Teratoma differentiated is composed entirely of mature or immature somatic elements. This tumour has an excellent prognosis in children, but in adults has been associated with metastatic disease and prognosis should therefore be more guarded. Malignant teratoma intermediate is the name applied to tumours containing a mixture of somatic elements and malignant tissue, regardless of the quantity of each component. Malignant teratoma undifferentiated is composed entirely of malignant tissues showing a variety of appearances ranging from a glandular pattern to solid sheets of anaplastic cells. Malignant teratoma trophoblastic contains cyto- and syncytio-trophoblasts forming villi with or without somatic elements or undifferentiated malignant tissue.

The classification used in America and largely adopted by the WHO is that of Mostofi and Price. It is important to be aware of this system when interpreting the American literature. Their classification includes an anaplastic seminoma, which is said to follow a more malignant course than the classical and spermatocytic varieties. For non-seminomatous germ cell tumours (NSGCT) they adopt a descriptive approach and all tissues present are listed. The term teratoma is only applied to tumours consisting entirely of somatic elements, and embryonal carcinoma is equivalent to the MTU of the British classification or the undifferentiated malignant areas of MTI neoplasms. Choriocarcinoma in contrast to MTT implies a tumour solely composed of syncytio- and cytotrophoblastic elements with or without villous formation.

At the time the British classification was introduced, when treatment of testicular tumours consisted of orchidectomy with or without radiotherapy, the groups TD, MTI, MTU, and MTT represented an ascending order of malignancy. The advent of chemotherapy has eroded these differences and prognosis now implies response to chemotherapy rather than the natural history of the disease. In therapeutic decisions clinical stage, as discussed below, is of major significance and the sub-types of teratoma are usually "lumped" together as NSGCT. Despite this, the maximum pathological information should still be made available to the surgeon and oncologist in a field where chemotherapeutic regimes are changing and the response and relapse rates of the different elements in these heterogeneous tumours have been shown to vary.

In recent years, following comparison between germ cell tumours in the ovary and testis and the advent of tissue and serum markers, yolk-sac tumour has been more widely reported in the adult testis. Formerly, it was only commonly recognized in children under a variety of synonyms including orchioblastoma and adenocarcinoma of the infant testis. This tumour is found within the MTI, MTU and embryonal carcinoma of the above classifications. However, as histopathologists are not in agreement regarding its morphological definition and biochemical markers are not specific (as discussed below), the prognostic significance of this element is unknown.

Tumour staging

In the United Kingdom, centres specializing in the treatment of testicular tumours use the Royal Marsden Hospital classification (*see* Table 24.2). This is mainly relevant to the teratomas, since seminomas rarely present with metastatic disease.

Over recent years, the relevance of tumour bulk to management of the disease has increasingly

Table 24.2 Royal Marsden Hospital staging classification.

Stage	*Tissue involved*
I	No evidence of disease outside the testis
II	Infradiaphragmatic node involvement This is subdivided according to the maximum diameter of metastases into the following substage categories: IIA – maximum diameter of metastases <2 cm IIB – maximum diameter of metastases 2–5 cm IIC – maximum diameter of metastases >5 cm
III	Supra- and infradiaphragmatic lymph node involvement This is subdivided as follows: Abdominal nodes: A, B, C as for Stage II Mediastinal nodes noted M+ Neck nodes noted N+ O = negative lymphogram
IV	Extension of tumour to extralymphatic sites The following suffixes define the extent and volume of metastatic spread: O, A, B, C, for abdominal nodes as for Stages II and III Mediastinal nodes noted M+ Neck nodes noted N+
	Lung substage L_1 metastases ≤ 3 in number L_2 metastases > 3 in number < 2 cm maximum diameter L_3 metastases > 3 in number > 2 cm maximum diameter H+ – hepatic involvement Other sites, e.g. bone and brain, are specified

been recognized, and this is taken into account in their system:

A P1 tumour is confined to the testis, the epidymis and cord being free of disease.
A P2 tumour has the lower cord involved, the upper being disease-free.
A P3 tumour has disease extending into the upper cord.

In the Tumour Panel series six per cent of the P1 cases had metastases at the time of surgery; these figures rose to 27 per cent of the P2 and 42 per cent of the P3 cases.

Work by Ray *et al.* (1979) has shown that tumour cells spread by lymphatic permeation and embolization through the rete testis and into the lymphatic centre cord which continue up along these lymphatic vessels and splay out to enter the

Table 24.3 UICC TNM classification for testicular tumours.

Stage	*Tissue involved*
T_1	Tumour confined to the body of the testis
T_2	Tumour extending beyond the tunica
T_3	Tumour involving rete testis or epididymis
T_4	Tumour invading spermatic cord and/or scrotal wall T_4a – tumour invading spermatic cord T_4b – tumour invading scrotal wall
N_0	No evidence of regional lymph nodes
N_1	Involvement of a single homolateral regional lymph node which, if inguinal, is mobile
N_2	Involvement of contralateral or bilateral or multiple regional nodes which, if inguinal, are mobile
N_3	Palpable abdominal mass is present or there are fixed inguinal nodes
N_4	Involvement of juxtaregional lymph nodes
M_0	No evidence of distant metastases
M_1	Distant metastases present M_1a – evidence of occult metastases based on biochemical and/or other tests M_1b – single metastasis in a single organ site M_1c – multiple metastases in a single organ site M_1d – metastases in multiple organ sites

retroperitoneal nodes at the point where the ureters cross. The chief spread is to the para-aortic nodes on both sides. Spread from the left testis tends to remain ipsilateral or at the most spread to the aorto-caval groups, whereas in advance cases some 20 per cent of right-sided tumours are found to have metastasized to the contralateral para-aortic nodes.

Lymphography and CAT scanning give an indication of lymph node size and a further subdivision of Stage II tumours is therefore possible. A similar notion of tumour bulk is indicated in the LI-III classification for Stage IV tumours (see Table 24.2). Ultimately, lymphatic spread will reach the thoracic duct and in advance cases nodes may be felt in the left cervical region. Spread by the blood stream is most commonly to the lungs, but the liver too may be involved.

Tumour markers

The two serum markers most widely used in the management of patients with germ cell tumours are *human chorionic gonadotrophin* (HCG) and *alpha fetoprotein* (αFP). Human chorionic gonadotrophin is a glycoprotein secreted by the syncytiotrophoblast of the placenta and is normally found in the serum during pregnancy. It contains two polypeptide subunits designated alpha (α) and beta (β). The α subunit is common to HCG and other glycoprotein hormones—luteinizing hormone, follicle stimulating hormone and thyroid stimulating hormone, immunological and biological specificity being conferred by the β subunit. Therefore, to reduce the possibility of cross-reactions in the radio-immunoassay of HCG, the antibody against the β subunit is used. Alpha fetoprotein is an α globulin and is the major protein found in the fetus, being synthesized by the yolk-sac, liver and gastrointestinal tract. It reaches a peak during intrauterine life, but has declined to adult levels by the time the infant is one year old.

Cells of origin

Human chorionic gonadotrophin The cells in germ cell tumours responsible for the production of HCG resemble, in their morphology, the giant cell forming the syncytiotrophoblast of normal chorionic villi. Predictably, all MTT tumours contain malignant syncytiotrophoblast in which HCG can be demonstrated immunocytochemically, but in addition solitary HCG positive giant cells are found in at least 60 per cent of MTIs, 50 per cent of MTUs and seven per cent of seminomas.

Malignant teratoma trophoblastic diagnosed histologically is known to have a highly malignant natural course. The survival rates for patients with other types of teratomas are unrelated to the presence or absence of HCG positive giant cells. Opinions are divided on the significance of HCG-containing cells in seminoma. Thus, tissue localization of HCG has not extended the prognostic value of conventional histopathology, and is not essential to the diagnosis. The major contribution of immunocytochemistry has been to demonstrate the neoplastic origin of a substance which can be measured in either urine or serum and reflects the presence of tumour.

Alpha fetoprotein Definition of the cell of origin of αFP is not so clear-cut as that of HCG. Alpha fetoprotein does not appear to withstand formalin fixation as well as HCG, thus precluding large retrospective series on wax-embedded tissue and necessitating the use of special acid fixatives or frozen material. Bearing in mind these reservations, αFP is said to occur in 75 per cent of NSGCTs in association with yolk-sac elements and immature tissue of gastrointestinal tract origin and is, therefore, found in MTI, MTU, MTT and embryonal carcinomas (*see* Table 24.1). Alpha fetoprotein has only been demonstrated convincingly in one seminoma. The prognostic significance of tissue localization of αFP has not been assessed, but the value of these investigations has been to demonstrate its derivation from tumour tissue.

Serum alpha fetoprotein and human chorionic gonadotrophin At least 75 per cent of patients in whom malignant teratoma is present have elevated serum levels of HCG, αFP or both. The fact that the levels of these two markers may be discordant is explained by their different cells of origin which are not necessarily both present in any one tumour. As indicated by the tissue localization studies discussed above, marker-producing tumours are not inherently more or less malignant than those that do not synthesize αFP or HCG. The finding that higher marker levels are associated with a poor prognosis probably reflects tumour volume and stage. It is essential to take blood preoperatively for the estimation of αFP and HCG in order to establish a baseline level so that, following orchidectomy, the rate of fall can be assessed and compared with the known half-life of the markers. Failure of the serum levels to fall after orchidectomy or to decline at a rate less than that predicted for the biological half-life (HCG—24 hours, αFP—five days) indicates metastatic tumour and, therefore, provides an adjunct to staging. During chemotherapy or radiotherapy, markers are used to monitor tumour response and, following the cessation of treatment, relapse may be indicated by elevation of markers before metastases are detected clinically, thereby, providing a valuable "lead time".

False positive elevation of αFP and HCG in patients with testicular germ cell neoplasms is virtually unknown, although it must be remembered that a variety of other tumours and inflammatory conditions may cause a rise in serum levels of these markers. Unfortunately, false negatives do occur when marker positive tumours are not associated with elevated serum levels on relapse.

The value of serum markers in the management of patients with germ cell neoplasia relates almost exclusively to teratomas. Few seminomas are HCG-producing and αFP-secretion by seminoma is anecdotal. Various other markers have been investigated but none are in established clinical use.

Summary

As soon as the diagnosis of malignant disease has

been confirmed by histological examination, arrangements must be made to refer the patient, together with all relevant clinical, radiological, and laboratory information, to a centre specializing in the management and follow-up of testicular tumour patients. There, lymphography and perhaps CAT scanning will allow of accurate staging, after which a decision can be made regarding the need for radiotherapy, chemotherapy or further surgery, either singly or in combination.

Cryptorchidism

The patient with one absent testis

Clinically these patients fall into several groups: the young child brought by parents worried about the possible risks of delayed puberty or the eventual failure of normal sexual development; the adolescent worried about "being different" from his school contemporaries; and the adult who, additionally, may have learnt of and become concerned about the possible risks of malignancy.

The first two groups are discussed in Chapter 29.

In the (otherwise normal) adult with one undescended testis, the main objective of clinical management is not so much the preservation of testicular function as the removal or reduction of the risk of tumour development. The increased liability of the undescended testis to become neoplastic is well recognized and the risk has been estimated to be of the order of 35 times that of the normally situated organ. Moreover, there is no good evidence that orchidopexy materially lessens this risk. It should also be recalled that tumour develops in the normally sited testis in about 20 per cent of cases of neoplasm arising in unilateral cryptorchids. The risk of tumour is higher in the intra-abdominal testis, though precise figures are difficult to obtain: the majority of tumours are seminomas but teratomas, which have a very much worse prognosis, also occur and occasionally rupture into the peritoneum, precipitating an acute abdominal emergency. Surgical opinion is divided upon the need to operate when the testis is in the groin and accessible to palpation. Some surgeons are content to leave it in situ and follow the patient, with regularly repeated marker studies. Others, probably the majority, favour exploration and orchidopexy or, preferably, orchidectomy. If no testicular tissue can be found in the groin, the question of laparotomy again arises and the indications for it are much more compelling than they are in the child.

Bilateral cryptorchidism in the adult

The management of these patients is governed by the same principles as outlined above. If secondary sex changes are present the patient must have testicular tissue somewhere.

Selective gonadal venography is a useful technique in the elucidation of this problem. Frequently testicular agenesis can be predicted, or at least strongly suggested, and operation thereby be avoided.

Selective gonadal arteriography may also be employed, as may CAT scanning.

These newer techniques even if they may not give the critical diagnosis as to whether neoplasm is present, will offer preoperative localization.

Male infertility

The investigation of the male partner must always be complementary to full investigation of the wife by a gynaecologist and should never be undertaken independently.

The clinical history should record the age, occupation, religion of the two partners, length of time they have been married and have been attempting to have a family. A previous history of mumps, tuberculosis, venereal disease, undescended testis and hernia operation may be relevant. Clinical evidence of endocrine or genetic disorder should be sought, but these are seldom found.

There is considerable variation of testicular size but a testis of good consistency is likely to have normal spermatogenesis. Sometimes a varicocele is present. The value of operating on these in order to restore fertility remains a matter of debate, but the usual practice (of JPW) is to operate if a varicocele of any size can be demonstrated. Any benefit may be psychological rather than physiological, but frequently an improved semen count results.

Basic investigations

These are complex and time-consuming. Three seminal analyses, each after three days' abstinence from sexual activity, are required. Specimens should be collected by masturbation in plastic containers and transferred speedily to a nearby laboratory, preferably one with a special interest in this problem. Collection by coitus interruptus is unsatisfactory since the sperm-rich fraction may be missed and condom specimens are unsatisfactory since a spermicide is frequently present.

The degree of liquefaction, pH, volume, sperm mobility and viability, morphology and number are all factors which may be of importance in diagnosis. The findings of numerous pus cells suggests infection in the prostate or vesicles. A post-coital test (PCT) of cervical mucus is the next step. If the results of the PCT and seminal analysis are within normal limits, it is necessary to exclude immunological causes by searching for agglutinating and immobilizing sperm antibodies. Somatic chromosome studies on buccal smears or leucocytes will exclude some anomalies, such as Klinefelter's syndrome.

Estimations of plasma testosterone and gonadotrophins (interstitial cell stimulating hormone (ICSH) and follicle stimulating hormone (FSH)) are essential in all patients, especially in those with small testes and complete azoospermia, where FSH levels of more than twice the normal indicate primary testicular failure.

Testicular biopsy

This has a place, admittedly a somewhat controversial one, in the series of investigations, but has the advantage of providing a precise assessment of the condition, and the potential, of the testis. We are of the firm opinion that biopsy of the testis has a place *only* in the study of the infertile male and that it should not be contemplated if there is any suspicion of neoplasia. The indications for biopsy are persistent azoospermia or severe oligospermia (which can be defined as less than ten million per ml) coupled with a high level of FSH, and when vasectomy reversal is undertaken. A small vertical scrotal incision is made. By gentle pressure between thumb and fingers the convex anterior surface of the testis is made to present. A small incision is made in the external tunica. After mopping away the fluid contained in the sac, the internal tunical is incised for 3 mm and continued pressure will cause a little testicular substance to protrude. This is snipped off with a pair of strabismus scissors and the material placed in a labelled jar containing fixative. The incision in the tunica is then closed with interrupted 3/0 catgut sutures and the external tunica closed in the same way. The scrotal incision is closed with two layers of fine catgut and a dressing applied. The patient is returned to the ward with a cotton wool pad surrounding the scrotum and held in place by a scrotal support.

Correct fixation of the specimen is vital: formol saline is **NOT** suitable and the fragment should be placed in Bouin's fluid. The Johnsen score technique is a very useful and convenient method of recording the results. The histologist should note whether the appearances are uniform throughout the specimen or if there is any evidence of interstitial scarring or tubular atrophy, such as might indicate focal damage secondary, for example, to an attack of mumps or a previous orchidopexy. Atypical germ cells should also be looked for: these occur in between ½ and 1 per cent of infertile men with atrophic testes and there is some evidence that there is subsequent primary testicular tumour development in a proportion of such patients.

Further reading

Buckman R. Tumour markers in clinical practice. In *Urology*, pp 9–20. Ed by JP Blandy. London: Blackwell, 1976.

Chisholm GD, Williams DI (eds). *Scientific Foundations of Urology*, 2nd edn. London: Heinemann, 1982 (General).

Hendry WF (ed). *Recent Advances in Urology—2*. Edinburgh: Churchill Livingstone, 1976 (Subfertility).

Hendry WF (ed). *Recent Advances in Urology/Andrology—3*. Edinburgh: Churchill Livingstone, 1981 (Subfertility).

Johnsen SG. Testicular biopsy score count. *Hormones* 1970; **I**:1–24.

Peckham MJ (ed). *The Management of Testicular Tumours*. London: Edward Anrold. 1981.

Pugh RCB (ed). *Pathology of the Testis*. Oxford: Blackwell, 1976.

Ray B, Hajdu SI, Whitmore WF. *Cancer* 1979; **33**:340.

Whitaker RH. Chapter title. In *Urology*, Chapter 44, pp 1153–1178. Ed by JP Blandy. London: Blackwell, 1976.

Whitaker RH. Torsion of the testis. *Br J Hosp Med* 1982; **Vol 27,** No. 1:66–9.

25

Benign Tumours and Non-Neoplastic Conditions of the Trachea, Bronchi, Lungs and Pleura

Section 1: Benign tumours R L Hurt and W F Whimster

Introduction

Benign tumours of the lower respiratory tract are much less common than malignant tumours. For example, at the Regional Thoracic Centre, North Middlesex Hospital, London, in the period 1951–1981, 130 benign tumours were resected compared with 3500 malignant tumours (see Hurt, 1984). As only about 30 per cent of malignant tumours are resectable, one benign tumour was seen for every 150 malignant ones. Nevertheless, it is important to be aware of the benign tumours and to recognize them when they do occur because, if they can be removed, the outlook for the patient is good. Although the clinical, radiological, and endoscopic appearances contribute to such recognition, histological examination, often initially of biopsies, but ultimately of the whole tumour, is needed to identify the tumour and to decide whether it has any potential for malignant behaviour.

Tumours are generally regarded as benign if there is no direct invasion of surrounding tissues and no metastatic spread. Unfortunately some tumour types cannot be absolutely categorized as benign or malignant. One of the commonest tumour types considered in this chapter, the carcinoid tumour, is usually benign, but some carcinoid tumours invade locally and/or metastasize. Examples of other tumour types discussed in this chapter also occasionally have malignant features.

When a tumour has been found in a patient, the clinician, pathologist, and the patient, all wish to give it a name. This allows the tumour to be accepted as something which has been experienced before, and gives some idea of how it is likely to behave and what can be done about it.

Since 'the cellular composition of all animal organisms' was established by Schwann in 1838 it has become customary to name each tumour according to the normal cell type(s) most resembled by the tumour cells. Such resemblances are, of course, closest in benign tumours. Whether or not the cells of the tumour have actually arisen, histogenetically, from the normal cells, and, if so, how and why, are questions that cannot be discussed here. Nevertheless, using this "histogenetic" approach to their classification, 26 types of benign tumour have been reported in the human trachea, bronchi, lungs and pleura as shown in Table 25.1. Their normal cell counterparts are to be found in the epithelia and connective tissues of the trachea, bronchi, bronchioles, alveoli, and bronchial glands. There are no reports of benign tumours of ciliated cells or of pneumocytes in humans, although benign tumours of type II pneumocytes have been reported to occur spontaneously in guinea-pigs and experimentally in mice, and malignant tumours of type II pneumocytes have been reported in humans.

Table 25.2, however, shows that the 130 benign tumours reported by Hurt (1984) included only 7 of the 26 benign tumour types, and also that, in practice, the thoracic surgeon has to deal principally with carcinoid tumours in the bronchi and hamartomas in the lung parenchyma.

The pathologist, on the other hand, must be aware of the histological differential diagnoses given in Table 25.1, although for some of these tumours there are very few convincing reports. Detailed descriptions of histological appearances are not included in this chapter; for these the reader is referred to *Diagnostic Tumour Bibliographies 1: Tumours of the trachea, bronchi, lungs, and pleura* (Whimster, 1983) in which these tumours are reviewed and references to the best pathological descriptions and illustrations are given.

Table 25.1 Benign tumours reported in the trachea, bronchi, lung and pleura (*see* Whimster, 1983).

	Trachea	*Bronchi*	*Lung*	*Pleura*
Adenoma, mixed differentiation		+		
Adenoma, mucous cell		+		
Adenoma, oncocytic		+		
Adenoma, pleomorphic	+	+		
Adenoma, serous cell	+	+	+	
Carcinoid tumour	+	+	+	
Chondroma	+	+	+	
Clear cell tumour			+	
Fibroma		+	+	+
Glomus tumour	+		+	
Hamartoma		+	+	
Haemangioma, capillary			+	
Haemangioma, sclerosing			+	
Haemangiopericytoma			+	
Histiocytoma		+	+	
Histiocytoma, fibrous	+	+	+	+
Intravascular bronchioalveolar tumour			+	
Leiomyoma	+	+	+	
Lipoma		+	+	
Lymphangioma			+	
Myoblastoma, granular cell	+	+		
Neurilemmoma			+	
Neurofibroma	+		+	
Papilloma	+	+		
Paraganglioma	+		+	
Teratoma			+	
(Total 26)	(11)	(15)	(20)	(2)

Table 25.2 Benign tumours of the lower respiratory tract seen at the North Middlesex Hospital 1951–1981 (*see* Hurt, 1984).

	Trachea	*Bronchi*	*Lungs*	*Pleura*	*Total*
Carcinoid		74*			74
Hamartoma		2	36		38
Chondroma	2		5		7
Fibroma				5	5
Lipoma		3			3
Leiomyoma		1	1		2
Papilloma		1			1
Totals	2	81	42	5	130

(* 3 initially reported as oat cell carcinoma on biopsy)

Finally, this section on benign tumours is divided into five parts: 1. benign tumours of the trachea and bronchi, all of which present and are treated in a similar manner; 2. benign tumours of the peripheral lung; 3. benign tumours of the pleura; 4. carcinoid tumours; and 5. hamartomas. The last two cover the commonest benign tumours of the lower respiratory tract and have certain features of interest to surgeons and pathologists.

Benign tumours of the trachea and bronchi

Introduction

Although the term "Bronchial adenoma" is still sometimes used to describe these tumours it should be abandoned, because it has come to include four different tumours. Indeed as long ago as 1937 Hamperl recognized that it encompassed both benign and malignant tumours. The latter, adenoid cystic carcinomas (formerly called cylindromas) and mucoepidermoid carcinomas, are not benign and are not considered in this chapter. The specific adenomas (*see* Table 25.1), which arise mainly in the large airways from the epithelial cells of the tracheobronchial glands, and carcinoid tumours should be specifically identified.

Benign tumours of the trachea are rare, but 11 benign tumour types have been reported in the trachea (Table 25.3). Only two benign tracheal tumours, both chondromas, were seen in the series of 130 benign tumours of the lower respiratory tract shown in Table 25.2.

Table 25.3 Benign tumours reported in the trachea (*see* Whimster, 1983).

Adenoma, pleomorphic
Adenoma, serous cell
Carcinoid tumour
Chondroma
Glomus tumour
Histiocytoma, fibrous
Leiomyoma
Myoblastoma, granular cell
Neurofibroma
Papilloma
Paraganglioma
(Total 11)

Benign tumours of the bronchi are also uncommon, but 17 tumour types (Table 25.4) have been reported. In most series, most of them are carcinoid tumours. Except for papillomas, benign tumours of the trachea and bronchi are usually solitary and are not associated with recognized aetiological factors, such as viruses.

Table 25.4 Benign tumours reported in the bronchi (*see* Whimster, 1983).

Adenoma, mixed differentiation
Adenoma, mucous cell
Adenoma, oncocytic
Adenoma, pleomorphic
Adenoma, serous cell
Carcinoid tumour
Chondroma
Fibroma
Hamartoma
Histiocytoma
Histiocytoma, fibrous
Leiomyoma
Lipoma
Myoblastoma, granular cell
Papilloma
Paraganglioma
Teratoma
(Total 17)

Benign tumours of the trachea and bronchi tend to grow slowly into the lumen from a broad base or a narrow pedicle, although carcinoid tumours may also grow into the bronchial adventitia or surrounding lung. They cause symptoms, signs and radiological changes by irritating the airway wall (cough), causing haemoptysis (especially carcinoid tumours), obstructing airflow (stridor, wheeze, exertional dyspnoea, obstructive emphysema), or by obstructing the upward passage of secretions (atelectasis, unresolved or recurrent consolidation, pleurisy, bronchiectasis).

Presentation

The patient, of whatever age, sex or race, complaining of a persistent cough, blood in the sputum, wheezing or otherwise noisy breathing, breathlessness (especially on exertion), pain in the chest (of pleuritic type), or recurrent chest infections, could have a benign tumour of the trachea or bronchi. On the list of diagnostic possibilities, however, this would come below infection, chronic bronchitis, emphysema, and malignant tumour. Bronchoscopy and biopsy are essential to establish the diagnosis. Cytology is unlikely to be of help.

Bronchoscopy

Most broncial tumours can be biopsied at bronchoscopy, especially now that the flexible fibreoptic bronchoscope allows more distal subsegmental bronchi to be examined. It may be difficult to obtain adequate tissue for diagnosis with the small fibreoptic bronchoscope biopsy forceps, especially if they are not sharp, and it may be necessary to repeat the bronchoscopic examination with a rigid bronchoscope to obtain a large enough biopsy for histological diagnosis.

It has been repeatedly stated in the literature, though with little statistical support, that biopsy of a suspected carcinoid tumour is associated with a risk of haemorrhage which may be difficult to control. This may be true of fibreoptic bronchoscopy, but is not true of rigid bronchoscopy through which any haemorrhage can always be readily controlled.

The interpretation of the biopsy will influence the extent of surgical resection.

The biopsy

Most of the benign tumours listed in Tables 25.3 and 25.4 are usually fairly easily recognizable on light microscopy, but because they are so uncommon the pathologist may doubt what he sees. Unfortunately the commonest tumour, the carcinoid, also presents the commonest problem in interpretation, namely its distinction from oat cell and undifferentiated carcinoma. In these circumstances, it can be very useful to have some tissue fragments fixed in cold glutaraldehyde solution and prepared for electron microscopy. As this is not done routinely in most hospitals, it may be necessary for the bronchoscopy and biopsy to be repeated if electron microscopy is subsequently required.

The tissue obtained with the biopsy forceps is gently floated or teased with a hypodermic needle (to avoid further crushing) into 10 per cent formal-saline as soon as it comes out of the bronchoscope. The specimen is then transferred to the histopathology laboratory and left to fix for a minimum of four hours and usually overnight. Then the macroscopic appearances, although seldom helpful, should be recorded, and the fragment(s) of tissue processed and embedded in wax in the usual way. If the epithelial surface can be identified, the biopsy should be embedded so that sections are cut at right angles to the surface because many benign tumours are covered by intact bronchial epithelium and it is useful to see this relationship. A series of sections should initially be cut for staining with haematoxylin and eosin, but the block should not be cut into too deeply because it may later be necessary to take further sections for special stains or to section right through the block if malignancy is suspected.

Management

The management of the tumour depends on the histological findings in the biopsy, in particular on whether there is any evidence of malignancy, on whether there is tumour outside the bronchus and within the lung substance, and on the degree of structural change that has occurred in the lung distally. If the tumour is entirely within the bronchial lumen and there are no distal changes, then removal by bronchotomy alone is indicated. But structural changes in the lung call for a segmental resection, lobectomy or pneumonectomy.

The specimen

A bronchotomy specimen is treated in the same way as a biopsy. Resected segments, lobes, or lungs, however, are best sent fresh to the histopathology laboratory to be inflated and fixed with 10 per cent formal-saline. This is easily done with a cannula (of appropriate size for the bronchi of the specimen—a Pasteur pipette can be used for the smallest specimens) and tube leading from a Winchester of formal-saline on a shelf about 45 cm (18 in) above the bench. The specimen should then be covered with a cloth and floated in a large container of formal-saline overnight. Dissection consists of removing all lymph nodes for histology and then carefully opening the bronchi longitudinally until the tumour and its attachment is fully revealed. Further dissection is then needed to see if the tumour extends into the surrounding tissues and to determine the extent of any pathology (particularly endogenous lipoid pneumonia or bronchiectasis) distal to the tumour. Appropriate blocks from which to confirm the nature of the tumour and its extent and any other pathology can then be taken for histology. A full macroscopic description with appropriate measurements must be made together with any photographs needed for record, teaching or research purposes. The histological recognition of benign tumours of the trachea and bronchi (Tables 25.3 and 25.4) after resection is seldom difficult. It is important to ensure that each tumour has been completely removed, so that recurrence is unlikely. This applies particularly with carcinoid tumours for which it is also important to be sure whether or not there are deposits in the lymph nodes.

Benign tumours of the lung

Introduction

Although Tables 25.1 and 25.5 show that 20 different types of benign tumour have been reported in the lungs, Table 25.2 shows that in practice few of these are seen at all often. Benign tumours in the lungs grow slowly and, unlike those in the large airways, seldom give rise to obstruction, haemorrhage or infection and thus rarely cause symptoms, although sensations of fullness or discomfort (but not usually pain) or movement in the chest may be reported by the patient.

Table 25.5 Benign tumours reported in the lung (*see* Whimster, 1983).

Adenoma, serous cell
Carcinoid tumour
Chondroma
Clear cell tumour (benign)
Fibroma
Glomus tumour
Hamartoma
Haemangioma, capillary
Haemangioma, sclerosing
Haemangiopericytoma
Histiocytoma
Histiocytoma, fibrous
Intravascular bronchioalveolar tumour (IVBAT)
Leiomyoma
Lipoma
Lymphangioma
Neurilemmoma
Neurofibroma
Paraganglioma
Teratoma
(Total 20)

Presentation

A benign tumour in the lung substance is usually seen first as a chance finding on a chest radiograph.

It usually appears as a well defined circular symptomless opacity, or "coin lesion", with or without calcification, whose anatomical site and pathological nature is then a challenge to the radiologist.

The radiologist usually tackles the anatomical problem by taking lateral radiographs, supplemented if necessary by tomography.

The differential diagnosis of a coin lesion includes malignant tumours (primary or secondary), benign tumours, particularly hamartomas, and miscellaneous benign lesions, such as plasma cell granulomas, rheumatoid nodules (especially if subpleural), infarcts, vascular abnormalities, foci of infection (e.g. tuberculosis), encysted effusions, and other pseudotumours. Sputum cytology is occasionally helpful in the diagnosis of peripheral lung lesions, particularly if they are malignant, but benign tumours are unlikely to be identified by this means.

Biopsy

The histological diagnosis of an intrapulmonary tumour may be obtained at bronchoscopy or by transpleural biopsy through the chest wall.

The transbronchial bronchoscopic biopsy technique was introduced by Anderson and his colleagues in 1965 and was further developed after the introduction of the flexible fibreoptic bronchoscope. The biopsy forceps are introduced into the appropriate subsegmental bronchus and then passed onwards under radiographic control into the lesion. A more recent development is the use of transbronchial needle aspiration, which is claimed to be more effective for peripheral lesions, especially in the upper lobe.

Transpleural biopsy of peripheral lesions is increasingly carried out under radiographic control by the radiologist himself using a wide-bore needle and syringe technique (for further details see Chapter 26 p. 334).

Tissue obtained by these methods is fixed in 10 per cent formal-saline and processed for histology in the usual way. The pathologist should be aware of the differential diagnostic possibilities listed above.

Management

If the diagnosis of a benign tumour is certain, it may be reasonable to leave it in situ, with follow-up examinations to ensure that it is not growing or changing in character. But if the biopsy diagnosis is not certain, and particularly if malignancy has not been confidently excluded, it is necessary to perform a thoracotomy to remove the lesion in order to identify it, provided that the patient is sufficiently fit.

Hamartomas (see p. 321) are the commonest benign tumours (Table 25.2) to be found in this way. At thoracotomy the appearance of an intrapulmonary hamartoma is quite characteristic—it feels hard, lobulation can often be detected and it is usually near the surface of the lung, more commonly in the lower lobe than the upper lobe. It is characteristically mobile in the lung substance, and is described as moving "like a piece of soap". The other benign intrapulmonary tumours (Table 25.5) are also usually well defined and easily excised.

The specimen

If the tumour is shelled out it should be fixed, described and examined, and blocks taken for histology in the usual way. If a lung, lobe, or segment is excised with the tumour inside it, 10 per cent formal-saline should be infused down the bronchus to inflate and fix the lung tissue and the tumour within it. It is then useful to lay the specimen on its pleural surface with the supplying bronchus uppermost and to slice it horizontally through the lung and the tumour. After inspecting the tumour and its relationship with the lung, a probe can be passed through the supplying bronchus to identify any bronchial connections of the tumour. Blocks of tumour, lung tissue, any other abnormalities and any lymph nodes are then taken in the usual way. The cartilage-predominant hamartomas (see p. 321) are readily recognizable macroscopically and microscopically. The histological features of the other benign tumours have recently been reviewed (Whimster, 1983).

Benign tumours of the pleura

Introduction

The pleural fibroma (also called a benign or localized mesothelioma) is the only benign tumour commonly found in the pleural cavity, although there is one convincing report of a fibrous histiocytoma of the pleura.

Presentation

Pleural fibromas occur equally in both sexes, usually over the age of 40 years. In over 50 per cent of cases the tumour presents as hypertrophic pulmonary osteoarthropathy, with pain in the joints of the hands, shoulders and wrists, in that order of frequency. When the tumour is removed these arthritic pains disappear and if it recurs, the arthritic symptoms also recur. In the remaining cases the tumour occurs as a well defined peripheral opacity found by chance on a chest radiograph. Further radiographs may be needed to identify its position in the pleural cavity.

Biopsy

Percutaneous biopsy may be carried out under radiographic control using a wide-bore needle and syringe technique (for further details see Chapter 26 p. 334). The tissue is fixed and processed in the usual way for histology. The histological appearances are usually those of benign fibrous tissue, but as the sample is small it is often difficult to exclude mesothelioma.

Management

In practice, thoracotomy is usually required because one may not be sure in advance whether the tumour is in the pleura or in the lung. But in either case excision is advisable. Pleural fibromas can usually be excised without difficulty. The pedicle is often narrow, but even when it is not it is usually easy to develop a plane of cleavage between the tumour and the chest wall. Rarely, the tumour appears to infiltrate the lung substance itself.

The specimen

A pleural fibroma is uaually a spherical, somewhat lobulated, firm mass with a whorled cut surface which resembles that of a uterine fibroid. Briselli and his colleagues reviewed the features of 360 reported cases in patients aged between 5 and 87 years in 1981 and found that 80 per cent were attached to the visceral pleura and 20 per cent to the parietal pleura. Many were pedunculated and this was a good prognostic feature. They measured between 1 cm and 36 cm (mean 6 cm) and weighed up to 4972 g. By contrast, only 5 were seen at the Regional Thoracic Centre, North Middlesex Hospital, London, between 1951 and 1981 (Table 25.2); of these 3 were attached to the visceral pleura and 2 to the parietal pleura. There is one report of multiple localized pleural mesotheliomas.

The histology varies according to how cellular the fibrous tissue is and whether glandular areas, which may be papillary, are present. Pleural fibromas are usually benign, but malignant cases have been reported.

Carcinoid tumour

This tumour is the commonest benign tumour reported in the lower respiratory tract and this is confirmed by personal experience (Table 25.2). It is also worth further discussion because of its histogenesis, variable histological appearance, occasional difficulties in histological diagnosis, and reported malignant behaviour in some cases—3 of the 74 in Table 25.2 behaved in a malignant way.

Carcinoid tumours of the bronchus were first described by Mueller in 1882. They were later reported to be capable of causing the carcinoid syndrome, but rarely do so.

Carcinoid tumours are believed to arise from cells of the APUD (amine-precursor uptake and decarboxylation) series which have distinctive membrane-bound granules in their cytoplasm. These granules can sometimes be identified with argentaffin and/or argyrophil stains, but are best seen electron microscopically.

Such granular cells were first observed in intestinal epithelium by Kultschitzky in 1897, but in the bronchial epithelium, where they are sometimes called Feyrter cells, they were not reported until 1949. Their presence has been confirmed electron microscopically in the human bronchial glands, in the bronchiolar epithelium, and in the segmental bronchi.

Although carcinoid tumours have been reported in the trachea, the majority occur in the large bronchi. They probably originate from the submucosal glands and the epithelium over them is often intact. A few are seen in the peripheral airways and parenchyma. They may be multiple.

The minute multiple "tumourlets" reported in the lung parenchyma are also believed to be of APUD cell origin and are usually found incidentally at port mortem. Tumourlets are not a surgical pathological problem.

Histologically, trabecular, insular, glandular and papillary patterns may be seen. A spindle cell component may be present, particularly in peripheral carcinoids. The atypical variety reported by Arrigoni and his colleagues in 1972, although uncommon, is the variety most likely to metastasize and may be difficult to distinguish from small cell undifferentiated carcinoma. None of the 74 cases reported in Table 25.2 had an atypical pattern.

Both central and peripheral carcinoids can be argyrophil and/or argentaffin positive or negative. In 1981 Sorokin, Hoyt and McDowell described a light-microscopic staining sequence which revealed ten "distinct cytochemical signatures", i.e. cells with different staining combinations. Electron microscopy, by revealing the characteristic cytoplasmic granules, is diagnostically rewarding in carcinoid tumours.

It thus seems likely that carcinoid tumours may be further subtyped by electron-microscopic, histological and also immunochemical differences in the granules. It remains to be seen whether such subtyping will be of clinical value.

The carcinoid tumour may metastasize. The reported incidence of metastases varies, with 10 per cent thought to be the usual figure in the USA. Malignant behaviour cannot be predicted reliably from the clinical or the histological features, although the atypical appearance should be treated with suspicion. Of the 74 cases shown in Table 25.2, lymph node metastases were found in one, but the patient was subsequently lost to follow-up. Two carcinoid tumours recurred—8 and 16 years after resection. The former developed widespread metastases 9 years after the recurrence had been resected. The latter was found to have widespread metastases at the time of the recurrence. In these two cases the histology was confirmed as typical on review of all the slides including the initial biopsies.

A carcinoid may be misdiagnosed as carcinoma at the light-microscopic level, and it may sometimes be impossible to differentiate carcinoid tumours from undifferentiated carcinomas without electron microscopy. Fisher, Palekar and Paulson thoroughly examined the points of differential diagnosis from oat cell carcinoma in 1978.

Carcinoid tumours of the respiratory tract have been reported in patients of all ages including children, the youngest being 6 years old. The age range of the cases in Table 25.2 was 14 to 75 years (mean 49 years). No causative or predisposing factors have been identified.

Hamartoma

Albrecht coined the term "hamartoma" in 1904. It is applied to tumour-like malformations "in which the various tissues of a part are present in improper proportions of distribution, with prominent excess of one particular tissue . . . Malformations have no powers of excessive uncoordinated growth" (Willis). If such a mass does not show uncoordinated growth or histological evidence of malignancy, there is no objective way of determining whether it is a tumour-like malformation or a benign neoplasm.

Most thoracic surgeons and surgical pathologists see such masses in the lower respiratory tract from time to time. They usually consist predominantly of cartilage, although rarely masses occur in which smooth muscle predominates.

The cartilaginous type of hamartoma is usually seen in the periphery of the lung, but has been reported in the bronchus. Both consist of islands of cartilage, separated by clefts lined by respiratory epithelium, together with varying amounts of connective tissue. These tissues are histologically benign, but calcification and ossification are sometimes seen. Cartilage-predominant hamartomas are usually only a few centimetres in diameter, but one large one 30 cm in diameter, has been recorded. The youngest case reported was 13 years old. The one report of multiple cartilaginous hamartomas is not convincing.

It is difficult to determine whether chondromas exist separately from cartilage-predominant hamartomas. Liebow (1952) believed that chondromas consisted solely of cartilage and occurred only in the large bronchi, and that hamartomas contained a mixture of tissues and occurred mainly in the periphery, although they could occur in large bronchi. By this definition chondromas are so rare that there is only one reported convincing example. Bateson showed that the peripheral chondromatous masses were usually associated with small bronchi, and finally decided that they were neoplasms rather than hamartomas. We agree with the conclusion that they are neoplasms rather than developmental abnormalities because they are usually seen in adult patients and may enlarge during a period of observation. The two endotracheal and five intrapulmonary chondromas shown in Table 25.2 consisted solely of cartilage.

There have been several reports of hamartomas becoming malignant or being associated with malignancy, but in none of them is the relationship very convincing.

Conclusions

1. The clinician's role is to recognize benign tumours of the lower respiratory tract at the earliest opportunity so that the tumour may be excised

completely with the least damage to the respiratory tract. The pathologist's role is to distinguish between benign tumours and other lesions, particularly malignant tumours, in biopsies and resected specimens. It is of less importance to the patient to classify the benign tumour into one of the 26 types reported in the lower respiratory tract.

2. Benign tumours of the lower respiratory tract are far less common than malignant tumours, but surgeons and pathologists must be aware of their occurrence so that the patient is treated correctly.

3. Modern radiological, bronchoscopic, and pathological techniques have improved their recognition.

4. Carcinoid tumours, which occur mainly in the bronchi, but also in the trachea and lung, are the commonest benign tumours of the lower respiratory tract, but a few behave in a malignant manner. Their variants and differential diagnosis should be known to both surgeons and pathologists.

5. Cartilage-predominant hamartomas, the second most common of the benign tumours in the lower respiratory tract, are usually seen in the periphery of the lung. There is some doubt as to whether they are neoplastic, but they are entirely benign and present no threat to the patient. The risk is that less innocent masses may be left in the belief that they are hamartomas.

6. Fibromas (localized mesotheliomas) are virtually the only benign tumours of the pleura. Over 50 per cent of patients suffer arthritic pains which are relieved when the tumour is recognized and removed. It is therefore important that pleural fibromas should not be overlooked.

Section II: Non-neoplastic conditions of the lung and pleura of surgical importance M Bates and K J Jarvis

Introduction

This section deals with those conditions of the lung and pleura, other than tumours, which may require surgical intervention. The introduction of antibiotics in 1944 has had a profound effect on the incidence of many pleuropulmonary infections, so that a condition such as acute lung abscess has become uncommon and consequently the operation of open drainage for lung abscess, a rarity.

Nevertheless, there are congenital and acquired conditions of the lung causing acute mediastinal displacement by cyst, emphysematous bulla or tension pneumothorax which require urgent surgical intervention to save life. Due to the ease of intercontinental travel, diseases which had been uncommon in this country, such as hydatid disease or drug-resistant tuberculosis, are now being diagnosed and knowledge of the correct surgical treatment is necessary.

Congenital conditions of the lung which present with respiratory distress

Congenital bronchogenic cysts

These arise singly and may cause respiratory distress and attacks of cyanosis shortly after birth. If a cyst has a bronchial communication, air becomes trapped and the effect is similar to a tension pneumothorax, causing marked mediastinal shift.

Pathology

The cysts are lined by respiratory epithelium or by flattened endothelial-like cells. They result from a "pinching off" of respiratory tissue in the early stages of development. They may be paratracheal, carinal, hilar or para-oesophageal in position. They can exert extrinsic pressure and cause lobar obstruction and collapse.

Treatment

Thoractomy and excision of cyst. If a cyst has become infected and the epithelial lining destroyed, treatment as for a lung abscess is indicated.

Congenital pulmonary cysts

These occur within the lung parenchyma and are lined by cuboidal or ciliated epithelium. No cartilage or mucous glands are present in the wall. Symptoms arise from air trapping, and acute complications of pneumothorax, haemorrhage and infection may result. These cysts often arise in the middle or upper lobes.

Treatment

Urgent cystectomy or lobectomy is required.

Congenital infantile lobar emphysema

This presents with acute symptoms of dyspnoea and cyanosis in the first three months of life. The upper lobes, particularly the left upper lobe, are most commonly affected and cause marked mediastinal displacement.

Pathology

Examination of the bronchial wall concerned may show deficient cartilage formation or a redundant fold of bronchial mucosa, so allowing air trapping from a collapse of the bronchial wall.

Treatment

Urgent lobectomy is required.

Hypoplastic lung associated with congenital diaphragmatic hernia

This condition—which should be distinguished from congenital cysts, congenital emphysema and tension pneumothorax—gives rise to severe respiratory distress shortly after birth. The chest X-ray shows one pleural cavity, generally the left, to be full of abdominal contents, with marked mediastinal shift and compression of the right lung. The herniation occurs through a patent pleuroperitoneal canal, which normally closes at the third month (Bochdalek hernia).

Treatment

In spite of urgent surgery, there is a high mortality to this condition. Ventilation may be required as is urgent decompression by a nasogastric tube. The best approach for a right-sided hernia is by thoracotomy, but on the left side, a transverse subcostal incision is ideal as malrotation of the gut, if present, can be corrected while reducing the hernia and closing the defect.

This condition may be associated with a hypoplastic lung which expands only slowly to fill the large pleural cavity previously occupied by the intestines. Difficulty may also be experienced in closing the abdomen.

Congenital cystic adenomatoid malformation

This is a rare cystic or solid lung malformation found in premature infants. Acute respiratory distress occurs within a few hours of birth. Enlarging cysts may rupture and cause a pneumothorax. A solid variety is also recorded composed of glandular tissue. The condition is associated with a high incidence of other congenital abnormalities.

Treatment

Although the prognosis is very poor, it it not necessarily hopeless and lobectomy may result in normal development.

Congenital conditions of the lung which present with cough and infective symptoms

Pulmonary sequestration

This congenital abnormality occurs during the fifth week of development and results from an accessory lung bud which arose from the foregut in addition to the right and left lung buds.

There are two varieties, the *extralobar* or lower accessory lung, which is surrounded in its own pleural envelope and gives rise to no symptoms, and the *intralobar* which forms 85 per cent of these sequestrations and gives rise to infective symptoms early in life. It is characterized by partial or complete separation from one segment of the lung, generally the medial basal of either lower lobe. It receives its blood supply from a systemic artery which arises from the thoracic or upper abdominal aorta and passes to the sequestrated cystic mass through the pulmonary ligament.

If, as a result of bronchial communication, infection of this mass occurs, it will give rise to cough, infected sputum and occasionally haemoptysis.

Diagnosis

Diagnosis is suggested by the chest X-ray showing an irregular cavitating mass which can be mistaken for a malignant lung abscess. Bronchogram shows an abnormal pattern, often with an extra segmental bronchus in the lower lobe, and retrograde aortogram confirms the diagnosis by demonstrating a large aortic branch passing directly into the cystic mass.

Pathology

The alveoli and alveolar spaces are infected and areas of bronchiectasis are present. The walls of the pulmonary arteries are muscular, similar to systemic vessels.

Treatment

Segmental resection or occasionally lobectomy is required. Careful dissection and division of the aortic vessel is an important first step in the operation.

Acquired pleuropulmonary conditions resulting from bacterial infections

Acute empyema

The collection of infected fluid in the pleural cavity results either from an infective process in the lung, such as pneumonia, or from direct haematogenous infection. Acute empyema may also result from other infective conditions in the mediastinum, liver or subphrenic space.

The infected fluid may quickly thicken to form pus, depending upon the organism concerned. Pneumococcal and staphylococcal infections produce thick pus, while the pus remains thin in a haemolytic streptococcal empyema. Anaerobic infections result in marked foetor and anaemia.

Diagnosis

Diagnosis is made by chest aspiration and culture of the pus obtained. Antibiotic sensitivity tests are of great importance.

Complications

A bronchopleural fistula is the only serious complication of an acute empyema.

Treatment in children

By repeated aspiration and intrapleural antibiotic replacement. Systemic antibiotics are not effective in crossing the pleural barrier. If large quantities of fibrin are present, then intrapleural streptokinase is required to liquefy the clots. Rib resection and open drainage is never required, but intercostal intubation and closed drainage may be.

Treatment in adults

Rib resection and open drainage under local anaesthesia is the treatment of choice, particularly if a bronchopleural fistula is present. In a young nervous patient, general anaesthesia may be necessary, provided no fistula is present.

Care must be taken to ensure dependent drainage and post-drainage physiotherapy and general acitivity are essential for quick expansion of the lung. The length and position of the drainage tube is decided by weekly sinograms and only when the cavity is seen to be healed can the tube be removed. This process generally takes between four and six weeks.

Following influenzal pneumonia, a patient may become extremely toxic with bilateral streptococcal empyemas, when intercostal intubation and closed drainage is a matter of urgency.

If an empyema can be sterilized by intrapleural antibiotics, and no bronchopleural fistula is present, then a formal thoracotomy and complete excision of the cavity is the treatment of choice.

Acute lung abscess

This results from suppurative pneumonitis and is generally a single cavity, but multiple cavities may be associated with blood-stream infections.

Due to antibiotics, specific bacterial abscesses are uncommon, and most would follow the aspiration during sleep, or following an excessive intake of alcohol, of material from infected teeth, tonsils or cranial sinuses.

Abscess formation can also occur distal to bronchial obstruction by a tumour or retained foreign body.

Diagnosis

Diagnosis is by chest X-ray, the most common sites being in the axillary segments of the upper lobes, or the apical segments of the lower lobes.

Treatment

Bronchoscopy should be performed at some stage in the course of treatment to ensure that there is no bronchial obstruction. Sputum culture and sensitivity tests are essential so that the appropriate antibiotic may be given. A search for acid-fast bacilli should always be made.

Postural drainage and weekly X-rays should ensure gradual diminution in the size of the cavity. Very occasionally an abscess will fail to heal with this treatment and if the patient is still expectorating large quantities of foetid sputum, then rib resection and open drainage is required.

Rib resection is performed under local anaesthesia as for drainage of an empyema, but 5 cm (2 inches) of two adjacent ribs should be resected subperiosteally together with the intervening intercostal bundle. The ribs chosen are those closest to the abscess cavity and careful inspection of the pleura is required. If it is opaque and no lung movement can be seen, then the cavity can be explored with a large-bore needle before incising with the diathermy needle. The cavity should be packed with a gauze roll for the first ten days and then tube drainage can be instituted. If, however, lung movement can be seen, then the wound is closed over an iodine swab in order to encourage adhesions and allow of drainage in one week's time. It is most important to avoid producing an empyema when draining a lung abscess, and for this reason aspiration must not be attempted except at operation.

If a lung abscess is not healed within three months, then the cavity will be lined by respiratory epithelium and lobectomy will be required.

Multiple lung abscesses These can be treated only by intravenous antibiotics.

Complications

Cerebral abscess may result from haematogenous spread of infection, or by way of the chest wall and spinal veins. This is particularly liable to occur with a micro-aerophilic infection.

Bronchiectasis

This is less common as the aetiological factors are largely prevented by prophylactic vaccination in childhood: whooping cough, measles and primary tuberculosis. The clinical picture of cough, purulent sputum and occasional haemoptysis results from infection of pre-existing dilated bronchi whose walls have already been damaged by inflammation. This dilatation, which may be cylindrical, fusiform or saccular in nature, is due to collapse and fibrosis of the surrounding lung.

Partial or complete bronchial obstruction rapidly leads to accumulation of bronchial secretions, and if these are not removed they quickly become infected.

Congenital saccular bronchiectasis This has been reported and is generally associated with cystic fibrosis.

Acquired bronchiectasis In this condition the symptoms are particularly liable to occur following a common cold in winter. Aspiration of infected material from cranial sinuses may also be associated with recurrence of bronchiectatic symptoms. Chronic sinusitis, associated with situs inversus and bronchiectasis, is known as Kartagener's Triad.

A foreign body, if retained for any length of time, can result in *distal bronchiectasis*, as can an innocent bronchial tumour. If the bronchial dilatation is only cylindrical in nature, then the condition is reversible, provided the obstruction is removed early in the history.

Brock's middle lobe syndrome In this syndrome bronchiectasis is confined to the middle lobe. The wall of the middle lobe bronchus is thin and deficient in cartilage and therefore becomes easily compressed by swelling of the peribronchial lymph nodes as a result of tuberculous infection.

Upper lobe bronchiectasis This is generally associated with tuberculosis or sarcoidosis.

Diagnosis

The patient may present with clubbing of the fingers and coarse rales at the bases.

Complete bilateral bronchograms are essential to diagnose the extent of the disease, which may well be bilateral and often affects the middle and lower lobes on the right side, and the lingula and lower lobe on the left. Bronchograms are performed under general anaesthesia in children and under local anaesthesia in adults, unless bronchoscopy is indicated at the same time.

Sputum examination and culture is essential before commencing treatment and, as in all chronic pleuropulmonary infections, careful search should be made for acid-fast bacilli.

Treatment

Postural drainage, physiotherapy and appropriate antibiotics should first be instituted in all cases.

If the disease is extensive and bilateral, medical treatment only is indicated.

Surgical treatment can be considered after a course of medical treatment and when the disease is unilateral and unilobar, with expectations of a good result.

When haemoptysis is a predominant and worrying symptom and is associated with enlarged bronchial arteries, this alone will fully justify resection, provided one is first certain of the source of the bleeding.

Tuberculosis

Due to effective drug therapy, surgical treatment is required only occasionally for pulmonary tuberculosis. Persistent cavitation and bronchostenosis associated with drug-resistant organisms are the main indications for surgery.

Collapse therapy by thoracoplasty is indicated where the bronchus concerned is patent and persistent cavitation and resistant organisms make resection surgery dangerous due to the risk of post-resection bronchopleural fistula.

Thoracoplasty is a staged procedure generally involving the removal of five to seven ribs in two stages at two to three weeks' interval. At the first stage, the first and second ribs are resected completely, together with the posterior half of the third rib. Apicolysis is also performed in order to produce concentric relaxation of the cavity. At the second stage, the anterior half of the third rib is removed together with diminishing posterior parts of the fifth to seventh ribs as required.

Bronchostenosis is an absolute indication for resection surgery, as no cavity will collapse if the draining bronchus is obstructed.

Excisional surgery is also indicated where a healed tuberculous cavity is involved in opportunistic infection by *Aspergillus fumigatus* and causing troublesome haemoptysis.

Patients, usually from abroad, with very advanced disease and total lung destruction, possibly associated with a tuberculous empyema and bronchopleural fistula, will require pleuropneumonectomy.

Acquired cysts of the lung causing dyspnoea

Simple cysts or blebs

Situated at the extreme apices of the lung, simple cysts are liable to rupture and give rise to a *spontaneous pneumothorax*.

This common condition occurs in young people, particularly males, between the ages of 18 and 30. They are often of tall and thin physique. This type of pneumothorax is very liable to recur, is often bilateral but only very occasionally so simultaneously. The patient may experience pain in the chest and slight dyspnoea, but it is rarely associated with exertion.

Emphysematous cysts or bullae

These occur in middle-aged and older patients, are always associated with generalized emphysema and often give rise to severe dyspnoea. They are often bilateral and generally occur at the lung apices. They may enlarge to occupy nearly all of one pleural cavity, causing mediastinal shift. Occasionally they may rupture and cause a spontaneous pneumothorax which, due to the underlying disease, may persist for several months as a *chronic pneumothorax*. Very occasionally haemorrhage can occur into such a cyst, simulating a bronchial carcinoma on chest X-ray.

Pathology

No specific histological picture has been found to account for cyst formation in the lung apices of *young patients*. These cysts have a thin fibrous wall lined by cuboidal epithelium. They are small in size and rarely exceed 1 cm in diameter. Areas of atelectasis, fibrosis and chronic inflammation are constant findings in wedge resection specimens, but no evidence of healed tuberculosis has been seen.

In older patients, bullous cysts are often large and bilateral and associated with generalized destructive emphysema.

Management of pneumothorax

In young patients with spontaneous pneumothorax, *conservative measures* may be employed in the first instance, depending upon the size of the pneumothorax and symptoms. A small pneumothorax can be observed under X-ray control until there is full lung re-expansion. Air aspiration may be desirable for a large pneumothorax and the potential danger of penetrating the lung with the aspirating needle can be avoided by inserting a teflon catheter. Where there is any degree of mediastinal shift and tension pneumothorax, then the insertion of an intercostal tube to water-seal is mandatory.

Chemical pleurodesis or poudrage is no longer considered advisable due to its high recurrence rate.

Surgical treatment is indicated in *young patients* when the pneumothorax presents on the second or third occasion, or on the first occasion when a causative cyst can be seen on the chest X-ray.

The disease area at lung apex, be it a cyst or area of fibrosis, is best managed by wedge resection. Some surgeons consider this to be sufficient treatment, but many prefer in addition some form of pleural abrasion or parietal pleurectomy, to ensure permanent lung adherence to the chest wall. Pleurectomy is performed through a limited thoracotomy, the chest wall pleura and the upper mediastinal pleura down to the level of the azygos arch or arch of the aorta being removed. Recurrence rarely follows this operation.

In *older patients* with large emphysematous cysts, surgical excision is indicated when such a cyst occupies at least half of one pleural cavity and is causing increasing dyspnoea. Thoracotomy and excision will benefit the patient by allowing the compressed and more normal lung tissue to expand. At thoracotomy many small emphysematous cysts may be found in addition to the larger cyst and a lobectomy may be indicated.

When bilateral cysts are to be excised, and the patient is severely restricted, it will be safer from the anaesthetic point of view, and of greater benefit to the patient, if vertical sternal split is employed and both sides are dealt with at the same operation.

Spontaneous haemopneumothorax This is a less common but much more serious condition which generally results from the tearing of an apical adhesion in which there is a small vein, but could follow the rupture of an emphysematous bulla. The patient experiences considerable dyspnoea and pain and his general condition rapidly deteriorates due to the accumulation of large quantities of blood in the pleural cavity. Urgent blood transfusion and intercostal drainage are essential before performing thoracotomy.

A pneumothorax may also occur as a complication of general surgical operations such as nephrectomy or partial thyroidectomy. Routine chest X-ray should follow such procedures and immediate arrangements made for the aspiration of air should a pneumothorax be detected.

Hydatid cysts

Hydatid cysts of the lung may cause cough and dyspnoea, although they can be found on routine chest X-ray and produce no symptoms. They have a sharply defined outline with an ovoid shape, and may be multiple and bilateral.

Hydatid cysts may rupture either into the bronchial tree or pleural cavity. Pleural contamination may result in anaphylactic shock and sudden death. If communication with the bronchial tree occurs, the cyst wall can collapse and be coughed up with spontaneous cure. Calcification can result, but is more commonly seen when the cyst is in the liver.

Diagnosis

The diagnosis is suggested if the patient should come from the Middle East, Australia, South Africa or Wales. On no account should transpleural needling be attempted for fear of rupturing the cyst when the scolises would be spilled into the pleural cavity. In the majority of cases the compliment fixation test and the Casoni test are positive. Eosinophilia may also be found in the peripheral blood.

Pathology

Hydatid cysts are the intermediate larval (cystercercal) stage of the dog tapeworm (*Echinococcus granulosus*). Man may become infected by ingesting eggs which are present in the faeces of a dog carrying the parasite. The embryos within the eggs are released in the stomach and upper small intestine by the shell being dissolved. The released embryos penetrate the wall of the intestine and are carried by the blood stream to the liver and lungs, where one may develop into a hydatid cyst.

A cyst comprises the pericyst which is a layer of fibrous tissue formed by the host, the ectocyst, a thick laminated structureless coat, and the endocyst, an inner one-cell-thick syncytial germinal layer. The scolises form in the brood capsules which develop from the endocyst. Daughter capsules also develop from the brood capsules and endocyst. These are lined by a germinal layer and grow into the cavity and lie free in the parent cyst.

Treatment

The aim of surgical treatment is the complete removal of the cyst or cysts while retaining all lung tissue. Lobectomy, and very occasionally pneumonectomy, is performed only when the cyst has become complicated by infection from bronchial communication.

The chest is opened and the lobe containing the cyst is packed off from the pleural cavity by gauze rolls soaked in 50 per cent saline solution. With a very sharp knife, the fibrous ectocyst is incised over the full extent of the cyst, so exposing the glistening white surface of the true endocyst. The anaesthetist then slowly inflates the lung, gradually extruding the cyst which can be collected in a kidney dish and removed with great care from the chest cavity. The remaining space in the lobe is obliterated by mattress sutures before closing the chest with drainage.

Further reading

Section I: Benign tumours of the trachea, bronchi, lungs and pleura

Carter D, Eggleston JC. Tumors of the lower respiratory tract. In *Atlas of Tumor Pathology*, Second series, Fasc. 17. Armed Forces Institute of Pathology, Washington DC. 1980.

Hurt RL. Benign tumours of bronchus and trachea 1951–1981. *Annals of the Royal College of Surgeons of England*, 1984, 66, 22–6.

Hurt RL, Bates M. Carcinoid tumours of the bronchus: a 33 year experience. *Thorax* **39:** 617–23.

Liebow AA. Tumors of the lower respiratory tract. In *Atlas of Tumor Pathology*, Sec. 5, Fasc. 17. Armed Forces Institute of Pathology, Washington, DC. 1952.

Whimster WF. *Diagnostic Tumour Bibliographies 1: Tumours of the trachea, bronchi, lungs, and pleura*. London: Pitman Books, 1983.

Section II: Non-neoplastic conditions of the lung and pleura

"Further reading" as for Chapter 26 "Cancer of the Lung".

26

Cancer of the Lung

M Bates and K J Jarvis

Introduction

Malignant lung tumours have become one of the main terminal diseases of Western civilization. They are the commonest cause of death from malignancy in men, and in women are the third commonest to carcinoma of the gastrointestinal tract and to carcinoma of the breast. The ratio of men to women with the disease is 4.6:1. It occurs commonly between the ages of 45 and 70 and is rare under the age of 20. Patients with malignant lung tumours may present with symptoms referable to many organs of the body. They may therefore be seen not only by chest physicians and thoracic surgeons, but also by specialists in other fields. A pathologist may see material for cytological or histopathological diagnosis from a number of sites in the body. A close cooperation between the clinician and pathologist is therefore required for the diagnosis and management of patients with this disease.

Clinical presentation

Thoracic symptoms

Patients may present with symptoms referable to the chest. A persistent cough always needs to be explained in a patient at risk, and a normal chest radiograph is no safeguard against an endobronchial tumour. Sputum production commonly accompanies the cough. Profuse expectoration may accompany a bronchiolo-alveolar carcinoma.

Dyspnoea may arise for several reasons. The Hering–Bruer reflex may be brought into operation even with the smallest of tumours. Bronchial obstruction causing total or partial lung collapse will cause dyspnoea. A pleural effusion of large size, either inflammatory or neoplastic in nature, will give rise to breathlessness. Very occasionally, a spontaneous pneumothorax develops due to a peripheral tumour rupturing into the pleural space.

Persistent pneumonia is often a complication of bronchial obstruction and requires further investigation.

Unilateral wheeze may well be noticed by the patient, particularly at night, and is due to air passing through a partially obstructed main bronchus.

Haemoptysis from surface ulceration of the tumour is an important symptom when it occurs daily and generally first thing in the morning. Occasionally, a single haemoptysis can occur and then several months elapse before a further haemoptysis, by which time the condition may well be inoperable.

Chest pain may be caused by pleurisy of inflammatory origin or by tumour invading the pleura, ribs, sternum or vertebrae. Pain from bone involvement is much worse during the night than during the day.

Dysphagia may result from compression of the oesophagus due to mediastinal lymph node involvement.

Extra-thoracic symptoms

Patients may be seen with symptoms referable to organs other than those in the chest.

They may present to the Ear, Nose and Throat Department with a hoarse voice due to recurrent laryngeal nerve involvement. This is usually left-sided.

The Rheumatology Department may see patients with hypertrophic pulmonary osteoarthropathy. In this condition, patients present with marked clubbing of the fingers and toes and joint pain particularly affecting the ankles, knees and wrists. The radiographic appearances are those of subperiosteal new bone formation in the metaphyseal regions of the radius, ulna, tibia and fibula.

Patients may present to the Neurological Department with Pancoast's syndrome due to tumour involvement of the heads and necks of the upper three ribs, the lowest trunk of the brachial plexus and the inferior cervical sympathetic ganglion giving rise to Horner's syndrome. They may also be seen with sensory neuropathy, subacute cerebellar degeneration or pseudomyasthenia.

The Endocrinology Department may see patients with endocrine syndromes due to hormone production by lung tumours, particularly small cell carcinoma but also squamous cell carcinoma and giant cell carcinoma. Such endocrine syndromes are Cushing's syndrome due to adrenocorticotrophic hormone (ACTH) production and inappropriate antidiuresis due to antidiuretic hormone (ADH) production. The patient may have non-metastatic hypercalcaemia due to parathyroid hormone (PTH) or osteolytic substances being formed by the tumour. Gynaecomastia may result from production of gonadotrophins or human placental lactogen (HPL). Hyperthyroidism may occur due to thyroid stimulating hormone (TSH) production. The carcinoid syndrome may result from 5-hydroxytryptamine (5HT) formation. There may be skin pigmentation due to melanocyte stimulating hormone (MSH).

Addison's disease may occur due to adrenal destruction by metastatic tumour.

Patients with lung tumours may present to the Skin Department with dermatomyositis or with skin nodules due to secondary tumour.

The Department of Cardiology may see patients with pericarditis or pericardial effusions due to direct involvement of the pericardium by tumour. Patients may also present with superior vena caval obstruction due to compression by metastases in anterior mediastinal and paratracheal lymph nodes.

Departments of General Medicine may see patients with pyrexia or cachexia. Patients may also present with epigastric pain and jaundice due to hepatic metastases. Thrombosis of peripheral veins may occur with lung tumours.

Pathological fractures or bony metastases from lung tumours are likely to be seen by the Department of Orthopaedics.

Patients with cerebal metastases may present initially to the Neurosurgical Department. This occurs particularly with small cell carcinoma.

General surgeons may see patients with cervical lymphadenopathy due to metastases, or metastatic subcutaneous nodules.

Lung tumours may present as a symptom-free shadow seen on a routine chest X-ray or a mass miniature X-ray.

Aetiological factors

A knowledge of the aetiological factors is important in history-taking.

Smoking

All the large series have shown that heavy smoking is associated with lung cancer. Cigarette smokers are at higher risk of developing lung cancer than pipe or cigar smokers. The risk increases with the number of cigarettes smoked daily and decreases to that of a non-smoker 13 years after cessation of smoking. The tumours associated with smoking are squamous cell carcinoma and small cell carcinoma.

Occupation

Workers in certain industries are more likely to develop lung cancer. Workers exposed to asbestos, either in the manufacture or handling of asbestos, are at risk of developing malignant mesothelioma of the pleura and carcinoma of the lung, particularly adenocarcinoma. The dimensions and physical characteristics of the various asbestos fibres are important. Chryosotile may not penetrate the lungs deeply and those fibres that are retained are liable to the natural process of elimination including dissolution. The amphoboles (crocidolite and amosite) penetrate readily into terminal air spaces and remain within the lung. Workers exposed to asbestos in the form of amphoboles are at greater risk of developing malignant tumours than those exposed to chrysotile.

Workers in mines exposed to radioactive gases, together with those exposed to arsenic, nickel and chromates during the course of their employment, are also at risk of developing lung cancer. Gas workers and those chemical workers exposed to chloromethyl-methyl-ether have an increased risk of developing lung cancer.

Other

There is a higher incidence of lung cancer in towns than in rural areas; this may be related to atmospheric pollution.

Chronic bronchitis and lung scars may precede the development of malignant lung tumours.

Diagnostic procedures

Once a presumptive diagnosis of cancer of the lung has been made from the history, clinical findings and possible radiographic changes, then at this stage the help of a pathologist is usually enlisted.

Sputum cytology

Sputum cytology is a non-invasive procedure that is used in the investigation of patients with a presumptive diagnosis of primary or secondary lung cancer and can be carried out while the patient is still an outpatient. Full instruction should be given to the patient to collect three early morning specimens of sputum on three successive days. The patient must be told to expectorate sputum into the containers given and not to spit saliva. No fixative is added to the specimen which should be brought to the laboratory on the morning that it is produced. In the laboratory, two smears are taken of each specimen of sputum which are fixed in 95 per cent ethyl alcohol and stained by the Papanicolaou method for examination.

The advantages of sputum cytology are that the specimen can be obtained easily and gives a good representative sample of the entire respiratory tract. It has disadvantages in that in only approximately 52 per cent of cases of lung cancer is it positive with one specimen. This rate rises to 63 per cent with three specimens. It is time-consuming, taking approximately one hour for three specimens to be examined, apart from preparation time. It also does not provide localization of the lesion.

Bronchial carcinomas that are not apparent on a chest radiograph can, however, be diagnosed on cytology.

The report of the pathologist with regard to the sputum cytology specimen should include whether or not the specimen is satisfactory and whether it is entirely negative or shows squamous metaplasia. Any atypia of the cells should be noted in the report and if carcinoma cells are present they should be classified as to their type.

Bronchoscopy

Bronchoscopy by the rigid Negus instrument is the most important single investigation. This can be performed either under local or general anaesthesia. With modern techniques the latter method is entirely safe. The vocal cords are first examined for weakness or paralysis and the trachea is examined for compression or the presence of tumour. The state of the main carina is the most important point regarding operability and it should be sharp and mobile. Rigidity or rounding of the carina indicates underlying involved lymph nodes and signifies inoperability. The main and lobar bronchi can be examined with direct and indirect telescopes and biopsy material obtained. However, only the orifices of the segmental bronchi can be seen, and biopsied.

The introduction of the flexible fibreoptic bronchoscope has been of great value in adding to the important basic information obtained by the rigid instrument. The fibreoptic bronchoscope enables small peripheral tumours at subsegmental levels to be seen and biopsied often with the aid of radiographic screening.

Bronchial biopsy

Biopsy material should be obtained from the main body of tumour present in the bronchus. Biopsy of overlying necrotic debris or blood clot often does not produce sufficient material to allow an adequate histological diagnosis. The biopsy should be taken with care to prevent crushing of the specimen. This is particularly important with small cell carcinomas where crushing artefact readily occurs. The material should be placed immediately in fixative, which for most histopathology departments is 10 per cent buffered formol saline. The specimen container and request form should be labelled and the request form completed as to the site of the biopsy and as regards to clinical details.

Processing of biopsy specimens

It is often possible to process bronchial biopsy specimens in 4 hours using heat and vacuum on the Autotechnicon ultra and enclosed single-chamber tissue-processing machines. This enables a bronchial biopsy taken in the early part of the morning to be reported during the late afternoon. If such an urgent report is required, then the specimen should be sent to the histopathology laboratory immediately.

A 16-hour cycle, using heat and vacuum, is also available on the Autotechnicon ultra and enclosed single-chamber tissue-processing machines, which allows biopsy specimens taken during the afternoon to be reported the following day.

Such rapid processing and reporting enables those patients for whom operative treatment is contemplated to be put on the next operating list.

Non-urgent bronchial biopsies can be processed after adequate fixation on a routine 16-hour overnight cycle which allows a report to be given approximately 24 to 48 hours after receipt of the specimen in the laboratory.

Once the biopsy has been processed, the tissue is embedded in paraffin wax in a block and sections are cut from this and stained using haematoxylin and eosin. For biopsies taken via the Negus bronchoscope, most histopathologists examine three sets of sections taken 50 μm apart (levels). If these show no abnormality, then further sets of sections taken 50 μm apart are examined until either an abnormality is detected or it is obvious that there is no abnormality in the submitted bronchial biopsy.

The smaller biopsies taken via the fibreoptic bronchoscope can be examined by taking ten sets of three serial sections which are cut into the block for 150 μm. Alternate sets of these serial sections are stained with haematoxylin and eosin and examined. The unstained sets of serial sections are available for haematoxylin and eosin staining if necessary or for special histological stains to be carried out.

Reporting of biopsy specimens

The histopathology report should state the amount of bronchial wall included in the specimen. Abnormalities of the bronchial epithelium should be described. These can range from goblet cell metaplasia to squamous metaplasia. There may be dysplasia of the metaplastic squamous epithelium or in-situ squamous cell carcinoma may be present. Infiltrating carcinoma in the submucosa should be classified. The presence of other disease changes in the bronchial biopsy should also be noted.

Histological classification of lung tumours

An agreement as to which histological classification of lung tumours is to be used in surgical reporting should be made between the thoracic surgeon and the histopathologist. A commonly used classification is that of the World Health Organisation which was published in 1967 and which was revised in 1982. This more recent revised classification with examples is set out in Table 26.1. Benign tumours which occur in subgroup A of each group have been omitted, together with Group VII (Tumour-like lesions).

Table 26.1 Histological classification of malignant lung tumours. (Based on the World Health Organisation histological typing of lung tumours. Second edition (1982). "Benign tumours", which occur in subgroup A of each group, have been omitted, together with Group VII ("Tumour-like lesions").)

I EPITHELIAL TUMOURS

B. *Carcinoma-in-situ*

C. *Malignant*

1. Squamous cell carcinoma
   (epidermoid carcinoma)
   Variant:
   (a) Spindle cell (squamous) carcinoma
2. Small cell carcinoma
   (a) Oat cell carcinoma
   (b) Intermediate cell type
   (c) Combined oat cell carcinoma
3. Adenocarcinoma
   (a) Acinar adenocarcinoma
   (b) Papillary adenocarcinoma
   (c) Bronchiolo-alveolar carcinoma
   (d) Solid carcinoma with mucus formation
4. Large cell carcinoma
   Variants:
   (a) Giant cell carcinoma
   (b) Clear cell carcinoma
5. Adenosquamous carcinoma
6. Carcinoid tumour
7. Bronchial gland carcinomas
   (a) Adenoid cystic carcinoma
   (b) Mucoepidermoid carcinoma
   (c) Others
8. Others
   Basal cell carcinoma of bronchus

II SOFT TISSUE TUMOURS

Fibrosarcoma, Neurofibrosarcoma, Haemangiosarcoma, Leiomyosarcoma, Malignant haemangiopericytoma, Malignant fibrous histiocytoma, Chondrosarcoma, Rhabdomyosarcoma, Kaposi's sarcoma.

III MESOTHELIAL TUMOURS

B. *Malignant mesothelioma*

1. Epithelial
2. Fibrous (spindle cell)
3. Biphasic

IV MISCELLANEOUS TUMOURS

B. *Malignant*

1. Carcinosarcoma
2. Pulmonary blastoma
3. Malignant melanoma
4. Malignant lymphoma
5. Others
   Intravascular sclerosing bronchiolo-alveolar tumour (IVSBAT)

V SECONDARY TUMOURS

VI UNCLASSIFIED TUMOURS

Incidence of primary malignant lung tumours

About 95 per cent of primary malignant lung tumours are bronchogenic carcinomas. There is a variation in the incidence of bronchogenic carcinomas between series. However, approximately 35 per cent are squamous cell carcinomas, 30 per cent adenocarcinomas, 20 per cent small cell carcinomas and 10 per cent large cell carcinoma and its variants.

Secondary malignant lung tumours

The possibility that the tumour is a secondary should always be considered by the histopathologist examining the sections. The histopathologist reporting a squamous cell carcinoma of the lung can be certain that it is a primary when evidence for a local origin of the tumour is present in the form of in-situ squamous cell carcinoma in the overlying bronchial epithelium. Small cell carcinoma of the bronchus has sufficiently distinctive histological features as to be reasonably certain that it is a primary lung cancer.

Lung tumours which are unlikely to be metastases are bronchial gland carcinomas (adenoid cystic carcinoma and mucoepidermoid carcinoma), basal cell carcinoma of bronchus, carcinosarcoma and pulmonary blastoma.

In a recent series, 0.95 per cent of pulmonary tumours were found to be metastases, and approximately 20 per cent of these were from patients with no previous history of malignant disease. The commonest primary sites for unsuspected pulmonary metastases are gastrointestinal tract, kidney, prostate, testis, breast and thyroid. The majority of these metastases are adenocarcinomas. A histopathologist diagnosing an adenocarcinoma of the lung on cytology or on bronchial biopsy cannot be certain that the tumour is not a metastasis and should always alert the surgeon to this possibility.

Use of special histological stains Special histological stains may be of help in differentiating primary from secondary adenocarcinomas in a bronchial biopsy. A periodic acid-Schiff (PAS) stain with and without diastase should be carried out. This special stain will demonstrate the present of glycogen and mucin. Treatment with diastase will remove the glycogen and therefore following this a periodic acid-Schiff stain will demonstrate only mucin.

Adenocarcinomas of the lung contain little if any mucin, whereas those from the gastrointestinal tract often contain much. A periodic acid-Schiff stain may therefore be of help in differentiating these tumours.

The presence of glycogen in a clear cell adenocarcinoma suggests that the tumour may be of renal origin. A clear cell carcinoma of the lung does not contain glycogen. A benign clear cell tumour of the lung however does.

Other possible secondary lung tumours

The possibility that malignant melanoma in a bronchial biopsy is a metastasis should be considered and evidence of local origin sought in the biopsy.

The possibility that a carcinoid tumour is a metastasis should also be considered.

Malignant soft tissue tumours of the lung may also be metastases.

Diagnostic rate of bronchial biopsies

The diagnosis of a malignant lung tumour can be made in about 51 per cent of cases with biopsies using the rigid Negus bronchoscope and in 72 per cent of cases using the fibreoptic bronchoscope. Where the tumour is seen and accessible to biopsy, this rate increases to 84 per cent with the rigid Negus bronchoscope and 91 per cent with the fibreoptic bronchoscope.

Methods of increasing the diagnostic rate

Cytology may be used in conjunction with biopsy at the time of bronchoscopy to increase the diagnostic rate. Bronchial aspirates may be obtained using suction during the course of the bronchoscopy and sputum collected in a trap. The sputum is treated in the same way as an expectorated specimen for cytological examination.

Bronchial washings are obtained using normal saline which is instilled via the bronchoscope and re-aspirated. The material is again collected in a trap and sent to the cytology laboratory, where after centrifugation smears are prepared from the sediment on glass slides. These are fixed in 95 per cent ethyl alcohol and stained using the Papanicolaou method, after which they are reported.

Bronchial brushings may be taken via the bronchoscope and cytology preparations made by smearing the brush material directly onto glass slides in the operating theatre. These are fixed at once in 95 per cent ethyl alcohol. The slides are sent to the cytology laboratory where they are stained using the Papanicolaou method and reported. Alternatively, the bronchial brush can be dropped into 10 per cent buffered formol saline for sending to the histopathology laboratory. The brush is processed in the same way as tissue and embedded in paraffin wax. Sections are then cut from the block and stained with haematoxylin and eosin for reporting.

Bronchial brushings have a diagnosis rate of 59–65 per cent. Bronchial brush cytology combined with bronchial biopsy via the fibreoptic bronchoscope increases the rate of diagnosis to 80 per cent. Needle aspiration cytology may be used via the fibreoptic bronchoscope and material aspirated and cytology preparations made. With this technique the rate of diagnosis is 80 per cent. It is of use where forceps biopsy is difficult as in upper lobe tumours, in submucosal tumours and where the tumour is producing external compression of the bronchus.

Other diagnostic procedures

Needle and drill biopsy

For tumours that are too peripheral for bronchial biopsy, then transpleural biopsy using a large-bore needle and syringe, or by Steel's high-speed drill, should be carried out. The needles for these procedures are inserted under television fluoroscopic control.

The biopsies obtained using the large-bore needle and the Steel's high-speed drill are needle biopsies of tissue which should be placed into 10 per cent buffered formol saline for sending to the histopathology laboratory. In the laboratory, the pieces of tissue are processed and embedded in paraffin wax. Sections of 5 μm are cut for 150 μm into the block. Sets of three serial sections are placed on slides and alternate slides are stained with haematoxylin and eosin and examined.

Fine-needle aspiration cytology

Transthoracic fine-needle aspiration cytology of peripheral lung shadows can be carried out using a 15 cm long, 22 gauge needle on a 20 ml syringe. The needle is inserted under television fluoroscopic control into the lesion. The syringe has a special holder and suction is created by traction on the piston of the syringe. With suction the needle is moved to and fro within the lesion. The suction is released and the needle withdrawn. The aspirated material is expressed onto glass slides and fixed in 95 per cent ethyl alcohol. The slides are then sent to the cytology laboratory where they are stained using the Papanicolaou method for examination. Approximately 82 per cent of malignant tumours can be diagnosed on the first aspiration using this method.

Diagnostic and staging procedures

Mediastinoscopy and mediastonotomy with lymph node biopsy

Mediastinoscopy and mediastonotomy are used for the detection of spread of tumour to mediastinal lymph nodes. In mediastinoscopy, the anterior group of subcarinal and paratracheal lymph nodes may be reached and biopsied under direct vision through a mediastinoscope. In mediastonotomy, the approach is via the second costal cartilage on either side. The non-invasive method of computerized tomography (CAT scan) is most effective in the demonstration of mediastinal lymph nodes and may supercede mediastinoscopy and mediastonotomy.

It is assumed that any mediastinal node of 1 cm or more in diameter is likely to be neoplastic rather than inflammatory in nature.

Scalene lymph node biopsy

Scalene lymph node biopsies should be taken in those patients with palpable supraclavicular lymph nodes.

Handling of lymph node biopsies where secondary tumour is suspected

The lymph nodes should be placed in 10 per cent buffered formol saline for transport to the histopathology laboratory where, following adequate fixation, blocks of tissue are taken from the lymph nodes and processed. The tissue is then embedded in paraffin wax and sections cut for staining with haematoxylin and eosin for reporting.

Handling of lymph node biopsies where lymphoma is suspected

Biopsies of lymph nodes are of particular importance where a lymphoma of the lung is suspected on histological or cytological grounds. It is not possible to diagnose with certainty a lymphoma on bronchial biopsy, needle biopsy or cytology. A larger amount of tissue than is produced by these procedures is required for diagnosis. An involved lymph node should be biopsied. Excision of the area of lung infiltrated by lymphoma is not necessary unless it is required for diagnosis in cases where there are no involved lymph nodes.

It is important that lymph nodes, where a diagnosis of malignant lymphoma is suspected, should be properly fixed. They should be sent to the histopathology laboratory in 10 per cent buffered formol saline as soon as possible after they are removed. The lymph nodes are then cut into 2–3 mm-thick slices and are left in 10 per cent buffered formol saline to receive further adequate fixation before processing. If this procedure is not carried out then only partial fixation of an enlarged lymph node occurs, as formalin is only able to penetrate a short distance beneath the capsule of such a lymph node before autolysis begins in the more central areas. This results in difficulty in diagnosis.

Diagnosis of pleural tumours

There may be pleural involvement by tumour with pleural thickening or effusion. Cytology of the effusion is helpful in confirming pleural involvement. At aspiration, the fluid is collected and sent to the laboratory where it is centrifuged and smears made from the sediment on glass slides. These are fixed in 95 per cent ethyl alcohol and stained by the Papanicolaou method for examination. The diagnosis rate is approximately 54 per cent.

Closed pleural biopsy can be performed using an Abram's needle. A diagnosis is only possible in about 40 per cent of cases using this procedure. An open biopsy produces a diagnosis in about 78 per cent of cases.

It is often not possible to be certain of the diagnosis of a malignant mesothelioma on cytological grounds, and a closed biopsy or needle biopsy of the pleura may not produce sufficient material for this diagnosis. Thoracoscopy and biopsy can be performed when a pleural effusion is present. Open pleural biopsy will produce sufficient material for a histological diagnosis. It does, however, carry the theoretical risk of tumour involving the wound.

Biopsy of distant metastases

Where metastic spread of the lung tumour has occurred, then biopsies can be taken at the sites of suspected metastases. A needle biopsy of the liver can be carried out where there is liver enlargement or where liver metastases are suspected. A biopsy may be taken from the site of a pathological fracture.

Where the diagnosis of a small cell carcinoma of the bronchus is made, a trephine biopsy of bone marrow can be undertaken as part of the routine staging of the tumour, as bone involvement may be as frequent as 50 per cent at the time of initial presentation.

Handling of biopsies

Pleural and other biopsies should be placed into 10 per cent buffered formol saline for transport to the histopathology laboratory, where they are processed and sections cut and stained with haematoxylin and eosin for reporting. Specimens containing bone require decalcification before processing.

Management

The management of a patient with lung cancer depends on the histological type of tumour, its spread, and the general condition of the patient.

Table 26.2 Staging and TNM classification of malignant lung tumours.

Staging of lung carcinoma

Stage I	– The growth is confined to the lung
Stage II	– Involvement of bronchopulmonary nodes at the hilum
Stage III	– Involvement of mediastinal nodes
Stage IV	– Spread outside the chest

TNM classification

T	– Primary tumour
T1	– Tumour is 3 cm or less in diameter and not seen on bronchoscopy
T2	– Tumour is more than 3 cm in diameter and can be seen on bronchoscopy, but it must lie at least 2 cm distal to the carina
T3	– Tumour of any size with direct extension to adjacent structures such as chest wall, diaphragm or mediastinum
N	– Regional nodes
N0	– No evidence of regional lymph node involvement
N1	– Evidence of involvement of peribronchial nodes
N2	– Evidence of mediastinal node involvement
M	– Distant metastases
M0	– No evidence of distant metastases
M1	– Evidence of distant metastases

The tumour can be staged according to its spread, as in Table 26.2.

Malignant lung tumours spread by direct infiltration of the lung and adjacent structures such as the pleura, pericardium, mediastinum and chest wall.

There is lymphatic invasion and spread to lymph nodes. The main groups to be involved are tracheobronchial, cervical, supraclavicular, abdominal, retroperitoneal, axillary, and peripancreatic.

Invasion of pulmonary veins leads to blood-borne metastases. The organs usually involved by this route are liver, adrenals, brain, skeletal system, kidneys and spleen.

It is usual for patients with lung cancer to present late in the course of the disease and in about one third of the patients the presenting symptom is due to metastasis. The expectation of life in such patients is only about nine months from the time of diagnosis.

One third of the patients are fit only for palliative treatment due to adverse general conditions, such as emphysema, chronic bronchitis or cardiac ischaemia.

One third of the patients are fit for radical treatment either by surgery, radiotherapy, chemotherapy, or a combination of these treatments.

In order to detect lung cancer at an earlier stage, the possibility of using sputum cytology combined with chest radiography as a screening method in patients at risk has been considered. Sputum cytology is more likely to detect the centrally placed intrabronchial squamous carcinoma rather than the peripheral adenocarcinoma, which is more likely to be detected by a chest X-ray. The results of screening have been disappointing and at the present time does not appear to be economically worthwhile.

The radiographically occult bronchogenic carcinoma

A patient may, however, be seen in whom malignant cells have been detected in the sputum and in whom there is no radiological evidence of tumour. The malignant cells are usually from a squamous cell carcinoma which is either *in situ* or showing early invasion of the bronchial wall. Localization of the radiographically occult bronchogenic carcinoma is therefore required. The carcinoma may be visible on bronchoscopy, however if no abnormality is noted then bronchial brush cytology is carried out on each segmental bronchus and as many subsegmental bronchi as possible. Each of the bronchial brush specimens needs to be smeared onto separate glass slides which are labelled as to the site of the brushing and fixed at once in 95 per cent ethyl alcohol for sending to the cytology laboratory.

The area of the tumour is localized using this procedure and a bronchial biopsy from the area can be used to confirm the cytological findings. Excision of the involved area by lobectomy or pneumonectomy may then be carried out.

Infiltrating lung tumours

For patients with infiltrating lung tumours, excision of the involved lung still remains the best form of treatment giving the patient a good chance of a long-term result. A lung tumour becomes inoperable when:

1. There is pleural involvement with malignant cells in the pleural fluid.
2. There is recurrent laryngeal nerve involvement.
3. There is superior vena caval obstruction.
4. There are contralateral mediastinal lymph node metastases.
5. There is involvement of the trachea, carina or contralateral main bronchus due to mediastinal lymph node infiltration.
6. There are metastases in lymph nodes above the arch of the aorta from tumour in the left lung or metastases in the highest mediastinal lymph nodes on the right.
7. There are distant metastases.

Preoperative radiotherapy

Preoperative radiotherapy may be given to operable small cell carcinomas of the bronchus. It is advisable that a low dosage such as 1750 rads is employed. Larger doses will lead to radiation pneumonitis when lung tissue is being preserved after a lobectomy, or to a bronchopleural fistula following pneumonectomy.

Lung resection

The amount of lung tissue that has to be removed is essentially decided by the position of the growth in the bronchus and the extent of lymph node involvement. Conservative resection is performed whenever possible and the whole lung is never removed when a lobectomy or segmental resection will suffice.

When the growth lies in the main bronchus, then the whole lung will need to be removed in nearly every case. The tumours arising in the main bronchus are usually squamous cell carcinomas. If the main vessels, particularly the pulmonary veins, are involved close to the surface of the pericardium, they will need to be ligated and divided within the pericardium. Many growths can be removed only by intrapericardial resection as they are involving the pericardium. This adds to the complications and mortality of the operation. The hospital mortality rate for the operation of pneumonectomy remains in the region of 12 per cent, while the rate for lobectomy is around 4.5 per cent. A patient who would not tolerate pneumonectomy, who has an upper lobe tumour encroaching on the main bronchus, can be treated by sleeve lobectomy. In this operation the lobe is removed together with a cylinder of the main bronchus. The right middle and lower lobes or left lower lobe are then anastomosed to the trachea. Segmental resection is fully justified and gives good long-term results for small peripheral lesions where there is no peribronchial lymph node involvement. These tumours are more likely to be adenocarcinomas.

Pleuropneumonectomy and pleurectomy

Malignant mesothelioma of the pleura can be excised by pleuropneumonectomy. Pleural effusions due to this tumour can be controlled by pleurectomy.

Frozen section diagnosis

On occasions, the patient may present with a clinically resectable lung tumour in which a preoperative histological diagnosis has not been possible. An exploratory thoractomy is required and a frozen section may be helpful in diagnosis. The technique does however have limitations in that it is not possible to diagnose with certainty some tumours such as malignant lymphomas on a frozen section. Where a frozen section may be needed, the thoracic surgical department should make arrangements with the histopathology laboratory prior to the operation so that a histopathologist and a medical laboratory scientific officer are available. The surgeon should take a representative sample of the tumour or a lymph node containing tumour and send the labelled specimen without fixative to the histopathology laboratory immediately.

In the laboratory, a suitable block is cut by the histopathologist and placed on a chuck in embedding medium. The material is immediately frozen using an aerosol spray of dichlorodifluoromethane. The chuck is then clamped in a microtome in a cryostat which is usually refrigerated at −20°C. Sections of the tissue are then cut, placed on slides and stained with haematoxylin and eosin for examination by the histopathologist.

This technique may also be used to determine whether there is tumour present at the line of resection of the bronchus at the time of operation.

Handling of specimens of lung in the operating theatre

Following removal, the pneumonectomy, lobectomy or resection specimen should be inflated with 10 per cent buffered formol saline. The inflation is most easily carried out using a 10-litre, or larger, polythene container on a shelf 75–100 cm above the specimen. The polythene container should have a tap at the lower end to which is connected approximately 100 cm of rubber tubing with an adaptor at its lower end. A Mohr's clip is used to control the flow of 10 per cent buffered formol saline. With the specimen in a suitable container, the adaptor is placed within the bronchi and formol saline allowed to flow into the bronchi inflating the specimen. The specimen, covered in fixative, should then be sent to the histopathology laboratory.

Handling and reporting of specimens of lung in the histopathology laboratory

After approximately 48 hours' fixation, the specimen is examined by the histopathologist. If there is no palpable tumour, then the bronchi require careful opening using scissors. If there is a palpable tumour, then parallel slices of the lung may be taken using a brain knife cutting in a axial plane towards the hilum of the lung.

The pathologist will note in the naked-eye report the relation of the tumour to bronchi, its size and position and involvement of other structures such a pleura, chest wall or pericardium.

Blocks of tissue for processing for sections will need to be taken of the tumour. In order to determine the spread of the tumour, blocks will need to be taken of the pleura, if the tumour is close to this, and if an intrapericardial pneumonectomy has been performed, a block of pericardium. Blocks will also need to be taken of bronchial and hilar lymph nodes if present in the specimen. Other lymph nodes, such as paratracheal and mediastinal, may also have been removed by the surgeon at the time of operation. In order to determine excision of the tumour, a block should be taken of the line of resection of the bronchus. Blocks may also be taken of the lung away from the tumour if there is a naked-eye abnormality.

The histopathological report should classify the tumour and give its differentiation. The report should state whether or not there is involvement of pulmonary veins or arteries. Spread of the tumour to pleura or pericardium should be noted. Involvement of lymph nodes should be described. The report should state whether or not the bronchial line of resection is clear of tumour.

Any other pulmonary disease such as emphysema should also be noted.

The prognosis as regards survival following resection is most favourable with squamous cell carcinomas, followed by large cell carcinomas. The survival figures for adenocarcinoma are little better than those for small cell carcinoma, which are the worst. There is a better survival rate where lymph nodes are not involved.

Involvement of pulmonary blood vessels carries a poor prognosis.

There is a possibility of recurrence if the tumour is present at the line of resection of the bronchus or has penetrated the pleura.

Radiotherapy

Radiotherapy may be used for primary curative treatment either alone or in combination with surgery or chemotherapy for such highly radiosensitive tumours as small cell carcinomas. A total dose of 4000–5000 rads is required for curative treatment and this may cause oesophagitis, pericarditis or even coronary artery occlusion.

The main use of radiotherapy is in the palliation of such complications as persistent haemoptysis, superior vena caval obstruction, and pain due to bone erosion.

Radiotherapy may also be used for recurrent tumour in the bronchial stump following resection.

Cytotoxic drugs

There are now many cytotoxic drugs for use in the treatment of malignant tumours and with highly sensitive tumours the initial response may be dramatic. Such drugs are lomustine, doxorubicin hydrochloride, nitrogen mustard, vincristine sulphate, bleomycin and cyclophosphamide. Systemic chemotherapy is the treatment of choice for malignant lymphomas. Chemotherapy may be used for the treatment of malignant mesothelioma of the pleura, either by intrapleural instillation or systemically.

Immunotherapy

Immunotherapy has also been attempted to stimulate the patient's resistance to remaining tumour cells. Intrapleural injection of *Bacillus Calmette-Guerin* (BCG) following lung resection has been of benefit. It has not been so where the BCG has been given intradermally.

Use of lasers in treatment

A new method of treatment of bronchial tumours by a laser beam passed along a flexible endoscope is now being considered. Such lasers are the argon laser and the neodymium-yttrium aluminium garnet laser.

Palliative treatment

Palliative treatment may be needed for advanced tumours. Where there is a persistent bronchial infection and haemoptysis, continuous antibiotics can be given. Chlorpromazine is effective in controlling the nausea and vomiting associated with hepatic metastases. Steroids and the Brompton cocktail are invaluable in the relief of pain and mental distress. Intense headache due to cerebral metastases can be alleviated by dexamethazone. Heroin is required for the most severe forms of pain.

Conclusion

A knowledge of the pathogenesis and behaviour of malignant lung tumours is necessary for diagnosis and treatment. There is, however, a depressingly low 10-year survival rate of 15.6 per cent and 20-year survival rate of 5.5 per cent for resected lung tumours. Preventive measures will lower the incidence of these tumours in the general population. However, there still remains the necessity to improve the survival either by earlier detection or other treatment methods. An understanding of the pathology of malignant lung tumours is likely to have an important role in the development of these methods.

Further reading

Bates M. Surgical treatment of bronchial carcinoma (Hunterian Lecture). *Annals of the Royal College of Surgeons of England* 1981; **63**:164–7.

Bates M (ed) *Bronchial Carcinoma. An integrated approach to diagnosis and management.* Berlin: Springer-Verlag, 1984.

Dunnill MS. *Pulmonary Pathology.* London: Churchill Livingstone, 1982.

Leigh Collis J, Clarke DB, Abbey Smith, R. *d'Abreu's Practice of Cardiothoracic Surgery*. London: Edward Arnold, 1976.

Rees LH, Ratcliffe JG. Ectopic hormone production by non-endocrine tumours. *Clin Endocrinol* 1974; **3**:263–99.

Spencer H. Carcinoma of the lung. In: *Pathology of the Lung*, pp 773–859. Oxford: Pergamon Press, 1977.

Spencer H. Rare pulmonary tumours. In: *Pathology of the Lung*, pp 861–936. Oxford: Pergamon Press, 1977.

Spencer H. Pulmonary reticuloses. In: *Pathology of the Lung*, pp 936–72. Oxford: Pergamon Press, 1977.

The World Health Organisation histological typing of lung tumours, 2nd edn. *Am J Clin Path* 1982; **77**:123–36.

27

Endocrine System

T L Kennedy, K D Buchanan and E F McKeown

The adrenal glands

Introduction

Although some adrenal tumours both benign and malignant have no apparent biological effect, the majority of lesions of interest to the surgeon present with either hypertension, the features of Cushing's syndrome or virilization. Non-functioning adrenal cortical adenomata have long been recognized as a relatively common post-mortem finding. With the advent of CT scan and real-time ultrasound, small adrenal tumours are now being found by chance. These "incidentalomas" may cause trouble to the surgeon. Although the majority are harmless there is always the worry that they may be malignant. It is generally safe to watch these tumours if they are small, but larger tumours are likely to be malignant and to metastasize. Non-functioning medullary tumours, phaeochromocytoma or ganglioneuroma may also be found.

Cysts or pseudocysts of the adrenals are not uncommon. Their origin is uncertain, but they may be due to haemorrhagic degeneration of a benign tumour. Occasionally they have a parasitic origin. Secondary deposits in the adrenals from primary tumours of bronchus, breast and other sites are not uncommon, but have little relevance to the endocrine surgeon, though they may cause hypoadrenalism.

The adrenal cortex

Cushing's syndrome (Fig. 27.1)

The clinical features of this syndrome are well known. The face becomes florid, hirsute and rounded. There is obesity of the trunk often associ-

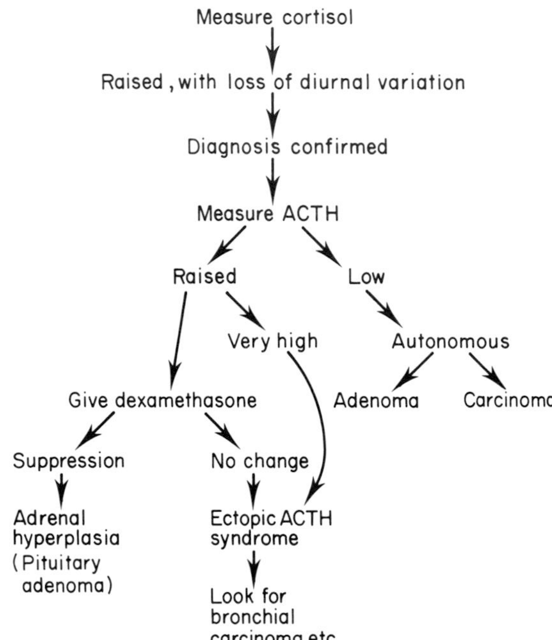

Fig. 27.1 The investigation of Cushing's syndrome.

ated with striae around the hips and a "buffalo hump"; the limbs are spared and may be quite thin due to muscle wasting and there is associated weakness. Pathological fractures may occur, particularly of ribs and vertebral bodies, due to osteoporosis. Spontaneous bruising is often found due to increased capillary fragility, and simple wounds heal poorly. Amenorrhoea, impotence and sterility are usual. Hypertension of varying severity is common. Moderate degrees of hyperglycaemia often occur and there may be frank diabetes. A moderate degree of hypokalaemic alkalosis is common and sodium and water retention may lead to cardiac failure. Mental disturbance and psychotic symptoms are occasionally seen.

It is not necessary to find more than a few of

these symptoms and signs to be alerted to the possibility of cortisol excess. The causes are:

1. *Iatrogenic* It is always important to determine whether the patient is on topical or systemic steroid therapy for rheumatoid arthritis, asthma or some other chronic complaint.
2. *Adrenal cortical hyperplasia* Associated with
   (a) hypothalamic pituitary hyperfunction
   (b) pituitary adenoma
   (c) other tumours—ectopic adrenocorticotrophic hormone (ACTH) syndrome
3. *Adrenal cortical tumour*
   (a) adenoma
   (b) carcinoma

Having excluded iatrogenic causes, it is important to prove that there is adrenal cortical hyperfunction and this is done by measuring plasma cortisol. As there is considerable diurnal variation, measurements are made at 8.00 a.m. and 10.00 p.m. The morning level is normally in the range 400–760 nmol/litre and in the evening it is in the range 60–200 nmol/litre. In Cushing's syndrome this diurnal variation is lost and levels are raised.

It is now necessary to determine whether the cortical hyperactivity is autonomous. Measurements are made of plasma ACTH which is normally less than 70 ng/litre in the morning specimen. In the presence of an adrenal tumour, benign or malignant, ACTH levels are low, as high circulating cortisol levels inhibit the release of ACTH from the pituitary. Dexamethasone is a synthetic glucocorticoid which inhibits ACTH release and thus the secretion of cortisol in normal patients and those with pituitary tumours. In the presence of an adrenal tumour, dexamethasone has no effect on cortisol levels.

Adrenal cortical hyperplasia

In the great majority of patients, Cushing's syndrome is due to bilateral adrenocortical hyperplasia as a result of excessive stimulation by ACTH. A basophil or chromophobe pituitary adenoma may be responsible. These tumours may be microscopic in size and it is therefore difficult to assess the frequency with which they occur in Cushing's syndrome, but in our experience it has been 80 per cent. In those patients without pituitary tumours, a disturbance of the feed-back mechanism at the hypothalamic level is suspected, with insensitivity to circulating cortisol levels. A specific peptide with corticotrophin releasing factor (CRF) activity has recently been identified which acts specifically on the anterior pituitary stimulating ACTH release directly. In the future this may form the basis for a clinical test to differentiate between pituitary and hypothalamic causes of disorders of ACTH secretion.

In the normal adult the average combined weight of the adrenals does not exceed 13 g. In over 50 per cent of ACTH-dependent Cushing's syndrome patients each gland weighs less than 8 g and in only 12 per cent do they weigh more than 12 g. The hyperplasia may be described as simple or nodular. In the latter, heavier weights are usually encountered. The association of Cushing's syndrome with an adrenal gland of normal weight (6 g) is universally accepted.

In simple hyperplasia, the adrenal is typically yellowish in colour, with rounded edges and a widened cortex which may show a prominent inner brownish zona reticularis. When the glands are only marginally enlarged, the compact cells of the zona reticularis are particularly prominent. In nodular hyperplasia, small focal yellow nodules up to 2.5 cm in size are found in the cortex. They may not be apparent to the surgeon at operation, being only visible after sectioning the gland. Histologically they resemble small functioning adenomas but, unlike the gland in Cushing's syndrome, due to an adenoma the attached cortex is hyperplastic rather than atrophic.

Diagnosis depends upon the finding of raised cortisol levels, with loss of diurnal variation. The raised cortisol levels are usually suppressed by high doses of dexamethasone and associated with normal or high levels of ACTH.

This type of Cushing's syndrome is generally treated today by pituitary microsurgery. In the past, bilateral total adrenalectomy gave good initial results, but in about 10–15 per cent of patients a pituitary adenoma revealed itself postoperatively, either by local signs or by the excessive production of both ACTH and melanin stimulating hormone (MSH) leading to gross pigmentation—Nelson's syndrome.

Ectopic ACTH syndrome

Cushing's syndrome may be due to ACTH produced by tumours other than pituitary adenomas. The commonest of these is oat cell carcinoma of the bronchus, but many others have been described including bronchial carcinoid, thymoma, medullary carcinoma of thyroid and islet cell tumour of the pancreas. The syndrome in these patients is rapidly progressive and usually fatal within a few weeks or months. Adrenocorticotrophic hormone levels are usually very high, much greater than with pituitary-dependent Cushing's syndrome and are not suppressed with dexamethasone. The adrenals are generally very much larger than in pituitary-related hyperplasia and weights of over 20 g are not uncommon. The thickened cortex has a distinctive brownish colour and shows great prominence of compact cells which extend from medulla to capsule with only isolated clusters of clear cells.

Removal of the primary tumour producing ACTH is rarely possible and the patients are usually too ill to tolerate bilateral adrenalectomy. Some benefit may result from the drug metyrapone which interferes with the release of cortisol from the adrenal cortex, substance S being released instead.

Adrenal adenoma

About 5–10 per cent of Cushing's syndrome are due to an adrenal adenoma. The biochemical findings are similar to those with carcinoma, but the smaller size of the adenoma on ultrasound or CAT scan may be helpful in the differential diagnosis. Its weight is usually within the 5–20 g range and encapsulation is the rule. The cut surface is yellow with brownish areas or foci of haemorrhage and necrosis. Most lesions have a well differentiated structure with proliferation of fasciculata and reticularis-type cells in varying proportion. Even in the benign lesion, nuclear pleomorphism may occasionally be a marked feature, and on histological criteria the future behaviour of the tumour may be unpredictable. It is for this reason that the pathologist may express some difficulty in interpreting frozen sections during surgery. Bilateral cortical atrophy accompanies the lesion and it may be many months before the patient becomes independent of exogenous cortisol after the tumour is removed. The long-term prognosis, however, is excellent: virtually all patients ultimately becoming cortisone-independent.

Adrenal carcinoma

This tumour accounts for a few cases of Cushing's syndrome and is usually considerably larger than an adenoma (100–1000 g), but the syndrome is not necessarily more severe as large malignant tumours are often biologically relatively inefficient. Macroscopically, the growth may appear lobulated, well encapsulated, soft in consistency and with a greyish yellow colouration. It tends to invade neighbouring structures and metastasizes to lymph nodes, liver and lungs. Histologically, there is variation in the degree of differentiation; some tumours showing a close resemblance to the normal gland structure, yet recurring after removal, whilst others with a bizarre pleomorphic appearance may behave less aggressively than their histological appearance would suggest. Large size, necrosis, mitotic activity and capsular invasion are the most valid criteria of malignancy. Electron microscopy cannot distinguish with certainty between benign and malignant tumours.

Localization of adrenal tumours is simple and precise with modern radiological techniques, the CAT scanner being of particular value. Isotope-labelled iodocholesterol is selectively concentrated by the adrenal cortex and readily demonstrates a tumour. The prognosis in carcinoma is poor, nearly all cases ultimately recurring. Some benefit may be derived from the use of Orthopara DDD, a drug which specifically causes necrosis of the adrenal cortical cells. Unfortunately it has a high degree of systemic toxicity.

Hyperaldosteronism

When hypertension is associated with low levels of potassium—less than 3 mmol/litre—an excess of aldosterone secretion must be suspected, provided other causes can be excluded, in particular, treatment with diuretics, Cushing's syndrome and the use of steroid-like drugs, in which aldosterone levels remain normal.

Primary aldosteronism

In Conn's syndrome or primary aldosteronism, the degree of hypertension is usually only moderate and is accompanied by muscular weakness, intermittent tetany, polyuria and polydipsia. In the great majority of cases the cause is a benign cortical adenoma which is generally small, frequently less than 3 cm in diameter. It may project above the surface of the gland or be deeply buried within its substance, making its recognition at operation difficult. The cut surface of the adenoma is characteristically orange-yellow in colour. In a few cases there may be bilateral cortical hyperplasia with or without nodules, or very rarely a carcinoma. Rarely, the gland may appear normal macroscopically. The histological structure of an adenoma is difficult to correlate with its functional activity, the cells often appearing fasciculata in type, but ultrastructurally glomerulosa, fasciculata and hybrid cells have been identified, the latter showing the mitochondrial features of the other two cell types. In the apparently normal gland, focal proliferations of glomerulosa-type cells may be identified. A renal biopsy should be taken at operation since there is evidence, especially in the older age groups, that renal vascular changes, if well established, may perpetuate the hypertension postoperatively.

Aldosterone can be measured by immunoassay of peripheral blood or samples obtained by catheterization of the adrenal veins and it is extractable from the tumour. Adrenal vein sampling is not entirely safe; it may lead to infarction of the gland. Aldosterone secretion can be suppressed by spironolactone. A low plasma renin is usually demonstrable following moderate volume depletion with frusemide.

Secondary hyperaldosteronism

Secondary hyperaldosteronism is due to renin-angiotensin stimulation as a result of hypovolaemia or renal ischaemia, for example in renal artery stenosis. Some renal tumours, including renal carcinoma, Wilm's tumour and haemangiopericytoma, may secrete renin and thus activate aldosterone. In secondary hyperaldosteronism, renin levels are raised, but they are normal or low with primary aldosteronism. Deoxycorticosterone acetate (DOCA) inhibits aldosterone secretion in normal individuals and those with secondary aldosteronism, but has no effect on those with tumours. This drug forms the basis of a test to differentiate primary from secondary aldosteronism.

Spironolactone is a useful drug as it inhibits aldosterone. It is therefore not necessary to operate on all small benign tumours or on patients with hyperplasia. If hypertension is not relieved by large doses of spironolactone, removal of a tumour is probably not worthwhile as the hypertension is irreversible.

Virilism

The adrenogenital syndrome

In infants and young children this is generally due to adrenal cortical hyperplasia and the adrenals may be greatly enlarged, up to or above 30 g in weight. Macroscopically, they have a typical convoluted appearance, and most of the enlarged cortex is brownish in colour, correlating histologically with a proliferation of reticularis-type cells. The appearances are those of an ACTH-stimulated gland, which is indeed the case, since there is lack of a specific hydroxylating enzyme, with defective production of cortisol and accumulation of androgens. In the infant male this results in macrogenitosomia praecox—the infant Hercules—and in the female infant, pseudohermaphroditism. The condition can be controlled by cortisone therapy. In older children, virilism is more likely to be due to tumour, either an adenoma or carcinoma, which secretes androgens autonomously, the effects depending on the age and sex of the patient. Adenomas range in weight from 30–300 g and are generally reddish brown in colour, due to proliferation of compact cells. Unlike the adenomas of Cushing's syndrome there is no atrophy of the iso or contralateral adrenal cortex. There is an increased secretion of 17 ketosteroids and testosterone, which in these cases will not be inhibited by cortisone therapy.

Very rarely an adrenal carcinoma may secrete oestrogen leading to feminization and testicular atrophy in adult males.

The adrenal medulla

Phaeochromocytoma

Phaeochromocytoma is a rather rare tumour of the medulla which is usually benign, but may be malignant and may metastasize to lymph nodes and lungs. About 10 per cent of tumours are malignant, but they may be slow-growing and patients often live for many years. Whilst usually single, about 10 per cent are multiple or bilateral, and as many as 20 tumours have been described in a single patient. There may be an association with other endocrine abnormalities, notably medullary carcinoma of the thyroid. When the latter is accompanied by mucocutaneous lesions of neuromatous type, especially around the tip of the tongue and sometimes in the gut, the condition is known as Sipple's syndrome.

About 20 per cent of all phaeochromocytomata arise in chromaffin tissue outside the adrenal glands, in the organ of Zuckerkandl, related to the origin of the inferior mesenteric artery, or at the hilum of the kidney, in the bladder wall and sometimes even in the thorax or the neck. There is a greater risk of malignany in extra-adrenal tumours.

The tumour secretes catecholamines, usually a mixture of adrenaline and noradrenaline, but the latter tends to predominate. Extra-adrenal tumours, if active, generally secrete only noradrenaline. The dominating clinical feature is hypertension. In about half, the hypertension is sustained, but in the remainder it is episodic; episodes being associated with headache, sweating and sometimes intense vasospasm causing peripheral cyanosis. The hypertension may be sufficiently severe to cause cerebral haemorrhage or cardiac failure.

Paroxysmal hypotension may be the only blood pressure abnormality in rare cases, related to excess adrenaline secretion. The diagnosis depends upon the measurement of catecholamines or their metabolites in urine or blood. The most generally used test is measurement of total catecholamines in a 24-hour specimen of urine. In the normal individual, catecholamines should be less than 1.0 μg per 24 hours. Since secretion is episodic, there is advantage in measuring catecholamines in a 24-hour specimen, thus diminishing the risk of a false negative; it is advisable to repeat the estimation at least three times. When the patient is manifestly in an attack, it is useful to be able to measure the blood levels. These measurements should not be made when patients are taking methyldopa or other antihypertensive drugs. Many clinicians prefer to measure the excretion of the degradation products, particularly vanylmandelic acid (VMA), but also occasionally the phenylglycols. It is important to note that high levels may be due to the consumption of large quantities of bananas, coffee, tea, chocolate, vanilla flavouring, aspirins, sulphonamides and tetracycline.

Two more sophisticated tests have been introduced, a radio-enzymatic assay and high-pressure liquid chromatography; these methods may be particularly applicable to small blood samples obtained by venous sampling from the vena cava, renal or adrenal veins. These new tests are complicated and available only in a few biochemical laboratories in the more specialized centres.

In the past, localization of phaeochromocytoma depended mainly on angiography, venography and venous sampling, but these are now largely replaced by CAT scan and ultrasound. Symptomatic tumours are almost always 2 cm or more in diameter and easily demonstrated. A recent

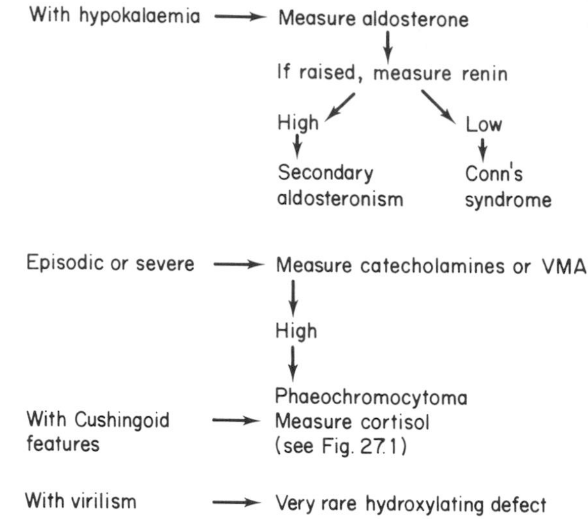

Fig. 27.2 The investigation of hypertension.

localizing technique involves the use of I^{131} metaiodobenzylguanidine (MIBG). This isotope is selectively concentrated by medullary tissue, and scans are particularly valuable in the detection of ectopic tumours. This isotope may also be used therapeutically in malignant tumours with metastases.

The tumour presents as a rounded discrete mass of variable size, but with an average weight of 100 g. The cut surface is light brown in colour, perhaps showing areas of fibrous trabeculation, haemorrhage or cystic degeneration. When surgery is contemplated, close collaboration between surgeon and pathologist is essential to ensure proper processing of the tissue. The tumour assumes a deep mahogany colour after formalin fixation and the cells have an affinity for chromate salts, which can be demonstrated by appropriate fixation in a chromate—dichromate solution. Histochemical methods may be used to identify catecholamines and assay of tumour tissue generally reveals a high concentration, with noradrenaline usually predominating. Noradrenaline and adrenaline secreting cells can be distinguished from each other electromicroscopically by the structure of the catecholamine granules. There are no absolute histological features which would justify a diagnosis of malignancy, not even the presence of vascular invasion. Nuclear and cellular pleomorphism is quite common in benign lesions and may be lacking in malignant variants. The only criterion of malignancy is the finding of metastases in sites not normally occupied by chromaffin tissue.

As in Conn's syndrome, it is of some value at

operation to take a renal biopsy to evaluate the degree of vascular change secondary to the hypertension. If this is severe, hypertension may be perpetuated despite the removal of the tumour and its persistence need not be indicative of recurrence.

Adrenal medullary hyperplasia

The existence of bilateral medullary hyperplasia is now accepted. It may occur as an isolated entity. In multiple endocrine adenomatosis (MEA) Type II with a gross tumour in one adrenal, there may be hyperplasia on the other side so bilateral adrenalectomy is advocated even when there is no gross abnormality in one gland. When no phaeochromoctyoma is found at operation, the tail of the gland should be examined by frozen section to identify medullary tissue which is normally absent in this zone.

When hyperplasia is suspected, morphometric studies should be carried out on the resected gland to confirm a significant decrease in the corticomedullary ratio. Cellular pleomorphism has been noted in some cases.

The pancreatic islets and gut hormones

Introduction

The normal pancreatic islets produce insulin, glucagon, somatostatin and pancreatic polypeptide. Tumours of islets can produce not only these hormones, but several others including gastrin. These tumours, and endocrine-secreting tumours arising from the gut, have been called "apudomas", a term derived from the histochemical properties of the constituent cells—Amine Precursor Uptake Decarboxylase. The cells of origin are derived from the neural crest.

Although some islet cell tumours such as insulinoma and gastrinoma present with dramatic symptoms, others such as glucagonoma, somatostatinoma and pancreatic polypeptideoma may present with minimal symptoms. Some of these patients may undergo laparotomy, the surgeon believing the tumour to be an ordinary adenocarcinoma. It is important that the possibility of an endocrine origin should always be borne in mind. This can be proved or refuted by fasting hormone screens to include all the known peptides secreted by islet cell and gut endocrine tumours. At laparotomy, even though the tumour is inoperable, a biopsy should always be taken. This, in a skilled pathologist's hands, should differentiate between an exocrine and an endocrine tumour. This is important as the prognosis and management of endocrine tumours are entirely different from exocrine cancers and even those with liver metastases may live for several years because the rate of growth is often slow.

Investigation and diagnosis

Many surgeons regard the pancreas as a treacherous organ and are reluctant to take biopsies lest a fistula should result. With a properly taken needle biopsy this risk can be almost eliminated. If the tumour is in the head of the pancreas, the needle should be passed through both lateral and medial duodenal walls. If a pancreatic duct is inadvertently opened, any fistula caused will drain harmlessly into the duodenal lumen.

The criteria for the diagnosis of an endocrine tumour are:

1. The presence of the clinical syndrome.
2. Demonstration of high levels of the appropriate hormone in peripheral blood.
3. Demonstration of the tumour either radiologically or at operation.
4. A characteristic histological appearance.
5. The demonstration of hormone in the tumour by specific immunohistochemistry or assay of hormone in the tumour tissue.
6. Demonstration of characteristic secretory granules by electron microscopy.

It is unusual for all these criteria to be satisfied, but all should be attempted as this will lead to improved understanding and management. Inadequate investigation can lead to misdiagnosis and inappropriate management. Correct diagnosis requires close collaboration between the clinician and the laboratory. Proper technology for endocrine diagnosis is not available in every hospital laboratory so contact may have to be made with supraregional assay services. It is helpful if the laboratories involved prepare protocols which the clinicians can easily follow. The conditions for taking blood and the handling of tissue samples should be strictly followed, otherwise results may be invalid.

Blood samples for hormone assay

The conditions of sampling vary from hormone to hormone so no single set of instructions can be given. Hormone levels can be altered by many factors including fasting, feeding and diurnal rhythm. It is important, therefore, that standard basal conditions for the hormone under study should be adopted. Many hormones are subject to degradation and require careful handling to prevent loss; this may require storage and transport at 0°C in special containers.

In some tumour syndromes, peripheral circulating levels of hormone may show wide fluctuation and on occasion may be normal. Several samples, perhaps a minimum of three, should therefore be taken when there is a strong suspicion of a syndrome. Various dynamic and stimulatory tests can add further information and sharpen the diagnosis. These include the influence of feeding, fasting and stimulation or suppression by various drugs.

Table 27.1 Table of normal fasting values for hormone assays in our laboratory.

Insulin	3–15 mU/litre
Gastrin	< 100 ng/litre
Glucagon	
N terminal assay	< 250 ng/litre
C terminal assay	< 100 ng/litre
Pancreatic polypeptide	< 100 ng/litre (rises with age)
Somatostatin	< 100 ng/litre
Vasoactive intestinal polypeptide	< 150 ng/litre

Usually it is practicable only to obtain samples of peripheral venous blood. It is, however, sometimes possible to obtain regional venous samples from around the site of the suspected tumour, either before or at operation. The finding of gradients of hormone levels in the veins draining the tumour may help localization. At operation, regional venous sampling with rapid (half to one hour) assay may help the localization of tumours which are too small for the surgeon to palpate.

Handling of the tumour

Tissue removed at operation is normally fixed in formalin, but this makes comprehensive investigation of hormone-secreting tumours impossible. It is suggested that tumour tissue should be handled in the following four ways:

1. Part should be routinely fixed for conventional histopathology.
2. Part should be fixed appropriately for endocrine-specific histochemistry. The fixatives used vary from centre to centre, so the surgeon should consult the specialist pathologist. This tissue must not be frozen since freezing destroys its immunoreactivity.
3. Part should be appropriately fixed for electron microscopy, in an attempt to assess the type of secretory granules present in the tumour.
4. Part should be frozen as rapidly as possible, i.e. in liquid nitrogen. This tissue can be subsequently extracted for hormone assay. Various parts of the tumour, both primary and metastatic, should be sampled, as hormone levels vary markedly from one site to another, and there may even be different hormones in different areas.

If tissue samples are to be dealt with correctly, it is important that the surgeon should contact the laboratory before operation, and that a member of the laboratory staff should be present at operation to collect tumour tissue and process it appropriately.

Hypoglycaemia

Reactive hypoglycaemia is not uncommon in postgastrectcomy patients and is often described as "late dumping". Hypoglycaemia also occurs after ingestion of alcohol; neither has any known endocrine background. It may also be due to anterior pituitary or adrenal hypofunction, hepatic disease or, rarely, to the action of certain mesodermal tumours, such as retroperitoneal fibroma, mesothelioma or haemangiopericytoma, which secrete an insulin-like growth factor.

Insulinoma

Insulin excess of pancreatic origin may be due to an islet cell tumour, arising from the beta cells, and it is this tumour that is of great interest to the surgeon. About 90 per cent of insulinomas are benign and 90 per cent are single. Benign tumours are seldom more than 1–2 cm in diameter. Multiple tumours are found in multiple endocrine adenomatosis (MEA) Type I, and are often associated with parathyroid adenomata.

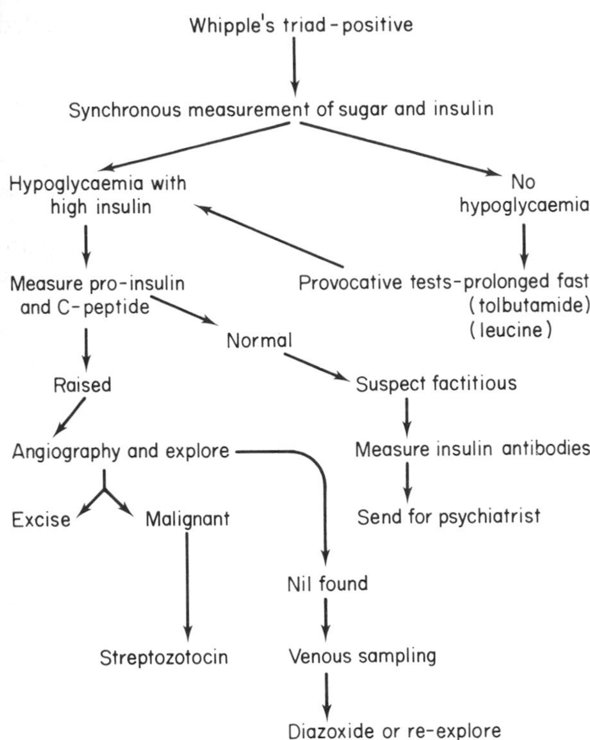

Fig. 27.3 The investigation of spontaneous hypoglycaemia.

The diagnosis of insulinoma is based on Whipple's triad: the symptoms of hypoglycaemia associated with fasting, a low blood sugar level, and relief of symptoms by intravenous or oral administration of glucose. The symptoms of hypoglycaemia are varied and often bizarre: clouding of consciousness, strange behaviour and difficulty in rousing are common.

The investigation of organic hypoglycaemia hinges on the linkage of blood sugar with insulin levels measured by immunoassay. Normally, low blood sugar is associated with low insulin levels and high blood sugar with high insulin levels. With insulinomas, however, the insulin level remains high and is inappropriate to the blood sugar level. This finding is the key to diagnosis. An inappropriately high insulin level does not prove the presence of an insulin-secreting tumour of the pancreas. There have been many instances of factitious hypoglycaemia in individuals, usually nurses, doctors or paramedicals who inject themselves with insulin for obscure reasons. They will develop antibodies to commercial insulin. A more sophisticated test is to measure pro-insulin and C-peptide. C-peptide is that part of the pro-insulin molecule that is split off to leave active insulin, but is also secreted as a separate entity in equimolar amounts with insulin. Both are precursors of insulin produced freely by tumours but not associated with injected commercial insulin. Hypoglycaemia may also be factitiously produced by the sulphonylurea group of drugs, for example tolbutamide. It is possible in suspicious cases to estimate blood levels of these drugs.

It is not always easy to demonstrate hypoglycaemia. The most effective measure is prolonged fasting—up to 72 hours in some cases—with vigorous exertion at the end of the fast to accentuate any lowering of blood sugar. Many other tests have been used, but most are now only of historical interest. Tolbutamide has been used to precipitate hypoglycaemia, but may be dangerous; l-leucine, glucagon and calcium infusion have all been recommended to stimulate release of insulin and hence hypoglycaemia, but none is widely used today. (*see* Fig. 27.3.)

Estimation of glycosylated haemoglobin (HbA_1) has been suggested as a measure of hypoglycaemia at some time during the weeks preceding sampling, but is probably of no clinical value. Suppression of endogenous insulin can be achieved using fish insulin. The assay specifically detects endogenous insulin, which is not suppressed in insulinoma, whereas fish insulin does not react with the antibodies.

As most insulinomas are small, they may be difficult to find. With good angiography nearly all can be located, but some still elude detection. In the past, blind distal pancreatectomy was advocated on the assumption that there are more islets in the tail of the pancreas than in the head, but insulinomas are in fact equally distributed throughout the pancreas.

If liver metastases occur, the problem will be the control of hypoglycaemia. Diazoxide which suppresses insulin release is often helpful and there may be good results from the use of streptozotocin, a drug which is specifically toxic to the islet cells; it is also nephrotoxic and must be used with great care.

The great majority of insulinomas are benign, and only about 15 per cent are malignant. Multiple tumours are found in MEA and are often associated with pituitary and parathyroid adenomata. Benign tumours are seldom more than 1–2 cm in size. They may be deeply buried in the pancreas or present superficially as grey to pink nodules which feel soft, firm or even hard, according to the amount of collagenous stroma. Malignant variants are usually softer and more haemorrhagic than benign lesions. The surgeon may get the impression that the tumour shells out easily, but it is rarely well encapsulated and at the microscopic level tends to engulf the surrounding acini, an appearance which must not be interpreted as malignant infiltration. Indeed, the evaluation of malignancy is often impossible in the absence of metastases in lymph nodes, liver or elsewhere. When malignant, the rate of growth is often very slow.

Pancreatic and gut endocrine tumours have been divided into four main histological groups in an attempt to correlate light microscopic findings with granule staining, immunocytochemical reactions and electron-microscopical findings.

The insulinomas commonly present a trabecular or ribbon pattern of growth, but the cells may be arranged in solid alveoli. Beta granules can usually be demonstrated in the cells with differential staining. The amount of granulation is variable and there may be mixed populations of cells in those tumours which secrete more than one hormone. For localization of insulin, immunofluorescence may be used, and with electronmicroscopy, granules in the cells have a specific structure. The results of radioimmunoassay are the final arbiter of the function of the tumour.

Nesidioblastosis

In infants, diffuse islet cell hyperplasia, with or without microadenomas, causes severe hypoglycaemia, neuroglycopenia and brain damage. Subtotal pancreatectomy gives good results. There is some doubt whether true beta-cell hyperplasia exists in adults, though islet cell adenomatosis is recognized.

Hyperglycaemia

Glucagonoma

Glucagon is secreted by the alpha cells of the islets. Tumours secreting this hormone are rare. They are characterized by mild diabetes, anaemia and a curious painful skin rash particularly affecting the lower abdomen and the perineum. This necrolytic migratory erythema often leads to the patient being first seen by a dermatologist. The rash may improve spontaneously with bed rest and its cause is unknown. The majority of tumours described have been malignant. Diagnosis depends upon the finding of raised levels of glucagon in the blood. Occasionally this syndrome may not have been recognized when a pancreatic tumour is found by chance at laparotomy.

Although most glucagonomas are malignant, the macroscopic or light microscopic appearances do not differ essentially from those of insulinoma and other islet cell tumours. Alpha-secreting granules may be identified by differential and immunostaining, and electromicroscopy may confirm their nature. Radioimmunoassay gives a positive result for glucagon, but as with other functional islet cell tumours, glucagon may be only one of several hormones produced.

Aggressive peptic ulcer

The Zollinger–Ellison syndrome (ZES)

Aggressive, often multiple, peptic ulcers sometimes in unusual sites such as the distal duodenum and jejunum, may be associated with very high acid levels due to an excess of gastrin. Classically, this is due to an islet cell tumour which may be large, often with metastases in local lymph nodes or liver; occasionally the tumour is found in the duodenal wall and may be quite small. The diagnosis depends upon awareness and appropriate biochemical investigations.

Usually the diagnosis is not made until ulceration has recurred after one or more operations, but it is obviously desirable to make the correct diagnosis before the first operation. This can only be guaranteed if acid studies and gastrin assay are performed preoperatively in every patient with peptic ulcer. Except perhaps in a few specialized centres this is scarcely practicable. Nevertheless, a careful assessment of the clinical features often leads to a suspicion of ZES (*see* Fig. 27.4).

Acid levels, in the basal state, greater than 15 mmol/hour will lead to suspicion, and levels around 100 mmol are virtually diagnostic. Between these levels the diagnosis depends upon the ratio of basal to stimulated acid, using the conventional pentagastrin test. If the basal acid level is as much as 60 per cent of the stimulated level, there is almost certainly a tumour. Acid levels only infer the presence of the syndrome; proof depends upon estimation of gastrin. Sometimes, however, these levels are close to the normal range and repeated sampling may be required before a definite result can be obtained.

Provocative tests tend to be more misleading

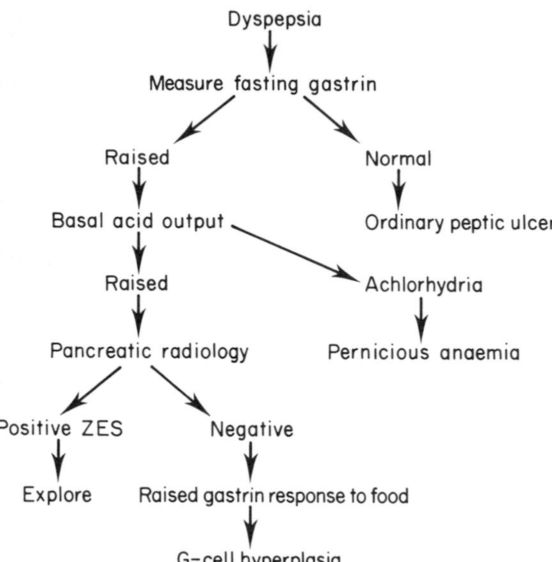

Fig. 27.4 The investigation of dyspepsia.

than useful. Secretin is said to produce a sharp rise in gastrin in ZES, but in our experience secretin often gives rise to false negatives and false positives and is therefore unreliable. Stimulation by a standard mixed meal usually shows little increase of gastrin levels in ZES, but there is considerable overlap with the normal and the test is probably not of great value.

Localization is largely by ultrasound and CAT scanning. Angiography is of little benefit as these tumours do not blush like insulinomas. The reason is not clear as there is no obvious difference in the vascularity of the two types of tumour.

About 90 per cent of Zollinger–Ellison tumours are malignant and ultimately metastasize. They may arise primarily in other sites such as the stomach or duodenum. Multiple tumours are frequently a component of the MEA syndrome. Histologically, they do not differ in structure from other islet cell tumours, despite their high rate of malignancy. There is controversy about the cell of origin; some tumours contain cells with secretory granules typical for human antral G-cells, which could be explicable embryologically on the foregut origin of pancreatic endocrine tissue. Immunohistological investigation not infrequently demonstrates the production of other hormones, for example pancreatic peptide, and electron microscopically the cell population is often mixed. Gastrin production is confirmed by radioimmunoassay of the tumour tissue.

G-cell hyperplasia

There is a group of patients with aggressive peptic ulcers and high levels of acid and gastrin in whom no tumour can be found, even at laparotomy. In some, at least, of these cases, there may be excess production of gastrin by the G-cells of the antrum and the ulcer diathesis may be cured by antrectomy. The diagnosis rests on finding hypergastrinaemia and high basal secretion of acid similar to the Zollinger–Ellison Syndrome. Usually, however, the levels of fasting gastrin and acid secretion are not as great as in the ZES. Characteristically they show dramatic rises in gastrin levels after food. Unfortunately, it is usually histologically impossible to prove the existence of G-cell hyperplasia, or "hyperfunction" as Morton Grossman insisted that it should be called, prior to surgery, as G-cells are randomly distributed in the antrum so that biopsies give a patchy distribution. If the diagnosis is strongly suspected, then the logical approach is antrectomy which should result in reduction of gastrin levels to very low levels. The antrum can then be examined for the presence or absence of excessive numbers of G-cells.

Diarrhoea

There are a number of endocrine causes of persistent and often severe diarrhoea. Diabetes mellitus, thyrotoxicosis and medullary carcinoma of thyroid are all important causes, but will not be further considered in this chapter. Diarrhoea may be prominent in the Zollinger–Ellison syndrome which has already been considered. Tumours secreting vasoactive intestinal peptide or serotonin are rare but important causes and will now be considered. (Fig. 27.5.)

The Verner–Morrison (WDHA) syndrome

This is a rare clinical syndrome in which a tumour, usually arising in the pancreas, causes Watery Diarrhoea, Hypokalaemia and Achlorhydria. The diarrhoea characteristically is profuse but inoffensive; the term "pancreatic cholera" has been used. Potassium levels are low and gastric acidity is low or absent. The causative tumours of islet cell type secrete vasoactive intestinal peptide (VIP) which also causes dilatation of the gall bladder, palmar erythema and spider naevi.

As with other apudomata, these tumours, though usually malignant, are slow-growing even after metastasis to lymph nodes and liver. They

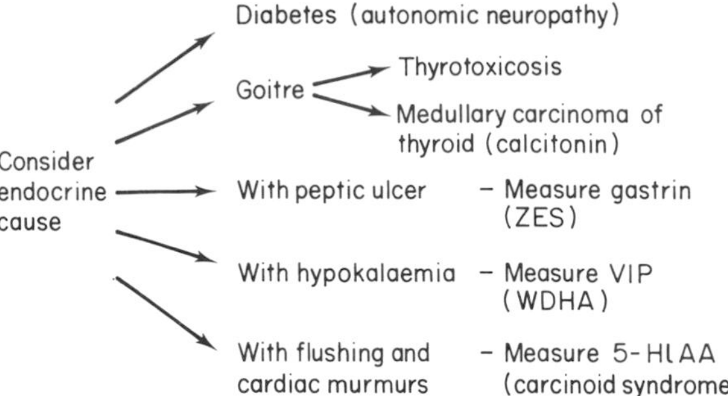

Fig. 27.5 The investigation of prolonged and unexplained diarrhoea.

often secrete pancreatic polypeptide in addition to VIP. These hormones can be demonstrated immunohistologically and by extraction. The tumours are particularly sensitive to treatment with streptozotocin.

Carcinoid tumours

These tumours arise from neuroendocrine cells in the gut, bronchial tree and, rarely, other sites. They are usually yellowish in colour and quite small; those greater than 2 cm in diameter have a much higher malignant potential. An association with other malignant neoplasms has been reported.

The commonest site of origin is the appendix where the tumour presents as a small firm yellowish nodule and very seldom metastasizes. Appendicular carcinoids, especially if proximally situated, may cause symptoms due to obstruction and appendicitis, but some are an incidental finding. The second commonest site is the ileum where the tumours are generally quite small and often multiple, 20 or more nodules sometimes being found. These nodules are usually submucous but, rarely, may ulcerate and cause gross haemorrhage or may lead to intussusception. The tumour infiltrates the muscle coat and there is associated muscle hypertrophy, fibrosis and elastosis, leading to distortion and intestinal obstruction. Carcinoids of stomach and rectum may cause symptomless nodules or present with metastases. In the latter site the carcinoid syndrome is very rare, and metastatic spread is less common than with ileal tumours.

Malignancy is demonstrated by local invasion especially of perineural lymphatics, and metastases to lymph nodes and liver eventually develop. Occasionally there are metastases to lung, bone and brain. Carcinoid tumours are often extremely slow-growing and survival for five or even 10 years after the appearance of liver metastases is in no way exceptional. Apart from those cases which produce appendicitis or small bowel obstruction, these tumours are seldom detected until they produce the carcinoid syndrome. Carcinoids have the capacity to liberate 5-hydroxytryptamine and kinins, but these substances are metabolized in the liver. It is only when they are secreted directly into the inferior vena cava, as with liver metastases, or the systemic circulation, as in bronchial carcinoids, that the syndrome occurs. Even in the presence of liver metastases the syndrome only develops in about half the cases.

The salient features of the syndrome are attacks of flushing of the face, neck and chest, bouts of diarrhoea with frequent watery stools and lesions of the right heart. The latter consist mainly of fibrosis of the tricuspid and pulmonary valves with associated murmurs. The syndrome ultimately leads to cardiac failure.

Unfortunately, the various chemical diagnostic tests are not very reliable. 5-hydroxyindoleacetic acid (5-HIAA) only becomes elevated when malignant tumours have metastasized to the liver, and even then it is not invariably elevated. For this reason, other markers of the tumour have to be sought. The estimation of plasma serotonin is probably more valuable and accurate than that of urinary products, but is only available in a few specialized centres. In a search for peptide markers, substance P may be the most promising.

Most carcinoids present a histological structure which is readily identifiable by the pathologist and in some cases is similar to that of the islet cell tumours already described. Various histochemical and other techniques are of value in their further study. These include the argentaffin and argyrophil reaction, the tissue requiring to be freshly fixed in formalin, the alkaline diazo-coupling reaction, formaldehyde-induced fluorescence, ferric ferricyanide reduction and electronmicroscopy. The most consistently positive reactions are found with appendicular and ileal tumours.

Other endocrine tumours

Other tumours have been described, for example somatostatinoma and pancreatic polypeptideoma, but no characteristic clinical syndrome has been defined. Adrenocorticotrophic hormone, antidiuretic hormone and calcitonin may all be ectopically secreted by islet cell tumours. There remain a number of endocrine tumours as yet uncharacterized with respect to their hormonal secretion and clinical syndrome. There seems little doubt that further syndromes will be recognized in the future.

Further reading

The adrenal glands

Montgomery DAD, Welbourn RB. *Medical and Surgical Endocrinology*. London: Edward Arnold, 1975.

Rabin D, McKenna TJ. *Clinical Endocrinology and Metabolism*. New York: Grune and Stratton, 1982.

Sloper JC, Fox B. The adrenal glands. In: *Systemic Pathology*, 2nd ed., Vol. 4. Ed by W. S. Symmers, Edinburgh: Churchill Livingstone, 1978.

Symington T. *Functional Pathology of the Human Adrenal Gland*. Edinburgh and London; E. & S. Livingstone, 1969.

Brennan MF, Keiser HR. Persistent and recurrent phaeochromocytoma. *World J Surg* **6**:397.

Thompson NW, Surgery for Phaeochromoctyoma-Invited Commentary. *World J Surg*, 1982; **6**:397.

Van Heerden JA, Hamberger B, ReMine WH. Phaeochromocytoma. *Surgery* 1982; **91**: 367.

The pancreatic islets and gut hormones

Bloom SR, Polak JM. *Gut Hormones*. Edinburgh: Churchill Livingstone, 1981.

Stoward PJ, Polak JM. *Histochemistry the Widening Horizons*. Chichester: Wiley and Sons, 1981.

Buchanan KD. Gastrointestinal hormones: general concepts. In: *Clinics in Endocrinology and Metabolism. Gastrointestinal Hormones*, 8 (2), 249–63. Ed by K. D. Buchanan. London: W. B. Saunders, 1979.

Buchanan KD. Gut hormones and gut endocrine tumour syndromes. *Br J Hosp Med*. 1980; **24:**190–97.

Modlin I. Endocrine tumours of the pancreas. *Surg Gynecol Obstet*. 1979; **149**:751.

Kennedy T. The management of the hypoglycaemic patient. *World J Surg*. 1982; **6**:718–24.

McCarthy DM. Zollinger–Ellison syndrome. *Ann Rev Med*. 1982; **33**:197–215.

Marks C. *Carcinoid Tumours*. Boston: Hall, 1979.

28

The Skeletal System

P M Yeoman, A W F Lettin, A N Henry and P D Byers

Surgical pathology of the skeletal system

Introduction

There are two different situations in which a knowledge of pathology can contribute: (i) establishing a diagnosis; (ii) treatment. In the first, what is required is an awareness of the similarities that may exist between different classes of lesion, and what constitutes the critical difference between them. In the second, decisions are governed, in part, by an understanding of the pathogenesis and how it is manifested. The surgeon's encounter with a bone lesion is macroscopic: by inspection and palpation, and representation by imaging techniques. If diagnosis is the object, then the widest range of possible explanations of the observations should be considered so that appropriate steps may be taken in refutation or corroboration. If treatment and management are in hand, then it is necessary to know what may be expected in that class of pathology, and of the specific entity.

The classical approach to morbid anatomy and histopathology is through the delineation of pathological processes, mainly by visual means. Their classification and the attention they have attracted has varied according to circumstances and interest over the years.

The surgical pathology of the skeletal system retains the same basic philosophy of the coordination of initial examination and a knowledge of the possible basic underlying pathology which leads to a diagnosis. It varies from elective soft tissue surgery in two ways:

1. Radiology plays a major part in the initial diagnosis.
2. Biopsy may not be conclusive.

Procedures for handling biopsy tissues

The pathologist aims to minimize distortion of tissues in the course of making histological preparations. The two most deleterious factors are rough handling and delay in preservation, both of which are in the control of the surgeons. Normal care of tissues, i.e. gentle handling and early immersion in fixative, are sufficient for conventional histological procedures. To undertake electron microscopy requires that small (a few millimetres) samples of tissue are put quickly and gently into fixative. For many electron microscopists the speed with which this happens is far more important than the fixative, and many find that buffered formalin does very well.

Some histochemical and immunocytochemical procedures require fresh tissue or special fixatives, and to carry out these procedures the pathologist needs to receive the tissue unfixed as soon after removal as possible. Since the histopathologist cannot always know in advance what procedures are eventually going to be required, fresh tissue can be frozen for later reference. But it is also possible to keep a reserve of frozen sections and of tissue imprints.

Frozen section technique is useful not only for the rapidity with which sections can be prepared, but also for the minimal interference with chemical structure and activity, especially of enzymes. Tissue imprints offer similar advantages. The technique of their preparation is simple: the cut surface of the tissue is touched on a clean glass slide and the adherent cells are immediately dried by waving the slide in air. Many samples can quickly and easily be prepared and stored for later use. A variety of procedures for cell identification can be applied to these cytological preparations, just as to frozen sections.

Diagnostic procedures

The histological contribution to tumour diagnosis is to establish the identity of the tissue with that of one item of a tumour classification. The basic technique is by histological study of paraffin-embedded tissue, which necessitates decalcification. Two components in the section are of principal interest: the cells, and the intercellular matrix, if any. Sections are conveniently and traditionally visualized in the first instance by haemotoxylin and eosin staining. The attributes of the individual cells are established (in a manner similar to cytological examination), and, if indicated, special stains are used to determine cell content, structure or activity. The methods for this are traditional dyes, histochemical and immunocytochemical methods.

In general, the object is successively to categorize the cell: epithelial versus connective tissue, haematopoietic, or endothelial, and to proceed further to identify within these categories.

Alternatively, or additionally, the intercellular component can be examined. This might be no more than the supporting reticulin fibre network which sometimes can suggest the nature of the tissue, e.g. epithelial versus connective tissue. Intercellular collagen can belong to bone, fibrous tissue or cartilage. The organization of the material, its collagen content and fibre structure (visualized most simply and readily by polarized light), mucopolysaccharide content (a number of stains are sensitive to these) and the tendency to mineralize (in paraffin sections this can only be inferred from the staining characteristics) are all helpful.

In this Chapter the whole subject will be considered under sectional headings; some conditions dealt with are rare, but must be included in order to provide an overall clinical picture leading to recognition, adequate investigation and the eventual proper treatment. The patient will present with pain, swelling, deformity and loss of function, all of which may occur separately or in combination and yet are derived from the various and separate components of the skeletal system.

Bone pain

Bone pain may arise from a wide variety of pathological entities as in the Fig. 28.1 which also incorporates the clinical investigation and management.

Infection

Inflammation is a defensive response to an injurious agent. The response may be classed by its aetiology or its pathogenesis. The former are living organisms, ranging from viruses to protozoa,

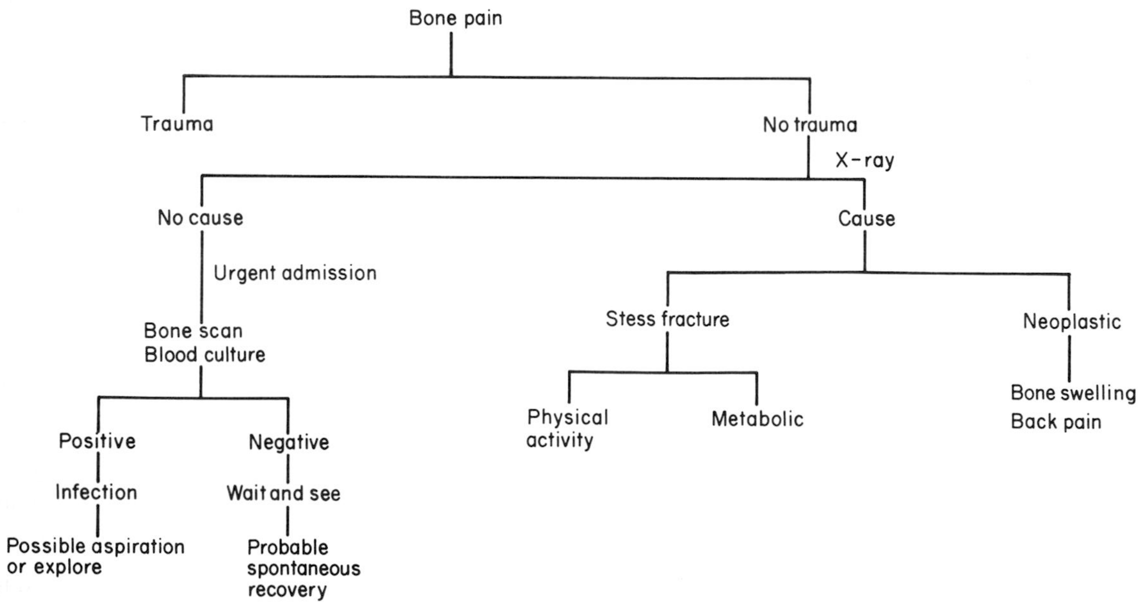

Fig. 28.1 Bone pain.

physical and chemical agents. The latter are:

1. Acute—exudative, pyogenic
2. Chronic—proliferative, granulomatous

Acute, exudative and pyogenic are synonyms. This reaction gives rise to the cardinal signs of inflammation: redness, heat, pain and swelling. The most usual cause is pyogenic bacteria, but some physical and chemical agents may produce a similar picture. The reaction to staphylococci is the prime example of acute inflammation. There is an interval of some hours after penetration of the bacteria in which there is little visible response and when the organisms can multiply and spread; they may even enter the circulation in appreciable numbers without giving rise to other foci. In this interval the bacteria elaborate their toxins and these lead to the release of mediators from cells in the vicinity, in particular from mast cells, and these set in motion the reaction. Existing humoral antibodies in the circulation will assist in containing the organism through bacteriostatic and bactericidal mechanisms. Nevertheless, organisms have a tendency to get into the blood stream throughout the progressive stages of the inflammation, giving rise to the possibility of distant foci of inflammation; trauma is a cause of localization of the circulating bacteria, presumably because of the vascular response.

Osteomyelitis is caused by many organisms and the inflammatory response varies from acute pyogenic to an indolent granulomatous reaction. Occasionally, infection is implanted from an external wound, but the usual route is through the circulation from an already established lesion; the local reaction will follow one of the established patterns of inflammation depending on the toxicity of the organism and the resistance of the host. An isotope bone scan will determine an early lesion, whereas an X-ray will not reveal any abnormality for 2–3 weeks until there is a degree of bone resorption or necrosis.

In the course of the inflammation focal tissue necrosis occurs accompanied by the death of bacteria and of polymorphs. The enzymes released from the cells liquefy the tissue to form pus. The progressive entry of polymorphs and tissue fluids into this leads to extension of the tissue necrosis towards a surface where the pus escapes. The process of resolution and healing then comes to the fore.

The mediators of inflammation are neurogenic and chemical. The former occur quickly in response to physical stimulus—the triple response of Lewis—and finally result in vasodilatation, and escape of fluid from capillaries. The chemical mediators are derived from the plasma or tissues (cells), are numerous, not all of them significant, and are interrelated to some degree. Agents are also present which limit or inhibit the response. The following classes of mediators are recognized:

1. Vasoactive amines—histamine (mast cells, basophils, platelets) serotonin
2. Plasma proteases and polypeptides—kinins, complement, coagulation/fibrinolytic system
3. Prostaglandins and related compounds
4. Products of leukocytes

The osteolytic region is filled with pus or granulation tissue and may later contain a fragment of dead bone known as a sequestrum. The response is non-specific except that an active osteolytic area is more likely in the acute lesions from staphylococcal and haemolytic streptococcal infection. Granulomatous areas are fairly common in tuberculous lesions. The cell pattern at the periphery of an infected area of bone is non-specific and similar to the reaction invoked by neoplastic tissue (see Biopsy, p. 352).

Stress fracture

Repetitive activity which produces an abnormal load on one part of a bone may lead to a stress fracture. It may occur in the tibia in cross-country runners or in ballet dancers; in the humerus in javelin throwers; and classically in the second metatarsal in army recruits, "march fracture", which, in fact, is more common in hikers and in those patients with a short first metatarsal and a relatively long second metatarsal. The physical weakness immediately before stress fracture of a compact bone is not comparable to "metal fatigue" which retains its strength almost to the point of fracture; bone responds by micro-fractures not only of the trabeculae but of the reinforcing fibres.

Metabolic bone disease

In ordinary practice, radiography is used in a qualitative fashion. Quantitative histomorphometry gives reasonably accurate assessments of bone samples. The difficulty with this, as with any other method which samples the skeleton, is to know how representative it is of the whole. In particular, there may be disparities between the axial and appendicular skeleton.

Osteoporosis

Pain in the back particularly in the thoracic region may be associated with idiopathic or secondary osteoporosis. Age-related reduction in bone mass is accompanied by a reduction in bone surface activity (see Other metabolic disorders p. 356). All our understanding points to osteoporosis as the resultant of imbalance between resorption and formation of bone: more is removed than is replaced. As a consequence, the bone becomes less able to sustain the demands upon it. The result may be microfractures, or fractures that are clinically evident. The former lead to callus formation around the individual trabeculum and the complete cycle of healing in miniature. Macroscopic fractures, crushed vertebrae or femoral necks, call forth a healing reaction but progress through the complete cycle is slow and sometimes inefficient.

Localized osteoporosis, such as that which follows immobilization of a limb or in Sudek's atrophy, can develop very rapidly. Histological examination shows a considerable vascular response and substantial osteoclastic activity. In some cases there is even minimal fibrous replacement of bone. There is little associated osteoblastic activity. The appearance in radiographs may be quite striking because of the rate, severity and pattern. Only part of the bone may be affected, especially in long bones where a metaphyseal band can occur. In more diffusely affected parts, multiple discrete small foci give a "raindrop" picture. There may be a problem in neoplastic cases in distinguishing the changes from extension of tumour. As a material, the bone can only be described as soft. It does not present the resistance of normal bone, and may be easily crushed by pressure.

Collapse of one or more vertebral bodies may occur insidiously or as an acute episode, often associated with a minor injury when the pain is frequently severe. There is often an associated kyphosis, especially when more than one vertebral body collapses. There is frequently localized tenderness and the onset is acute.

Diagnosis is usually made radiographically. Generalized loss of bone density and thinning of the cortex of the vertebral bodies is characteristic. The serum calcium, phosphorus and alkaline phosphatase are usually with normal limits. If the diagnosis is in doubt, trephine biopsy of the iliac crest can help to resolve the matter by establishing the fact of reduced bone volume and the absence of other causes (best see opening paragraph). Acute or insidious vertebral collapse does not lead to vertebral instability or pressure on the spinal cord and treatment is symptomatic.

Osteomalacia

Osteomalacia and rickets are brought about by failure in the mineralization of osteoid, which is continually produced at different sites on the bone surfaces as part of the turnover process (see Other metabolic disorders, p. 356). A wide range of causes underly this failure. Moreover, in well developed osteomalacia there is an associated muscle weakness, giving rise to complaints, such as difficulty in rising from a chair and a waddling gait. Symptoms may be complicated by the development of secondary hyperparathyroidism. The mechanism of mineralization has been the subject of much enquiry, which has uncovered a complex system in which the metabolites of vitamin D play a crucial role in the absorption and secretion of calcium and its availability to osteoblasts to implement the mineral deposition. The growing understanding of what happens in the matrix, where mineralization occurs, provides a fascinating story.

In both osteomalacia and rickets the bone changes are similar. What distinguishes rickets is the effect on the epiphyseal plate of vitamin D-deficiency. The growth plate is a coordinated system for production of cartilage matrix, i.e. growth, and its conversion to bone. Interference with any part disturbs the whole. Thus, the failure to mineralize slows the matrix production, retards cell maturation (a prelude to making way for osteoblasts), reduces osteoid apposition on the cartilage lattice by osteoblasts, and upsets the remodelling process of already formed bone. The result is a thick epiphyseal plate, readily visualized by X-ray and a disordered plate structure found on histological study.

The bone changes are explained by continuation of the remodelling/turnover activity of bone cells which results in the production of osteoid that fails to be mineralized. Thus, as the condition continues, the bone (i.e. the mineralized tissue) is progressively resorbed to be replaced by osteoid. This reduced bone density is eventually evident in radiographs. However, the total skeletal tissue (bone + osteoid) is not infrequently greater than normal, so that successful treatment results in a skeleton more dense than normal, a state of affairs subsequently corrected by remodelling.

The reduced radiographic density of the skeleton is usually not distinguishable from that of generalized osteoporosis. The diagnosis is biochemical and histological. The low serum calcium and phosphorus and the usually raised alkaline phosphatase are important features, with other alterations according to stage and first cause.

Histological signs of failure of mineralization are the hallmark of osteomalacia. The most obvious feature is usually the excess of osteoid. This is recognized in undecalcified sections (although it is possible to stain bone first by silver precipitation techniques and then to decalcify, leaving the silver behind as the mineral substitute) as a layer of osteoid on bone. Usually this is so substantial that the abnormality is readily recognized. However, since osteoid seams are a normal aspect of healthy bone a quantitative assessment of minimal abnormality may be required to establish the diagnosis. There are several techniques for doing this, some of which are quick and simple, once the section has been prepared, itself a somewhat slow procedure. But it is also possible to assess and quantify the mineralization process: at the junction between osteoid and bone is the site where mineral is deposited. Tetracycline is incorporated here when the process is active. If a gram of tetracycline is given orally two days before a biopsy, then a fluorescent line will be found in undecalcified sections viewed in ultraviolet light wherever mineral was being deposited. This provides a means of quantitative assessment, which is of great use when the amount of osteoid is on the borderline of normal.

Other metabolic disorders

The conditions generally included under metabolic bone disease are:

- Osteoporosis (*see above*)
- Osteomalacia (*see above*)
- Primary hyperparathyroidism
- Renal osteodystrophy
- Paget's disease of bone
- Fibrogenesis imperfecta ossium

These conditions present problems which ordinarily bring the patient to medical clinics. However, because of some musculoskeletal complaint the first referral may be orthopaedic. This is particularly the case in osteoporosis and Paget's disease. Additionally, a resorptive lesion of hyperparathyroidism, the so called "brown tumour", may present as a bone tumour. Presenting complaints of osteoporosis and osteomalacia have already been referred to. Since these are metabolic disorders, diagnosis and management are based on biochemical analysis. Biopsy is resorted to as an aid to diagnosis, as a means of monitoring progress, and as a research procedure.

The pathogenesis of all these depends on the activity of osteoclasts and osteoblasts. Throughout life, although at rates diminishing with age, a proportion of the available bone surface is undergoing resorption or formation. This activity is generally referred to as bone turnover, a concept which implies a "skeletal half life", estimated at about 10 years (but clearly with a wide variation according to age and constitution). Just as osteoporosis comes about through modification of turnover, and osteomalacia through this and interference with mineral deposition (in which osteoblasts have a key role), so the other disorders are made manifest through skeletal modification by osteoclast and osteoblast activity. These activities can be recognized and quantified in histological sections as can the resulting modification in the architecture and structure of bone. Because osteoclasts can only remove bone (rate, duration and extent of bone surface acted on, are variable), and because osteoblasts can only form bone (rate, duration surface area, osteoid quality (lamellar or woven) are variables) the specificity of the resultant tissue pattern is limited, and must be interpreted in the light of clinical and biochemical findings. Thus, both hyperparathyroidism and Paget's disease are the result of high bone turnover, and may not be histologically distinguishable: the mosaic pattern is brought about by resorption/formation producing small, irregular, packets of new bone, much of which may have an irregular (woven) collagen pattern (as opposed to the usual lamellar structure). Demarcation of a phase of resorption from ensuing apposition is by a very fine line of stainable material, as yet unidentified, referred to as the reversal or cement line. The other features which are used for assessment of metabolic bone disease are the presence of bone cells, if any, on surfaces; fibrous replacement; and features relating to osteocytes.

Neoplasm

It is apparent that what makes a tumour (or any

other bone lesion) visible in a radiograph is a change in bone density. An appreciable alteration, at least 15 per cent, must occur to be detectable on a film. If a process is invasive but does not lead to any bone cell activity then it will not be visible: an excellent example, but not neoplastic, is the population of marrow by lipid-laden macrophages in Gaucher's disease. One of the consequences of this condition may be an infarct of the bone, when the reactive changes involving the bone cells that is thereby induced produce an X-ray image. Neoplasia in bone usually provokes bone resorption, although degrees of the bone formation, which may be dominant occur, but some tumours can permeate marrow with little disturbance of bone cells, e.g. leukaemias and lymphomas, some metastatic carcinomas. In consequence it may be some while before the tell-tale difference in density, which may be an increase and/or decrease, is apparent.

Nothing is known of the control mechanisms that lead to bone cell activity, either in bone or in periosteum. The periosteal reaction roughly parallels that in bone, but a minimal response on the part of the former may well influence the interpretation of appearance in the latter.

Even though we know nothing of the control mechanisms, we do understand that it is the bone cells, osteoclasts and osteoblasts, which effect changes in the bone. Thus an expanding tumour induces osteoclasts to clear the way, and there may be an associated but substantial osteoblastic activity. The net effect is to produce radiographic appearances which allow assessment of the behaviour and character of the tumour. Taken in conjunction with clinical information it is possible to class a neoplasm according to one of the following categories:

1. Stable
2. Growing non-invasive
3. Slowly destructive with or without invasion
4. Rapidly destructive and invasive

Diagnosis

The diagnosis of a bone tumour is best established by a combination of clinician, radiologist, and pathologist who discuss the facts together in order to come to a conclusion. The presenting clinical picture should provide a pattern for subsequent detailed investigation. Bone tumours arise primarily in bone, but also in surrounding tissue or they may spread from other areas. An insidious onset of symptoms is common but the bone may be weakened by a cyst or tumour which may precipitate an acute onset from a pathological fracture. Occasionally, a bone tumour is suspected on a routine radiological survey.

Age

A bone tumour may arise at any age but malignant bone tumours represent 5 per cent of children's cancer. Under the age of five a malignant bone tumour is rare and more likely to be a metastatic neuroblastoma. Osteosarcoma is most common in teenagers: over the age of 50 metastatic tumours are more likely; occasionally malignant changes occur in elderly patients with Paget's disease of bone.

Symptoms

Pain

Relentless pain day and night of gradual onset, is typical of a malignant bone lesion, but it may be virtually asymptomatic until the bone breaks. A dull ache is common and usually confined to the side of the lesion unless there is referred pain from nerve root involvement. Aspirin characteristically relieves the pain produced by an osteoid osteoma, but otherwise pain from bone tumours is notoriously difficult to control by simple analgesia.

Swelling

A swelling arising in bone is most frequently due to a benign cause unless accompanied by unremitting pain. The history and careful clinical examination will provide the most useful information (*see* below); radiological examination is essential but not conclusive; biopsy is rarely necessary in suspected benign lesions.

Shape A spindle-shaped swelling indicates expansion of bone from a lesion inside, but fails to provide much positive proof of the identity of the lesion. By contrast, an eccentrically placed swelling is more in favour of a chondroma, particularly if it is situated near the metaphysis of a long bone. Previous swelling at the same site, or multiple but similar swellings, are again in favour of a cartilage tumour.

Rate of growth A sudden onset of a swelling

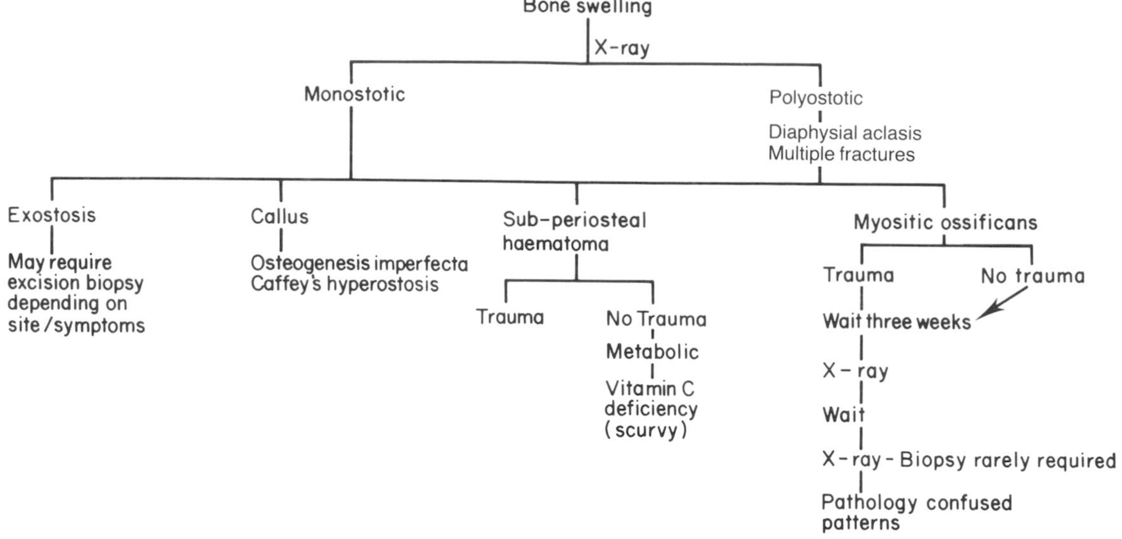

Fig. 28.2 Bone swelling.

does not necessarily indicate a rapidly growing lesion, but perhaps the patient's attention will have been directed to it by receiving a blow in that area. A chondroma often presents in that way, but generally a rapid onset is due either to a reactive lesion or malignant tumour. A recent increase in size of a bony swelling which has been present for many years, is typical of a sarcoma arising in a previous benign chondroma.

Site Associated swelling of a joint is more difficult. In young patients swelling of the knee, for example, may be due to trauma, infection or juvenile rheumatoid arthritis, but of more importance, an effusion may develop as a result of an adjacent osteosarcoma. Generalized swelling of a limb due to a bone tumour is evidence of malignant invasion through the bone cortex with involvement of the venous drainage.

Deformity Collapse of bone from cyst or tumour will cause angulation or gross deformity; previous bowing of limbs may be present in Paget's disease.

Inspection The skin overlying a malignant bone tumour will be stretched, shiny and contain engorged veins; occasionally a bone tumour may ulcerate the skin.

Palpation Most bone tumours feel uniformly firm or hard, depending on the covering soft tissue, but cartilage tumours may have an irregular surface. It is axiomatic that a general examination is made to exclude primary tumours in the thyroid, breast, kidney, and prostate.

Investigation

Pyrexia

A raised temperature for no apparent reason may occur in patients with a carcinoma of the kidney.

Blood

A complete blood picture is mandatory to exclude leukaemia, but a raised plasma viscosity or sedimentation rate indicates a general reaction which should lead to further examination of the plasma proteins and their electrophoretic pattern to exclude myelomatosis.

Urine

A 24-hour specimen is examined for catecholamines to exclude metastatic neuroblastoma.

X-ray

The radiological changes in and around a bone tumour reflect patterns on which a diagnosis can be determined. When a lesion is seen on conventional anterior/posterior and lateral views, it is essential to have further oblique views to ensure adequate inspection of the affected area.

Destruction Cortical bone is a tough structure and destruction of even a small part is usually an indication of a malignant lesion (Fig. 28.3).

Resorption A benign or malignant tumour arising adjacent to bone may cause resorption and a scalloped surface similar to the changes in vertebral bodies alongside an aortic aneurysm or para-aortic lymphadenopathy.

Expansion A localized expanding lesion in bone usually causes thinning of the cortex. It is invariably associated with a slowly growing lesion such as a giant cell tumour (osteoclastoma), but expansion of an entire phalanx or metacarpal is seen in a benign cartilage tumour (enchondroma) (Fig. 28.4).

Osteolysis Generalized loss of bone density is typical of osteoporosis or osteomalacia but a localized lytic lesion is seen in bone cysts (Fig. 28.5) where it is confined to an expanded area of bone. A giant cell tumour usually arises in the metaphysis of a long bone and has a unique predilection for an articular surface, thus causing an expanding lytic lesion advancing on the subchondral area of bone (Fig. 28.6). Multiple lytic, but clearly punched-out lesions, are seen in children with histiocytosis-X or in older patients with myelomatosis. Less well defined lytic areas are of sinister significance and often indicate bone metastases.

Osteosclerosis New bone is laid down around a stress fracture and this may not appear on the radiographs for a month or more after the onset of symptoms which is an indication of the slow turn of events. Dense areas inside the bone may be caused by an infarct. A "bone island" is a small dense bony focus without reaction, an innocent developmental lesion (Fig. 28.7). Areas of localized dense bone may arise on the cortex beneath the periosteum as a reaction to osteoid osteoma, which itself appears as a small round lytic area, possibly centrally mineralized (Fig. 28.8).

Increased density is usually due to deposition of bone by reacting osteoblast and not necessarily to bone formed by tumour cells which is found in osteosarcoma. Multiple areas of bone density are seen in metastatic tumours of which the prostate is the most likely source.

Periosteal reaction Elevation of the periosteum may arise at the margin of a lesion destroying the underlying cortical bone. Eventually new bone is laid down to give the "Codman triangle" seen in classical radiographs of osteosarcoma. Localized periosteal new bone formation occurs in the comparatively rare parosteal osteosarcoma (Fig. 28.9). Layers of periosteal new bone around a circumscribed lesion of the mid-shaft of a long bone gives an "onion-skin" appearance; often seen in Ewing's sarcoma; it is not diagnostic. Diffuse irregular periosteal reaction is more in favour of chronic infection.

Fracture

A pathological fracture is often transverse with smooth margins at the fractured bone ends, or lytic areas and destruction of part of the cortex. A history of comparatively trivial injury is common.

Trabeculation

A uniform coarse trabecular pattern with enlargement of bone, loss of distinction between cortex and medulla and a leading lytic area is typical of Paget's disease (Fig. 28.10). Coarse trabeculation is also seen in an haemangioma of a vertebral body.

Cartilage

Small flecks of mineral deposition are often seen in lytic areas in a chondroblastoma and in enchondromata.

Soft tissue

Expansion of a bone tumour into the surrounding soft tissue can be shown by different penetrations of the X-ray technique and this will be important not only in the diagnosis but future surgical management.

Skeletal survey

Multiple bone lesions may be revealed which will rule out many primary bone tumours except those arising from the cartilage cap of multiple exostoses in diaphysical aclasis. Multiple bone lesions are seen in fibrous dysplasia.

Chest X-ray

Bronchial carcinoma is common and must be excluded; a routine chest X-ray may reveal a pleural effusion or abnormality of the rib cage. Metastases from a primary bone tumour are usually multiple and typically rounded opacities giving a "cannonball" appearance.

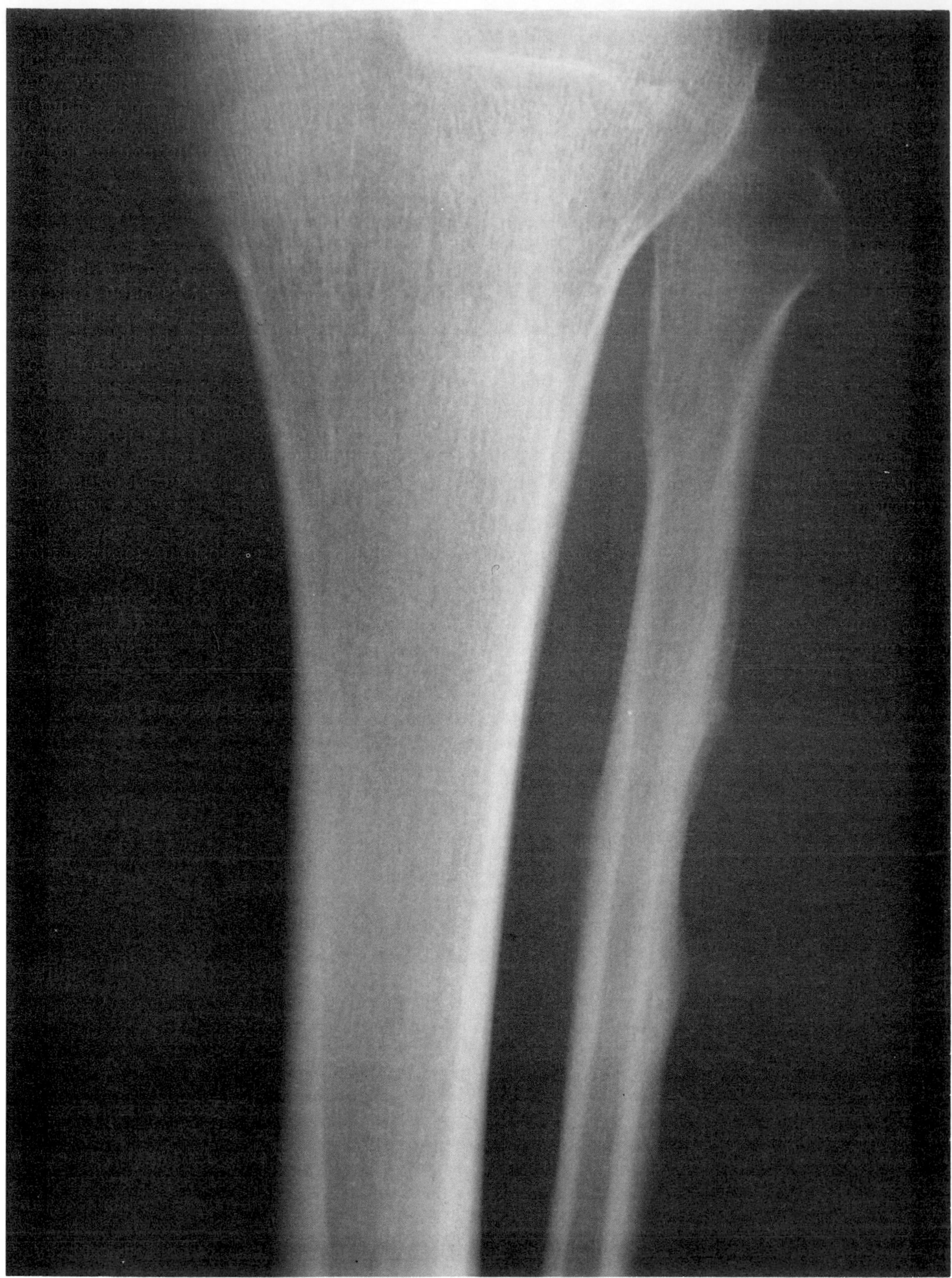

Fig. 28.3 Destruction of part of the cortex of the fibula due to a fibrosarcoma of the adjacent soft tissues.

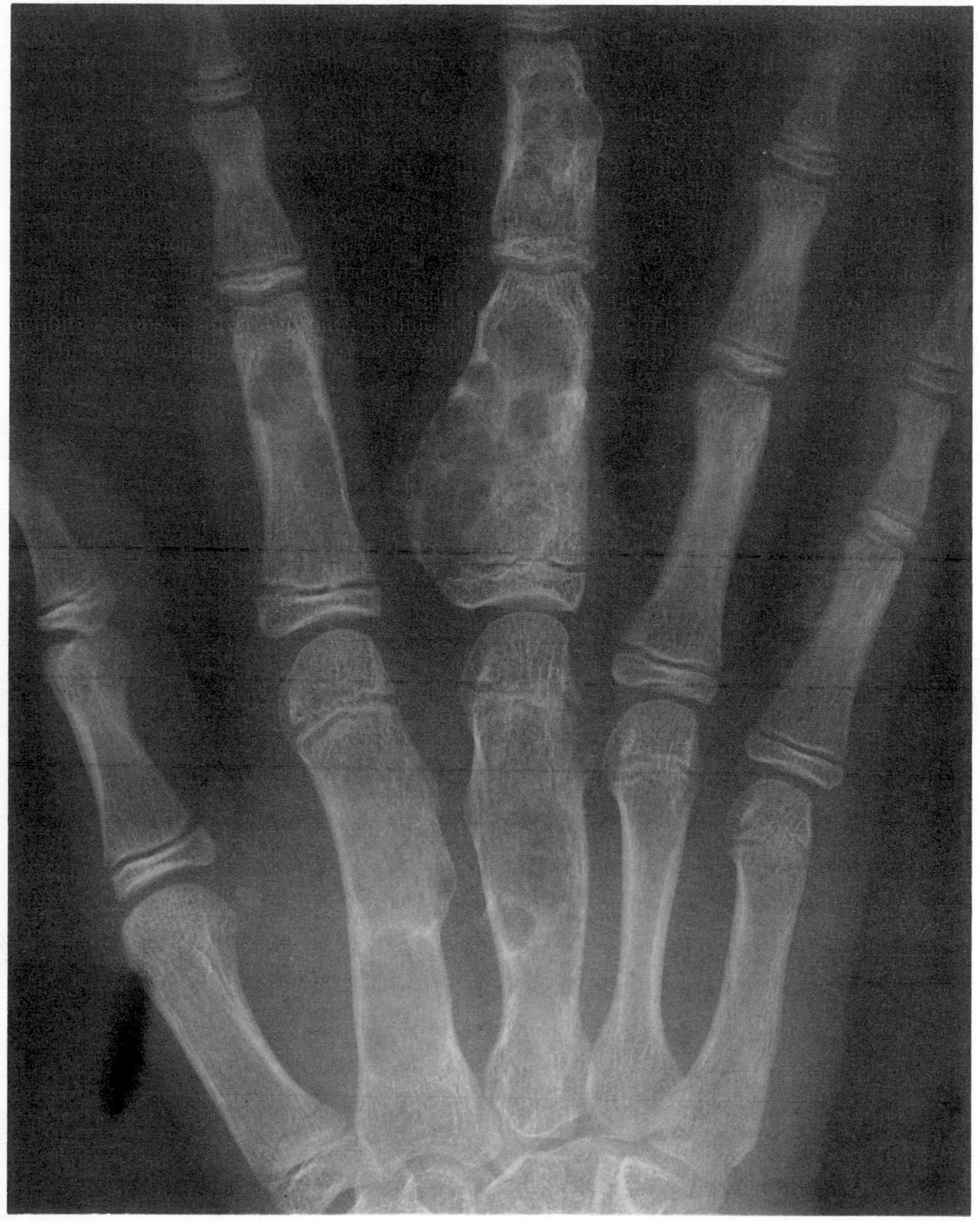

Fig. 28.4 Expansion of the proximal phalanx of the middle finger. Multiple enchondromata.

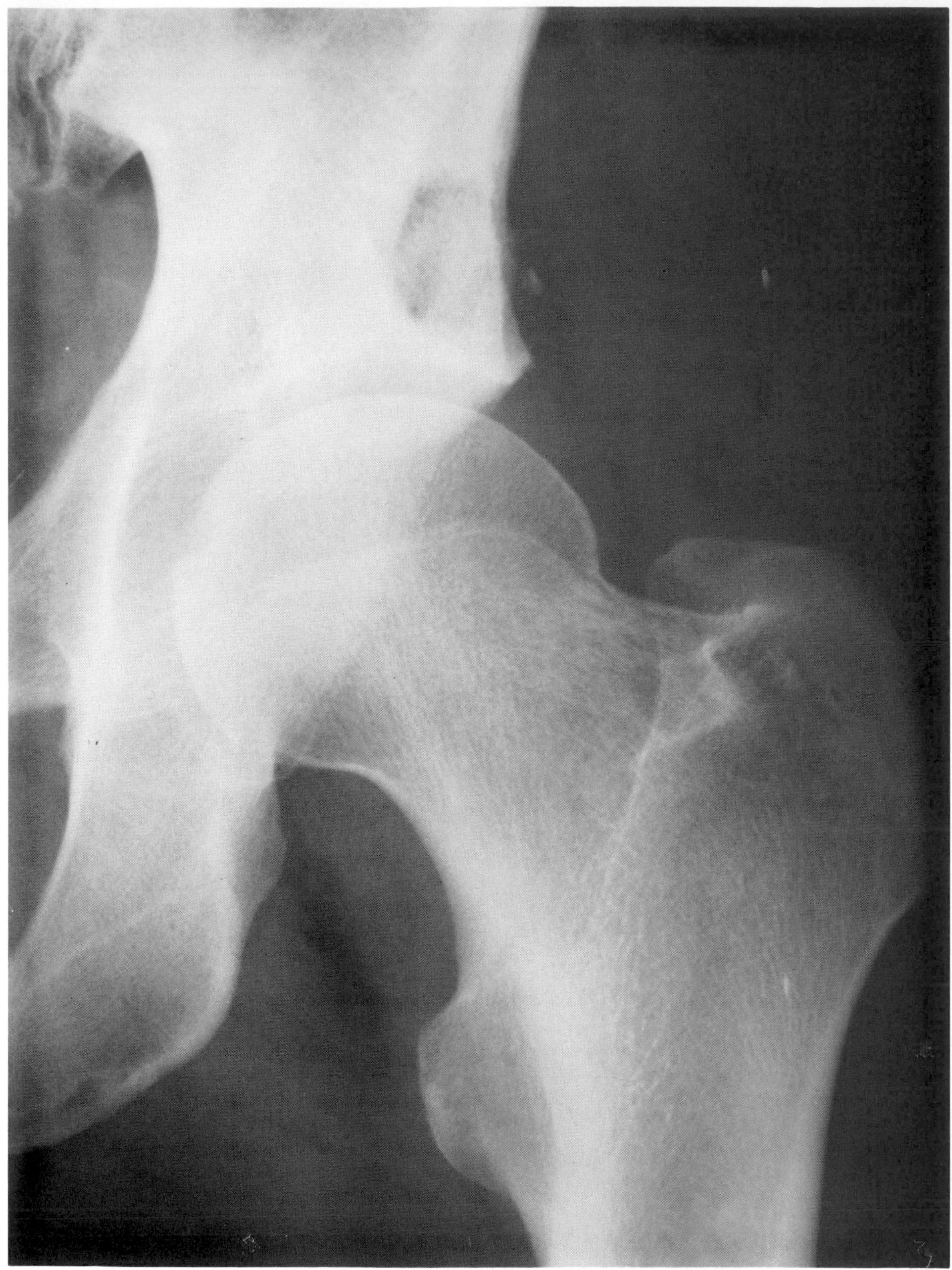

Fig. 28.5 An osteolytic lesion in the ilium due to a benign cyst.

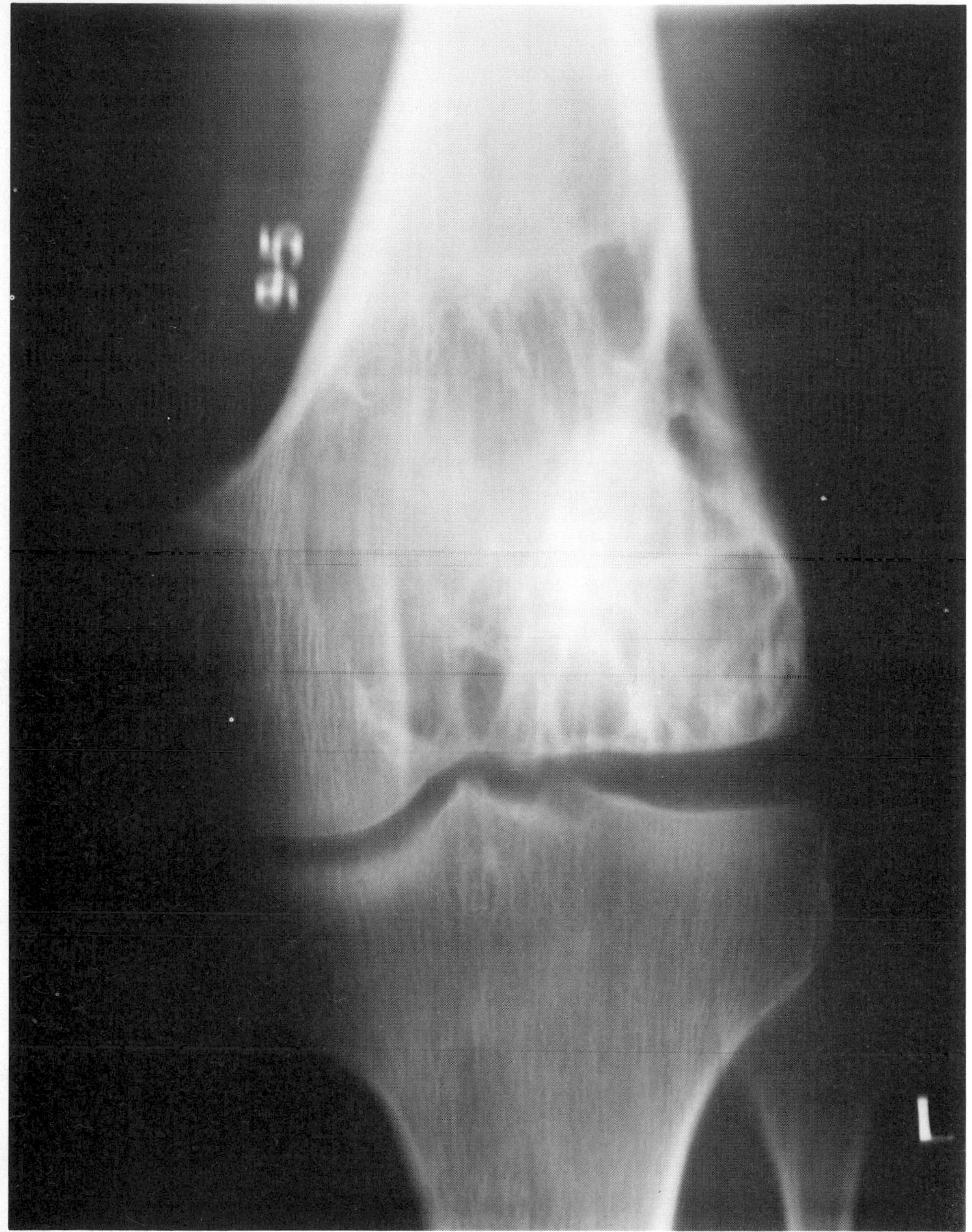

Fig. 28.6 A giant-cell tumour expanding the lower end of the femur and extending typically to the subchondral area.

Bone scan

Isotope scanning of the skeleton has become a routine examination for suspected bone tumours. It will not only determine a "hotspot" in the spine before any obvious changes on conventional radiographs but also multiple lesions.

Arteriogram

A detailed study of the blood supply of a bone tumour may reveal an intense vascular pattern associated with rapidly growing malignant tumours, or distortion of the normal blood vessels by tumour tissue. The main feeding vessels have been isolated for perfusion and others for embolization before excision.

Computerized axial tomography

This sophisticated and expensive examination is invaluable for the more inaccessible areas of the skeleton. In the spine it is combined with a radiculogram to obtain a precise extent of the tumour and this is of tremendous help to the surgeon planning any total excision. Likewise tumours of the pelvis can be accurately defined so that a combination of radiotherapy, excision and replacement can be attempted without resort to a mutilating hind-quarter amputation.

Biopsy—Surgical considerations

Open surgical biopsy is the preferred biopsy because it should provide sufficient material for the pathologist. The alternative is a needle biopsy which is often successful for spinal bone tumours, but certainly not adequate for tumours affecting the long bones and pelvis. If possible, a biopsy should be made before any treatment is given. A generous piece of material should be taken, to include the margin of the neoplasm. A lesion within a long bone should be approached through an oblong hole in the axis of the bone in order to prevent weakness and subsequent fracture. Details with regard to handling and examining the specimen have already been given (p. 353). Metastatic carcinoma is recognized by an epithelial organization of the tissue, which may only be possible to infer from the supporting reticulin network. But epithelial cells may be recognized by identifying a secretion product (e.g. mucus), an enzyme (acid phosphatase), ultrastructural morphology, or immunocytochemical reaction. Connective tissue sarcomas are often identified by their intercellular matrix production (e.g. osteoid) but enzyme reactions (e.g. alkaline phosphatase) or immunocytochemistry may give the answer. Where features are well developed and clear there is no problem; but as loss of differentiation progresses the difficulties increase and the pathologist is forced to use less specific diagnostic categories. No pathologist, any more than a radiologist, likes to feel he has "failed" to make a diagnosis; but to push categorization beyond objective supporting criteria is a false victory.

Since many of the techniques that can be employed in histopathological diagnosis require special preparation of tissue, some call for immediate treatment of fresh tissue. The only way in which to realize the full potential and benefits of the histopathology service is by advance notification of the intention to procure tissue.

It may be useful to the surgeon to know of the kinds of tumour that need to be considered under a given topic. A classification of bone tumours is given in Tables 28.1 and 28.2.

Table 28.1 Benign and malignant neoplasms of bone.

Benign	*Malignant*
Non-ossifying fibroma (fibrous histiocytoma)	Chondrosarcoma (primary and secondary)
Osteoid osteoma	Mesenchymal chondrosarcoma
Benign osteoblastoma	Dedifferentiated chondrosarcoma
Benign chondroblastoma	Fibrosarcoma
Chondromyxoid fibroma	Malignant fibrous histiocytoma
Osteochondroma	Osteosarcoma
Enchondroma	intraosseous (several types)
Fibroma	parosteal
Desmoplastic fibroma	periosteal
Lipoma	Giant cell tumour
Neurilemmoma	Haemangioendothelioma
Neurofibroma	Haemangiopericytoma
	Angiosarcoma
	Adamantinoma
	Plasmacytoma/myeloma
	Malignant round cell tumour
	Ewing's
	reticulum cell sarcoma
	Non-Hodgkin's lymphoma
	Hodgkin's disease
	Leukaemia
	Neurosarcoma
	Leimyosarcoma
	Liposarcoma

Table 28.2 Lesions relevant to the diagnosis of bone tumours.

Dysplastic	Fibrous dysplasia
Traumatic	Callus
	Traumatic periosteal resection
	Avulsion fracture
	Myositis ossificans
	? Epidermoid inclusion cyst (skull, phalanges, jaws, temporal bones)
Inflammatory	Pigmented villonodular synovitis
	Osteomyelitis
	? Paget's disease
Metabolic	Hyperparathyroidism – brown tumour
Circulatory	Infarct
Alternations in growth	Glomus
	Haemangioma
	Synovial chondromatosis
	Soft tissue tumours impinging on bone
Unknown pathogenesis	Ganglion – periosteal, intraosseous
	Aneurysmal bone syst
	Simple cyst
	Histiocytosis-X
	Mast cell disease

Giant cell tumour (GCT), aneurysmal bone cyst and brown tumour of hyperparathyroidism (HPT) are a triumvirate. If one is likely then the other two must be considered. As a matter of principle, hyperparathyroidism is a biochemical diagnosis. It may be that the possibility of that condition is so improbable that appropriate tests are unnecessary, but this must be a deliberate decision and not an oversight. Aware of these possibilities, the surgeon must be alert for a cystic structure at the time of biopsy. The probabilities are much influenced by age; GCT and HPT are highly unlikely in a child.

Classical osteosarcoma presents little problem; but as the lesion moves away from this other possibilities present themselves, at least to the pathologist. For him, the recognition of an osteoblastic tumour can present difficulties. If the histological sections reveal fibroblastic sarcoma, or poorly differentiated cartilage, or highly cellular sarcoma without differentiation the fact of osteosarcoma may elude him; this is a problem in sampling which is best seen against the background of the radiographic appearances. Osteosarcoma can be remarkably variable in its structure, and a variety of histological types are described.

1. Conventional (predominantly osteoblastic)
2. Fibroblastic
3. Chondroblastic
4. Giant cell rich
5. Telangiectatic
6. Intracortical

The first four are highly malignant tumours, and histological sections leave little doubt about this. Intracortical osteosarcoma is a rare, well differentiated neoplasm of long bones, and the problem becomes one of deciding aggressiveness. The alternatives are aggressive osteoblastoma and benign osteoblastoma. The distinction is of importance for the choice of treatment: the first two require the more aggressive surgery. This class of lesion calls for trained expertise in its diagnosis and assessment, and speaks for the specialist centre.

The expert osteoarticular pathologist insists on seeing X-rays in order to know the morbid anatomy of the lesion. The wise orthopaedic surgeon will do well to ensure that they are seen by the pathologist: the narrower the view of the case the more difficult diagnosis becomes.

Imaging techniques can tell much about the location of the lesion, but, beyond mineral content, they are not informative about content. However the surgeon can often supplement this information: what are the relationships of the neoplasm to adjacent tissues: is it in bone; is it on bone (arising from it, attached to it); is it in soft tissue; what are its relations to tissues and structures? A deliberate effort should be made to acquire this information. Most useful to know is whether a bone tumour is cystic or solid. Small cysts may survive in biopsy material; but large ones do not, and it can be difficult to recognize the wall of a cyst in the laboratory either macroscopically or microscopically.

The classification of bone tumours and tumour-like lesions is given in Table 28.1. A number of non-neoplastic lesions, which may be confused with bone tumours, are included in Table 28.2. The following discussion is not an attempt at a systematic portrayal of the subject, but an outline of some of the features that enter into the consideration of a case.

The following lesions can nearly always be recognized as benign, and can be categorized:

1. Fibrous dysplasia
2. Unicameral bone cyst
3. Osteoid osteoma
4. Benign chondroblastoma
5. Chondromyxoid fibroma

Difficulty may arise from some unusual feature: pathological fracture, an unusually large lesion, an uncommon location are instances, raising uncertainty and sometimes anxiety about malignancy. Very often the choice of treatment for a benign lesion is limited because of its location and the patient's age, as well as the fact that it is benign, and this may be an appropriate time at which to provide material for histological diagnosis. A great deal depends upon the confidence with which the categorization "benign to be treated surgically" can be made. The difficulty is that the sharp distinction between benign and malignant cannot always be made. Cartilage tumours are a case in point.

Cartilage tumours

Cartilage tumours can be set along a scale of tumour activity:

1. Inactive
2. Slowly growing
3. Slowly growing and invasive
4. Actively malignant

As has already been implied, the feature under assessment is the relationship between tumour and host. To have become a tumour (swelling) the neoplasm must have grown at some stage. But is it growing now, at the time of presentation? That can only be inferred from the patient's own assessment (which is only possible for lesions in some sites) and the interpretation of radiographs. These, taken serially, can give objective evidence. The fact of growing, however, is less important than an assessment of invasiveness, referred to on p. 357. When a biopsy has been performed, and if both tumour and adjacent bone have been removed, the pathologist can be of help by looking for invasion microscopically. There are pitfalls, too, in making this assessment; but it is important to realize that it is unlikely, in a slowly growing lesion, that there will be any of the conventional cytological criteria for malignancy. Thus, tissue from the body of the lesion may do no more than confirm the fact of cartilage; unless, that is, there are some surviving fragments of mature lamellar bone incorporated in the tumour, a sure sign of past invasiveness. It is of great importance to have confirmation of cartilage tumours, as failure to confirm invasion, whether by reason of inappropriate tissue or no evidence in a good sample, carries the problems of the negative result: the invasion may be taking place elsewhere. Failure to find cytological evidence of malignancy (again there is a sampling problem) is no bad thing either, for it means that there is ample time in which to assess and plan. In the end, however, every growing cartilage tumour in adults requires complete removal. The risks of leaving it are the complications of a local destructive growth, and the possibility of metastasis as and when the neoplasm becomes more malignant. It is difficult to quantify this possibility, but given a period of several years, particularly in recurring tumours, a small percentage will metastasize.

Enchondromas, benign cartilage tumours, are found in both children and adults, sometimes stationary and sometimes growing. Usually they are solitary, but may be multiple (see Fig. 28.4). The risk of malignancy in the latter condition is difficult to assess, but it is nothing like the incidence with which most orthopaedic surgeons frighten themselves. Nor is it an explosive event. A lesion will grow out of control and it is often difficult to know when to apply the term chondrosarcoma. Experience has shown that perfectly benign (as judged by behaviour) multiple lesions have cytological features that would be regarded as sinister in solitary lesions. But since there are no quantitative values for these features, an exercise in judgement is required, for which some degree of experience is necessary.

The invasive but still slowly growing cartilage tumours, to which the term "low-grade chondrosarcoma" can be applied (for reasons discussed above), occur in adults in long bones, in flat bones, or vertebrae. It is this class of lesion more than any other which tends to escape detection for a long time. It requires an alert radiologist or clinician to detect the minimal textural changes found in early stages.

There are also, however, highly aggressive chondrosarcomas, in which the question of malignancy is never in doubt. Radiologically, these present as malignant tumours. Their lack of differentiation renders them rather mucoid. Histologically, it may be difficult to know if the tissue is cartilage, but there is no doubt about sarcoma. Such neoplasms occur in both children and adults. Particularly in the former, there is always the question as to whether the neoplasm will turn out to be a chondroblastic osteosarcoma.

Cartilage tumours of hands and feet present a special problem because well established examples of chondrosarcoma are rare. Argument continues about this: are they rare or is it that they can be more effectively treated? The criteria for malignancy are hard to describe; but clearly as one moves up the scale of size, rate of growth, invasiveness and histological features of malignancy, sarcoma becomes more certain.

The discussion of osteochondroma naturally follows here. But it is well to discuss it in the context of "lesions on bone".

Lesions on bone

Traumatic: reactive and reparative tissues arising in stress fracture, detached ligaments and tendons, myositis ossificans, traumatic periostitis.

Neoplastic: osteochondroma, parosteal chondroma, parosteal chondrosarcoma, parosteal osteosarcoma, periosteal osteosarcoma.

Post-traumatic reaction can give rise to new bone formation in the periosteum and soft tissues, and this may be confused at times with neoplasis. A history of stress or trauma, and rapid appearance of the lesion are clues. The morbid anatomy differs from osteochondroma and juxtacortical neoplasia, but this depends on good X-ray views. The histological appearances can be confusing, since there may be nothing cytologically neoplastic in parosteal osteosarcoma; the pathologist is very dependent on history and radiological examination.

Osteochondroma is a distinctive benign neoplasm. It consists of a cartilage cap, taking origin from bone, which grows out from the parent structure. The product of its growth ossifies and remodels producing cortical and cancellous architecture which is continuous with that of the bone from which it arises. Persistent growth of the lesion in a child, or its resumption in an adult, especially where there are multiple lesions, always causes a sense of concern about malignancy. This is uncommon: figures from different centres vary considerably. If malignancy occurs, it is in the cartilage component, which grows in a lobulated fashion and becomes substantial in amount. Histological assessment for malignancy can be very uncertain. The problem is very much like that of enchondroma, but in this different location. Sessile lesions with an attenuated cap can present some confusion with parosteal osteosarcoma, whereas others may be confused with post-traumatic reaction.

Parosteal osteosarcoma is an uncommon lesion, but quite distinctive. Lying against the periosteum it can usually be seen in radiographs to be separated from the underlying cortex by radiolucent periosteum; but this may require rotational views. The problem lies in accepting that such a small slowly growing lesion with no histological features of malignancy (many are diagnosed as reactive or fibrous dysplasia) can be sinister. Recurrences following successive attempts at local removal are accompanied by increasing aggressiveness to the point of frank sarcoma and metastases.

Periosteal osteosarcoma is a predominantly cartilaginous lesion with whisps of neoplastic bone in lobules. This is an aggressive neoplasm amenable to local resection which, however, must be properly performed; chemotherapy may be useful.

Parosteal cartilage tumours There are both benign and malignant cartilage tumours so intimately related to periosteum that they seem part of the bone rather than of soft tissue. To recognize cartilage is not difficult, the problem of malignancy is of the same order as discussed above.

Soft tissue tumours are not the province of this section, but three are worthy of note in the context of the foregoing—pseudo malignant osseous tumour of soft tissue, soft tissue osteosarcoma, and mesenchymal chondrosarcoma. The first is a painful, rapidly growing, post-traumatic (from unaccustomed heavy gardening to vigorous sport), ossifying lesion whose characteristic is a shell of well differentiated bone enclosing cellular, growing spindle-celled tissue. The other two are both malignant lesions characterized by cellular tissue with bony or cartilaginous differentiation respectively; the matrix mineralizes and is evident on X-ray.

Thus, there is a range of reactive and neoplastic lesions on or adjacent to bone to be considered and differentiated. History, careful assessment of location and morbid anatomy, a choice between biopsy and excision, and only finally histological examination, are the steps to be taken.

Other malignant tumours of bone

The recognition of a malignant bone tumour, or the inclusion of that category as a possibility in consideration of a case, is generally not difficult. This should of course always include the possibility of metastatic carcinoma. Depending on the location of the lesion (i.e. the position in the

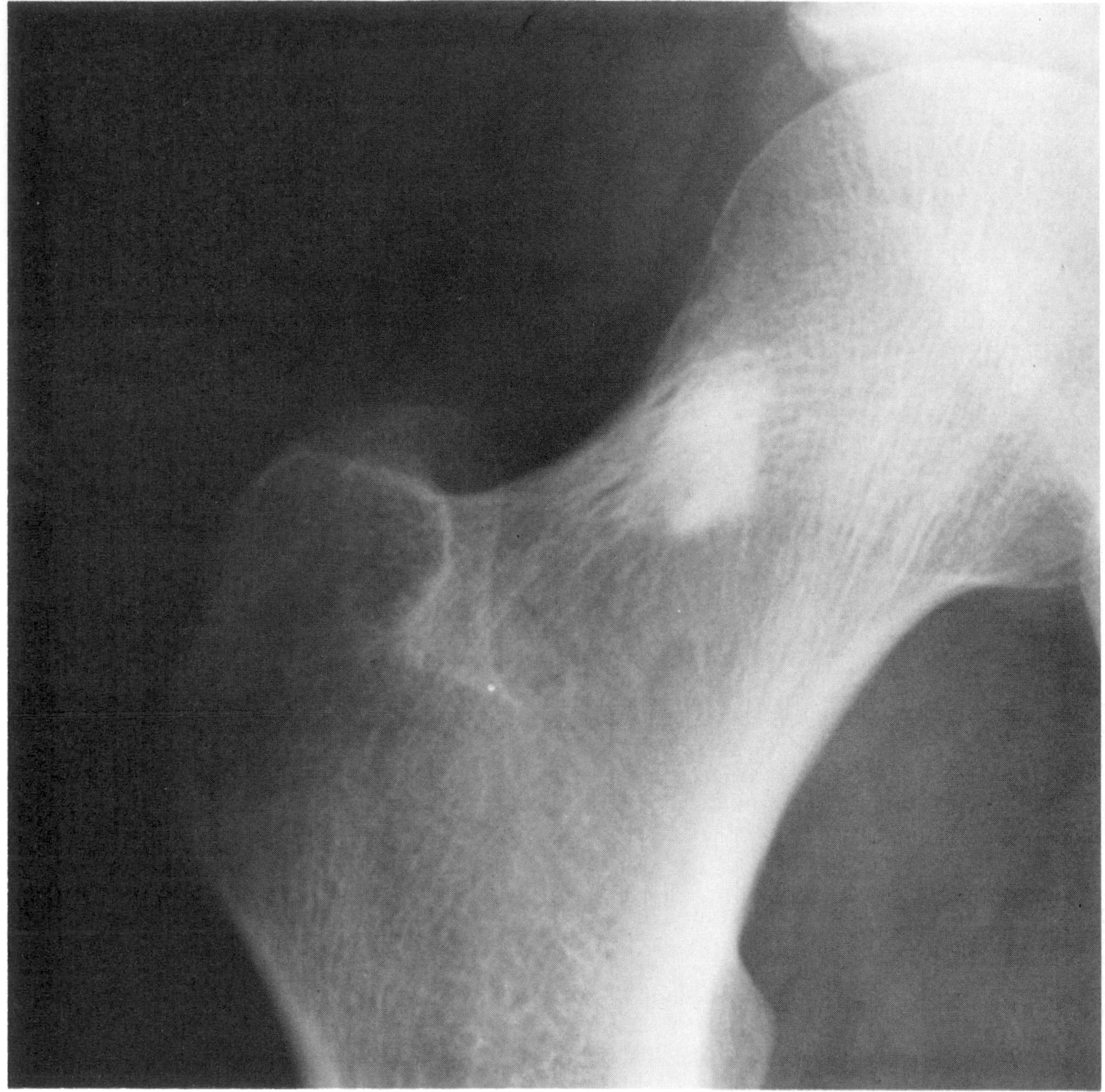

Fig. 28.7 A 'bone island' without surrounding reaction is an innocent developmental lesion.

skeleton—long bone, flat bones, vertebrae, hands and feet; and the localization in a tubular bone—epiphysis, metaphysis, diaphysis), the age of the patient, radiological features (amount of periosteal reaction), the content of the lesion (uniform, loculated, mineralized), associated conditions (Paget's disease, previous radiation, etc.), a provisional diagnosis or a selection of possible diagnoses may be made. These can be drawn from a hierarchical list, the last term of which can be expanded from the classification of bone tumours:

1. Malignant tumour unspecified
2. Primary malignant bone tumour unspecified
3. Metastatic carcinoma, unspecified or known
4. Specific primary sarcoma of bone

Malignant neoplasm that diffusely involve the bone with irregular destruction and some periosteal reaction must be distinguished from osteomyelitis, lymphomas, and leukaemias, and

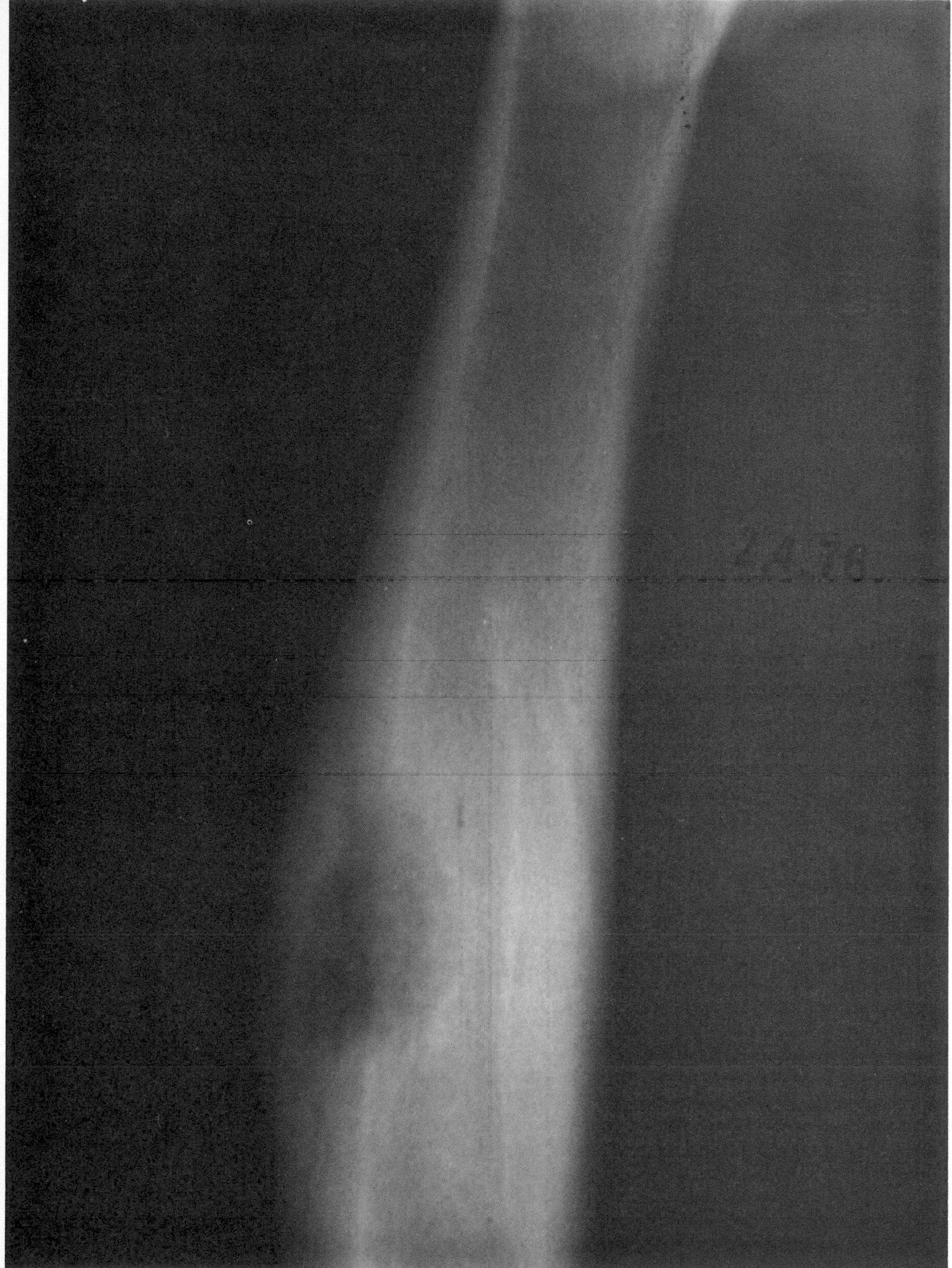

Fig. 28.8 Sclerosis around a lytic area in an osteoid osteoma.

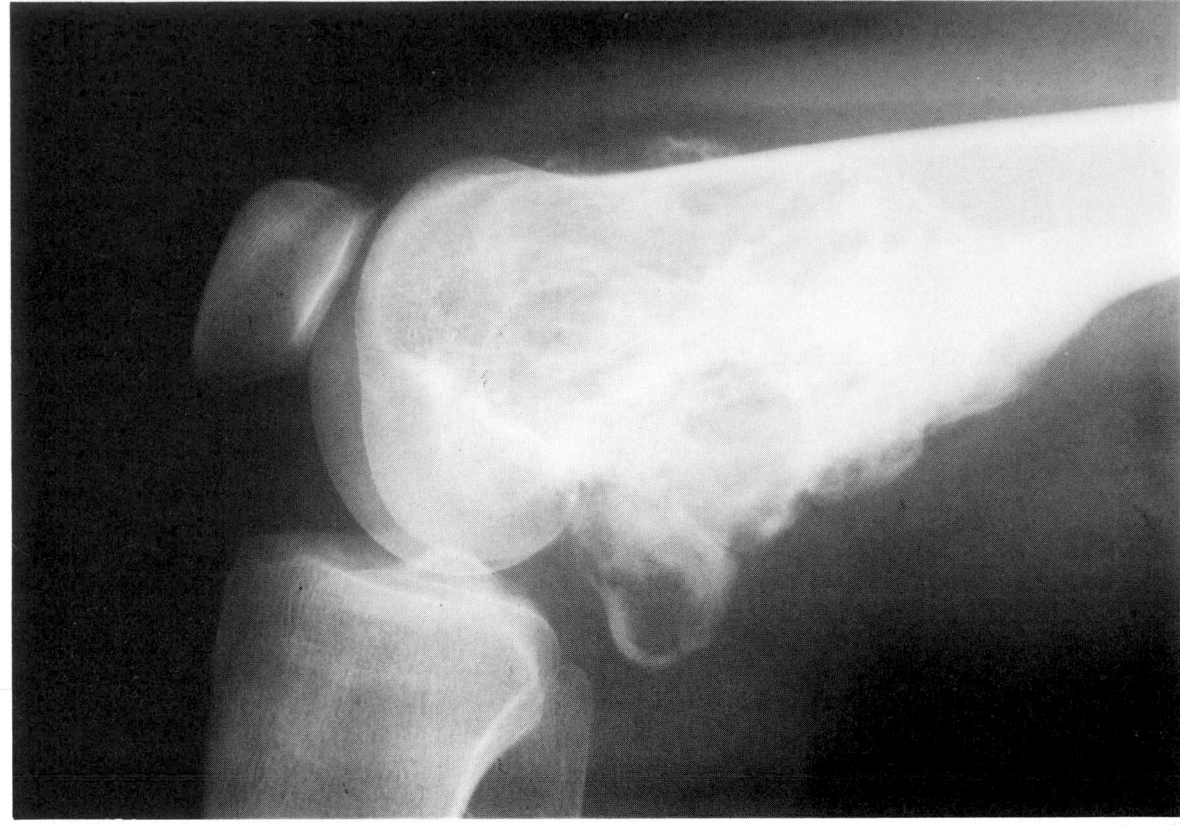

Fig. 28.9 Dense new bone formation in a parosteal sarcoma.

metastatic carcinomas. Obviously, the age of the patient, the history, the symptoms, the physical findings and laboratory results, will help to order the possibilities. This problem has been mentioned earlier, and the importance of tissue for bacteriological examination stressed, but these tumours can also be differentiated by electron microscopy and/or immunocytochemistry, and the histopathologist should be alerted in advance.

The concept of the histiocytic tumour has grown in popularity. Currently, "malignant fibrous histiocytoma" is a term frequently heard. It is a difficult diagnosis to make with confidence, and the prognosis to be attached to it is highly uncertain. There are immunocytochemical criteria for its recognition, but these require practice in their performance and experience in their interpretation.

Perhaps there is no more important message with which to end this section than to stress the necessity for *interdisciplinary discussion* when planning the management of a patient with either a malignant or benign bone tumour.

The spine

Introduction

Pain in the neck and the lower part of the back is a very common complaint with or without associated pain in the upper and lower limbs. It is often associated with unaccustomed physical activity, is shortlived and of no clinical significance.

Disorders of the abdominal and pelvic viscera such as the pancreas and kidneys may also give rise to pain in the back (see Chapter 11), the true nature of which will become apparent from other symptoms and signs and investigations, or by the failure to demonstrate an abnormality in the spine itself.

When the symptoms do arise from the vertebral column the cause may be in the body of the vertebra, the neural arches or the intervertebral disc and the synovial facet joints which link each

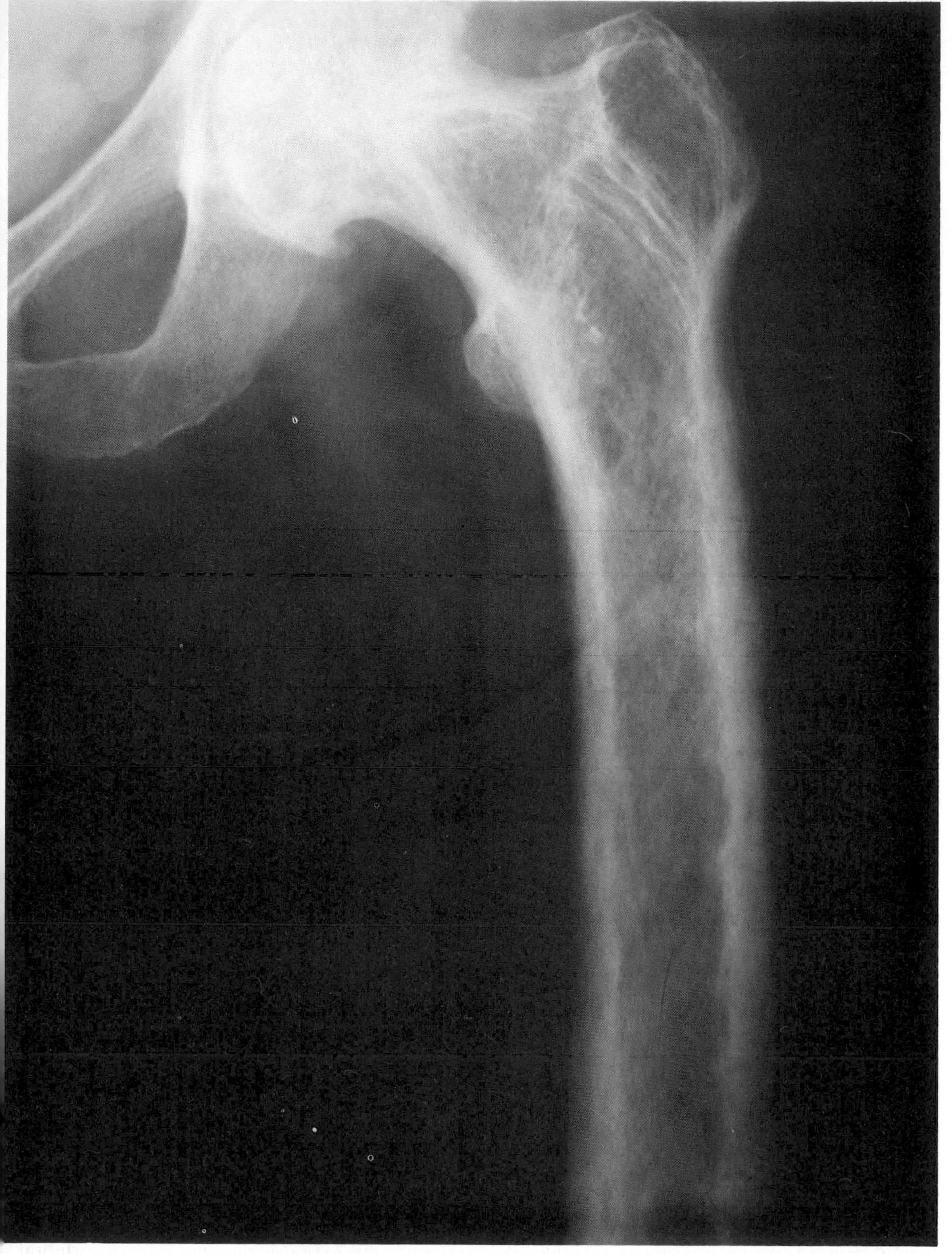

Fig. 28.10 Coarse trabeculation, sclerosis, bowing and multiple transverse stress fractures in Paget's disease.

vertebra, yet the patient is unable to distinguish pain from one or the other. Furthermore, the close proximity of the spinal cord and its coverings and the nerve roots may lead to radicular pain, paralysis and sensory loss in the trunk or limbs, the extent and nature of which is determined not by the precise nature of the underlying pathological lesion, but by its site and the speed at which the neural tissues are compressed (see "Weakness and Paralysis", p. 376).

Major injury

Acute pain following a major injury rarely causes diagnostic difficulty. Associated injuries to the spinal cord and nerve roots, resulting in motor and sensory deficiency and changes in the reflexes, are immediately apparent and demand priority in treatment.

A fracture, dislocation or fracture-dislocation will be apparent on radiographs of the injured region, and if the precise nature of the fracture is in doubt, tomography or computerized axial tomography may be necessary to determine whether the fracture is stable or unstable.

Rotational injuries producing fractures and fracture dislocations of the neural arch and facet joints are usually unstable and clearly represent a threat to the neighbouring neural tissue. Care is of paramount importance in handling the patient, and management is facilitated by operative stabilization of the unstable segment, although the ultimate outcome in the presence of paralysis is usually unaffected.

Stable fractures, which include the common crush or wedge fracture of the vertebral body, require no more than symptomatic treatment (bed rest and analgesics) and mobilization as soon as pain permits.

No major injury

Pain in the axial skeleton, as indeed elsewhere, is frequently attributed to a minor injury or strain by the patient, but such an injury is often coincidental.

In the absence of a major injury the pain will be broadly similar whether the cause be a specific pathological entity or a vague non-specific disorder, the precise pathology of which is ill understood. Management will depend to a large extent on excluding the more specific and potentially life-threatening disorders by radiography and laboratory investigations, and ultimately by biopsy and microscopic examination if the diagnosis remains in doubt.

Destructive bone disease

Infection of vertebral bodies with pyogenic or tuberculous organisms is the result of blood stream spread from a focus elsewhere. Pain at the level of the affected vertebra, is the predominant complaint, with subsequent deformity if there is extensive vertebral destruction, and with weakness and paralysis and sensory impairment below the level of the lesion should pressure on the spinal cord occur.

The diagnosis should be made before there is extensive bone destruction or neurological deficit but the early local symptoms and signs may be at this stage no more than non-specific local pain and tenderness at the affected level of the spine, with perhaps the general signs and symptoms of an infection.

The sedimentation rate will be raised markedly in the case of pyogenic infection and an increase in white blood count will in some measure assist in differentiating acute infection from other causes of vertebral destruction. Blood culture may lead to the identification of a pyogenic organism. Tubercle bacilli should be sought in the sputum and urine.

Radiographs will demonstrate a lytic lesion in the vertebral body usually adjacent to the disc in the case of infection. Characteristically, the disc will later be destroyed in tuberculosis as the infection spreads to the neighbouring vertebra and the vertebral bodies collapse but the neural arches are preserved.

Pyogenic infection more commonly results in new bone formation, peripheral to the destruction, but cannot be reliably differentiated from tuberculous infection on radiological grounds alone, especially in the early stages when the diagnosis should be made.

Similarly, an increased uptake of a bone-seeking isotope, such as technetium or gallium, indicates an increase in bone turnover, but will not unequivocally indicate its cause. Selective uptake of gallium is suggestive, but not conclusive, proof of infection, and ultimately biopsy may be required to establish the nature of the osteolytic lesion. Multiple lesions, however, are readily revealed by radionuclide scanning which is preferable to a skeletal survey.

Needle biopsy is more convenient than open

biopsy. A wide bore needle or, preferably, a small cutting trephine if hard bone is encountered, is inserted under local, or sometimes general anaesthesia, into the lesion using an image intensifier. A posterolateral approach is most appropriate for lesions in the thoracic and lumbar spine. The first to the third cervical vertebrae are best approached through the posterior pharyngeal wall in the midline, and the lower cervical vertebrae through a lateral approach behind the sternomastoid muscle.

Samples from the lesion are withdrawn in the cannula or trephine, some for culture and some for histological examination. The best procedure is to put all the material in a dry sterile vessel and deliver it without delay, but with full information, to the laboratory. Alternatively, the material can be divided, with a portion for culture and one for histology. From the latter, tissue imprints can be made on clean dry slides, and the remainder put into fixative as soon as possible.

Treatment will depend on the cause of the osteolytic lesion and its behaviour. Spinal osteomyelitis is primarily an infection of bone. The organisms arrive via the blood stream, usually the arterial supply; but occasionally the peripheral veins are implicated in transporting bacteria from the genitourinary tract.

Infections of the vertebral column are initially bone infections, i.e., osteomyelitis of the vertebral body. Pyogenic organisms lead to acute inflammation and hence to necrosis. The bone in the necrotic region is inaccessible to bone cells, therefore remains unaltered in the midst of the necrotic and purulent material and constitutes a *sequestrum*. The tissue response extends beyond the confines of the vertebra, causing swelling of the adjacent soft tissues; this can be visualized in radiographs. The inflammatory focus can extend up to the vertebral disc, which may then be subjected to gradual dissolution, and laterally into the soft tissues. An epidural abscess is a dangerous complication.

Tuberculous granulomatous inflammation develops more slowly and may not lead to destruction of the disc. However, disc destruction is an unreliable criterion for distinguishing pyogenic from the exudous inflammation.

Operative decompression of the spinal cord and fusion of the spine are required if there is severe weakness, spasticity or loss of sphincter control—either immediately, or if a mild neurological deficit fails to respond to antibacterial therapy and bed rest, within a few days of commencing treatment.

Spinal tumours

Neoplastic disease in bone is usually destructive, although osteoblastic responses occur. Pain is the usual symptom, and neural signs may accompany this or sometimes occur alone. The vertebral column is one of the most common sites for metastatic carcinoma. Multiple vertebral involvement is presumptive evidence of this in an adult: with a known primary site, further investigation is necessary. However, as at other sites, a solitary metastasis may be confused with primary neoplasia and even infection.

Primary neoplasms may also arise from any of the soft tissues of the spine, but rarely from adjacent tissues—with perhaps the exception of nerve tissue.

Of all primary bone tumours, 10–15 per cent occur in vertebrae or sacrum. Chordoma and myeloma account for half of them. The common benign lesions are chondroma, benign osteoblastic lesions (osteoid osteoma and benign osteoblastoma), angioma and aneurysmal bone cyst. The primary malignant tumours of the spine also include lymphoma, Ewing's sarcoma, chondrosarcoma and osteosarcoma.

The sites of involvement are vertebral body, neural arch or spinous process. When the vertebral body is affected, there may be mechanical instability of the spine which endangers the cord or nerve roots. Involvement of the neural arch less commonly causes loss of stability, but the cord and nerve roots are still at risk.

The benign lesions are amenable to surgery, and generally respond well. Benign osteoblastoma is sometimes more difficult to eradicate and recurrences are then a problem. Radiotherapy is indicated when parts of the tumour are inaccessible. Both chondrosarcoma and chordoma are treated by operation, but both are difficult to remove completely, so that recurrence is the rule with gradually extending tumour leading to death through local complications. The other malignant neoplasms, primary and secondary, are best treated by radiotherapy and chemotherapy, as indicated by the general principles of treatment that are applicable to other parts of the skeleton.

Osteoporosis

Pain in the back, particularly in the thoracic region, may be associated with idiopathic or secondary osteoporosis. *Osteoporosis* is a reduction in the amount of bone tissue associated with an attendant disability. Reduced bone volume associated with age is called *osteopenia.* The control mechanisms are not clear. Throughout life, some proportion of the bone surfaces (variously estimated to be in the range of 5–50 per cent, dependent on age and sampling) is being resorbed and formed. Thus, there is a constant renewal of bone substance, with a skeletal half-life in the range of 10 years. Bone mass generally rises steadily during growth and up to about 30 years, when it levels off; it declines from about 40 years onwards, and this feature is more marked in women. Accurate assessment of total bone mass is difficult, but computerized tomography or nuclear magnetic resonance may help. Measurements on histological sections of iliac crest biopsies are easy to perform accurately, but the sampling error can be large: the iliac crest may not reflect the state of the femoral neck or the vertebral column.

Microfractures, either localized to individual vertebrae or completely through the bone, are common in osteoporosis. Healing ensues, but the callus, owing to the age of the patient and the unresponsiveness of his tissues, is often inadequate.

Collapse of one or more vertebral bodies may occur insidiously or after minor injury, when the pain is severe. There may be associated kyphosis and localized tenderness.

The diagnosis is usually made radiographically on the characteristic appearances of generalized loss of bone density and thinning of the cortex. This is just as well because the usually measured biochemical indices are normal. There may be a negative calcium balance, but this requires careful assessment.

With regard to treatment, the collapse of a vertebral body does not lead to vertebral instability or pressure on the spinal cord and pain should be treated by simple analgesics. Anabolic steroids have no proven value. A corset or brace to hold the spine extended may be helpful if the pain is severe.

Bone formation

Ankylosing spondylitis

Back pain may occasionally be associated with *increased* bone formation. *Ankylosing spondylitis* characteristically results in ossification of the anterior and posterior longitudinal ligaments of the spine and the annulus of the disc. It is invariably associated with radiological changes in the sacro-iliac joint, the margins of which initially become indistinct and ill defined and later are obliterated altogether.

This disease is generally treated as a variant of rheumatoid arthritis (p. 383). The principal joints affected are the vertebral and sacro-iliac, and the patients are nearly all young males of HLA B27 type. Intervertebral discs become vascularized and ossified, with a minimal inflammatory component. Diarthrodial joints are sometimes involved, and the synovial changes are comparable with those of rheumatoid arthritis.

The treatment is essentially medical with anti-inflammatory drugs and exercises to improve and preserve mobility. Spinal deformity may be prevented by bracing, but occasionally deformities may become so severe that spinal osteotomy, although hazardous, may be the only way of preserving independence.

Paget's disease causes enlargement of individual vertebral bodies with coarse trabeculation visible in the radiograph. There may occasionally be encroachment on the canal and pressure on the spinal cord and nerve roots requiring operative decompression.

Osteoblastic secondary deposits from prostatic carcinoma are, like the primary tumour, usually responsive to stilboestrol, but if there is pressure on the spinal cord then decompression may be necessary.

Intervertebral disc disease

The intervertebral disc consists of a central gelatinous nucleus pulposus surrounded by a fibrous annulus. The annulus may rupture, allowing the disc to prolapse: this is the first stage in disc degeneration.

An acute disc prolapse may occur at any level of the spine, but most commonly at the lower lumbar levels and, less frequently, in the neck. A prolapsed thoracic disc is rare. The usual disc prolapse is characterized by sudden and severe pain, frequently associated with severe radiating pain down the arm and leg respectively, the result of pressure on a nerve root. As a result of this pressure there may be sensory loss, muscle weakness or reflex change in the distribution of the affected nerve roots.

Diagnosis is essentially made on clinical grounds, but contrast radiography will frequently demonstrate an extradural filling defect.

The treatment is initially conservative. The expectation is that the prolapse material will shrink and fibrose, relieving the pressure on the affected nerve roots. If, however, symptoms persist, and particularly if neurological signs increase, then operative decompression and removal of the prolapse material should be carried out.

Disc degeneration may follow an acute episode which has been treated conservatively or surgically, or the degeneration may occur without a specific acute episode and is the commonest cause of pain in the spine. The loss of disc substance allows the vertebral bodies to come closer together (a fact readily appreciated from lateral radiographs of the spine). This in turn alters the relationship of the posterior facet joints which in turn degenerate with the characteristic changes seen in the synovial joints generally (see "Joints", p. 382). The combination of disc and facet joint degeneration is termed "spondylosis".

The facets may sublux allowing a vertebra to slip forward (sometimes backwards) on the one below (degenerative spondylolisthesis), so upsetting the mechanical balance of that level of the spine. This throws an increased strain on the intervertebral ligaments and on the spinal muscles which leads to persistent pain in the back or neck, the usual symptoms of disc degeneration.

Spondylolisthesis in the lumbar spine may also be the result of a stress fracture in the pars interarticularis of the neural arch and, rarely, a congenital failure of the facet joints to develop which can be recognized on X-ray. The clinical manifestations and management are essentially the same whatever the cause of the spondylolisthesis.

Characteristically, the pain is aggravated by sitting or standing in one position for too long and is eased by changes in posture or activity, presumably by redistributing the stresses temporarily to other ligaments or muscles.

The intervertebral foramina, through which the spinal nerves emerge, may be reduced in size as a result of the narrowing of the disc and the subluxation of the facet joints, but also by osteophytes projecting into the foramen from the adjacent degenerating facet joints. The resulting irritation or compression of the nerve roots may cause pain in the limbs of a vague, illdefined nature, rather than the sharp shooting pain associated with acute pressure from a prolapsed disc. This is comparable to the compression of the median nerve in the carpal tunnel, and if left indefinitely may also cause sensory loss, muscle weakness and reflex change.

Furthermore, the spinal canal may be narrowed by osteophytes projecting from the posterior aspect of the vertebral bodies adjacent to the degenerative disc, or by the spondylolisthesis itself, or a combination of both. Compression of the cord in the cervical and thoracic spine leads to a spastic weakness of the limbs, while in the lumbar spine below the termination of the cord at L1 it is the cauda equina which is compressed. This initially reduces the blood supply to the cauda equina causing pain in the legs on exertion which clearly can be confused with intermittent claudication of peripheral vascular origin (p. 241) and has led to the name "intermittent claudication of the cauda equina".

Disc degeneration is evident on plain radiographs, but pressure on the contents of the spinal canal can only be demonstrated by injecting a radio-opaque contrast medium into the subdural space (myelogram). A water soluble contrast medium gives better definition and fills the dural extension around the nerve roots (hence the term radiculogram), but it is not suitable for the cervical spine. Even so, it is rarely possible to demonstrate compression of the more distal part of the nerve in the intervertebral foramen.

Narrowing of the spinal canal is easily demonstrable by myelography or computerized axial tomography.

The patient should initially be treated by rest if the onset is acute, followed by physiotherapy. When conservative treatment fails and symptoms become severe and unremitting, fusion of the adjacent vertebra abolishes movement of the painful level with relief of pain.

The pain from acute nerve root pressure often resolves with rest, as the inflammation associated with initial mechanical stimulation subsides. If not, the nerve root must be decompressed operatively.

Chronic nerve root pressure associated with disc degeneration may also require decompression, but this is more hazardous in the cervical region and should be contemplated with caution.

Acute cord compression should be relieved as a matter of urgency because, unlike peripheral nerves which can regenerate when the pressure on them is relieved, there is no capacity for regeneration in the central nervous system.

When neural compression of painful degenerative disc disease coexist, decompression and fusion may be combined.

Rheumatoid arthritis occurs predominantly in the upper cervical spine and at the atlanto axial level in particular, and is invariably associated with rheumatoid arthritis elsewhere and the diagnosis is rarely in doubt. The disease affects the synovial facet joints and the joints of Lushke and is associated with disc degeneration. There may be progressive anterior subluxation of one vertebral body on another as the disease becomes more severe. At the atlanto-axial level, this is the result of elongation of the transverse ligament of the atlas and erosion of the adontoid process which allows the atlas to sublux anteriorly. This can be recognized on lateral radiographs taken with the neck flexed and extended by an increase in the distance between the posterior surface of the arch of the atlas and the anterior surface of the adontoid, the distance does not normally exceed 4 mm.

The subluxation is usually gradual and the spinal cord accommodates to the gradual increase in pressure, so spasticity and weakness in the limbs are late manifestations. Pressure on the nerve roots, in particular C2 in atlanto-axial subluxation, occurs earlier, and is an indication for spinal fusion to prevent further damage to the neural tissue as well as for the relief of pain. This will be sufficient to prevent further damage to the cord, but if there is already significant weakness in the lower limbs, decompression of the cord will also be required.

Spinal deformity

Spinal deformity may be secondary to almost any disorder affecting the vertebrae or discs, or to weakness of the spinal musculature. The major developmental disorders are the dysplasias of the spinal cord and vertebral column, often referred to under the blanket term *spina bifida.*

Embryologically, the vertebral column arises from the folding of the neural crest to form a closed tube. Each vertebra is the result of fusion of the caudal and cephalic portions of adjacent mesodermal blocks. The opposing folds of the neural crest first fuse in the region destined to be thoracic. Closure extends cranially and caudally.

Degrees of failure are possible. *Anencephaly* is the most serious, but lesser degrees of involvement occur in children and may be compatible with life. The smallest defects are *diastematomyelia,* in which the cord is divided longitudinally over a short distance, usually in the lumbar segment. Occasionally a bony outgrowth from the vertebral body projects through it.

The distal segment atrophies to become the filum terminale. It can happen that the atrophic process is incomplete, with the result that the cord becomes tethered.

The manner of formation of vertebral bodies—midline fusion of lateral masses, and fusion in the horizontal plane with the mass above (or below)—opens the way to a range of developmental failures in their formation.

All these lesser anomalies of the cord and vertebrae may come to light as incidental findings, or because they give rise to symptoms and signs.

Scoliosis, whether idiopathic or the result of a structural abnormality (e.g. a hemivertebra) requires careful monitoring. If the deformity is rapidly progressive, it may be controlled to some extent by external braces. If the curve progresses to an unacceptable degree, operative correction and fusion of the affected vertebra may be necessary.

Kyphosis, most commonly occurring in children and young adults, is the result of a growth disturbance of the vertebral epiphysis (Scheurmann's disease) and causes wedging of several vertebrae. It may be associated with mild discomfort, but rarely enough to warrant bracing or rest and the deformity.

Wedging of a single vertebra (Calvé's disease) is usually caused by an eosinophilic granuloma (see p. 407 for pathology), rather than avascular necrosis of the vertebral body as previously thought. Needle biopsy to establish the diagnosis is followed by deep X-ray therapy.

Weakness and paralysis

Weakness and paralysis may arise as a consequence of intrinsic musculo-tendinous disease or of neurological disorders (which can be broadened to include the weakness sometimes associated with emotional disturbance) (*see* Fig. 28.11). Muscular disease is considered in Chapter 18.

Tendon rupture

This occurs in adults. When they are in good health it is almost always the achilles tendon that gives way. When they suffer from rheumatoid arthritis, extensor tendons at the wrist can be involved, and a tendon will rupture by attrition as it traverses a sharp piece of bone (usually the lower end of the ulna) or by ischaemia from the enveloping and invasive diseased synovial tissue. Like a piece of string, it is broken with little to show either macroscopically or microscopically except an attempt at repair with collagen tissue: within the tendon itself there is little reparative response and whatever occurs comes from adjacent tissues. Thus, in

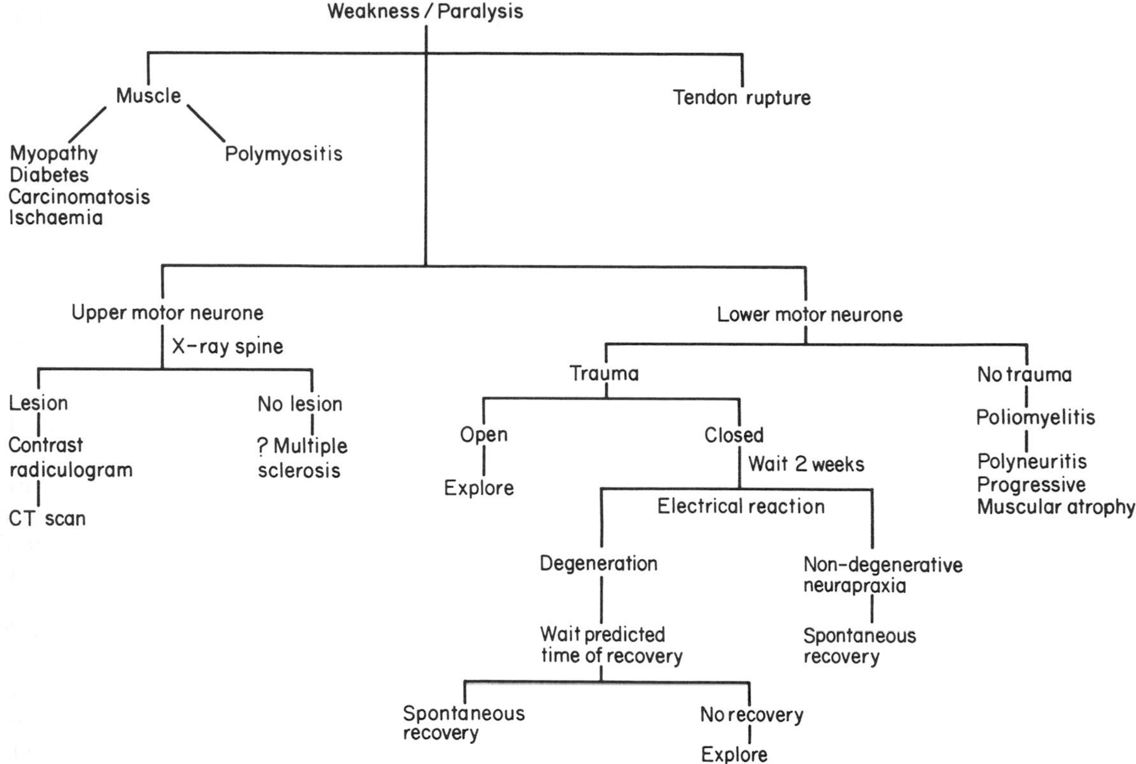

Fig. 28.11 Weakness and paralysis.

achilles tendon and rotator cuff rupture, the space will be filled by blood clot and granulation tissue originating from the soft tissue: this will organize and effect a repair by production and maturation of collagen fibres as in other situations.

Neurological disorders

Upper motor neurone lesions arising in the spinal cord produce a characteristic hypertonus leading eventually to spasticity. It is sometimes difficult to assess weakness in such patients but it is invariably present. Any space occupying lesion in the vertebra has to be excluded. The lesion will vary from a relatively benign area of cervical spondylosis to a malignant primary or secondary neoplasm. Similarly, intradural lesions also have to be considered together with motor neurone disease.

A lower motor nerve lesion involves the anterior horn cell or any part of the motor pathway directed towards and including the terminal muscle motor unit. By far the commonest cause is peripheral nerve injury.

Nerve injury

Introduction

A patient with a nerve injury is expected to present a clearly defined pattern of disability related to the loss of function in a particular nerve, but in practice the history and signs may be confused, which may lead to an incorrect diagnosis and poor management.

History

The history of the nature and site of the injury is important in order to focus the attention to one or more peripheral nerves. Laceration or open fracture indicates a severe injury; and the effect can be more confused when placed in the proximal part of a limb. Invariably there is a dramatic incident in the patient's history. An insidious onset of symptoms will warrant a full neurological assessment.

Nerve tissue may be damaged by direct trauma such as traction, laceration or compression. The site may be localized to the specific point of injury or widespread due to traction over a length of nerve. Associated injuries to surrounding or proximal tissue may cause further damage by ischaemia. Trauma is the most common cause of disruption of nerve conduction, but a nerve may be compressed or stretched by a swelling arising in adjacent tissue, such as a ganglion in the palm. Occasionally a nerve may be invaded and gradually destroyed by malignant tissue, as in Pancoast's tumour of the lung. Finally, nerve damage may be caused indirectly by irradiation and the effect may be delayed for many months after cessation of treatment for carcinoma of the breast and axillary irradiation.

Clinical signs

The presenting features are due to loss of function.

Motor paralysis

Paralysis is obvious in 'foot-drop' and the immediate conclusion is a lesion of the lateral popliteal nerve, but a detailed examination may reveal a wider pattern of weakness in the hamstring muscles, suggesting a proximal lesion of either part of the sciatic nerve or even a lumbar nerve root. Similarly, a "wrist-drop" may be caused by a lesion of the posterior interosseous nerve, the radial nerve, the posterior cord of the brachial plexus or the seventh cervical nerve root. Weakness may escape detection because of supporting unaffected muscle, trick movements or anomalous innervation; but wasting of muscle is a positive sign.

Sensory disturbance

Numbness and tingling may vary in severity from hypalgesia and hypoaesthesia to total analgesia and anaesthesia. The ultimate effect of loss of protective skin sensibility is illustrated in the infant with a complete lesion of the median nerve, due to previous injury by glass in the palm, who first presents with damaged pulps of the index and middle fingers due to chewing when finger sucking. The pattern is not always as clearly defined as in motor disturbance, but there is a very definite difference between a lesion of a nerve root and a peripheral nerve.

Pain

Subjective sensations described by patients will vary in severity from "pins and needles" to "agonizing" pain, but immediately after a nerve injury pain is not a feature unless there is superimposed muscle ischaemia. Pain at a later stage is invariably related to severe open injuries involving more than a peripheral nerve. It is customary to mention phantom pain and causalgia, both of which are separate and comparatively rare entities. Phantom pain is related to amputations, whereas causalgia is very rare and almost confined to gun shot injuries in the proximal part of a limb and not necessarily associated with an objective peripheral nerve lesion. The patient presents a sad dejected picture almost sobbing with pain, the affected limb protected by a damp cold cloth and all attempts at physical contact are avoided. A sympathetic nerve block usually provides an immediate diagnostic test with transient benefit. Causalgia, as a term, should be reserved for this rather special circumstance and not to be confused with common entities such as hyperpathia, hyperalgesia or hyperaesthesia, all of which mean increased sensitivity to touch occurring during reinnervation of the skin in the recovery phase after nerve repair or during spontaneous recovery in degenerative lesions in continuity.

Pain as a result of a severe traction lesion of the brachial plexus is continuous, burning in character and without any definite aggravating factor. The mechanism is not well understood, but it is not relieved by any local surgical procedure such as neurolysis, sympathectomy or even amputation. There is evidence of damage to the spinal cord in severe traction injuries of the plexus which provides the ultimate clue in determining the initial cause of the pain. Occasionally, nerve tissue is invaded by malignant lesions which cause intractable pain, but by contrast the rare primary tumours of nerves are not particularly painful.

Swelling

A localized swelling in a scar arising some months after an injury can be suspected to be a neuroma, which is painful, tethered and exquisitely tender to percussion. Tinel's sign is not considered to be a diagnostic test. Light percussion over a neuroma will cause tingling in the distribution of the affected nerve. When the percussion site is advanced distally along the course of the nerve and still evokes a response at successive intervals, it is an advancing Tinel's sign, which indicates regeneration. A stationary Tinel's sign at three to four weeks interval indicates lack of regeneration.

Vasomotor disturbance

The temperature, colour and nutrition of a limb may change as a result of an injury to a nerve responsible for major sensory areas such as the median or medial popliteal. By contrast, damage to predominantly motor nerves such as the radial or lateral popliteal rarely gives rise to trophic changes.

Temperature

The skin temperature of the affected extremity may feel warm immediately after a nerve injury, but within a month the main complaint is of coldness aggravated by cold weather and yet not particularly warm in hot weather.

Colour

Redness and cyanosis of the area of sensory loss are more apparent when the limb is cold and is dependent on the oxygenation of the capillary blood.

Skin atrophy

The natural texture of skin is altered in areas of sensory loss, and this is particularly evident in the pulps of fingers in lesions of the median nerve. The skin is shiny and feels smooth like the surface of paper compared with the normal velvety quality. There is wasting of the pulp and the nails become brittle.

Investigations

Electrical

The electrical excitability of tissue can be tested and compared by plotting a strength duration curve. The strength of current sufficient to produce a contraction of muscle is measured and, because nerve tissue is more electrically excitable than muscle, it is possible to determine the difference between normal and denervated muscle. This is the basis of the inaccurate single faradic/galvanic response which is superseded by the modern technique of employing stimuli of selected voltage and duration introduced by surface electrodes.

Electromyography

This method provides a sample of the electrical potential of muscle by a needle containing an electrode. Small muscles in the palm have only a few muscle fibres per motor unit when compared with bulky strong muscles of the leg. Normal muscle is electrically silent unless the exploring needle is near a motor end plate, but spontaneous and nonvoluntary electrical discharges are called fibrillations which occur in denervation. Further samples are taken in phases of muscle contraction.

Nerve conduction

The time taken to evoke a response in muscle is measured in milliseconds along various points of stimulation in a motor nerve. The nerve conduction velocity can be measured and compared with normal values which may reveal not only delayed conduction in a particular segment of the motor unit, but anomalous innervation. Sensory nerve conduction is usually measured in the opposite direction and thus it is possible to localize a nerve root lesion.

Diagnosis

In practice, the correct diagnosis of a nerve lesion can only be achieved by detailed analysis of the facts extracted from the history and clinical signs. This is a strict discipline based on definite anatomical pathways which vary very little.

Pathology

An understanding of the pathology is vital in the management of nerve injuries, indeed, the principles of repair are entirely dependent on these facts.

The nature and degree of damage in various circumstances is variable. Nevertheless, classification is possible; it would be more readily appreciated after reviewing nerve structure.

A single nerve fibre is an extension of the cytoplasm and cell membrane of a neuron, and is enclosed in turn by enveloping Schwann cells, their basement membrane and a mantle of collagen fibres produced by fibroblasts. This last forms a tube running from the neuron to the end organ of the axon, the endoneurium. On its way, the axon may branch many times, but each branch is enclosed by neural tube. Axons have the fluid property of cytoplasm, contain organelles, and have a transport system that runs in both directions. The principle organelles are protein structures—neurofilaments and neurotubules—which lend some body to the axon. The axon is, therefore, more than a simple impulse conductor on the analogy of a copper wire, and has a complex and incompletely understood biochemical activity of uncertain relationship to that of the Schwann cells. Every axon of whatever diameter is enfolded by Schwann cells: for axons below 1–2 μ diameter this is simple enclosure; but above this diameter the Schwann cell wraps itself around the axon to provide a multi-layer covering which we identify as a myelin sheath. The Schwann cell cytoplasm is excluded from the fully developed sheath, which consists then of only Schwann cell membrane; this is rich in lypoprotein which is responsible for the lipid-staining properties of myelin.

A variable number of nerve fibres are bundled together by an enveloping collagen sheath called the perineurium to form funiculi. The funiculi are bound together by an outer fibrous sheath, the epineurium, which blends with the perineurium where they are contiguous. Interstices in the nerve, whether within or around the funiculi are filled by small amounts of fibrofatty tissue. The funiculi divide, branch and coalesce in their course so that their transverse pattern is constant for distances only up to 15 mm. The perineurium and epineurium are both sufficiently substantial to withstand suture.

A blood supply to the nerve is by the extraneural and intraneural longitudinal vessels; some run alongside the nerve in a loose mesentery before penetrating it. These small vessels can be damaged by close dissection and their maximum intraneural length is not greater than 3 cm. They divide into short proximal and longer distal branches so that when a nerve is divided the proximal stump is usually well vascularized, but the distal stump may be ischaemic which can lead in turn to fibrosis. This could be a cause of failure in primary repair.

Classification of nerve injury

The terms *neurapraxia, axonotmesis* and *neurotmesis* are used as a simple classification with an histological basis and as such are better than loose descriptions such as contusion, compression or injury with intact nerve sheath. There is no easy classification of a traction injury of the brachial plexus which might well include all three types of lesion throughout the roots, cords, divisions and ramifications, but this injury is unique and requires separate study, although it does encompass the same pathological process as a peripheral nerve lesion.

Neurapraxia (non-action) is short-lived and predominantly a motor paralysis or paresis with associated but less pronounced sensory disturbance. The lesion is usually caused by local pressure which presumably temporarily affects the blood supply of a nerve segment or local demyelination may occur in larger fibres: details of the exact pathological process is not known because recovery is rapid and not longer than 2–3 weeks. Nerve degeneration does not occur in neurapraxia.

Axonotmesis implies damage to the AXON without disruption of the supporting stroma and collagen tubes. It is associated most commonly with closed fractures. For example, in seven out of eight closed fractures of the shaft of the humerus associated with a radial nerve lesion, the nerve will gradually recover without recourse to surgical repair. It will take time because the nerve fibre degenerates and will recover at a rate of 1 mm a day. Failure to recover after the expected date, which is estimated by measurement between the fracture and the first muscle to be innervated, is an indication to explore the nerve. This is sound advice for the management of closed nerve injuries at fracture sites and should prevent unnecessary meddlesome surgical procedures.

Neurotmesis (a cutting). The term describes the most serious lesion when the nerve may be completely divided or the contained nerve bundles and stroma are so disrupted that acceptable recovery is not possible.

Nerve degeneration

When a peripheral nerve fibre is severed there are three sites at which a reaction occurs.

The nerve cell The degree of the response is variable. For reasons not understood not all cells react; experimentally the proportion ranges from 10 to 90 per cent. Both the number of reactive cells and the degree of reaction are influenced by the severity and proximity of the injury. The reactions range from disorder and dissolution of Nissl substance to severe shrinkage, degeneration and eventual phagocytosis. In simple severence the cell reaction starts in 6 hours, and it is 2–3 weeks before recovery begins. This may be completed in up to 10 weeks.

The peripheral nerve Within hours of a severe nerve injury, Wallerian degeneration starts in both ends of the nerve. In those axons whose cell body maintains its integrity, the process extends proximally for only a few centimetres. But if neuron degeneration is severe or irreversible, then the whole of the axon disappears. The whole length of the distal portion of the nerve is affected by Wallerian degeneration. First the axoplasm breaks up, and within three days conduction has ceased. By the seventh day the myelin sheath begins to degenerate. The Schwann cells assume their phagocytic function and engulf the debris. They afterwards move out of the endoneural tube, mainly by migrating along its length, with the end result of empty neural tubes.

In addition to this specific axon response, there is the common reparative response of connective tissues to injury. Bleeding leads to blood clot, which in turn is the scaffold for granulation tissue, i.e. fibrovascular proliferation. Since funiculi tend to retract, there is a zone within the nerve ends where blood and epineural fibrous tissue are contiguous. The granulation tissue takes origin from the latter. This proliferating and developing fibrous tissue is augmented by the Schwann cells escaping from the neural tubes. Later on, when regenerating axons pass out of their neural tubes, they enter this reparative tissue; since the proliferating axons can branch extensively and their course is no longer guided, they add substantially to the bulk of the tissue at the end of the nerve. The usual end result is a bulbous swelling. But a reparative response also occurs at the severed end of the distal segment. This too is based on funicular retraction, blood clot, granulation tissue and a limited participation by Schwann cells. There are no axons unless the proximal stump is close enough for them to find their way to it. A much smaller swelling is produced; indeed, there may be none.

There is great variability in this reparative response, which, even when of substantial degree, does not necessarily impede restoration of axon continuity and some functional recovery. The regressive changes in the neuron and axon and the intense activity required to remove degenerate material and to effect repair is succeeded by the process of regeneration. The stimulus to this is thought to be biochemical; originating from the site of injury. It is difficult accurately to define the change of activity in the central parent cell from degeneration to repair, but restoration of Nissl substance is a major step in the latter. The proximal axon is stimulated to grow, a process associated with terminal enlargement, recognized as a growth cone. Numerous branches develop from each axon which explore the damaged territory in an attempt to make contact with the distal neural tubes. The stimulus, likely to be biochemical, is present within 4–5 days after injury, and is sustained by protein and later by lipids from the central cell. Any branch which grows down a distal neural tube will gradually increase the diameter of that shrunken tube. Myelination, that is the envelopment of the axon by Schwann cells, will occur later. Thus, there is an orderly method of repair in which an unknown factor attracts regenerating fibres into the distal nerve bundles. It is not recovery by chance, but there are serious hazards which can forestall the natural tendency to succeed. The pathway may be long, blocked by collagen tissue arising through infection or ischaemia, and at the distal end the tubes may be so shrunk by surrounding fibrous tissue as to render them incapable of expansion for the maturation of the regenerating nerve fibres.

It is not difficult to imagine the struggle that regenerating axons have to make to reach their goal. An impenetrable fibrous jungle perforated by nerve fibrils in a haphazard pattern is a fair description of a *Traumatic neuroma.* Spontaneous, but albeit very imperfect, recovery can take place, and if a secondary repair is to be considered, then the surgeon will have to balance this recovery against that which he hopes to achieve by resecting the reparative tissue and either closing the gap by suture or bridging it by graft.

Factors influencing regeneration

Age The younger the patient the better the quality of recovery. A child has rapid regeneration of axoplasm which flows faster than in adults. A limb of a child is comparatively short and the excursion between repair and end organ may be minimal.

Time The quicker the denervated end organs are reconnected to a central cell the better the recovery. A motor end plate will disappear within six months, but a sensory end organ may still be viable after two years. Moreover, denervated small muscle fibres shrink and become fibrous within six months, and their condition becomes irreversible.

Bulky muscle will survive much longer. There is sufficient evidence from the pathology of nerve injury to induce a sense of urgency in the surgeon. Nevertheless the biochemical changes in the central nerve cell and the probable, but not proven, chemotaxis which stimulate the growth cone, are not present for a few days after injury. The presumed moment of maximum biochemical activity might be the optimum time for repair. In all events, repair should not be delayed too long.

Joints

Introduction

The patient who refers his complaints to a joint will have one or more, perhaps all, of the following symptoms: pain, swelling, stiffness, deformity, locking, giving way, grating. All of these may have an abrupt or insidious onset, and may persist as a manifestation of a chronic disorder. In the basic approach to the patient's problem it is necessary to review the history and symptomatology in detail. A differential diagnosis is always made on the history, and is corroborated or refuted by clinical examination followed by investigation. It is therefore vital to take a very accurate history of the various combinations of the symptom complex. (See Fig. 28.12.)

It must be established at the outset whether the symptoms actually arise from joint involvement, and if more than one joint is affected. Soft tissue lesions such as bursa, ganglion, aneurysm and myositis ossificans may be confused with joint disease by the patient. The synovium may react in a quite non-specific way, and this will resolve when the condition is successfully treated.

Acute involvement of a single joint is nearly always due to a current traumatic episode or acute inflammation requiring immediate admission, further investigation, and treatment. Acute inflammation is suggested by the spontaneous onset of pain, swelling and limitation of movement through muscular spasm, and is often accompanied by a constitutional upset. Haematological investigation may suggest a generalized infective process with a local manifestation. X-ray of the joint will usually be negative. Aspiration of fluid for laboratory investigation for crystals, cells and organisms must be undertaken at an early stage to identify the organism for the most appropriate antibiotic treatment.

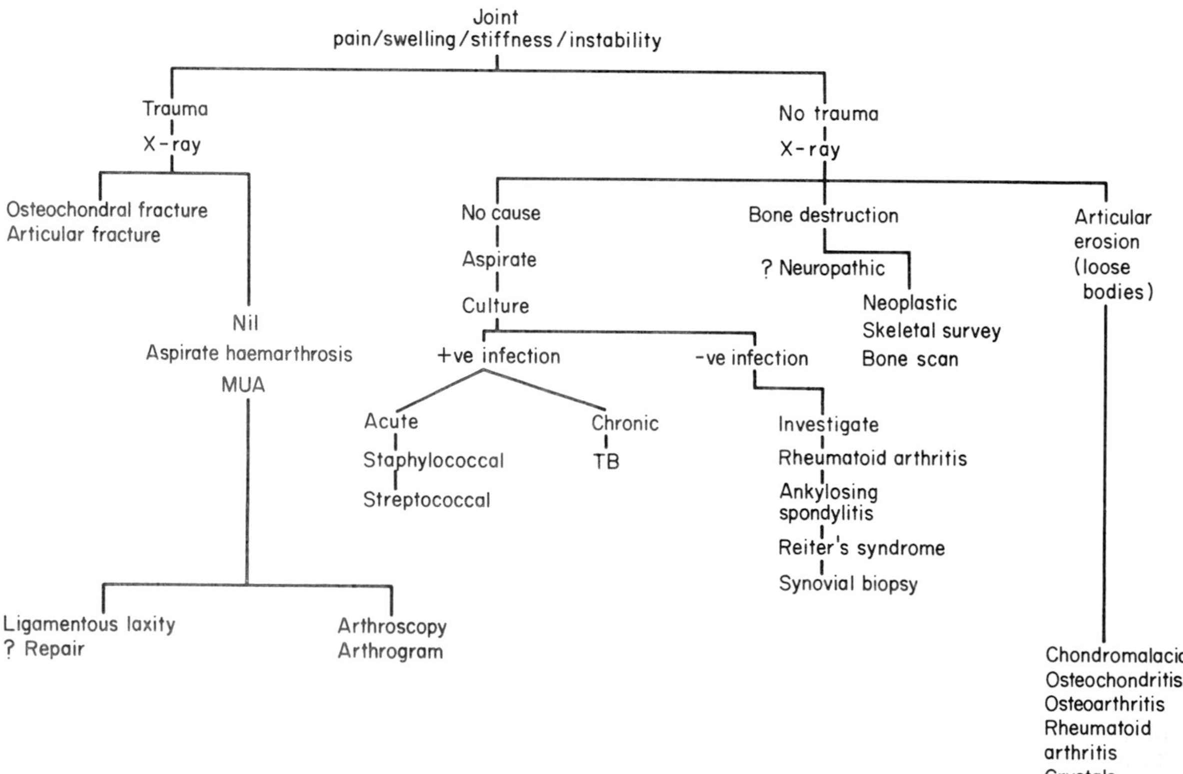

Fig. 28.12 Conditions arising in the joint.

Inflammatory joint disease

These diseases, mainly rheumatoid arthritis and its variants, are of major importance and are nearly always chronic in nature. There are acute inflammatory conditions due to pyogenic infection, which can occur alone or superimposed on chronic disease, such as rheumatoid arthritis. Additionally, inflammation of acute onset may be due to crystal deposition.

Underlying the aetiology and pathogenesis of much chronic arthritis is the HLA system, and its now widely recognized association with a number of diseases: for example, diabetes mellitus, ankylosing spondylitis, haemocromatosis and autoimmune diseases. At the moment this is expressed as the increased risk of disease in HLA types; for example, HLA B27 individuals have an 80 times greater risk of acquiring ankylosing spondylitis. The mechanism is not yet known.

Inevitably, the mechanism of the immune system is cell-dependent. Two main classes of lymphocytes, B and T, are recognized as the chief effectors, and there are two principle mechanisms: humoral and cell-mediated. B-lymphocytes are responsible for humoral antibodies, and T-lymphocytes for cell-mediated responses. Both cell types derive in the embryo from marrow stem cells. These migrate either to the thymus (T-cells) or the human equivalent (not yet identified) of fowl bursa of Fabricius (B-cells). Following maturation, both cell types migrate to lymphoid tissue from where they act, either *in situ* or by migration to a site of demand.

These two classes of cell act in concert with other mononuclear cells belonging to the monocyte series whose role is to present antigen to the effector cells. Moreover, the B and T effector cells have a number of subdivisions.

B-cells secrete immunoglobulins, of which there are five classes: IgM, IgA, IgD, IgE. Presentation of antigen by macrophages to the specific B-cell leads to its activation and to blast transformation with eventual production, through proliferation and maturation, of plasma cells which secrete antibody.

T-cells fall into a number of functional subcategories, either effector or regulatory. The former are responsible for T-cell-mediated immunity, which is activated through presentation of antigen by macrophages to the antigen-specific T-cell. This brings about blast transformation, cell division and differentiation into effector cells. Some of these are cytotoxic—so called killer cells—and some secrete mediators—the lymphokines, attractants of phagocytic cells. Regulatory T-cells are either helpers or suppressors. This is a reminder that the immune system is not an all-or-none response, but a complex system subject to regulation.

The expression of immune reactions in tissues has some or all of the features of an inflammatory process. The initial stages of acute inflammation are least influenced by immunologic factors. But their later stages, and chronic inflammation of whatever type, are very much involved with them. Auto-immune diseases also have a large element of the tissue pattern of inflammation in them. Such diseases are the consequence of a reaction against self-antigens. The concept, or hypothetical basis of these is far from fully corroborated. The body is complex with many antigenic components and is host to a highly organized system reacting to antigens. It remains a problem to know how the two are kept from interacting. Theory proposes that either or both of two methods operate: deletion of all lymphocytes bearing receptors for self-antigens; suppression of normally present autoreactive lymphocytes by T-suppressor cells.

Rheumatoid arthritis

The aetiology of the disease is unknown, but it is proposed that exogenous agents, mycoplasma and EB virus are favoured, initiate the immune reaction. Additionally, genetic factors play a part; individuals with HLA/DRW4, or DRW7, or DRW10 are more prone to the disease than others. Anti-IgG, the principle component of rheumatoid factor, is formed; and the antibody is mainly of the IgM class (80 per cent of patients are positive), but IgG, IgA, IgE antibodies are also found. Rheumatoid factor is found in a number of other diseases, and in some normal individuals. The IgG rheumatoid factor is found in joints, and since it is of itself an IgG molecule, self-association of rheumatoid factor molecules occurs forming complexes that can bind complement. The stage is set for the Arthus-type reaction: vasculitis, phagocytic infiltration, phagocytosis of complexes by these and by phagocytic synovial cells. Lysosomal enzymes are released which damage the tissues. The inflammatory response is proliferative in type: fibrovascular proliferation occurs and cellular infiltrate (lymphocytes, plasma cells, macrophages) accumulates. These cells may adopt a lymphoid tissue organization. The proliferative tissue thickens synovium, resorbs bone and extends over and beneath the articular cartilage which is resorbed. There then ensues progressive joint destruction, and either fibrous ankylosis or a secondary osteoarthritis. The majority of the lymphocytes are T-cells and there are grounds for believing that delayed hypersensitivity reactions are also involved.

Although the joints and periarticular tissues are principally involved, the disease is systemic and many other tissues may be affected: skin, arteries, nerves, heart, lungs and eyes.

Synovial membrane

As a vascularized tissue, the synovial membrane can undergo the range of inflammatory reactions described at the outset. But it is very rare to see acute pyogenic inflammation in the laboratory; and granulomatous inflammation is now an uncommon occurrence. Chronic inflammation is the class usually seen. A wide range of appearances is possible within that class, determined by the relative and absolute numbers of the different cells (lymphocytes, plasma cells, macrophages, multinucleated cells, and polymorphs), the reactive fibrosis, the degree of lining cell hyperplasia, and the amount of surface fibrin. Although there is no formal grading of this reaction, every pathologist uses a limited number of words with which to assess the inflammation. No degree of this inflammation is specific for any one disease. It is characteristic (not specific) for the synovium of some diseases to appear more frequently, but not exclusively, at one band in the range. Thus, there is a very limited predictive value in the reaction of synovial tissues, but as the inflammation becomes more severe, rheumatoid arthritis is more probable, and the converse for osteoarthritis. The overlap is extensive, and synovitis due to many other causes, including trauma and, for instance, adjacent osteoid osteoma, are not distinguishable. Plasma cells, often described as "rheumatoid cells", occur regularly in osteoarthritis. Small, superficially located multinucleated giant cells appear frequently in rheumatoid arthritis synovia, but they are not exclusive to it. The same is true of surface fibrin. There is nothing very surprising about this, since the inflammatory response is itself a pattern of activities inducible by a multitude of agents.

The one synovial reaction that does carry a good deal of specificity is pigmented villonodular synovitis. This is identifiable macroscopically by the brown/yellow pigmentation of the villous and nodular synovium. The condition can affect synovia at any site, the most common being the knees and the tendon sheath of the finger. The former is usually a diffuse involvement with villous, nodular and flat regions, all heavily pigmented. The membrane is thick and no longer supple. At points of contact with bone, erosion may occur, and this may be interpreted erroneously as neoplasia. In the tendon sheath of the finger, the lesion is generally a solitary pigmented nodule, and hence the concept of neoplasia or benign synovioma or even giant cell tumour of tendon sheath. Such solitary nodules may occur in any synovium, the tissues show a mixed cellular reaction in which macrophages and multinucleated giant cells are prominent. The pigment is haemosiderin and lipid, usually abundant and within macrophages.

Crystal deposition disease

Inflammation of connective tissue (excluding cartilage) is associated with crystal deposition disease. Two types of crystals are mainly responsible: monosodium urate and calcium pyrophosphate. The presence of the former invariably seems to cause disease, but the latter can be present without symptoms. When symptoms occur they resemble those of gout.

Both types of crystals are focally deposited in cartilage and synovium, where they appear as white chalky deposits. The mechanism of the deposition is not known; it is said of gout that during repeated acute attacks there is progressive deposition. The foci of urate crystals induce a foreign-body type of reaction. When the lesion is adjacent to or within bone, usually near joints, osteolytic foci result. There is, of course, no inflammation in cartilage, but it is believed that the deposits themselves render cartilage susceptible to its progressive loss and to osteoarthritis. On the other hand, there is little reaction to pyrophosphate deposits in the synovium. The pyrophosphate is more usually deposited in the cartilage, and this can be very extensive. Here, again, it is thought by some to predispose to osteoarthritis. But it is difficult to be certain whether the deposit occurred before or during, or at the end of the osteoarthritic process.

Pyrophosphate crystals can be associated with acute joint symptoms that are similar to those in gout. There is an acute inflammation of the synovium, presumably due to crystals formed by precipitation or released from deposits. The incorporation of crystals by neutrophils leads to disruption of the cells and release of lysosomal enzymes which are powerful mediators of acute inflammation. In addition, they can activate Hagemann factor, which also is a primary mediator of acute inflammation.

Primary gout is a generalized disease due to a hetrogeneous group of biochemical disorders affecting either production or excretion of uric acid, and transmitted genetically in several ways. It may also be a secondary complication in other metabolic disorders which affect uric acid metabolism. Hyperuricemia is the *sine qua non*. This may be present for some years before acute attacks occur. Any joint may be affected, but toe, ankle and knee are those usually involved. Later, urate deposits in the tissues are formed—the tophi of tophaceous gout: these occur most often in joints, periarticular tissues (ligaments, tendons, connective tissue), olecranon and patella bursae and ear lobes.

Cartilage and inflammation

Destruction of cartilage through inflammation is an enzymatic process, derived from cells or organisms. In pyogenic arthritis the enzymes are in the pus which bathes the cartilage and this is digested to allow the exposure of underlying bone.

In chronic inflammation the enzymes are released, it is believed, from cells in pannus. The latter is a fibrous or fibrovascular tissue taking origin from the synovium and extending over the articular surface. Although such a description is equated to rheumatoid arthritis, it is in fact a non-specific response of joints to a wide range of known and unknown stimuli. The classical example is the pannus in tuberculous joints. Another instance, but much less common, is the response to bone tumours occurring at the epiphyseal ends of bones, with or without treatment, which can include substantial amounts of pannus. Thus, the identification of pannus as an observation on its own is of limited value, and its significance is best judged in the context of the affected joint.

Further reading

Aegerter E, Kirkpatrick Jr. JA. *Orthopaedic Diseases; Physiology—Pathology—Radiology*, 4th edition. Philadelphia, London: WB Saunders, 1975.

Mirra Joseph M. *Bone Tumours: Diagnosis and Treatment.* Philadelphia, Toronto: Lippincott, 1980.

Robbins Stanley L, Angell Maria, Kumar Vinay. *Basic Pathology*. 3rd Edition. Philadelphia, London: Saunders, 1981.

29

Paediatrics

Section 1: L Spitz and J R Pincott

Vomiting in Infancy

Introduction

Although the regurgitation of milk and even the occasional actual vomiting of a feed is generally regarded as a normal occurrence in the infant, persistent vomiting or the presence of bile in the vomitus requires urgent investigation. Non-bilious vomiting may be either projectile or non-projectile in character (see Fig. 29.1).

Non-bilious vomiting

Hypertrophic pylonic stenosis

A potent cause of projectile vomiting is hypertrophic pyloric stenosis, a relatively common condition which is seen in one of every 200 boys, and one of every 800 girls. There are clinical grounds for believing that neuromuscular pyloro-spasm is the first step in the development of this condition. This is, however, followed by a marked hypertrophy of all three layers of the pyloric muscularis propria, but particularly the outermost circular layer. Submucosal inflammation and oedema also contribute to the obstruction. No specific cause for the condition has been found, though secondary degenerative changes in the pyloric neuronal plexuses have been seen. To the naked eye, the end result of the hypertrophy is in a spindle-shaped pyloric mass which ends abruptly at the pyloroduodenal junction—a fact of great surgical importance when relieving the obstruction surgically.

Vomiting in hypertrophic pyloric stenosis commences between 2 to 4 weeks of age, but may be present from birth. The vomiting occurs within 30 minutes of a feed and may contain "coffee-ground" material. The source of the blood loss has been ascribed to a concomitant gastritis, but recent studies have shown it to be due to reflux oesophagitis. The infant fails to thrive, is constipated and, on physical examination, visible gastric peristalsis and a palpable "pyloric tumour" can be found.

Gastro-oesophageal reflux

Vomiting from gastro-oesophageal reflux may closely mimic that of pyloric stenosis, but is usually less forceful and may even be regurgitant in type. The lower oesophageal sphincter is relatively immature at birth and most infants with gastro-oesophageal reflux will respond to conservative treatment such as upright posture, thickened feeds and antacids, while gradual maturation of the sphincter occurs. Indications for surgical treatment include stricture formation and failure of intensive conservative treatment with persistent failure to thrive, oesophagitis or respiratory problems. Apnoeic attacks and recurrent bronchitis may be particularly troublesome.

Other causes of non-bilious vomiting

These include feeding problems, infections (urinary tract infections, meningitis, or pneumonia), neurological conditions such as cysts, tumours and hydrocephalus, which cause intracranial hypertension.

Bilious vomiting

The presence of green bile in the vomitus of a newborn infant should be regarded as pathological and indicative of mechanical intestinal obstruction, unless an alternative diagnosis can be established. Obstructions in the upper intestine will be associated with epigastric fullness only, while the lower in the intestine the obstruction, the greater the degree of abdominal distension.

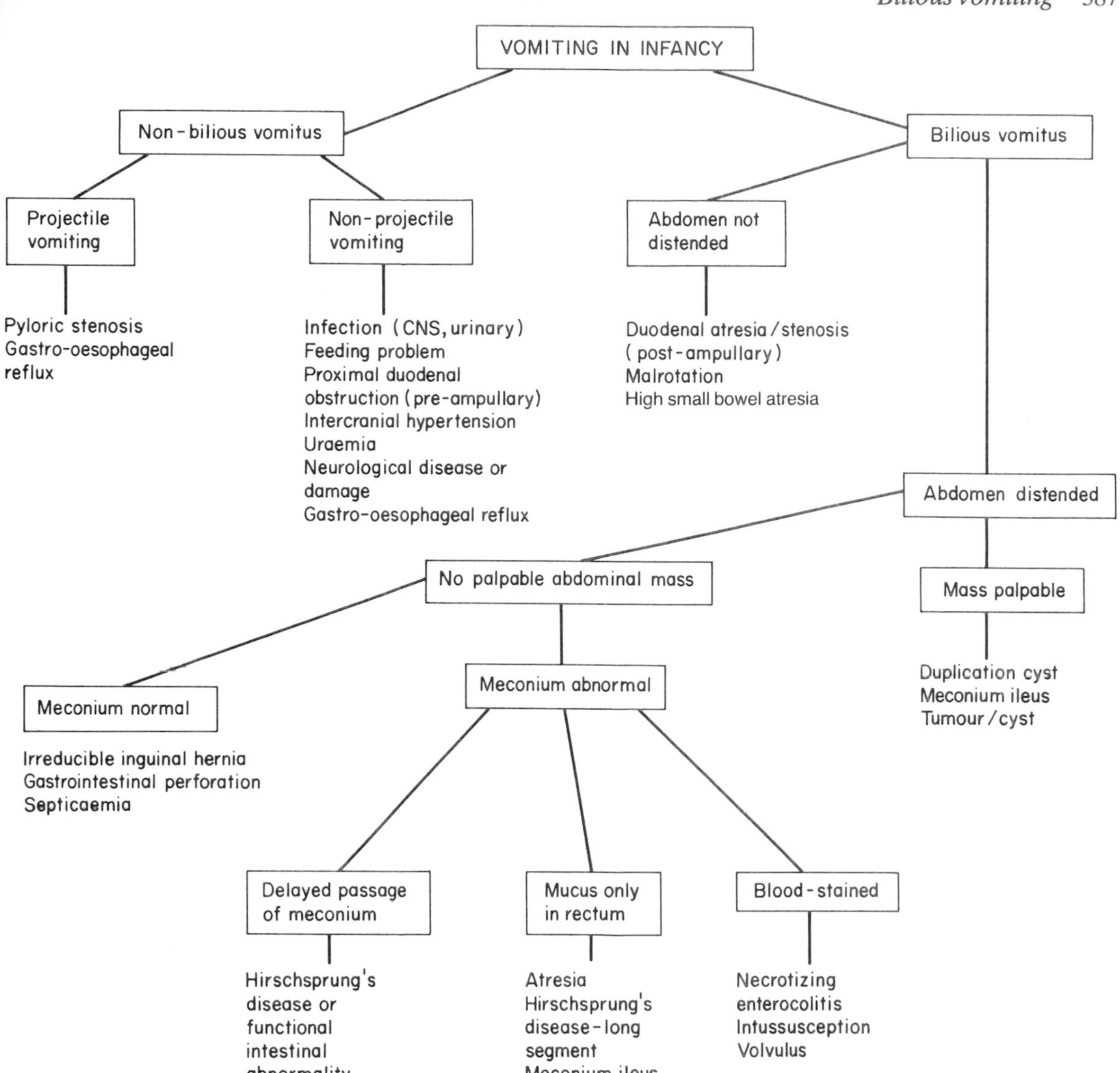

Fig. 29.1 Causes of vomiting in infancy.

Duodenal obstructions

Duodenal obstructions may be caused either by intrinsic or extrinsic lesions. Duodenal atresias and stenosis are frequently associated with additional anomalies such as Down's syndrome, congenital cardiac malformations, oesophageal atresia and anorectal anomalies.

In atresias of the duodenum, the gap between the proximal and distal is frequently occupied by the pancreas, giving the impression of an annular pancreas. Stenosis of the duodenum may be due to a narrowing of the lumen, but is frequently caused by a diaphragm with a central aperture. As the malformation is usually found at the junction of the second and third parts of the duodenum, the vomiting is bile-stained. Atresias of the oesophagus and anus are sufficiently common in association with the duodenal lesion to require careful assessment routinely. The treatment in all cases is by a duodenoduodenostomy without dissection of the ampullary region.

In midgut malrotation causing extrinsic compression in the duodenum, there is a significant risk of volvulus, particularly in the neonatal period. This may result in massive intestinal necrosis. A constrast study of the upper gastrointestinal tract will demonstrate the abnormal configuration of the duodenum. Alternatively, a contrast enema may demonstrate the abnormally placed caecum. In atresias of the upper intestine, the plain erect abdominal X-ray will demonstrate air-fluid levels in the dilated proximal intestine—this is the origin of the "double-bubble" in duodenal atresia, with an opaque appearance in the rest of the abdomen. In early infancy, until 6 months of age, it is difficult to differentiate large from small intestine on the plain abdominal radiograph.

Small intestinal atresias

In small intestinal atresias, it is more common to find discontinuity of intestine, though the proximal and distal blind ends may be connected by a fibrous cord. A segmental deficiency is often found in the adjacent part of the mesentery with associated anomalies in the vascular arcade. Small intestinal atresias are so frequently multiple—in an estimated 15 per cent of cases—that detailed examination of the remainder of the intestine is mandatory in surgery for this condition. In rare cases, multiple small intestinal atresias may be arranged spirally around a central mesentery—the so-called "apple-peel intestine".

Abdominal mass

An abdominal mass causing extrinsic compression on the intestine produces bilious vomiting and abdominal distention. The mass may be either *intraperitoneal* (duplication or mesenteric cyst, meconium ileus, ovarian cyst, hydrometrocolpos, etc.) or *extraperitoneal* (hydronephrosis, multicystic kidney, mesoblastic nephroma, etc.) and will be palpable on abdominal examination. Intestinal duplications are most commonly found in the terminal ileum, and may be enclosed with the small intestine in a single muscularis propria. Alternatively, tubular or cystic duplications may be found within the mesentery at its junction with the intestine.

Other causes of bilious vomiting

There remains a large group of infants in whom bilious vomiting and abdominal distension are not associated with a palpable abdominal mass. In these cases attention should be focused on the character of the meconium. The complete absence of meconium or the presence of mucus alone in the rectum is suggestive of an intestinal atresia or meconium ileus. Delayed passage of meconium, that is in excess of 24 hours after birth, should alert the suspicion of Hirschsprung's disease (see "Constipation"). The presence of blood mixed in the meconium or stool, particularly in the distressed premature infant, is suspicious of necrotizing enterocolitis. The presence of pneumatosis intestinalis on the plain abdominal X-ray is diagnostic. Necrotizing enterocolitis characteristically involves the terminal ileum, ascending and descending colon in a distinctly focal fashion. The affected areas show severe vascular congestion and oedema, gas bubbles within the bowel wall and, ultimately, necrosis, perforation and peritonitis. Ischaemic intestine due, for example, to volvulus or intussusception, will also produce blood in the stools.

As inguinal hernias are liable to strangulate in 50 per cent of cases in the first three months of life, examination of the inguinal canal should never be omitted in the obstructed infant. Infection, as indicated above, frequently causes vomiting in infants. When the infection progresses to a septicaemia, ileus supervenes and the clinical picture may closely resemble a mechanical obstruction. The clue to the diagnosis is that the infant appears much more lethargic and ill than is compatible with the degree of obstruction. In addition, there is often jaundice and thrombocytopenia. Blood cultures, urinalysis, cerebrospinal fluid and skin swabs are submitted for laboratory investigations, culture and sensitivity, but broad-spectrum antibiotic (pencillin, gentamicin and metronidazole) administration should not be delayed pending the results of these investigations.

Respiratory Distress

Introduction

Respiratory distress in the neonate is present when there is a tachypnoea in excess of 60 per minute, a tachycardia of over 160 per minute, cyanosis and/or evidence of the use of accessory muscles of respiration.

Cardiac failure in infancy presents predominantly with respiratory symptoms such as dyspnoea, particularly during feeding, and tachycardia. Peripheral oedema is unusual and signs of pulmonary

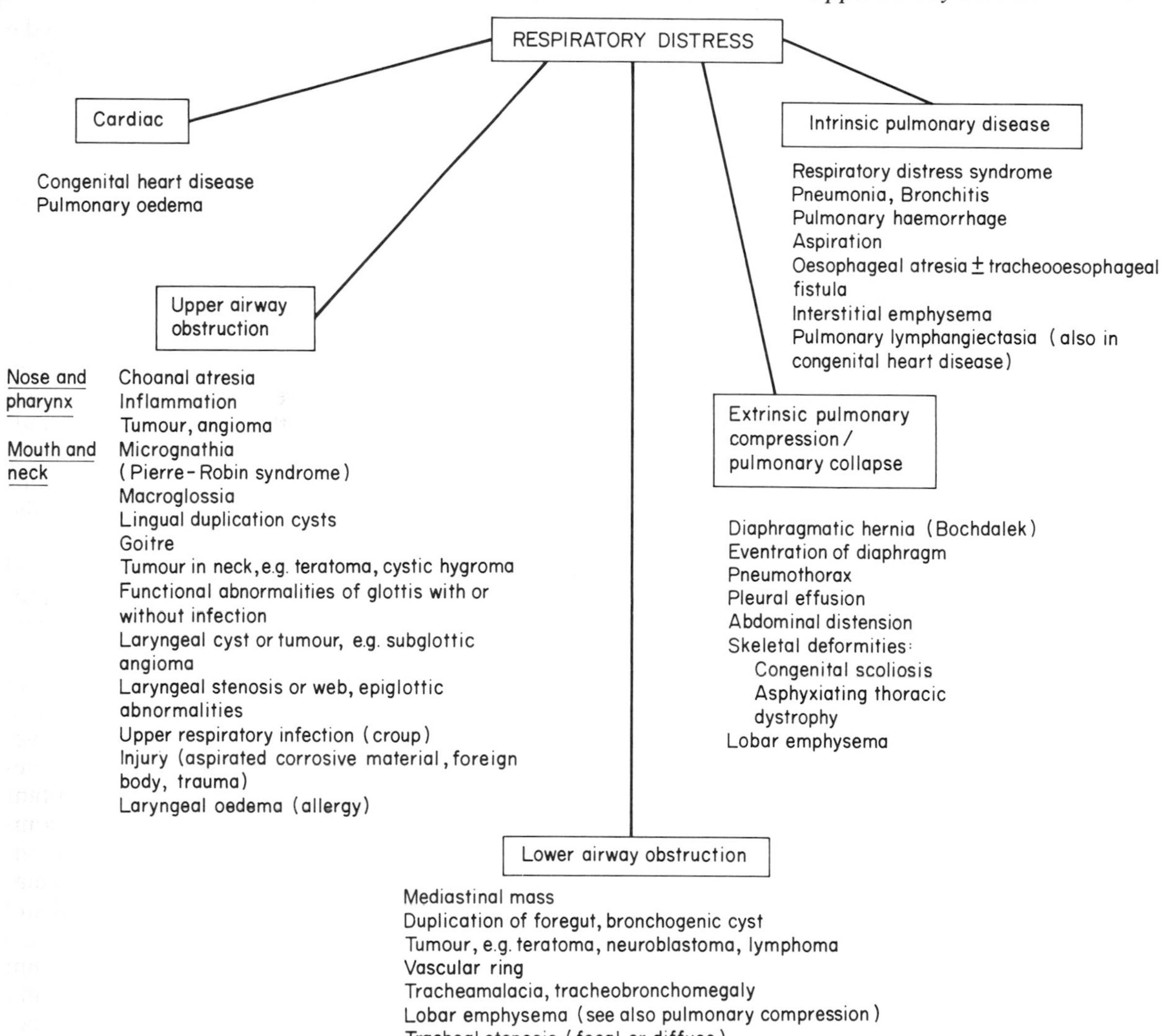

Fig. 29.2 Causes of respiratory distress in the neonate and infant.

congestion are late manifestations. Hepatomegaly is invariably present to a greater or lesser extent.

Upper airway obstruction

Causes of upper airway obstruction may be obvious on external inspection, for example micrognathia, goitre, cystic hygroma, etc., or may only be discovered after endoscopic examination of the upper air passages, for example laryngeal cysts, epiglottitis. Choanal atresia may be either unilateral or bilateral and may result from membranous or osseous obstruction. There is a failure of the normal dissolution of the choanal membrane. The newborn infant being an obligatory nasal breather will suffocate unless the patency of the airway is established. The diagnosis of choanal atresia is made by failure to pass a nasal catheter or by contrast nasopharyngography. Definitive treatment consists of resection of the obstructing membrane or bony spur, combined with prolonged stenting to prevent stenosis of the nasal passages. Obstructing lesions, such as cysts or tumours, are treated by excision, while inflammatory causes of upper airway obstruction may necessitate the use of temporary endotracheal intubation pending a response to antibiotic therapy, for example epiglottitis.

Lower airway obstruction

Lower airway obstructions result from compression on the air passages by tumours or cysts arising in the mediastinum or from intrinsic abnormalities in the structure of the wall of the main airways, for example tracheomalacia. Mediastinal masses are best classified according to their anatomical location. The most common anterior mediastinal masses encountered in this age range are lymphomas, teratomas, dermoid cysts, cystic hygromas, thymic masses, pericardial cysts and anterior diaphragmatic hernias (Morgagni). In the middle mediastinum, lymphomas and congenital anomalies of the heart and great vessels predominate. All tumours of the mediastinum should be submitted for histological examination after consultation with the pathologist. The tumours should be provided fresh, with no fixative, so that investigations such as tumour markers may be performed. Most of these tests, though essential for accurate diagnosis and treatment in modern oncology, cannot be carried out on fixed tissues.

Vascular rings, for example abberant right subclavian artery and double aortic arch, may cause either dysphagia or stridor. The diagnosis is established at contrast oesophagogram and angiography and treatment consists of division of the constricting ring. Posterior mediastinal masses consist mainly of foregut duplication cysts and neurogenic tumours, particularly neuroblastomas. Duplication cysts usually do not communicate with the organ of origin but may contain ectopic mucosa. Excision is generally accomplished fairly easily, but the larger duplication cysts may communicate through the diaphragm with the upper small intestine. Thoracic neuroblastomas do not appear to carry the same serious prognostic indications as do the abdominal neuroblastomas, possibly because early compression of mediastinal structures leads to earlier presentation.

Posterolateral diaphragmatic hernia

An important surgical cause of respiratory distress in the newborn requiring urgent intervention is the posterolateral diaphragmatic hernia through the foramen of Bochdalek. It presents with progressive respiratory distress, displacement of the heart and mediastinum to the right and a scaphoid abdomen. The left side is more frequently involved than the right in the ratio of 9:1. The defect is in the posterolateral area of the diaphragm at the site of the pleuroperitoneal canal (foramen of Bochdalek) which normally is obliterated by the 12th week of intrauterine life. The herniated intestine compresses the developing lung resulting in a varying degree of pulmonary hypoplasia. It should be remembered that the contralateral lung will also be hypoplastic as a result of its compression by the shifted mediastinum.

Malrotation of the midgut invariably accompanies the anomaly and for this reason an abdominal surgical approach is generally recommended so that the malrotation can be corrected simultaneously with the hernia repair. The diagnosis is established on plain X-ray of the chest and abdomen which reveals intestinal gas shadows on the ipsilateral side of the chest, a shift of the mediastinal structures to the contralateral side and minimal intra-abdominal bowel gas.

The emergency treatment consists of nasogastric decompression, nursing in a high-oxygen environment and endotracheal intubation with mechanical ventilation if respiratory distress fails to respond. The prognosis is directly related to the degree of pulmonary hypoplasia. Infants presenting within the first 6–12 hours of life have severe pulmonary hypoplasia which is responsible for the 40–50 per cent mortality rate. Presentation after 12 hours of life is rarely associated with a significant degree of pulmonary hypoplasia and most of these infants should survive.

Eventration of the diaphragm

Eventration of the diaphragm may result from trauma to the phrenic nerve during a difficult delivery or may be acquired during surgery in the thorax. It may also be congenital in origin as a result of muscular hypoplasia of the developing diaphragm. Clinically, the condition may present in the neonatal period with respiratory embarrassment or may only be diagnosed following recurrent bouts of pneumonia. Straight X-ray of the chest reveals an elevated leaf of the affected diaphragm with paradoxical movement on screening. The mediastinum is displaced to the opposite side.

The condition is poorly tolerated by the young infant, particularly if the paralysis of the diaphragm is bilateral. If there is a possibility that the damage to the phrenic nerve is reversible, the acute situation can be managed conservatively with continuous positive airway pressure ventilation (CPAP) for a period of 4–6 weeks. Where there is a relapse following the conservative regimen, or where the phrenic nerve is permanently damaged, surgery is recommended. The aim of surgery is to splint the paralysed diaphragm in the inspiratory position, thereby minimizing paradoxical movement. This is best achieved by means of a plication-type procedure.

Congenital lobar emphysema

Congenital lobar emphysema is the result of massive overinflation of one lobe of the lung (most often the left upper lobe), caused by obstruction by a congenital anomaly of the bronchus to the affected lobe. The anomaly is most commonly a hypoplasia, dysplasia or even total absence of the bronchial cartilages which allows bronchial collapse on expiration and prevents escape of air. The overinflated lung compresses the adjacent pulmonary lobes, causes displacement of the mediastinum to the contralateral side and produces increasing respiratory distress.

Oesophageal atresia

Oesophageal atresia may be associated with a tracheo-oesophageal fistula from the upper pouch, the lower pouch, both or neither, but the commonest by far is a fistula from the lower pouch, this occurring in 90 per cent of cases.

The diagnosis may be suspected before birth by the presence of maternal polyhydramnios. At birth the infant is excessively mucous and requires repeated oropharyngeal suction to clear the upper air passages. A large nasogastric tube (No. 10 French) fails to enter the stomach—arrest of the tube commonly occurs 10 cm from the lower gum margin. An X-ray will confirm the high position of the tube in the upper oesophagus and air in the gastrointestinal tract will indicate the presence of a tracheo-oesophageal fistula.

In 5 per cent of cases in which there is an isolated oesophageal atresia, no gas can enter the stomach, and the entire abdomen appears opaque on X-ray examination. Associated malformations in combination with oesophageal atresia are common. These include congenital heart anomalies, duodenal atresia and the VATER association (Vertebral, Anorectal, Tracheal, "Esophageal", Radial and Renal anomalies). The majority of cases can be successfully corrected by ligation of the tracheo-oesophageal fistula and end-to-end oesophago-oesophageal anastomosis. A survival rate in excess of 90 per cent can be expected where there are no major associated anomalies.

Constipation

Introduction

Constipation refers to the presence in the rectum of hard stools which are difficult to evacuate. Contrary to popular belief, it is not synonymous with infrequent or irregular bowel actions, Basically, the causes of constipation can be grouped into two categories according to the presence or absence of normal intestinal innervation. This in no way inplies that histopathological examination should be carried out in every case as the differentiation may frequently be made on clinical grounds.

Hirschsprung's disease

Hirschsprung's disease most frequently presents in early infancy with delayed passage of meconium, i.e. failure to pass meconium within the first 24 hours after birth. It is almost invariably associated with abdominal distension, while bilious vomiting develops in relation to the degree of intestinal obstruction. Digital rectal examination may reveal a relatively "tight" anus and frequently results in the passage of a plug of inspissated meconium followed by large quantities of normal meconium. Although the obstructive symptoms may be relieved by this manoeuvre or by a subsequent rectal washout, the relief may be only of a temporary nature and investigations to exclude Hirschsprung's disease should proceed. The barium enema examination is notoriously misleading during the neonatal period and the only positive feature may be prolonged retention of the barium over a 24-hour period. In the older infant and child, the classical picture of a contracted irritable lower aganglionic segment with proximal dilatation is seen in over 75 per cent of cases. Electromanometric studies in Hirschsprung's disease reveal failure of the internal sphincter to relax in response to proximal stimulation. This examination is unfortunately also unreliable in the neonatal period.

Biopsy

The most reliable method of diagnosis of Hirschsprung's disease is by means of tissue diagnosis of suction rectal biopsies. For adequate pathological examination at least three specimens—2, 3 and 4 cm from the anal verge—should be obtained. The procedure can safely be carried out without

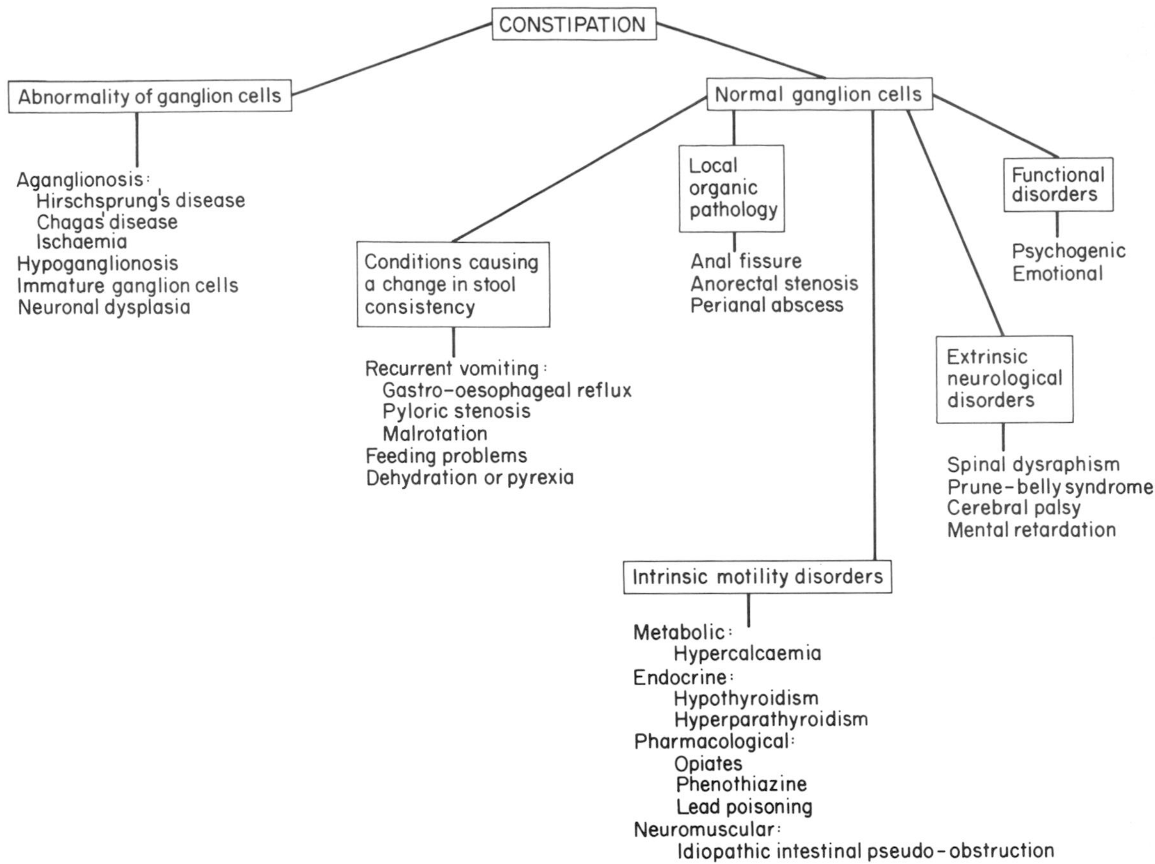

Fig. 29.3 Causes of constipation in the neonate and infant.

an anaesthetic, and in practised hands the risk of intestinal perforation is negligible.

The suction rectal biopsies may be dealt with in one of two ways—paraffin wax-embedded serial sections or the acetylcholinesterase method. A decision has to be made before the time of biopsy as to which of these techniques will be employed, because the former method requires the specimen to be fixed promptly in formalin, and the latter can only be performed on snap-frozen material. Any doubts on this or other questions can usually be solved by a short consultation between the surgeon and the pathologist.

The rectal biopsies, once taken, are orientated gently, submucosal side downwards on a piece of card to be fixed or frozen immediately, or transferred directly to the laboratory for these procedures to be carried out as soon as possible.

The fixed specimens are embedded in paraffin wax and serial sections taken from the submucosal surface. It is essential that adequate numbers of these sections be available for examination, so 60 are cut at first, in ribbons of 10 sections, two ribbons per slide. This method provides maximum information from any biopsy with minimum effort and a few slides for storage. The slides are examined for submucosal ganglion cells or nerve trunks: the presence of ganglion cells excludes the diagnosis of Hirschsprung's disease at the level of that biopsy, and the presence of large abnormal nerve trunks in the absence of ganglion cells on the serial sections confirms the diagnosis of Hirschsprung's disease. Difficulties may arise with biopsies from the terminal 1–2 cm of rectum where ganglion cells are normally sparse, and occasional nerve trunks normally found in the submucosa, but these problems are usually solved by the examination of adequate numbers of serial sections.

For the acetylcholinesterase technique, the frozen material is sectioned perpendicularly to the surface and sections prepared by the method of Meier-Ruge et al. (1972) or the modification of Lake et al. (1978). The sections are examined for evidence of Hirschsprung's disease, namely an increase in acetylcholinesterase-positive nerve fibres in the lamina propria, muscularis mucosae and submucosa, and the absence of submucosal ganglion cells.

In those rare cases of total colonic aganglionosis there may be considerable variation in the number or distribution of mucosal and submucosal nerves whichever method is used for their demonstration, and it may even be impossible to demonstrate any at all in some biopsies. In these cases, the presence or absence of ganglion cells is the only criterion of any value in assessing the length of the aganglionic segment.

Occasionally, an emergency situation arises where it is essential to confirm the diagnosis of Hirschsprung's disease for the purpose of immediate surgery. This can usually be achieved rapidly by haematoxylin and eosin staining of frozen sections of suction rectal biopsies, though the technique is best reserved for emergencies as it can provide difficulties for the pathologist not experienced in this field.

Where experienced histopathological assistance is lacking, a full thickness rectal biopsy may be necessary. This is a more difficult and potentially hazardous procedure in the newborn requiring general endotracheal anaesthesia. The pathological findings in a full-thickness biopsy are very similar to those in a suction biopsy. The aganglionic segment will be found to end at almost exactly the same point in the myenteric as in the submucosal plexus.

Should the diagnosis have been overlooked in the neonatal period, there is a 70 per cent mortality rate and a 30 per cent risk of the infant developing enterocolitis. This presents with profuse diarrhoea in association with abdominal distention and bilious vomiting. Urgent resuscitation and gentle mechanical evacuation of the large intestine is mandatory prior to the establishment of a colostomy.

The older child who presents with chronic constipation and mild malnutrition almost certainly represents a "missed" case in the neonatal period. Over 80 per cent of these children will have a positive history for delayed passage of meconium in the neonatal period.

Premature infants, especially those with perinatal problems such as respiratory distress, commonly failed to pass meconium for 48–72 hours. In the absence of other features of intestinal obstruction, a conservative approach should be adopted. Immature ganglion cells may be demonstrated in those cases in which a rectal biopsy is taken. The immaturity of the appearance of the ganglion cells may reflect an immaturity of function, leading to failure to pass meconium, but this is not proved.

When performing a colostomy for aganglionosis, it is desirable to have frozen-section facilities available in order to ensure that the colostomy is performed in normally innervated intestine. The barium enema may give an indication of the extent of the aganglionic segment and at laparotomy a transition from dilated proximal ganglionic bowel to narrow, contracted aganglionic intestine may be evident. The biopsy for frozen section should contain both layers of muscularis propria, so as to ensure that part of the myenteric plexus is present. Frozen sections are cut and ganglion cells and nerve trunks sought between the two layers of muscularis.

Other causes of constipation.

The majority of cases of constipation in older infants and children are due to a variety of conditions other than aganglionosis. These include conditions which cause an alteration in stool consistency, such as a poor diet, recurrent vomiting, local organic pathology causing pain on defecation (the most important of which is a simple anal fissure), and extrinsic neurological disorders such as spinal dysraphism and mental retardation, especially Down's syndrome. These conditions are relatively simple to diagnose, though may themselves be associated with abnormal nerve trunks with ganglion cells in the neural plexuses. The diagnosis of intrinsic motility disorders requires special investigations, such as serum calcium for hypoparathyroidism and idiopathic hypercalcaemia and plasma triiodothyronine (T_3) for hypothyroidism. Drugs such as opiates and phenothiazide may also induce constipation. By far the largest group of constipation cases in children result from emotional psychogenic causes. These are particularly refractory to treatment and the resulting megacolon may require prolonged periods of bowel training before the problem is alleviated.

Finally, mention must be made of the technique of handling the colon and rectum removed at the time of the pull-through procedure for Hirschsprung's disease. The specimen is opened longitudinally and pinned out mucosa upwards for fixation in the usual manner. After fixation is complete, a full thickness strip of bowel is taken from one end of the specimen to the other, the strip being approximately 0.5 cm wide. This is cut into pieces, each as long as will comfortably fit on a microscope slide, and the orientation of the pieces preserved. They are labelled alphabetically from distal to proximal and a mucosal nick taken from the distal end of each piece. After routine paraffin wax processing, it is then possible to determine precisely the length of the aganglionic segment removed and ensure that normally innervated bowel is present at the proximal cut end.

Jaundice

The investigation of hyperbilirubinaemia is simplified by classifying the various causes into two main groups—unconjugated and conjugated forms.

Unconjugated hyperbilirubinaemia

Unconjugated hyperbilirubinaemia is defined biochemically as an increased total serum bilirubin with less than 15 per cent in the conjugated form. It is frequently physiological in the neonatal period where levels of up to 200 μmol/litre are recorded on the second to fourth day and which gradually return to normal by the eighth day. Haematological disorders, rhesus and ABO incompatibility in particular, are fairly common causes and are responsible for the majority of the cases of kernicterus. This complication, which results in permanent brain damage, is due to the deposition of unconjugated bilirubin in the basal ganglia. A serum bilirubin of 340 μmol/litre in a full-term infant, and proportionately less in the premature or ill neonate, constitutes a significant risk. Early treatment with phototherapy or exchange transfusion is essential. Genetic and metabolic causes of jaundice in this category are rare.

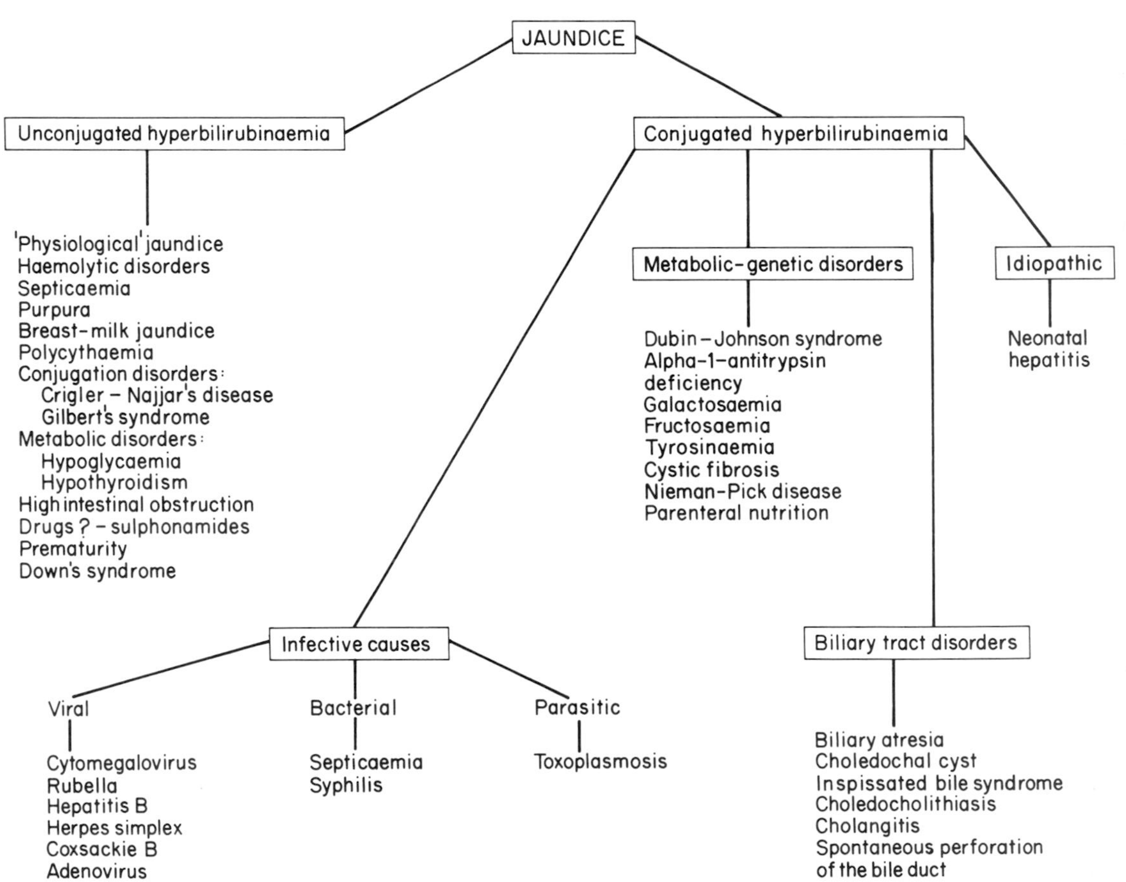

Fig. 29.4 Causes of jaundice in the neonate and infant.

Conjugated hyperbilirubinaemia

Conjugated hyperbilirubinaemia is *always* pathological in infancy and demands urgent investigation. It is most commonly due to either inflammatory lesions of the liver or to obstructive causes in the biliary tract. Differentiation in early infancy on clinical and biochemical grounds between these two conditions is extremely difficult, but, if surgically correctable lesions are to be successfully managed, operative treatment must be carried out within the first three months of life, i.e. prior to the development of irreversible liver damage. It is also important for prognostic reasons to recognize the metabolic genetic disorders even though effective treatment may not be available.

Biliary atresia/neonatal hepatitis

Although laparotomy with operative cholangiography and wedge liver biopsy will ultimately establish a definitive diagnosis of biliary atresia, a number of biochemical, radiological and pathological studies have been shown to be of value in differentiating between biliary atresia and neonatal hepatitis. Serological tests should be undertaken to exclude all known causes of hepatitis in this age-group. Of particular importance is the alpha-l-antitrypsin estimation. The rose-bengal faecal excretion test has been shown to be of diagnostic value when less than 10 per cent of the injected dose in excreted in the faeces in 72 hours. This result would indicate severe cholestasis compatible with the diagnosis of biliary atresia. Radioisotope scans of the liver, ultrasonography and percutaneous transhepatic cholangiography may be of diagnostic assistance.

In the differentiation of extrahepatic biliary atresia from neonatal hepatitis, which is the most common diagnostic dilemma in this area, a percutaneous needle biopsy is invaluable. It is also useful in diagnosing other, rarer causes of jaundice. Certainly the great majority of cases may readily be categorized accurately by this investigation.

The hall-mark of biliary atresia, as with most other forms of extrahepatic bile duct obstruction is a striking degree of bile duct proliferation within the portal tracts of the liver; very little bile duct proliferation is seen in giant cell hepatitis. As might be expected, the liver of biliary atresia can show considerable bile stasis, though a little bile may also be detected in the liver of giant cell hepatitis. Other histological features are less reliable in the differential diagnosis, though commonly seen. In the portal tracts there is a progressive fibrosis in biliary atresia which progresses to linking of adjacent tracts and ultimately a portal cirrhosis. The fibrosis of giant cell hepatitis is more diffuse, less severe, and often involves the hepatic parenchyma in addition. Although inflammatory changes are common in both conditions, neutrophils are more common in association with atresia, and lymphocytes with hepatitis.

Finally, multinucleate hepatocytes—"giant cells"—though apparently a non-specific response of the infant liver to almost any injury, are found far less frequently in atresia than giant cell hepatitis. In this condition they are seen in association with such other signs of liver injury as hepatocellular "ballooning" degeneration and rosette formation. As neonatal giant cell hepatitis has been described in association with a wide variety of bacterial, viral and other infections, it is a wise precaution to submit a piece of the biopsy for culture.

It is essential to complete all the above investigations as soon as possible so that surgical correction of those infants with biliary atresia can be carried out before 2–3 months of age. Correctable types of extrahepatic biliary atresia are treated by means of a Roux-en-Y enterobiliary anastomosis, while the Kasai type of procedure, or one of its many modifications, is performed in infants in whom no patent biliary channel can be isolated outside the porta hepatis. Bile drainage has been achieved in 80 per cent of patients with biliary atresia when the correction is performed before 60 days of age, while the "success" rate falls to below 20 per cent if surgery is delayed beyond 90 days.

Gastrointestinal haemorrhage

Introduction

The presence of blood in the stools is an alarming symptom which is promptly brought to the attention of the doctor. Once a bleeding diathesis such as thrombocytopenia, vitamin K deficiency or haemophilia has been excluded, there remains a wide spectrum of conditions to be aetiologically implicated. Close enquiry should be made as to the nature and quantity of blood lost as well as to additional physical signs, such as bilious vomiting, hypovolaemic shock, chronic anaemia. The anus

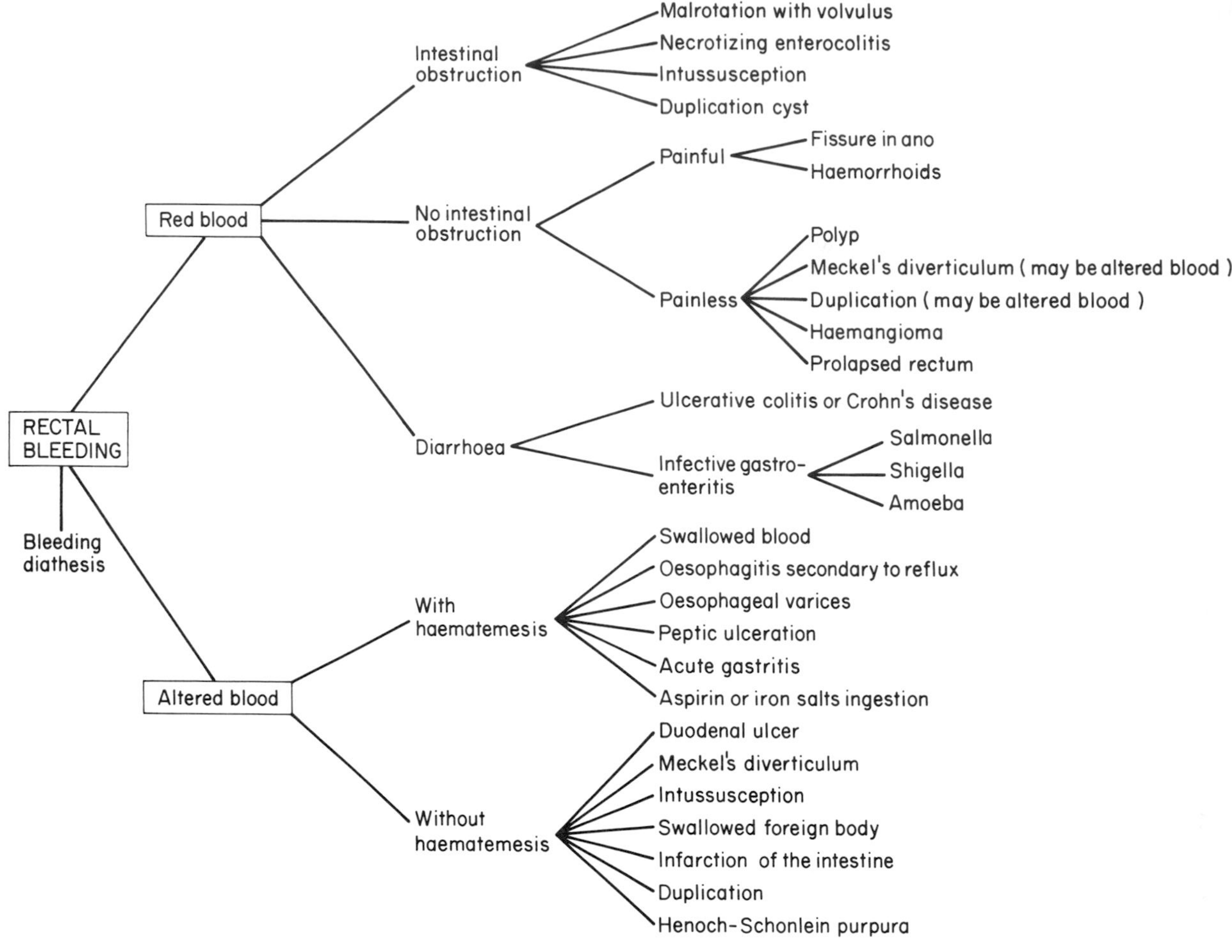

Fig. 29.5 Causes of gastrointestinal haemorrhage.

should be carefully inspected for fissure before a digital rectal examination is performed. The age of the patient is also important as certain conditions are virtually confined to limited age ranges: for example midgut volvulus, necrotizing enterocolitis, Meckel's diverticula and intussusception are common causes of bleeding in infants under two years of age, while oesophageal varices, chronic peptic ulceration, colonic polyps and inflammatory bowel disease are conditions found in older children.

The passage of red blood per rectum should lead to an enquiry regarding any alteration in bowel habit. In the neonatal period in particular, bilious vomiting associated with blood in the stools is highly suspicious of either a malrotation with midgut volvulus or of necrotizing enterocolitis. The plain abdominal X-ray may be helpful in distinguishing the two conditions—pneumatosis intestinalis is diagnostic of necrotizing enterocolitis, while the "gasless abdomen" will favour a diagnosis of midgut volvulus.

Intussusception characteristically presents with episodes of colicky abdominal pain, the passage of "red-currant-jelly-like" stools (60 per cent) and a "sausage-shaped" abdominal mass (60 per cent). Vomiting is frequent, but persistent bilious vomiting occurs as a result of delayed diagnosis. Barium enema may be diagnostic as well as therapeutic. In the vast majority of infants no obvious cause of the intussusception is found. The hyperplastic lymphoid tissue found in these cases is as likely to be the result of the disorder as its cause, though it is of interest that most intussusceptions occur in the ileo-caecal region where lymphoid tissue is most abundant. In older children there may be a readily definable cause, and specific efforts should be made to identify inflammatory tissue, a tumour or even a Meckel's diverticulum. Henoch–Schonlein disease should also be considered, as abdominal pain, gastrointestinal petechial haemorrhages and intussusception are integral features of this condition. Operative reduction and occasionally resection is indicated in those cases which fail to reduce with hydrostatic barium enemas as well as in patients presenting with manifestation of ischaemic intestine (peritonitis, shock, intestinal obstruction).

Anal fissure

The most frequent cause of painful passage of bright red blood is an anal fissure. The blood usually coats the surface of the stool producing a streak-like effect and invariably follows a bout of constipation. Unless treatment consisting of laxative, local analgesic ointments and digital dilatation are promptly and vigorously executed, a vicious circle of recurrent fissures and constipation results in the development of secondary megacolon.

Polyps

Polyps of the large intestine in childhood are usually of the "juvenile" variety. They are hamartomatous in nature and in no way precancerous; the removal of those which do not amputate themselves is advocated solely for symptomatic reasons. They frequently bleed, when red blood is found admixed with mucus in the stool, though these episodes are painless. It has been estimated that juvenile polyps occur in about one per cent of children and the great majority are single. Though they are rarely found under the age of one year, their frequency increases in later childhood. Eighty per cent of the polyps are within reach of the sigmoidoscope, and double contrast barium enema or colonoscopy is diagnostic in the remaining 20 per cent of cases. If auto-amputation does not occur, endoscopic resection should be performed where the facilities exist. Examination of the resected specimen will reveal a smooth rubbery lesion comprising cystically dilated mucus-filled crypts embedded in an oedematous inflamed stroma.

Other causes

Meckel's diverticulum and duplications cause rectal bleeding secondary to peptic ulceration in the bowel adjacent to the ectopic gastric mucosa. Blood loss varies from small quantities to exsanguinating haemorrhage. Tc^{99} pertechnetate scan may demonstrate the ectopic gastric mucosa. An infective cause should always be sought where there is diarrhoea with blood in the stools. Chronic inflammatory bowel disease, although affecting predominantly young adults, presents in approximately 15 per cent of cases during childhood and specific efforts should be made to seek the diagnostic features of both chronic ulcerative colitis and Crohn's disease.

Altered blood in the stool results from the conversion of haemoglobin to haematin by acid-pepsin digestion. It is frequently accompanied by haematemesis. Reflux oesophagitis may occur at any age, but in young infants in particular it is a common cause of chronic blood loss with resultant hypochromic anaemia. Failure to thrive and persistent vomiting are usually also present. Oesophageal varices may develop secondary to extrahepatic causes, such as portal vein thrombosis, or liver cirrhosis. There is generally an associated splenomegaly which may be accompanied to a varying degree by hypersplenism. Peptic ulceration is relatively uncommon in infancy and childhood. Acute gastric erosions or acute peptic ulceration occur secondary to stress, particularly trauma, burns and neurological disease, while chronic ulcers may be found in older children and adolescents.

Minimal rectal bleeding

Minimal rectal bleeding of short duration in the small infant, even in the absence of an anal fissure, can quite safely be ignored and ascribed to superficial mucosal erosions. It is generally unproductive to embark on a series of investigations such as contrast studies of the upper and lower gastrointestinal tract, upper and lower gastrointestinal endoscopy, technetium scans, etc. unless the bleeding persists, is recurrent or results in profound hypochromic anaemia. Angiography to localize the bleeding site is generally unrewarding unless haemorrhage is actively occurring at a rate in excess of 1–2 ml per minute.

Section II: J. D. Atwell and A. G. MacIver

Visible Anomalies

Many of the congenital anomalies found in the neonatal period are not difficult to diagnose but may be difficult to manage, for example high and low anorectal anomalies. The malformation is easily seen provided the neonate is examined carefully.

Abdominal wall defects

Omphalocele major and minor, syndrome and non-syndrome; gastroschisis

The important findings are the presence of a sac, the size of the defect and the contents. Exomphalos major contains liver and intestines with a defect over 5 cm in diameter. In gastroschisis, the sac is absent and the swollen matted and shortened mid-gut lies on the surface of the abdomen. The umbilical cord has a normal origin which contrasts with exomphalos where the umbilical vessels run over the surface of the sac.

Other major syndromes are often found with exomphalos major: Beckwith–Wiedemann syndrome, macroglossia, diaphragmatic hernia, ectopia cordis.

If the sac is intact, the only initial investigation required is a straight X-ray of the abdomen to exclude intestinal atresia.

Number of umbilical vessels

The umbilical cord should always be examined in the newborn to determine the number of vessels present (normally two umbilical arteries and a single umbilical vein). A single umbilical artery may be associated with congenital anomalies, especially those of the genito-urinary system. This observation can be confirmed by histological examination.

Umbilical, supraumbilical and epigastric hernia

Protruberance of a skin-covered defect at the umbilicus which bulges on crying indicates an umbilical hernia. This must be differentiated from a supraumbilical defect. Small umbilical herniae undergo spontaneous closure by 5–7 years, but surgical treatment is required for large defects. Supraumbilical herniae are similar to epigastric herniae and are due to a split in the interlacing fibres of the linea alba and the defect usually contains extraperitoneal fat. Spontaneous resolution does not occur.

Umbilical granuloma

Low-grade inflammation at the umbilicus may cause an umbilical granuloma (pyogenic granuloma). The granuloma should be removed and the base cauterized. Histological examination is necessary to exclude vitello-intestinal remnants such as ectopic gastrointestinal or pancreatic tissue, but the commonest cause is a foreign-body reaction to talc.

Umbilical dermoid

Small cystic lesions are sometimes seen at the base of the umbilicus. Excision and histological examination is required. This is a variant of congenital or acquired inclusion dermoid.

Patent vitello-intestinal duct and vitello-intestinal remnants

Occasionally, following separation of the umbilical cord, milk is seen to leak from the umbilicus. This is followed by prolapse of intestinal epithelium at the umbilicus. Surgical excision of the entire duct to the point of origin from the terminal ileum is required.

Patent urachus and urachal remnants

Leaking of urine from the umbilicus suggests the presence of a patent urachus. This observation can be confirmed by the intravenous injection of methylene blue which then appears on the dressing at the umbilicus.

Urachal cysts can present with a tender swelling at the umbilicus.

Treatment for the urachal cyst is excision and ligation from the obliterated urachal remnant. Intravenous pyelography is indicated in patients with a urachal fistula as they may be associated with outflow tract obstruction such as posterior urethral valves, bladder-neck obstruction and the prune-belly syndrome.

Ectopic bladder, ectopia vesicae, bladder exstrophy and vesico-intestinal fissure

In exstrophy, the bladder mucosa is exposed below the umbilicus in the midline with separation of the pubic symphysis. There is an associated exomphalos; in males there is an epispadias and in females the labia minora and clitoris are bifid.

Vesico-intestinal fissure is a rare variant with separation of the extrophy into two by an everted caecum with a prolapsing ileostomy. There are two appendices and the hind gut is absent. Limb anomalies may be found in association with this severe defect.

Inguinal herniae are commonly seen with these defects because of the anatomically abnormal inguinal canal. Other associated defects include renal, vaginal and uterine anomalies.

Anomalies of the genitalia

Hypospadias

This common condition with an incidence of 1 in 300 live born males may be either a minor or a major malformation. The external urethral orifice opens on the ventral aspect of the penis and may be glandular, coronal, penile, peno-scrotal, scrotal or perineal. Associated stigmata include a hooded prepuce, external urethral meatal stenosis and chordee which results in bowing of the penis and is aggravated in the erectile state. In coronal examples there may be plugging of the external urethral meatus with epithelial debris.

There is an increased incidence of other congenital anomalies higher in the urinary tract, which increases with severity of the hypospadias. Therefore in peno-scrotal, scrotal and perineal hypospadias, intravenous pyelography and cysto-urethroscopy are indicated. In patients with an undescended testis, chromosome analysis is indicated.

Epispadias

In the male: a rare anomaly which is part of the spectrum of bladder exstrophy. Incontinence due to a short urethra and wide bladder neck is found in the majority of patients. The urethra opens into the dorsal surface of the shortened penis with a split glans.

In the female: rare but often missed on cursory examination of the genitalia as the clitoris and labia minora are bifid. The urethra is short and the bladder neck is open and the majority of patients present with urinary incontinence.

Full urological investigations are required; intravenous pyelography, micturating cystography and cystourethroscopy.

Intersex

The new infant who presents with ambiguous genitalia is a medical emergency. Rapid diagnosis and appropriate treatment will determine the success of the outcome for the infant and his family.

The assignment of sex is based upon anatomical factors which determine future sexual function. Naming of the infant should be withheld until a decision is taken about the sex of the infant. In order to make a definite diagnosis full investigation and surgical treatment may have to be performed before the age of 6 weeks. Statutory registration of the infant's birth is required by this age.

A full explanation must be given to the family of the internal and external anatomy of the genitalia, histology of the gonads, hormonal defect and analysis of the chromosomal karyotype.

The following investigations are usually necessary as there are many different types of intersex:

1. Evaluation of the external genitalia including endoscopy.
2. Sex chromatin and chromosomal analysis.
3. Evaluation of the internal genitalia including laparotomy.
4. Gonadal biopsy.
5. Hormonal studies and evaluation of enzyme deficiencies.

Maldescent of the testes

Diagnosis should be made on the routine examination of the newborn infant and then confirmed at the 6-week and 4-monthly examinations.

An empty scrotum is a common finding. In such patients it is important to determine whether the gonad is palpable, and its position. An impalpable gonad can be intra-abdominal or an inguinal undescended testis. A testis which is intermittently palpable is probably emergent, i.e. it can be "milked" out of the inguinal canal. A testis which is palpable in an abnormal position is ectopic (superficial inguinal, perineal, femoral, penile). If palpable and if it can be manipulated into the scrotum, it is either a high retractile or retractile (normal) testis. Clinical evidence of an inguinal hernia should be sought.

The scrotum is normally developed in ectopic testes, but is small and hypoplastic in undescended testes.

Absence of the testis may be due to intrauterine torsion (blighted testis syndrome). Exploration of the inguinal canal and laparoscopy are indicated.

Ano-rectal anomalies

Congenital anorectal anomalies are subdivided into two main groups depending on where the rectum ends. This may be either above the level of the pelvic floor with a fistulous communication to the viscus lying anteriorly, i.e. bladder and posterior urethra in the male and vagina in the female; or in low anomalies, the rectum passes through the pelvic floor and opens onto the surface in an abnormal position but usually anterior to the normal anus, i.e. ectopic anus in the female and the "covered" anus in the male. A rare variant is membranous obstruction at the junction of the proctodeum and the hind gut.

Diagnosis of an anomaly is visual and easy. Evaluation of the anatomical type is more difficult and depends upon the experience of the examiner and further investigations. These may include an inverted radiograph, needle exploration of the perineum with the injection of contrast, ultrasound and computerized tomography. Air in the bladder or meconium on the tip of the penis is indicative of a high fistula.

In infants with congenital anorectal anomalies there is a high incidence (50 per cent) of other serious defects (VATER—see p. 417).

Sacrococcygeal teratoma

The presence of a cystic lobulated tumour attached to the coccyx with distortion of the perineum suggests the diagnosis of a sacrococcygeal teratoma. They can be large and cause an obstructed delivery. In others, the pelvic and intra-abdominal portion is larger than the visible external skin-covered lesion. Histological sections confirm the presence of multiple tissues from all three germ layers with squamous and columnar epithelium, neuroglia and connective tissues. Sarcomatous tumours have a bad prognosis and so do yolk sac tumours, many of which have detectable alphafetoprotein in the serum and the tumour. Neuroblastic areas do not necessarily imply a poor prognosis in infants. Nodules of cartilage may be derived from the coccyx and not from the tumour. Tumours which present after 1 year of age have a worse prognosis and have a high (60 per cent) local recurrence rate.

Central nervous system malformations

These interrelated malformations are the commonest serious congenital defects of infancy. They often have a familial incidence.

Anencephaly

The cranial vault is absent in anencephaly. Haemorrhagic neural tissue is recognizable on the top of the head. The male:female sex ratio is 1:4.

The diagnosis is suspected with a history of maternal polyhydramnios and in recent times is confirmed by ultrasound and raised alphafetoprotein levels in maternal serum and amniotic fluid.

Spina bifida and neural tube defects

Minor defects have no neurological deficit whilst major defects have severe paralysis, hydrocephalus (secondary to the Arnold–Chiari malformation) and associated deformities such as kyphosis, talipes and paralytic dislocation of the hips.

The defects are classified on a positional basis, i.e. occipital, cervical, thoracic, thoracolumbar, lumbar, lumbosacral and sacral. They range from occulta to meningocele, meningomyelocele or myelocele which is dependent upon the coverings of the nervous tissue. In some patients with a meningomyelocele there may be an associated lipoma and diastematomyelia (10–20 per cent).

Full neurological investigations are required before treatment and include radiographs of the spine and skull, myelography, ventriculography, and computerized tomography of the skull. Urological investigations include intravenous pyelography, micturating cystography and urodynamic studies of bladder function. Orthopaedic assessment is also required. On the basis of full investigations and their results, a decision is made about active surgical intervention. At operation, excised tissue is sent for histological examination to determine whether neural tissue is present.

Encephalocele

Clinically it is important to differentiate the occipital meningocele or meningomyelocele from the "true" encephalocele which contains part of the cerebrum. Transillumination, ventriculography, ultrasound and computerized tomography are indicated in selected patients.

In some children there is marked neurological deficit and mental retardation.

Hydrocephalus

The diagnosis of hydrocephalus is dependent upon the size of the head as measured from the occipital-frontal circumference. Progressive hydrocephalus requires treatment and the diagnosis is dependent upon serial measurements plotted against the chronological age of the infant on a skull circumference chart. The severity of the hydrocephalus can be assessed by transillumination, ultrasound sonography, computerized tomography and air ventriculography. Causes of hydrocephalus in the neonatal period include intrauterine infections such as toxoplasmosis, birth trauma with a resulting basal block, congenital aqueduct stenosis (often sex-linked and occurring in males), meningitis, the Arnold–Chiari malformation and the rare choroid plexus papilloma. Other rarer conditions are exit foramina blockage of congenital origin (Dandy–Walker syndrome) and porencephalic cysts. Subdural effusion following injury or birth trauma may similarly present with progressive hydrocephalus. Tumours are rarely a cause of hydrocephalus in the first three months of life.

Orofacial malformations

The following list includes major syndromes of surgical significance:

Special syndromes

1. Pierre–Robin syndrome
2. Treacher–Collins syndrome
3. Klippel–Feil syndrome
4. Potter facies
5. Laurence–Moon–Biedl syndrome
6. Prader–Willi syndrome
7. Sturge–Weber syndrome
8. Tuberose sclerosis (Bourneville's disease)

Syndromes of chromosomal origin

1. Down's syndrome (trisomy 21)
2. Patau's syndrome (trisomy 13)
3. Edward's syndrome (trisomy 18)
4. Turner's syndrome (45 XO)
5. Klinefelter's syndrome (47 XXY)

Cleft lip and palate

The following classification of cleft lip and palate is in common use:

Group I Cleft of the anterior (primary) palate:
- (a) lip
- (b) alveolus

Group II Clefts of the anterior and posterior (primary and secondary) palate:
- (a) lip
- (b) alveolus
- (c) hard palate
- (d) soft palate

Group III Clefts of the posterior (secondary) palate:
- (a) hard palate
- (b) soft palate

Facial clefts occur at other lines of fusion but these are rare.

Swellings of the neck

MIDLINE

1. Submental lymph mode
2. Thyroglossal cyst and fistula
3. Adenoma of the isthmus of the thyroid
4. Congenital dermoid cysts

LATERAL

A. *Anterior triangle of neck*
   1. Lymph node
      - (a) submandibular
      - (b) deep cervical
   2. Branchial cyst: fistula
   3. Thyroid adenoma and carcinoma
   4. Sternomastoid tumour
   5. Cystic hygroma
   6. Salivary gland
      - (a) submandibular
      - (b) parotid

B. *Posterior triangle of neck*
   1. Lymph node

Clinical presentation (Fig. 29.6 and Table 29.1)

Swellings of the neck are extremely common in children and usually follow a viral or streptococcal

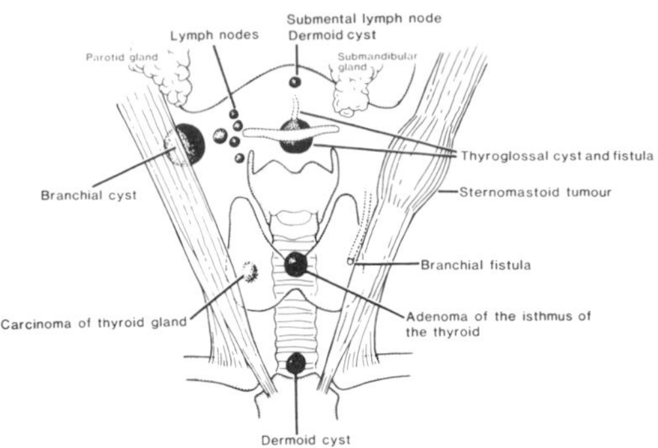

Fig. 29.6 Swellings of the neck.

throat infection. Other swellings such as thyroglossal and branchial cysts are less common and follow upper respiratory tract infections due to the hyperplasia of the lymphoid tissue which they contain. Thyroglossal cysts usually arise above and below the hyoid bone and have a tract extending upwards to the foramen caecum at the junction of the anterior two thirds and posterior third of the tongue. Characteristically, such swellings move up and down on swallowing or with protrusion of the tongue. Branchial cysts although believed to be congenital in origin are extremely rare in infancy and childhood. They lie partially beneath the sternomastoid muscle at the junction of the upper quarter and lower three quarters.

An enlarged and palpable submental lymph node is uncommon, but usually results from a local pyogenic infection.

Swellings of the thyroid gland are not common, but if present are either due to a papillary carcinoma or a follicular adenoma which can even occur in the very young, i.e. 4 years of age. Uniform enlargement of the thyroid gland is occasionally found at puberty and resolves spontaneously in the majority of patients.

Congenital dermoid cysts are usually found at lines of embryological fusion and common sites are sublingual, upper and lower midline cervical, internal and external angular. They may also overlie the skull bones or lie between the tables of the developing calvarium and even extend intracranially. The skin is always freely mobile over the surface of these cysts which may cause erosion and condensation of bone (epidermoidoma). The mobility of the skin overlying the cyst allows differentiation from sebaceous cyst or pilomatrixoma (calcifying epithelioma of Malherbe).

Swelling of the sternomastoid muscle (usually middle or lower third) results in torticollis. When presenting in the neonatal period it has usually followed a difficult or forceps delivery. Rarely, there are structural changes in the cervical vertebrae to account for a torticollis. It may lead to facial asymmetry later.

Cystic hygroma due to congenital maldevelopment of the lymphatic and angiomatous tissues in the neck varies enormously from the giant lesions with a significant mortality due to respiratory obstruction. Smaller lesions often resolve spontaneously. The majority of lesions contain mixed haemo- and lymphangiomatous elements.

Swellings of the parotid gland may be intermittent due to inflammation associated with sialectasis or calculi. Intermittent parotid enlargement without infection may resolve at puberty. Swellings of the parotid gland must be distinguished from enlargement of the lymph node within the parotid.

Cervical lymphadenopathy

Full recognition and classification of inflammatory reactive lymphadenopathies and lymphomas requires careful history-taking and clinical examination, with particular attention being directed to history of contact with infective diseases and with animals. Note must be taken of other sites of lymphadenopathy and hepatosplenomegaly. A full blood count is performed and absolute counts of lymphoid and granulocyte cells should be calculated. Bone marrow aspirate or trephine biopsy may often be necessary as part of the work-up. Immunological tests are required to detect circulating monoclonal populations of lymphocytes in blood or bone marrow and the presence of monoclonal paraproteins (Bence-Jones protein) in the urine, both of which indicate lymphoma.

If there is any suspicion of tumour, one or more lymph nodes should be carefully removed without crushing. Little information can be gained from macroscopic inspection of the node, which should be sent unfixed and intact to the laboratory. Frozen section may often be desired by the surgeon, but it may be difficult to interpret unless the local pathologist is experienced in this particular field. In most cases it is advisable to wait for a paraffin section report. Other techniques which can be used to aid pathological diagnosis include fresh node imprints for cytology, microbiological culture for bacteria and viruses, and preparations of cell suspensions for immunological marker studies to distinguish T-lymphocytes and their subsets from B-lymphocytes and monocytes. Most important of all, the node must be fixed soon after

Table 29.1 Investigations and pathology of swellings in the neck.

Pathology	*Investigation*	*Comment*
Cervical lymphadenopathy	Examination to exclude generalized lymphadenopathy and splenomegaly Haematological indices	
1. Infection		
(a) Acute	Search for local inflammatory focus	Especially tonsils, teeth and skin
(b) Chronic	Chest X-ray	
	Heaf Mantoux test	Human and non tuberculous (atypical) should be excluded, especially avian strains
2. Neoplastic		
(a) Lymphoma	Immunological indices	Excludes immunodeficiency
(b) Metastatic	Lymph node biopsy	Differentiation reactive lymphadenopathy from Hodgkin's disease, non-Hodgkin's Lymphoma and metastatic tumours, especially thyroid carcinoma
Thyroid and thyroglossal remnants		
1. Goitre		
(a) Neonatal		Caused by antithyroid drug therapy during pregnancy
(b) Pubertal		Transient goitre due to hormonal changes at puberty
(c) Dyshormonogenic	Thyroid function tests e.g. T4, T3, thyroid scan, thyroglobulin	Multiple varieties dependent upon the stage of blockage in thyroglobulin synthesis
2. Nodule		
(a) Single	Thyroid function tests	Solitary thyroid nodules in children are usually neoplastic
(b) Multiple	Chest X-ray Thyroid scan	
3. Thyroglossal cyst/fistula and ectopic thyroid	Thyroid scan	Excludes ectopic thyroid
Congenital dermoid (epidermoid) cysts	None	Occur in certain classical sites, e.g. external angular dermoid
Branchial remnants		
1. Fistula		
2. Cyst	None	
3. Cartilagenous remnants		
Sternomastoid 'tumour'	X-ray cervical spine in selected patients	Exclude bony anomalies in patients without a history of birth trauma
Cystic hygroma	X-ray root of neck Haematological indices	Detects tracheal compression and deviation Platelet trapping in large haemangiomas may cause thrombocytopenia
Salivary gland		
1. Calculi	Straight X-ray	Confirm calculus and its position
2. Inflammation	Sialogram	Demonstrates duct system and obstruction
3. Neoplasm	Biopsy/excision	Determines diagnosis

receipt in the laboratory in an adequate amount of formalin for good light microscopic histology in paraffin-wax and resin-embedded sections.

Acute lymphadenitis and specific chronic infections such as tuberculosis, other mycobacterial infections, yersinial infections, fungal diseases and actinomycosis are easily recognized in histological sections as they show the usual typical features, as in adults. An attempt should always be made to identify the offending microorganism if the cell reaction suggests a particular cause: i.e. digested PAS stain or Grocott stain for fungi; Ziehl–Neelsen stain for mycobacteria. Organisms and foreign bodies may often be visible within cell cytoplasm using careful inspection with oil-immersion lens for agents such as *Toxoplasma gondii* and X-polarized light for foreign particles. In other disorders, the histological appearance may be highly suggestive, but other investigations are required for confirmation, for example serology to confirm yersinial infection, "second-look biopsy" for microbiological culture, careful history-taking for postimmunization lymphadenitis, skin test for cat-scratch disease, antibody test for toxoplasma, monospot test for infectious mononucleosis, etc. In many cases no cause is established despite intense investigation.

Non-specific reactive nodes show either follicular hyperplasia (which must be distinguished from follicular lymphoma) or sinus hyperplasia as, for example, in nodes draining infected and inflamed local foci. A wide range of different histopathological features may be seen in the varying reactive lymphadenopathies which are well described in standard text books. Both giant lymph node hyperplasia, an important mediastinal lesion, and sinus histiocytosis with massive lymphadenopathy, are found in childhood.

Recognition of lymphoma is straightforward in most cases, although confusion can arise in conditions such as infectious mononucleosis (Epstein–Barr virus infection), drug reactions and autoimmune diseases. Lymphoma must be first defined as either Hodgkin's disease or non-Hodgkin's lymphoma. Table 29.2 shows the incidence of lymphomas in childhood in one series and emphasizes the predominance of leukaemia. This is agreement on the sub-classification of Hodgkin's disease (Table 29.3) and there is emerging agreement on non-Hodgkin's lymphoma based on the Kiel classification (Table 29.4). Staging laparotomy is

Table 29.2 Relative incidence of different types of lymphoma and leukaemia in black and white children in the USA. (Young and Miller, 1975.)

Leukaemia		
Acute lymphoblastic leukaemia		438
Chronic lymphoblastic leukaemia		2
Acute myeloid leukaemia		125
Chronic myeloid leukaemia		16
Monocytic leukaemia		7
Others and unclassifiable		124
	Total	712
Malignant lymphoma		
Hodgkin's disease		103
Burkitt's lymphoma		10
Non-Hodgkin's lymphoma		123
	Total	236

Table 29.3 Incidence of different forms of Hodgkin's disease in children. (Figures derived from series reported by Jenkin *et al.* (1975), Norris *et al.* (1975), Smith *et al.* (1977).)

Lymphocyte predominant	48	(18%)
Mixed cellularity	59	(22%)
Nodular sclerosing	152	(57%)
Lymphocyte depleted	5	(2%)
Unclassifiable	1	(<1%)

Table 29.4 Kiel classification of the non-Hodgkin's lymphoma (Lennart *et al.*, 1983.)

Low-grade malignancy
Lymphocytic
  B-chronic lymphocytic leukaemia
  T-chronic lymphocytic leukaemia
  T-zone lymphoma
Lymphoplasmacytic
  lymphoplasmacytic
  polymorphic
Plasmacytic
Centrocytic
Centroblastic-centrocytic
  follicular pattern
  diffuse pattern
  mixed follicular and diffuse patterns
High-grade malignancy
Centroblastic
  diffuse
Lymphoblastic
  B-lymphoblastic
  B-lymphblastic – Burkitt type
  T-lymphoblastic
  T-lymphoblastic – convoluted cell type
Immunoblastic
Histiocytic
Unclassifiable

carried out for Hodgkin's disease with biopsies of lymph nodes, liver and splenectomy being performed and tissue is sent fresh to the laboratory.

As recognition, classification and treatment of lymphomas and leukaemias is changing rapidly, it is essential that as much information as possible is gained from each individual, including the patient's immune status at time of diagnosis. The demonstration that primary immunodeficiency states such as Wiskott–Aldrich syndrome and ataxia-telangiectasia may subsequently lead to the development of non-Hodgkin's lymphoma, indicates that some lymphomas may be detected at an early stage by screening and biopsy of affected subjects.

Thyroid and thyroglossal remnants

Lymphocytic thyroiditis, Hashimoto's disease and other forms of inflammatory thyroiditis are all rare in childhood.

Diffuse smooth and nodular thyroid enlargement is found in colloid goitre and adenomatoid hyperplasia. Both these conditions may occur in euthyroid and hyperthyroid subjects as well as in endemic hypothyroidism. Dyshormonogenetic glands show diffuse multinodular enlargement with cysts and haemorrhage and may result from several different genetic defects in iodine incorporation and thyroglobulin synthesis. Microscopic examination usually shows a microcystic pattern with poor colloid formation. Worrying areas of papillary formation and atypia may occur. Examination of multiple blocks will be necessary to distinguish this disease from a thyroid carcinoma.

A solitary nodule in the thyroid of a child is a follicular adenoma or a carcinoma, usually papillary type. The presence of papillary proliferation within thyroid glands may also be found in hyperthyroidism and in solitary adenomas following haemorrhage, but the presence of calcified psammoma bodies within tumour cells and stroma is a useful diagnostic pointer for carcinoma. Capsular and vascular invasion are not usually detected but, if present, are important features of malignancy. In a number of instances, the tumour is only recognized after excision of an adjacent lymph node containing metastatic carcinoma, this being a more usual clinical presentation of thyroid cancer than thyroid enlargement alone.

Cysts of the thyroglossal duct are a common cause of swellings in the neck, usually in the region of the hyoid bone. They have smooth walls and are lined by squamous or ciliated columnar epithelium. Inflammation and scarring are common. Surprisingly, it is unusual for them to contain ectopic thyroid tissue.

Congenital dermoid (epidermoid) cysts

These cysts occur at embryonic lines of closure, often in the eyebrows, nose and jaw, and have a similar appearance to the implantation epidermal cysts. They have a wall of squamous epithelium and are filled with keratinous debris.

Branchial cysts, sinuses and fistula and cartilagenous remnants

Branchial cysts have a thick fibrous wall with a lining of non-keratinizing squamous epithelium or ciliated columnar epithelium. They are filled with keratin or colloid debris unless there is associated infection. Prominent lymphoid infiltrates, often with large follicles, characteristically lie immediately beneath the epithelium.

Branchial fistulae form small elongated communications between skin and the pharynx. They are usually lined by squamous epithelium and probably represent remnants of the first and second branchial arches.

Solitary cartilagenous nodules are sometimes found in the soft tiisues of the neck and also represent further branchial cleft remnants. They do not contain other branchial tissues and have no communication with normal bony and cartilagenous structures.

Cystic hygroma: lymphangioma and haemangioma

The cysts of a hygroma vary in size and form a ramifying network of thin-walled channels lined by flattened endothelial cells. The presence of blood indicates a vascular malformation (haemangioma), whilst the absence of red blood cells and a lymphoid infiltrate suggests lymphangioma.

Salivary gland lesions

Chronic inflammatory disorders with destruction and dilatation of the salivary duct system and an associated lympoid infiltrate are characteristic of sialadenitis. The changes may result from obstruction to the duct by calculus, fibrocystic disease, or may occur spontaneously (benign lymphosialoadenopathy).

Epithelial tumours mostly occur in the parotid gland and are pleomorphic adenomas. Others are infrequent but include adenolymphoma, epidermoid carcinoma, adenoid cystic carcinoma, acinic cell carcinoma and undifferentiated tumours.

Skin lesions and soft tissue swellings

Vascular and pigmented naevi are obvious on inspection. Some, such as the strawberry naevus, disappear spontaneously, others may require removal often without a clear idea as to their origin. Histological examination is required for these to determine their exact nature, behaviour and prognosis, and for subsequent management. Small lesions should be completely excised with a clear margin of uninvolved tissue, larger lesions should have an adequate biopsy with tissue being sent fresh to the pathologist. Multiple blocks are taken for histological examination. Sometimes both electron microscopy and immunohistological examination are necessary.

Skin tumours, malformations and scars

Naevi

Naevi may be flat, elevated, pedunculated or papillomatous. Most are pigmented and some contain hairs. On histological examination they are either junctional, intradermal or mixed (compound). Junctional activity is common before the age of 10 years, but malignant change is rare.

Naevi may enlarge, particularly close to puberty, but this does not imply that they are melanomas. Nevertheless, it is prudent to observe them carefully.

Benign juvenile malanoma, better known as Spitz naevus (spindle-epithelioid naevus) is a sparsely pigmented, pink, dome-shaped tumour. Most are readily recognized, but some still cause diagnostic problems.

The rare congenital hairy naevus may be extensive and can also enlarge, sometimes quite rapidly. There is an increased risk (5 per cent) of the subsequent development of melanoma.

Other naevi which may be encountered include the halo naevus, the simple blue and cellular blue naevus and the sacro-coccygeal Mongolian spot which disappears in most races (except Mongoloids) by 3–4 years of age. Nodular melanoma is rare.

Vascular malformations and tumours

Vascular hamartomas include port-wine stain, the dermal capillary haemangioma or strawberry naevus, and the cavernous haemangioma. The strawberry naevus may be absent at birth but appears between the 3rd and 5th week, often with rapid enlargement up to 1 year and subsequent spontaneous regression. Interpretation of the histological appearances of occasional vascular lesions in children can be difficult, and distinction between the malignant haemangioendothelioma and the benign cellular angioma of infancy and infantile haemangiopericytoma is not easy.

Multiple vascular tumours and malformations may occur in assorted syndromes (*see* Table 29.5).

Table 29.5 Vascular tumours and malformations occuring in assorted syndromes.

Sturge–Weber syndrome	Naevus flammeus of skin (port-wine stain) Vascular malformations of meninges and sometimes retina
Maffucci syndrome	Cavernous haemangioma of skin and soft tissues Osteochondromas and defects of ossification
Blue rubber – bleb naevus	Subcutaneous, oral and intestinal cavernous haemangiomas
Hereditary haemorrhagic telangiectasia	Multiple telangiectasis in the skin, nose, mouth and liver. Autosomal dominant inheritance
Bourneville's disease (tuberous sclerosis)	Angiofibroma of skin (adenoma sebaceum), sclerotic patches of glial proliferation in the brain and retina, angiomyolipoma of kidney, peri-ungual fibroma
Von Hippel–Lindau disease	Haemangioblastoma of brain, angiomata of retina, sometimes skin and liver involvement. Also adenomas and cysts in pancreas, liver and kidney

Keloids and hypertrophic scars

Wound repair in the dermis results in the production of collagen by fibroblasts. The persistence of foreign bodies will encourage chronic inflammatory reaction and increase the local formation of collagen.

Excessive amounts of coarse collagen fibre are seen in keloids. They are found particularly in the face, ears, neck and arms and have a high recurrence rate. Keloids never occur in the skin of the penis, scrotum or labia.

Pilomatrixoma (calcifying epithelioma of Malherbé)

These are nodular benign tumours arising from the hair follicle and are often found in childhood. They have characteristic histological features which include the presence of basal cells, ghost cells, necrosis and calcification.

Soft tissue tumours and associated lesions (Table 29.6)

Xanthoma, xanthogranuloma, reticulohistiocytosis and histiocytosis-X

Although these lesions are not directly related, they all contain a similar form of macrophage—the tissue histiocyte. In histiocytosis-X it is likely that the predominant histiocyte is the Langerhans cell, normally found in the skin.

Xanthomas are nodules of foamy histiocytes occurring in the skin of people with hyperlipoproteinaemia, either as part of a primary metabolic disorder or as a result of liver disease. Xanthogranuloma is a localized dermal lesion of infants and young children which is rarely multiple. The lesion is a mixture of histiocytes, eosinophil polymorphs and reactive giant cells of Touton type. The reticulohistiocytoma, in contrast, is composed almost entirely of multinucleate giant cells. Both of these locally infiltrative lesions must be distinguished from histiocytosis-X, the generic name for Letterer–Siwe disease, Hand–Schüller–Christian disease and eosinophilic granuloma. The most serious and aggressive form is Letterer–Siwe disease, in which the dermis contains a diffuse infiltrate of histiocytes, often showing atypia and increased mitoses. Lymph nodes, spleen and bone marrow are also involved. In Hand–Schüller–Christian disease and eosinophilic granuloma, most involvement is seen in lungs and bone.

Table 29.6 Soft tissue tumours with an inherited or familial basis. (After Enzinger and Weiss, 1983.)

Glomus tumour	Occasionally autosomal dominant
Neurofibromatosis	Autosomal dominant. Also gliomas, meningiomas, neuroblastomas, café-au-lait skin lesions
Chemodectoma	Sometimes autosomal dominant
Leiomyoma	Occasionally autosomal dominant
Basal cell naevus syndrome	Autosomal dominant inheritance Also neurofibromas, fibrosarcoma of jaw, ameloblastoma, ovarian fibroma, medulloblastoma of brain
Xanthoma tuberosum	Familial, hyperlipidaemia.
Lipoma and angiolipoma	Familial in 5% patients
Palmar and plantar fibromatosis	Occasionally familial
Mesenteric fibromatosis	Autosomal dominant Associated with polyposis coli and Gardner's syndrome
Myofibromatosis (musculoaponeurotic fibromatosis, hyaline fibromatosis)	Familial on occasion

Dermatofibroma, malignant fibrous histiocytoma, fibroxanthosarcoma, infantile fibrosarcoma, fibromatosis, neurofibroma and neurofibrosarcoma

Dermatofibroma (also called histiocytoma) occurs as a solitary benign nodule within the dermis, whereas malignant fibrous histiocytoma is a locally aggressive tumour composed of cells with similarities to fibroblast and histiocyte. Both are rare in children. Malignant fibrous histiocytoma has a wide range of behaviour from low-grade infiltration to highly malignant metastasizing variants, which include the fibroxanthosarcoma or pleomorphic malignant fibrous histiocytoma. A cartwheel or storiform pattern of spindle-shaped cells is characteristic and immunohistological techniques reveal alpha-1-antitrypsin and alpha-1-antichymotrypsin in the cytoplasm of the tumour cells.

Infantile fibrosarcoma seems to be a different tumour from that arising later in life and it has a better prognosis. The tumour is composed of spindle cells and is often quite vascular and this may cause confusion. Infantile fibromatosis has a similar histological structure, particularly so-called "aggressive fibromatosis" which is better considered as a low-grade fibrosarcoma. A further group of poorly understood fibrous proliferations include the benign fibrous hamartomas of infancy which may be solitary or multiple (infantile fibromatosis). The solitary lesion is composed of fibrous tissue, mucopolysaccharide and fat and arises most often in the axillary region, arm and thigh and almost never in the digits. Thus it should not be confused with infantile digital fibromatosis.

Desmoid-type fibromatosis is the equivalent of muscular aponeurotic fibromatosis of adult life. The lesions vary in behaviour from a highly primitive cellular form arising in infancy to a more mature collagenized form after 5 years of age.

Von Recklinghausen's disease is diagnosed in children by the café-au-lait spots. Pedunculated neurofibromas of the skin and subcutaneous tissue are rare but may be painful, enlarging and causing compression of vital structures when in visceral sites. Occasional lesions may subsequently become malignant (neurofibrosarcoma, malignant Schwannoma).

Lipoma, hibernoma, lipoblastomatosis and liposarcoma

Lipomas are quite uncommon in children unless associated with a neural tube defect. Hibernoma is a rare benign tumour of children with an origin from cells which form brown fat. Lipoblastomatosis produces a benign lobulated fatty and myxoid tumour in the limbs, mediastinum or retroperitoneal region which is probably derived from white fat and nearly always occurs before the age of 3 years. Liposarcomas are rare.

Embryonal, pleomorphic and alveolar rhabdomyosarcoma

Rhabdomyosarcoma is an important malignant soft tissue tumour of childhood and three types exist: embryonal, pleomorphic and alveolar. Embryonal rhabdomyosarcoma (sarcoma botryoides) arises in soft tissues and viscera, particularly orbit, nose, bile ducts, bladder, prostate and vagina. A gelatinous myxoid appearance gives rises to the title sarcoma botryoides, but does not affect the diagnosis or prognosis. The tumour is composed of small dark cells, but skeletal muscle differentiation should be demonstrable by the presence of cross-striations on light microscopy or by immunohistological detection of myoglobin, actin or desmin. Otherwise, the cells may appear similar to those of Ewing's tumour, neuroblastoma and malignant lymphoma. Most tumours are detected between 3 and 5 years of age. There is a slight predominance of males.

Alveolar rhabdomyosarcoma occurs in somewhat older children and usually arises in the soft tissues of the upper limb or perineum. The tumour may be initially confused with an epithelial neoplasm as it is composed of sheets of cells in an alveolar pattern with surrounding bands of fibrous tissue. Multinucleate tumour cells may be prominent. Unfortunately, skeletal muscle differentiation is rarely observed. Metastasis is to lymph nodes.

Pleomorphic rhabdomyosarcoma is very uncommon in childhood but usually arises within skeletal muscle.

Other tumours

Other tumours include granular cell myoblastoma, nasopharyngeal angiofibroma, nasopharyngeal carcinoma, Kaposi sarcoma and synovial sarcoma.

Ewing's tumour is an undifferentiated tumour arising in bone and bone marrow, but it may present as a soft tissue mass. It may also arise as a primary soft tissue neoplasm. It is composed of small cells with no evidence of differentiation. The pathologist usually finds difficulty in distinguishing Ewing's tumour from malignant lymphoma, leukaemic deposits, neuroblastoma and embryonal rhabdomyosarcoma. Metastatic retinoblastoma and nephroblastoma may also appear similar if no differentiated areas are present. The only positive distinguishing feature is the presence of cytoplasmic glycogen.

Ganglion cyst

This is a degenerative cystic lesion filled with mucoid material which occurs in relationship to tendons often on the dorsum of the hand, wrists or feet. Incomplete excision is followed by recurrence. It is not a tumour and its causation is not known.

Swellings in the Groin

Lymph nodes

Hernia and hydrocele
1. Inguinal
2. Femoral

Varicocele

Epididymis
1. Infection
   (a) acute bacterial
   (b) chronic

2. Cysts
3. Appendages

Testes
1. Maldescent
   (a) undescended
   (b) ectopic
   (c) absent
   (d) retractile
2. Torsion: neonatal infarction
3. Trauma
4. Tumour
   (a) rhabdomyosarcoma: leiomyoma
   (b) yolk sac tumour
   (c) teratoma
   (d) seminoma
   (e) Leydig cell tumour: Sertoli cell tumour
   (f) lymphoma and leukaemia

Clinical presentation (Table 29.7)

There can be few sites in the body where the pathology is so visible and palpable as in the inguino-scrotal region. Despite this, the physical findings are often misinterpreted with serious consequences.

Minor enlargement of the inguinal lymph nodes in infants and children of all ages is a common occurrence. This and further enlargement is usually related to local infections such as a nappy rash, eczema or fungal infections. Further investigations in such patients are not required. Differentiation from the other inguinal swellings is not difficult unless the glands are beginning to suppurate, which can be confused with an incarcerated inguinal hernia. Redness of the skin, localized tenderness and fluctuation do not differentiate these two conditions, but the site and the presence of associated abdominal signs suggests a hernia.

The question to be answered with other swellings in the groin is "are they confined to the scrotum", i.e. can one palpate above them? The non-scrotal lesions are inguinal, femoral herniae, and varicoceles. All have a cough impulse. Demonstration of this in the infant is not necessary if the history has been precise. Differentiation of inguinal from femoral herniae depends upon the relationship of the swelling to the public tubercle; above and medial for inguinal, and below and lateral for femoral hernia. It must be remembered that femoral herniae are rare (1–2 femoral: 150 inguinal hernias) in infants and children. If the swelling is not palpable, useful additional signs are the thickening and silken feel of the spermatic cord.

A varicocele is not an infrequent finding in the older child. The 'bag-of-worms', a cough impulse and the bluish discolouration are characteristic.

A swelling localized to the scrotum may be in the cord, the body of the testis or the epididymis. Persistence of the processus vaginalis in infancy as a patent canal allows fluid from the peritoneal cavity to track along the cord and into the tunica vaginalis to produce a hydrocele. Transillumination of the swelling is essential to differentiate the hydrocele from a yolk sac tumour of the testes, which can feel similar on palpation. Communicating cysts of the cord characteristically move downwards when the testis is manipulated into the scrotum and, conversely, on moving the cyst upwards the testis follows. Primary (idiopathic) hydroceles do not occur in the young and hydroceles secondary to trauma and infection are uncommon unless associated with torsion.

Careful clinical examination of the patient with maldescent of the testis is important if unnecessary alarm and surgery is to be avoided. Undescended testes in the abdominal cavity and inguinal canal are impalpable; an emergent testis is intermittently palpable. Other palpable testes must be classified as ectopic in either the superficial inguinal, perineal, femoral or pubo-penile position. This group must be differentiated from the high retractile and the normal retractile testis. In practice it can be difficult to distinguish the high retractile from a lax superficial inguinal ectopic testis. Absence of a testis is unusual and can be due to torsion and infarction of the testes during intra-uterine life. Vascular infarction without torsion is seen in the neonatal period and causes blue discolouration of the testis. Pain in the scrotum and vomiting of sudden onset with swelling and tenderness herald torsion of the testes or hydatid of Morgagni in the older child. In some patients there are easily differentiated, but in others exploration of the testes is necessary. Acute epididymitis due to pyogenic organisms is easily confused with torsion and exploration is often required. Tuberculous epididymitis and congenital cysts of the epididymis are very rare in childhood. Any swelling of the body of the testes or change in consistency suggests a neoplasm and exploration is required for diagnosis and treatment.

Table 29.7 Investigations and pathology of swellings in the groin.

Pathology	*Investigation*	*Comment*
Significant inguinal lymphadenopathy (a) Infection (b) Inflammation	Haematological indices	Distinguishes inflammatory and neoplastic disease
(c) Lymphoma	Chest X-ray Abdominal ultrasound	Detects systemic lymphadenopathy and hepatosplenomegaly
	Lymph node biopsy	Determines diagnosis
Inguinal hernia	Herniogram	Unnecessary
Varicocele	IVP	Usually normal but excludes renal tumour
	In post-pubertal boys:	
	HCG stimulation	Testosterone reponse less than normal
	Clomiphene stimulation	Testosterone response less than normal
	Basal testosterone levels	Reduced
	Oestradiol levels	Increased
	Sperm counts	Counts reduced, less motile spermatozoa
Maldescent of the testis	(a) *Testis absent on clinical examination*	
	HCG stimulation test	Rise in testosterone levels confirms presence of testicular tissue
	Laparoscopy	Avoids laparotomy in blighted testis syndrome
	Laparotomy	Where orchidopexy is impossible the undescended testis should be removed if unilateral. Bilateral cases require conservation until after puberty
	(b) *At operation: inspection*	Undescended testis is often small and body of testis is separated from the epididymis by a mesorchium
	If testis absent, cord structures should be sent for histological examination	Confirms presence of vas deferens and epididymal remnants
Torsion of the tesis and neonatal infarction	*At operation: inspection* Non-viable testes excised Viable testes untwisted and fixed. Contralateral testis fixed	When the viability of the testis is doubtful, preservation may conserve hormonal function
Epididymis		
(a) Infection	(a) *Acute pyogenic*	
	MSU	Excludes urinary infection
	IVP Micturating cystogram Cystourethroscopy	Full urological investigation for other congenital urinary tract anomalies
	(b) *Tuberculosis* Chest X-ray Heaf/Mantoux test Early morning urine ×3	
(b) Cysts	Inspection	Confirms diagnosis
	IVP	Excludes congenital urinary tract anomalies
Tumours of the testis and appendages	*Preoperative*	
	Chest X-ray	Excludes pulmonary metastases
	Alpha-fetoprotein HCG levels	Markers of germ cell tumours
	At operation	
	Inspection of cord and testis	Confirms abnormality
	Excision of testis with cord	Histological examination confirms diagnosis and stages tumour (P1–3)
	Postoperative	
	Abdominal ultrasound Lymphangiography	Extent of lymphatic involvement determines staging and treatment
	Alpha-fetoprotein HCG Chest X-ray	Monitors progress of germ cell tumours

Pathology

Lymph nodes

One or more carefully dissected uncrushed fresh lymph nodes should be sent to the laboratory for the usual series of investigative tests, including frozen section.

Testis and appendages

Maldescended testes

The undescended testis is usually smaller than normal and contains a decreased number of small seminiferous tubules lined by primitive Sertoli cells and a few spermatogonia. Tubule size varies with age from 50 μ diameter in infancy to 170–250 μ in the adult. The diameter of the tubules should be measured carefully and compared with those from a child of a similar age. Histological examination of undescended and ectopic small testes from children under 5 years has produced conflicting results. Some studies claim that the tubules are smaller than normal with a reduction in spermatogonia, others suggest that they are normal. Orchidopexy can produce histological improvement in testicular morphology, whilst non-intervention causes progressive deterioration.

The significance of the histological differences between undescended and ectopic gonads is still undecided. The occurrence of these relatively minor changes in the testicular tubules is used to determine whether the testis is intrinscially abnormal (dysgenetic) or if changes have occurred as a result of maldescent. Ultrastructural studies suggest that abnormalities may be detected before 2 years of age, whilst later there is progressive intertubular fibrosis and tubular atrophy with an increasing rate of malignancy with intratubular carcinoma-in-situ.

Fibrosis of the epididymis and cord

This is found following inflammation or ischaemia, or with obstruction as in fibrocystic disease. Subfertility is a sequel. Testes may be absent in the blighted testis syndrome. In obstruction the changes range from active spermatogenesis to atrophy and intertubular fibrosis.

Torsion of the testis and appendages

Torsion results in swelling of the testis and epididymis. The dark red discolouration is due to venous occlusion. Infarction supervenes, the testis becomes paler and necrosis occurs with a surrounding inflammatory cell infiltrate. Necrotic testicular tissue is usually excised because of the risks of infection and auto-immune disease affecting the contralateral testis. Torsion of the hydatid of Morgagni (appendix testis) results in venous congestion and necrosis of this small cystic embryological remnant.

Testicular and paratesticular tumours and rests

Most (70 per cent) of the primary tumours in this area arise within the testis itself and are of germ-cell origin (Table 29.8). Secondary involvement by lymphomas, neuroblastomas, nephroblastomas and leukaemia can occur. The gross appearance of the tumour should clearly distinguish testicular from paratesticular neoplasms. Malignant tumours are likely to be larger and contain areas of necrosis. Multiple blocks must be examined from all tumours as some have mixed patterns, and it is essential that there is careful examination of the tunica for areas of penetration and of the lower cord for invasion. This helps to determine the prognosis. Further sections should be taken from the line of resection of the spermatic cord.

Table 29.8 Testicular tumours in children. (After Giebink and Ruymanin, 1974.)

Yolk sac tumour (167)	40%
Teratoma (113)	27%
Seminoma (11)	2%
Combined tumour (130)	31%

Histological examination is essential to determine the type of testicular tumour. Yolk sac tumour of the testis (embryonal carcinoma) has a cribriform pattern of tumour cells with duct-like or gland-like structures lined by columnar or cuboidal cells. Nuclei are irregular with prominent nucleoli. Tumour giant cells may be seen. Sometimes cells have clear, vacuolated cytoplasm which aids diagnosis. The stroma varies from myxoid to fibrous tissue.

Three germ layers should be identifiable in all teratomas although bone, cartilage and skin predominate. Differentiated teratoma (TD) are composed of mature tissues. Less differentiated areas indicate an intermediate grading and these tumours (malignant teratoma intermediate, MTI; malignant teratoma undifferentiated, MTU) tend

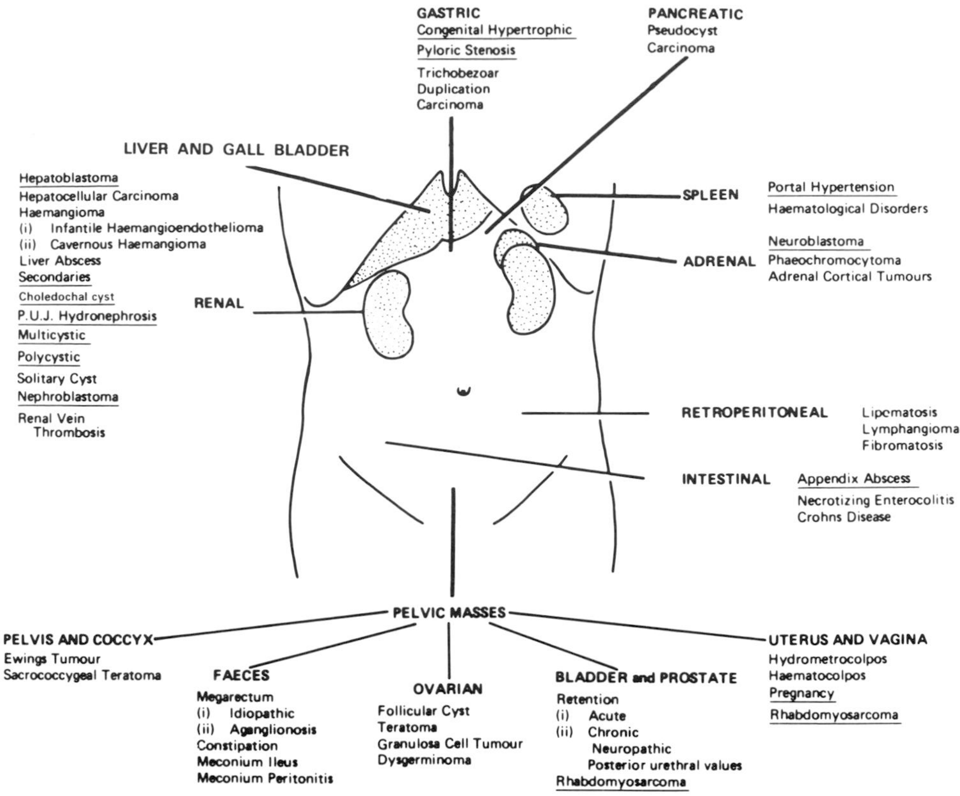

Fig. 29.7 Abdominal masses.

to occur after the age of 12 years. Clusters of neuroblasts are not considered to alter the prognosis in a neoplasm which is otherwise well differentiated, whilst the presence of areas of yolk sac tumour (embryonal carcinoma) indicates a mixed tumour (combined tumour, teratocarcinoma), which may also contain seminomatous areas. These have a worse prognosis. Choriocarcinoma (malignant teratoma trophoblastic, MTT) is virtually unheard of in children. Seminomas occur in older children and have the same homogeneous appearance as in the adult testis but are rare. Biopsies of the contralateral testis of patients with a seminoma has shown an increased incidence of carcinoma-in-situ.

Other rare tumours include those derived from Sertoli and Leydig cells. Lesions in the epididymis and cord include adrenal and splenic rests and soft tissue neoplasms, especially leiomyoma and rhabdomyosarcoma. Lymphoid infiltration occurs particularly in Burkitt's lymphoma and acute lymphoblastic leukaemia. It appears to be a favoured site for relapse during a period of bone marrow remission. Wedge biopsies of each testis are needed to show leukaemic infiltration. If only scattered leukaemic cells are present, relapse will be detected by the presence of specific enzymes which require special immunohistological techniques (Janossy et al., 1982).

Abdominal masses in infancy and childhood

An abdominal mass may be discovered as an incidental finding or following the development of symptoms or signs. Unfortunately in many instances the mass is noted late in the natural history of the condition. Clinical evaluation of the mass depends upon its shape, size, surface, consistency, mobility and relationship to other structures.

There are many causes of an abdominal mass and they are listed and tabulated in Fig. 29.7.

Full investigation is required to confirm the diagnosis as quickly as possible, i.e. within days and not weeks. Preliminary investigations such as

Table 29.9 Investigations and pathology of abdominal masses.

Pathology	*Investigation*	*Comment*
RENAL AND ADRENAL		
Pelvi-ureteric junctional hydronephrosis (unilateral or bilateral) Multicystic kidney Polycystic kidney	IVP	Differentiates a non-functioning unilateral multicystic kidney and renal agenesis. In neuroblastoma the kidney is displaced downwards
Nephroblastoma Neuroblastoma	Ultrasonography	Confirms: (a) Bilateral involvement in polycystic disease (b) Bilateral nephroblastoma (c) Coexistent renal agenesis (d) Patency of the renal vein
	Isotope renography	Routine investigation in PUJ hydronephrosis and in bilateral nephroblastomas
	Pressure flow studies	Indicated in PUJ hydronephrosis in equivocal diagnosis
	Chest X-ray and Skeletal survey	Excludes metastases
	24-hour urine collection for HVA and VMA	Differentiates neuroblastoma and can be used as a marker to detect recurrence
	Inferior venocavagram	Determines blockage of IVC by tumour
	Renal arteriogram	Essential in bilateral nephroblastoma
LIVER AND GALL BLADDER		
Hepatoblastoma Hepatocellular carcinoma	Liver function tests	
Choledochal cyst	Ultrasound	
	Liver imaging with isotopes	Determines whether hemihepatectomy is possible
	99.Tc^{m} labelled hepatobiliary agents	Demonstrates flow of bile into the alimentary tract
	Liver biopsy (open or closed)	Essential for diagnosis before starting treatment with irradiation or cytotoxic drugs
SPLEEN		
Leukaemia Lymphoma and portal hypertension	Haematological investigations	Excludes hypersplenism and thrombocytopenia
	Liver function tests	Differentiates prehepatic and hepatic disease
	Oesophagoscopy and barium swallow	Confirms diagnosis of oesophageal varices
	Liver biopsy	Diagnosis of cirrhosis
	Ultrasound	Determines whether portal vein is patent
	Splenoportogram	Measures portal venous pressure and demonstrates site and size of varices
STOMACH		
Congenital hypertrophic pyloric stenosis	Straight X-ray Barium meal Ultrasound	Only required in selected patients. Diagnosis and treatment are based on clinical findings
INTESTINE		
Intussusception	Straight X-ray	Fluid levels and gas-filled loops indicate intestinal obstruction. Mass sometimes seen
	Barium enema	Confirms diagnosis and used for therapeutic reduction
Duplication cysts and mesenteric cysts	Straight X-ray	Shows displacement of viscera
	Ultrasound	Confirms cystic nature of mass
	99.Tc^{m} labelled DTPA	Demonstrates ectopic gastric mucosa in duplication cysts and Meckel's diverticulum

the blood pressure, full blood count and sedimentation rate, serum electrolytes and creatinine, liver function tests, examination of the urine and a straight X-ray of the abdomen are required.

Specific investigations led to the correct diagnosis (Table 29.9). Treatment, i.e. laparotomy and definitive surgery, can be undertaken in some patients before the results are available, for example Homovanillic acid (HVA) and vanilmandelic acid (VMA) estimation on 24-hour urine collections.

Neuroblastoma

The commonest site of origin is in the adrenal medulla, but these tumours may arise from other sympathetic nervous tissue. They are the most common malignant tumour of the abdomen in childhood. Neuroblastomas arising in pelvis and thorax have a better prognosis and so do those in children of less than 1 year. Neuroblastomas form soft, white or haemorrhagic tumours. Necrosis and calcification are characteristic. They expand and invade local structures including liver and kidneys with metastasis to lymph nodes, lungs and bone. Undifferentiated tumours are composed of clusters of small blue cells with little surrounding stroma. A ring of neuroblasts with a central fibrillary mesh forms the characteristic Homer–Wright rosette. Evidence of differentiation and maturation occurs in ganglioneuroblastoma and ganglioneuroma. A lymphocytic reaction implies a good prognosis.

Electron microscopy should be used to confirm the characteristic dense neurosecretory granules in otherwise undifferentiated small cell tumours. The demonstration of neurone-specific enolase by immunoperoxidase methods may also be helpful.

Renal lesions

Hydronephrosis is most often due to a stenosis at the pelvi-ureteric junction of unknown aetiology. Intrinsic narrowing, adventitial kinks, aberrant vessels and a high ureteric insertion have all been implicated in some instances. The renal pelvis is distended with urine, the calyces are widened and there is progressive flattening of the tips of the renal papillae. Infection occurs in less than 30 per cent of patients.

Cystic dysplasia involving the whole kidney is known as multicystic kidney (multicystic dysplasia), and produces an enlarged irregular kidney with little resemblance to normal. Numerous fibrous-walled cysts occur, measuring up to 10 cm diameter; and the ureter often shows segmental atresia, particularly in the region of the pelviureteric junction.

Bilateral polycystic kidneys in infants (infantile polycystic disease) produces diffuse swelling of the kidneys with numerous small cysts whilst the ureters are normal. The condition is inherited as autosomal recessive.

Nephroblastoma (Wilms' tumour) is the second commonest abdominal tumour in infancy and childhood. Associated anomalies include hemihypertrophy, aniridia (often due to deletion of part of chromosome 11) and Beckwith–Wiedemann syndrome (macroglossia, omphalocoele and visceromegaly).

Other chromosomal abnormalities include elongation of the long arm of chromosome 16 and deletion of portions of chromosome 8. Occasional familial cases are described.

The tumour should be staged at the time of resection:

- Stage I: Tumour limited to one kidney and enclosed by capsule.
- Stage II: Tumour extends into perirenal fat, paraaortic lymph nodes or renal vein. Complete excision is possible.
- Stage III: Tumour extends into adjacent viscera, peritoneum or distant lymph nodes. Complete excision is not possible.
- Stage IV: Blood-borne metastases, usually in lungs.
- Stage V: Bilateral involvement at diagnosis (5–10 per cent).

Microscopic examination of multiple sections (at least one section for each centimeter diameter of tumour) reveals tubules, primitive but differentiating mesenchyme, and basophilic blastema. All three elements should occur in a typical nephroblastoma. Glomeruloid differentiation has no prognostic significance.

Histological variants which have a bad prognosis include anaplastic and pleomorphic forms, a rhabdoid form (with fibrillary whorls on electron microscopy and with PAS-positive cytoplasmic inclusions) and the bone-metastasizing renal tumour. These uncommon forms cause the majority of deaths.

Other less common variants include mesenchymal forms (rhabdomyomatous nephroblastoma, malignant mesenchymal tumour and clear cell tumour), cystic partially differentiated nephroblastoma and nephroblastomas occurring as a complication of nephroblastomatosis.

Congenital mesoblastic nephroma is a benign neoplasm causing unilateral renal enlargement in infants. Cut surface reveals a white firm tumour with the appearance of a uterine fibroid.

Other rare tumours in the kidney include angiomyolipoma and metastases.

Liver tumours

Hepatoblastoma occurs mainly in the first two years of life. Associated anomalies include hemihypertrophy, hyperglycaemia, renal malformations, osteoporosis and other hormonal changes. Rupture causes haemoperitoneum. Most tumours arise in the right lobe of the liver. Two histological types are recognized; epithelial and mixed type. Vascular invasion is common and leads to metastases in lungs and brain. Lymph node spread is also seen.

Hepatocellular carcinoma is less common in children than in adults. Histological examination shows either a trabecular or an adenoid variant and it may thus be confused with the epithelial type of hepatoblastoma although it usually arises after the age of 5 years.

Other tumours include malignant hepatic mixed tumour, malignant mesenchymona and embryonal sarcoma. Infantile haemangioendothelioma of the liver is a rare vascular tumour, but should be distinguished from the commoner cavernous haemangioma which is a hamartomatous malformation. In haemangioendothelioma, the liver is replaced by a mass of channels lined by a single or double layer of endothelial cells, many of which are plump and tufted. In contrast, the endothelial cells of the cavernous haemangioma are single and flattened.

Abdominal pain in infancy and childhood

Acute or recurrent abdominal pain is a common cause for emergency admission or for outpatient attendance. In clinical practice it is important to distinguish between these two clinical presentations although the pain may have a similar cause.

Acute abdominal pain

No cause is found in over 50 per cent of the children admitted to hospital with acute abdominal pain (Table 29.10). The symptoms and signs usually disappear within hours or days. Acute apendicitis is the suspected diagnosis in most of the others and operation is required.

In the management of acute abdominal pain in children it is essential to observe the child at regular intervals. The urine is examined to exclude

Table 29.10 Causes of acute abdominal pain in 416 patients (Drake, 1980).

Undiagnosed	186 (45%)		
Acute appendicitis	130		
Constipation	37		
Mesenteric adenitis	17		
Intussusception	9		
Urinary infection	7		
Other surgical causes (20)		*Other medical causes (10)*	
Appendix abscess	2	Pneumonia	3
Intestinal obstruction	3	Salmonella infection	1
Umbilical hernia	3	Diabetes mellitus	1
Inguinal hernia	1	Leukaemia	1
Torsion of the testis	1	Porphyria	1
Torsion of hydatid	1	Acute nephritis	1
Omental cyst	1	Iliac lymphadenitis	1
Biliary colic	1	Psychogenic	1
Renal colic	1		
Bilateral reflux	1		
Ovarian cyst	2		
Haematocolpos	1		
Salpingitis	1		
Ovulation	1		

diabetes and urinary infection. Straight X-rays of the abdomen are sometimes carried out to exclude intestinal obstruction and to detect appendicular faecoliths. A full blood count is only of value in making a decision about the cause of the abdominal pain in a limited number of patients.

In a recent study, 416 children were admitted during one year to the Wessex Regional Centre for Paediatric surgery with acute abdominal pain: 191 came to operation; of these 130 had acute appendicitis, 17 mesenteric adenitis, and 11 had no intra-abdominal pathology. Other medical and surgical causes of abdominal pain cover a wide range of diagnoses.

Recurrent abdominal pain

The clinical evaluation of the child with recurrent abdominal pain is difficult. A careful history is required with full details of the nature, site, duration and localization, radiation, relieving and aggravating factors, frequency and severity of the

Table 29.11 Investigation and pathology of urinary tract disease.

Pathology	*Investigation*	*Comment*
RENAL AGENESIS	IVP Ultrasound Isotope renography Cystoscopy	Differentiates non-function from absent kidney
RENAL HYPOPLASIA (hypoplastic dysplastic kidney)	IVP Isotope renography Renal biopsy	Determines individual renal function
CYSTIC DISEASE OF THE KIDNEYS		
1. Polycystic disease (a) infants (b) adult	IVP Ultrasound Renal biopsy	 Occasionally necessary
2. Cystic dysplasia (a) with ureteric anomalies	IVP Micturating cystogram Biopsy: excision	Associated with obstruction, i.e. upper pole of duplex with ectopic ureter, ureterocele and posterior urethral valves
(b) Multicystic kidney	IVP Ultrasound	Non-functioning kidney with a lobulated palpable mass
3. Solitary renal cyst	IVP Ultrasound	Used for diagnosis and treatment by aspiration
4. Pyelogenic cysts (microcalyx)	IVP Micturating cystogram	Excludes vesico-ureteric reflux
MALPOSITION, MALROTATION, FUSED AND ECTOPIC KIDNEYS		
1. Malposition and malrotation	IVP	Rarely of clinical significance
2. Horseshoe kidney; crossed renal ectopia and pelvic ectopia	IVP Micturating cystogram	Excludes associated vesico-ureteric reflux
OBSTRUCTIVE UROPATHY		
1. Pelviureteric junction hydronephrosis	IVP Isotope renography Micturating cystogram	Assesses renal function before and after surgery. 20% incidence of vesico-ureteric reflux in patients with PUJ hydronephrosis
2. Megaureter (uretero-vesical stenosis)	IVP Ultrasound Micturating cystogram Isotope renography	 Differentiates refluxing from non-refluxing megaureter
3. Posterior urethral valves	Biochemical evaluation of renal failure	Renal failure may require early treatment prior to surgery
	Isotope renography	
	Micturating cystogram	Confirms diagnosis
	Ultrasound	Confirms bilateral hydronephrosis and excludes renal agenesis
	Cystourethroscopy	Instrumentation for diagnosis and fulguration of valves
DUPLICATIONS OF THE URETER	IVP	
1. Complete (double ureters)	Cystoscopy Retrograde urethrography and pyelography	Confirms complete or incomplete duplication, ureterocele and ectopia. 25% of patients have contralateral reflux due to lateral ectopic ureteric orifice.
2. Incomplete (bifid renal pelvis, bifid ureter and blind ending ureter)		

ECTOPIC URETERS		
1. Urethral, vaginal and vestibular orifices	Inspection and catheterization of ectopic orifice IVP	Confirms single or more common duplex system. Renal segment may be non-functioning. Bladder shows filling defect with ureterocele
	Micturating cystogram	Excludes reflux – commoner in the male; rare in females
2. Ureterocele (including non-ectopic ureterocele)	Cystourethroscopy and retrograde catheterization	Confirms diagnosis and allows catheterization of ectopic orifice
VESICO-URETERIC REFLUX	IVP	Renal hypoplasia and ectopia are predisposing factors
	Micturating cystogram	Confirms diagnosis and severity of vesico-ureteric reflux (see above)
	Isotope renography	Monitors progression of renal scarring
	Cystoscopy	Evaluation of position and configuration of ureteric orifices
	Urodynamic studies	Required in difficult patients (detrusor overactivity)
URACHAL ANOMALIES		
1. Fistula	Intravenous methylene blue	Confirms leakage of urine at the umbilicus
2. Diverticulum	Micturating cystogram	
3. Cyst	Surgical exploration	
BLADDER		
1. Diverticulum	Micturating cystogram	A high incidence of reflux is associated with paraureteric diverticula
2. Duplication (incomplete and complete)		
ANTERIOR URETHRA		
1. Atresia of urethra	Inspection	Exceedingly rare
2. Meatal stenosis		May follow meatal ulceration and circumcision
3. Stricture	Anterior urethrogram	May follow urethral instrumentation
4. Anterior urethral valves and megalourethra	Urethroscopy	Very rare
ASSOCIATED ANOMALIES AND SYNDROMES		
1. Absent abdominal muscle syndrome (prune-belly)	All require full urological investigation	Cystic dysplasia is closely associated with prune-belly syndrome
2. Anorectal anomalies and oesophageal atresia (Vater syndrome)		A high incidence of associated urinary tract anomalies
NEUROPATHIC BLADDER	Biochemical evaluation of renal function IVP Micturating cystogram	
	Isotope renography	Differentiates different types of neuropathic bladder with low or high urethral resistance
CALCULI	Urodynamic studies	The majority of stones are of an infective origin
	Biochemical evaluation of renal function 24-hour urine collection for chromatography and calcium studies IVP Micturating cystogram Isotope renography	
	Stone analysis	Essential in all patients

pain. Disturbances of bowel and urinary habits are asscertained with particular reference to any relationship with the pain. Pain which wakes a child at night is usually significant. Details of any problems in the home and at school should always be sought.

The interpretation of central abdominal pain in the child under 7 years requires care, as pain of renal origin (e.g. hydronephrosis) is referred to the umbilicus. At later ages the pain is localized to the loin, as in adults.

A practical guide to management is to determine whether the history of pain suggests the diagnosis of recurrent attacks of acute appendicitis, intestinal obstruction or PUJ hydronephrosis. In many patients the cause of the pain may be psychosomatic or related to stress. Important factors are: parental separation and divorce, father working away from home, the presence of a chronically handicapped sibling and parental organic or psychiatric illness in the preceding three months (Crossley, 1982).

Two other diagnoses are important in patients with recurrent abdominal pain: constipation and non-specific mesenteric adenitis. These diagnoses are made on clinical grounds, rectal examination, straight X-ray and a barium enema to show a primary or secondary megarectum. Hirchsprung's disease can be exluded by suction rectal biopsy. Non-specific mesenteric adenitis is often related to viral infections. A history of sore throats with cervical lymphadenopathy coinciding or preceding the onset of the pain supports this diagnosis. Peptic ulceration, either in the duodenum or in Meckel's diverticulum and duplication, is another cause of pain. Barium studies and isotope scans are indicated.

In the majority of patients careful clinical assessment can avoid over-investigation. An accurate diagnosis can be made with only a few selective investigations. Operative intervention is seldom required and is not helpful in the long-term management.

Urinary Infection

Urinary infection in infancy and childhood requires full urological investigation as it heralds the existence of a congenital anomaly in the tract. The sex incidence varies with age, being commoner in boys under the age of 3 but thereafter being commoner in girls (male—0.17 per 1000; female—0.4 per 1000).

Anatomical factors such as the length of the urethra, obstruction, an intact epithelial surface and a competent uretero-vesical junction, all have an aetiological role. Vesico-ureteric reflux with an incompetent uretero-vesical junction is the single commonest cause of urinary infection in infancy and childhood, but there are other causes which need to be established in each patient. Physiological factors such as renal blood flow, urine flow, pH of the urine and vaginal secretions, all affect the incidence of infection in the young. The alkaline pH of vaginal secretions before puberty with vulvovaginitis and dysuria often leads to a mistaken diagnosis of urinary infection. Factors such as general health and constitution of the child, anaemia, constipation with or without faecal soiling, all increase the risks. Psychological stress with detrusor overactivity and an irritable bladder similarly predispose to infection and vesicoureteric reflux.

The diagnosis of infection depends upon the collection and culture of a suitable specimen of urine which contains more than 100 000 organisms per millilitre. Pyuria is a less reliable diagnostic feature. Midstream and clean catch specimens are usually adequate for diagnosis. Suprapubic aspiration and catheterization are used to confirm the infection in doubtful instances. Lower bacterial counts may sometimes be significant in these patients. Vaginal contamination in the female and from beneath the prepuce in the male may lead to difficulties in interpretation. Direct questioning about symptoms such as frequency, dysuria and hypogastric pain and also for systemic disturbances such as fever and vomiting, assist in the correct clinical diagnosis. Unfortunately, in the under-2-year age group the symptoms of urinary infection are vague so that diagnosis is difficult. They include non-specific symptoms such as vomiting, febrile convulsions and failure to thrive. In infants and children with recurrent infections, symptoms may be absent. This means that diagnosis depends upon the examination and interpretation of suitable collected urine samples, in itself a difficult undertaking. Biochemical assessment of renal function is essential at the outset of investigation in every patient. (Table 29.11).

Segmental cystic dysplasia, hypoplastic kidney and multicystic kidney all show a similar histological picture: abnormally formed glomeruli, dilated and atrophic tubules, peritubular rings of connective tissue and abnormal collections of interstitial mesenchyme. Cartilage is only found in

30 per cent of cases. Pyelonephritis may also be present when the ureter is patent.

References

Visible anomalies

Keen G. *Operative Surgery and Management*. Chapter 50. Bristol, London, Boston: Wright, 1981

Mustardé JC. *Plastic Surgery in Infancy and Childhood*. Edinburgh and London: E and S Livingston, 1981.

Norman AP. *Congenital Abnormalities in Infancy*. 2nd ed. Oxford and Edinburgh: Blackwell Scientific Publications, 1971.

Swellings of the neck

Jenkin, RDT, Brown TC, Peters MV, Sonley MJ. Hodgkin's disease in children. A retrospective analysis, 1958–1973. *Cancer* 1975; **35**:979–90.

Lennart K, Collins RD, Lukes RJ. Concordance of the Kiel and Lukes–Collins classification of non-Hodgkin's lymphoma. *Histopathology* 1983; **7**:549–59.

Norris DG, Burgert EO, Cooper HA, Harrison EG. Hodgkin's disease in childhood. *Cancer* 1975; **36**:2109–20.

Smith IE, Peckham MJ, McElwain TJ, Gazet J-C, Austin DE. Hodgkin's disease in children. *British Journal of Cancer* 1977; **36**:120–29.

Wright DH, Isaacson P. Biopsy pathology of the lymphoreticular system. *Biopsy Pathology Series*. London: Chapman and Hall, 1983.

Young JL, Miller RW. Incidence of malignant tumours in U.S. children. *Journal of Pediatrics* 1975; **86**:254–8.

Skin and soft tissue swellings

Enzinger FM, Weiss SW. *Soft Tissue Tumours*. St. Louis, Toronto and London: CV Mosby, 1983.

Favara BE, McCarthy RC, Mierau GW. Histiocytosis X. *Human Pathology* 1983; **14**:663–76.

Swellings in the groin

Berthelsen JG, Skakkebaek NE, Mogensen P, Sørensen BL. Incidence of carcinoma-in-situ of germ cells in contralateral testis of men with testicular tumours. *British Medical Journal* 1979; **2**:363–4.

Fonkalsrud EW, Mengel W. *The Undescended Testis*. Chicago, London: Year Book Medical Publishers Inc., 1981.

Giebink GS, Ruymanin FG. Testicular tumours in childhood. *American Journal of Diseases in Children* 1974; **127**:433–8.

Hadfield J, Hobsley M. *Clinical Surgical Practice*. Vol 3. Chapter 12. London: Edward Arnold, 1981.

Janossy G, Thomas JA, Eden OB, Bollum FJ. Nuclear terminal deoxynucleotidyl transferase (Tdt) in leukaemic infiltrates of testicular tissue. *Advances in Experimental Medicine and Biology* 1982; **145**:321–30.

Scorer CG, Farrington GH. *Congenital Deformities of the Testis and Epididymis*. London: Butterworths, 1971.

Abdominal masses

Darmady EM, Maciver AG. *Renal Pathology*. London, Boston: Butterworths, 1980.

Lauder I, Aherne WA. The significance of lymphocytic infiltration in neuroblastoma. *British Journal of Cancer* 1972; **26**:321–30.

Marsden HB, Lawler W. Bone-metastasizing renal tumour of childhood. *British Journal of Cancer* 1978; **38**:437–41.

Wright R, Alberti KGMM, Karran S, Millward-Sadler GH. *Liver and Biliary Disease*. London, Philadelphia, Toronto. WB Saunders Co, 1979.

Abdominal pain

Apley J. *The Child with Abdominal Pain*. 2nd ed Oxford: Blackwell Scientific Publications, 1975.

Crossley RB. Hospital admissions for abdominal pain in childhood. *J Roy Soc Med* 1982; **75**:772–6.

Drake DP. Acute abdominal pain in children. *J Roy Soc Med* 1982; **73**:641–5.

Urinary infection

Johnston JH. *Management of Vesico-Ureteric Reflux. Vol 10 International Perspectives in Urology*. Baltimore: Williams and Wilkins, 1984.

Williams DI. *Encyclopedia of Urology. Vol XV Urology in Childhood*. Berlin: Springer-Verlag, 1958.

Williams DI, Barratt TM, Eckstein HB, Kohlinsky SM, Newns GH, Polani PE, Singer JD. *Encyclopedia of Urology. Vol. XV supplement: Urology in Childhood*. Berlin: Springer-Verlag, 1974.

Williams DI. *Paediatric Urology*. London: Butterworth, 1968.

Further reading

Benn CD, Mintard WT, Rantch MM, Synder WH, Welch KJ. *Pediatric Surgery*. 2nd edition. Vol. 1 and Vol. 2. Chicago, London: Book Medical Publishers, 1979.

Berry CL. *Paediatric Pathology*. Berlin: Springer Verlag, 1981.

Dehner LP. *Pediatric Surgical Pathology*. St Louis: CV Mosby Co, 1975.

Filston HC. *Surgical Problems in Children: Recognition and Referral*. St Louis, Toronto, London: CV Mosby Co, 1982.

Gray SW, Skandalakis JE. *Embryology for Surgeons: The Embryological Basis for the Treatment of Con-*

genital Defects. Philadelphia, London, Toronto: WB Saunders Co, 1972.

Holder TM, Ashcroft KW. *Pediatric Surgery*. Philadelphia, London, Toronto: WB Saunders Co, 1980.

Jones PG. *Clinical Paediatric Surgery: Diagnosis and Management*. 2nd edition. Oxford: Blackwell, 1976.

Kissane JM. *Pathology of Infancy and Childhood*. 2nd Edition, St Louis: CV Mosby Co, 1975.

Potter REL, Craig JM. *Pathology of the Fetus and Infant*. 3rd Edition. Chicago, London: Year Book Medical Publishers, 1976.

Rickham PP, Lister J, Irving JM. *Neonatal Surgery*. 2nd Edition. London: Butterworths, 1978.

Willis RS. *The Borderland of Embryology and Pathology*. 2nd Edition. London: Butterworths, 1962.

30

Surgical Infection

M R B Keighley and D W Burdon

Introduction

Surgical sepsis can be classified as "established" infection which brings a patient into hospital, or "acquired" infection which occurs as a complication of a surgical procedure. Most established infections are a manifestation of disease and they usually require surgical drainage and sometimes antibiotic therapy, with treatment of the underlying pathology when appropriate. The incidence of postsurgical infections can be reduced by attention to surgical detail, aseptic techniques, and antibiotic prophylaxis in selected operations.

Established sepsis

Established infections include a variety of conditions such as soft tissue infections which are usually referred to casualty departments. This group includes patients with subcutaneous abscess, cellulitis, perianal sepsis, and contaminated traumatic wounds. Gas gangrene, synergistic infections of the abdominal wall and tetanus are occasionally seen. More serious established infections are cerebral abscess, mastoiditis and middle ear infections, bone and joint sepsis, and pelvic inflammatory disease. In general surgery the most frequent group of patients with established infections are those with acute gastrointestinal disease. Acute biliary disease is usually associated with infected bile and patients present with fever, rigors or acute abdominal signs. In contrast, there is little evidence that uncomplicated acute pancreatitis is bacterial in origin. Acute appendicitis is still the most frequent cause of acute admission to surgical wards and is often complicated by intra-abdominal sepsis. Intra-abdominal or retro-peritoneal abscess is also an important complication of Crohn's disease, diverticular disease and colorectal carcinoma. The presentation of established intra-abdominal infection is extremely variable. Clinical signs may be confined to the site of localized sepsis or they may be generalized in patients who present with septicaemia or septic shock.

Acquired sepsis

Hospital acquired infections are an important cause of prolonged hospital stay and serious morbidity. Specific infections include catheter-acquired urinary infection, surgical sepsis, post-operative respiratory sepsis, burns sepsis, intravenous catheter sepsis and infected surgical implants. After urinary infection, postsurgical sepsis is the most frequent and includes wound sepsis, intra-abdominal or pelvic abscess and septicaemia. The consequences of these potentially preventable complications include thrombo-embolism, malnutrition, anastomotic dehiscence, wound disruption and disseminated intravascular coagulation.

Diagnosis of infection

Clinical diagnosis

In most surgical infections, the causative organisms can be predicted and appropriate antibiotic therapy selected with a high degree of accuracy. Clues to the likely pathogen or pathogens are given by the clinical presentation of infection, by its site and by the nature of the bacterial flora of any adjacent mucosal surface. Reliable diagnosis depends therefore upon a working knowledge of the normal human bacterial flora as well as the types of organism associated with various clinical presentations of infection. For example, subcutaneous abscesses are usually caused by *Staphylococcus aureus*, except where they arise close to a mucous membrane such as the rectum, in which case a mixed anaerobic infection with *Bacteroides fragilis*, peptostreptococci and other anaerobes is probable. When the source of infection is the oropharyngeal cavity or the vagina, anaerobic infections are caused by different organisms, notably *Bacteroides melaninogenicus*. *Escherichia coli* commonly occurs with mixed anaerobic infections especially those in the lower half of the body. Mixed anaerobic infections of the head, neck and thorax are usually responsive to penicillin, in contrast to those at other sites which are mostly penicillin-resistant. Another clinically distinct type of subcutaneous infection is cellulitis in which beta-haemolytic streptococci are commonly incriminated. The clinical features of other infections will be described later in the appropriate sections.

Laboratory diagnosis

The accuracy of a provisional clinical diagnosis can be increased by immediate examination of a Gram film of pus, and of a Ziehl–Neelsen stained film if tuberculosis is suspected. This is best done by an experienced technician. Discussion of the result (taken in conjunction with the clinical findings) with a microbiologist, will generally provide the most reliable diagnosis. Nevertheless, the surgeon should be familiar with the staining and morphological classification of the principal pathogens (Table 30.1).

It is important to obtain a specimen for confirmatory bacteriological culture even though a clinical diagnosis and a decision on therapy may have been made. Bacteriological diagnosis is advised in every case for the following reasons: firstly the clinical diagnosis may be wrong, or the pathogen if correctly predicted may be unusually resistant to the antibiotic chosen; secondly, precise identification ensures that the data base upon which future clinical diagnoses are made is up to date; and finally, the isolation and identification of pathogens is an essential prerequisite for the recognition and control of cross-infection. Specimens for culture must be taken before antibiotic therapy commences. Specimens should be taken from the lesion itself, and when the illness is accompanied by a systemic reaction it is often helpful to take blood cultures as well. The request form accompanying the specimen should state the site from which the specimen was taken and the clinical diagnosis. If antibiotics are to be used they should be declared so that the laboratory can confirm their suitability.

Table 30.1 Morphological and staining characteristics of bacteria found in surgical infections.

	Bacilli (rods)	*Cocci (spheres)*
Gram-positive	*Clostridium perfingens*	*Staphylococcus aureus*
	Clostridium tetani	*Streptococcus pyogenes*
	Actinomyces israelii	*Streptococcus pneumoniae*
		Peptostreptococcus spp.
Gram-negative	*Escherichia coli*	*Veillonella sp.*
	Proteus mirabilis	
	Klebsiella aerogenes	
	Enterobacter cloacae	
	Pseudomonas aeruginosa	
	Haemophilus influenzae	
	Acinetobacter sp.	
	Bacteroides fragilis	
	Bacteroides melaninogenicus	

Infected lesions are commonly sampled with a swab, but it is preferable when pus is present to aspirate it into a syringe. Collection of a sample of pus rather than a swab is especially helpful in anaerobic infections because the pus provides a favourable reducing environment as well as giving protection from dessication. All specimens should be taken to the laboratory promptly because some fastidious organisms rapidly die, especially on a dry swab. The harmful effect of dessication and of atmospheric oxygen on anaerobes can be reduced by the use of special transport media. Most laboratories will provide these when their use is dictated by unavoidable delays in the delivery of swabs to the laboratory. Occasionally pieces of tissue are taken for culture. These should be sent to the laboratory in a dry sterile container or placed in transport medium if delay is unavoidable. On no account should they be placed in formalin. Since in many cases a specimen will also be needed for histological examination, it should be divided and the two portions placed in separate containers for the respective laboratories. Blood cultures should be taken according to the instructions on the bottle. Special care is needed to avoid contamination, by careful skin disinfection and use of a no-touch technique.

Origin of surgical infection

Infections arise either from the patient's own bacterial flora or from the hospital environment. Man is normally host to 10^{14} bacteria which comprise a complex flora of more than 500 different species. Only a few of these bacteria are pathogens with the potential to infect healthy tissue and cause disease. The bacterial flora varies according to the anatomical site and may be modified by disease.

Skin flora

The predominant bacteria on skin are staphylococci, corynbacteria and propionibacteria.

Staphylococcus aureus is the only important pathogen and is present in the nose of 20–50 per cent of normal adults. The incidence of skin carriage by *Staphylococcus aureus* increases after admission to hospital, or prolonged exposure to antibiotics, and is greater in patients who are nasal carriers. *Klebsiella aerogenes* may colonize the hands of hospital staff sometimes for prolonged periods. The skin adjacent to the perineum and on the thighs is usually contaminated by faecal organisms including *Clostridium perfringens*, and coliforms.

The gastrointestinal tract

The gastrointestinal tract is an extremely important reservoir of pathogenic bacteria. However, the frequency of bacterial species depends upon the site within the intestinal tract and the presence of disease. In the normal oesophagus there are no resident bacteria and contamination by swallowed oral commensals is transient. Similarly, stomach contents in patients with normal acid secretion are usually sterile. However, in patients with neutral gastric contents, as occurs in pernicious anaemia, gastric carcinoma, and after gastric resection, counts of bacteria often exceed 10^6 organisms/ml. The bacteria present include streptococci, coliforms, bacteroides, clostridia and occasionally anaerobic streptococci. As far as is known, bile and pancreatic secretions are normally sterile, but there is a 60–80 per cent incidence of infection in bile 12 hours after an acute attack of cholecystitis. Bile is infected in approximately 30 per cent of patients requiring biliary operations. The highest incidence of infected bile is amongst patients with choledocholithiasis and bile duct stricture, being over 80 per cent, whereas the incidence is only 33 per cent in malignant jaundice and less than 15 per cent in patients with stones confined to the gall bladder. The predominant bacteria include *Escherichia coli, Klebsiella spp*. and *Streptococcus faecalis*. Anaerobic bacteria are uncommon and if present are either streptococci or clostridia.

The upper small intestine is often sterile, but there is a transient increase in bacteria after meals. Organisms isolated from the jejunum include strepotococci, lactobacilli and yeasts. The number of bacteria increases towards the ileocaecal valve and the bacterial flora becomes more like that of the large intestine. Increased numbers of small bowel organisms are found in patients with duodenal diverticulae, after small bowel bypass, in regional ileitis and in acute small bowel obstruction. Distal to the ileo-caecal valve there is a striking change in the number and type of bacteria present. The anaerobes, particularly *Bacteroides spp*. and *Bifidobacterium spp*. are increased in number, but also include *Peptostreptococcus spp., Clostridium spp*. and *Fusobacterium spp*. The predominant aerobes are *Escherichia coli*, streptococci, staphylococci, proteus and *Pseudomonas spp*. There is no change in the bacterial flora throughout the colon or rectum and the numbers of bacteria are not increased in large bowel obstruction.

The respiratory tract

Apart from *Staphylococcus aureus*, the organisms which can be isolated from the nasopharynx include *Streptococcus pyogenes, Streptococcus pneumoniae, Haemophilus influenzae* and neisseria. By contrast, the lower respiratory tract is usually sterile.

The urinary tract

Urine is usually sterile, but the urethral meatus may become colonized by staphylococci, lactobacilli, corynebacteria and non-haemolytic streptococci. In the female urethra, *Escherichia coli* may be found intermittently.

The female genital tract

The bacterial flora of the vagina varies with the menstrual cycle. The predominant resident vaginal flora before the menopause are lactobacilli, but streptococci, *Escherichia coli, Proteus spp., Bacteroides spp.*, anaerobic streptococci, bifidobacteria, and yeasts including candida, are also represented. Before puberty and after the menopause, the vaginal secretions are alkaline and anaerobes are less frequent.

Environmental sources

Many of the bacteria which contaminate the hospital environment originate from the patients, staff and visitors. These organisms are widely distributed on laundry, washing facilities and food. Gram-positive bacteria (streptococci and staphylococci) remain viable for relatively long periods, whereas Gram-negative bacilli rapidly die unless they contaminate a moist environment. Spore-forming organisms such as clostridia can remain viable for a long time. In operating theatres, airborne staphylococci shed from the skin of theatre personnel are the major source of environmental contamination of surgical wounds.

Susceptibility to infection

Susceptibility to infection is related to the patient's constitution, the presence of underlying disease and exposure to drugs (Table 30.2).

Table 30.2 Susceptibility to infection.

Patient factors	
Age: elderly and children	
Malnutrition	
Obesity	
Immunological deficiency: humoral – hypogammaglobulinaemia	
cellular – leucopaenia	
impaired function (a) hereditary (b) acquired	
Disease	
Burns	Anaemia
Trauma	Renal disease
Malignancy	Arterial insufficiency
Diabetes	
Therapeutic agents	
Steroids	Antimitotic agents
Immunosuppressive agents	Ionizing radiation
Antimetabolites	Antimicrobials

Patient factors

Sepsis is more common in the extremes of life. Infection is also more common in the malnourished patient, as well as in the obese. Deficiencies in both humoral and cellular immunity will render the patient more susceptible to infection. For instance, hypogammaglobulinaemia is associated with recurrent episodes of sepsis. Failure of the cellular immune response is termed anergy and is associated with an increased incidence of postoperative infection and septicaemia. Anergic patients may be detected by failure to respond to a series of skin test antigens and their anergy may be reversed by nutritional therapy. Numerical deficiency of neutrophils, as in aplastic anaemia and leukaemia, is another predisposing factor for bacterial infection. There are also certain rare hereditary disorders in which the antibacterial function of neutrophils is impaired.

Underlying disease

There is an increased risk of sepsis in malignancy, poorly controlled diabetes, burns, trauma and anaemia associated with acquired defects of neutrophil function. In addition, the incidence of infection in patients with chronic renal and arterial disease is increased.

Therapeutic agents

Various forms of therapy may exert a profound influence on susceptibility to infection. Long and short-term steroid therapy causes a depression of the inflammatory response. Immunosuppressive agents and cytotoxic drugs depress phagocytosis, impair reticulo-endothelial system function and reduce the generation of immuno-competent and phagocytic cells by the bone marrow. Radiotherapy has a similar effect, but will also cause epithelial ulceration. Antimicrobial agents which suppress the normal bacterial flora may allow overgrowth of other organisms. This phenomenon is extremely dangerous in hospital if normal commensal organisms are replaced by multiresistant bacteria which can be difficult to treat.

Established sepsis

Principles of surgical therapy

Treatment of established infection relies upon attention to surgical principles combined with intelligent use of antimicrobial therapy. The principles of surgical management are drainage of pus and debridement with secondary suture of heavily contaminated wounds. Antimicrobial agents alone cannot be expected to succeed if there is dead tissue or a collection of pus within a walled-off cavity into which antibiotics cannot diffuse. By contrast, surgical drainage is rarely necessary if infection is not accompanied by pus, as in leucopaenic patients, in patients with cellulitis or in patients with an inflamed segment of acute diverticular disease without abscess.

Principles of antimicrobial therapy

Antimicrobial therapy is not required for the majority of surgical infections in which a localized abscess has been surgically drained. If the abscess is multiloculated, shows signs of extension, is surrounded by extensive cellulitis or is accompanied by signs of septicaemia or a toxic state, then antibiotics should be started at once. Therapeutic antimicrobials should be given in full dosage for no less than 5 days. The dose given should be sufficient to achieve a peak serum concentration of at least five times the minimum inhibitory concentration of the antibiotic for the infecting organism. If there is no clinical response, the organism may be resistant to the antibiotic or there might be a collection of pus requiring more efficient surgical drainage. Combined antimicrobial therapy is unnecessary except for some mixed infections or for the treatment of tuberculosis. Topical antimicrobial therapy is undesirable because of the risks of hypersensitivity and because it tends to select resistant bacteria at sites exposed to many bacteria. Antiseptics are therefore to be preferred in patients with superficial sepsis requiring local treatment.

Examples of established sepsis

Staphylococcal sepsis

Staphylococcus aureus is responsible for a variety of clinical syndromes including furuncle, carbuncle, acute infections of the hand such as paronychia, infected web space and suppurative tenosinovitis. It is the most frequent isolate from subcutaneous abscess and acute osteomyelitis. In most cases, localization of infection is determined by direct inoculation at the site of local trauma or a penetrating wound, but sometimes the source of infection may be haematogenous. Cloxacillin is the antibiotic of choice for most of these syndromes, and early therapy may render surgical drainage unnecessary. A swab or sample of pus should be cultured in all cases, because infections by other pathogens may mimic the clinical features of staphylococcal lesions. In patients with osteomyelitis blood cultures should also be taken. If the infection has proceeded to formation of pus, drainage is mandatory. There is some evidence to support the concept of early drainage and immediate primary skin closure if the patient is given high doses of an appropriate antibiotic for 5 days. The advantages of this technique are that there is minimal morbidity and daily dressings are unnecessary.

Streptococcal sepsis

It is remarkable how the incidence of acute streptococcal infection has declined. The most important syndromes are cellulitis and erysipelas. Both conditions are due to a spreading subcutaneous infection without pus formation and may progress to lymphangitis and septicaemia. Localization by natural defences is inefficient, possibly because of the production by *Streptococcus pyogenes* of hyaluronidase, streptokinase and anti-leukocyte toxins. There is a rapidly expanding diffuse red swelling of which examples are orbital cellulitis, Ludwig's angina and pelvic cellulitis. There may be localized complications due to expanding tissue planes or venous thrombosis. Unlike staphylococcal sepsis, drainage is rarely necessary or appropriate and high doses of penicillin should be used.

Sepsis in open wounds

Open wounds are invariably contaminated by bacteria originating from the patient's own flora or from the environment. Infection is common when there is extensive necrosis of muscle following road accidents or agricultural injury. Occasionally, infection in wounds may be complicated by gas gangrene or tetanus. The principal infecting organisms are *Staphylococcus aureus*, streptococci and faecal aerobic and anaerobic bacteria. The management of traumatic wounds involves complete excision of all devitalized tissues and delayed skin closure. This is because the natural defences against infection are impaired in tissues with a deficient blood supply due to interference with the migration of phagocyte cells and transfer of antibody and plasma proteins. Furthermore, devitalized tissues provide the conditions required by anaerobic bacteria for multiplication, and this is aggravated by the presence of foreign bodies and soil which has reducing properties. These principles have had to be relearned during the early years of almost all armed combat. Wounds must be thoroughly cleaned and fasciotomy may also be required. Primary wound closure should never be performed in the presence of foreign material or devitalized tissues. Antibacterial therapy with penicillin is also advised.

Tetanus

Tetanus is a potentially lethal complication of wounds which are contaminated by *Clostridium tetani*. The organism itself is not responsible for localized infection, but elaborates an exotoxin which becomes fixed to neural tissue. The organism will only multiply under anaerobic conditions and hence the complication is rare if wound debridement has been satisfactory. The neurotoxin blocks the release of glycine, a neurotransmitter that prevents the contraction of opposing muscles. Early symptoms are stiffness of the jaw and muscle spasms starting in the neck and extending to the trunk and limbs. Death is usually from respiratory complications. Treatment of established tetanus includes local debridement to remove the source of the toxin, administration of human tetanus immunoglobulin, respiratory support and intravenous fluids.

Prevention of tetanus is by early appropriate wound toilet and administration of a booster dose of tetanus toxoid in previously immunized persons who have not received toxoid within the preceeding 5–10 years. In a heavily contaminated wound of a patient who has never been previously immunized, penicillin should also be given and human tetanus immunoglobulin is often advised.

Gas gangrene

The term "gas gangrene" implies gangrene from gas-forming bacteria and includes synergistic gangrene. However, most clinicians associate the term specifically with *Clostridium perfringens* infection. Although *Cl. perfringens* is an important cause of synergistic gangrene, it is by no means the only bacterium responsible. Other species include certain gas-forming coliforms: peptostreptococci, fusobacteria, bifidobacteria, bacteroides and other clostridia. Gas gangrene from *Cl. perfringens* is a rare complication of any infected abdominal wound. The organism may arise from the biliary tract or large bowel. Gas gangrene is more common following lower limb amputation for peripheral vascular disease and, as the mortality is over 40 per cent, penicillin prophylaxis should be given to all such patients even though the risk of infection is low. The onset of clostridial gas gangrene will only occur if there is a focus of devitalized or anaerobic tissue. This need only be small, but once clostridial growth starts, exotoxins are released into the surrounding tissues. These cause necrosis, increased capillary permeability and accumulation of fluid with impairment of the venous return. The clostridia invade and multiply in the expanding area of necrotic tissue. The terminal stage of the infection is marked by septicaemia with shock, haemolysis and renal shutdown. Treatment of established gangrene is by extensive debridement and systemic penicillin. The value of antiserum and hyperbaric oxygen is questionable.

Non-clostridial infective gangrene

A variety of clinical syndromes have been described in patients with non-clostridial gangrene. The most common pathogens are anaerobic streptococci, *Escherichia coli*, *Fusobacterium fusiforme* and sometimes other anaerobes. There is usually a mixed bacterial synergistic infection in a debilitated host which compound to produce a necrotizing fasciitis and rapidly spreading gangrene. In some examples of these clinical syndromes a causative organism has not been incriminated. Precipitating factors include traumatic open wounds, recent surgical operations, viral infections and diabetes. Table 30.3 lists the types of non-clostridial infections which may be seen in surgical practice.

Table 30.3 Clinical varieties of non-clostridial gangrene.

Name	*Site*	*Comments*
Calcrum oris	Mouth	Often malnourished, previous viral disease
Norma vulva	Vulva	Slow relentless necrosis
Meleney's postoperative gangrene	Peritoneal sepsis	Bright red – gangrene, microaerophilic streptococci might be responsible
Meleney's ulcer	Abdomen/scrotum	Postoperative undermined ulceration
Fournier's gangrene	Scrotum	Extensive scrotal necrosis due to anaerobic streotococci
Necrotizing fasciitis	Subcutaneous fat	Streptococcal
Anaerobic non-clostridial wound infection	Limb amputations/ abdominal wall	Profound toxaemia, 35% mortality

Urinary tract sepsis

Repeated urinary tract infections particularly in the male subject, usually indicate an anatomical or physiological abnormality in the urinary tract causing inadequate drainage. Stenosis at the pelviureteric junction, at the ureteric orifice, the bladder neck or the urethra, and bladder or renal stones, are the most common abnormalities and often require surgical correction. Vesicoureteric reflux or neuromuscular abnormalities at the pelviureteric junction account for physiological stasis with bacterial overgrowth. The most frequent pathogens are *Escherichia coli, Klebsiella spp., Streptococcus faecalis, Proteus spp., Pseudomonas aeruginosa* and *Staphylococcus aureus*.

Pelvic inflammatory disease

Pelvic sepsis usually presents as an unexplained fever, abdominal pain, urinary frequency and vaginal discharge. There is an expanding cellulitis in the parametrium which may later form a tubo-ovarian or pelvic abscess. The condition is often secondary to salpingitis and may be complicated by septic thrombophlebitis and septicaemia. The organisms usually responsible are anaerobic species, coliforms and *Neisseria gonorrhoeae*. Treatment should be by antimicrobials using metronidazole and a cephalosporin. Operation is only required for drainage of pus.

Abdominal sepsis

Many aspects of abdominal sepsis, such as acute cholecystitis, acute appendicitis, acute diverticular disease and the complications of granulomatous bowel disease, cannot be dealt with in detail here. Abdominal sepsis may also present as an unexplained septicaemia or pyrexia of unknown origin. Careful clinical and radiological investigation will then be necessary to exclude a pelvic abscess, an infected abdominal viscus or intra-abdominal abscess. The latter include subhepatic and subphrenic abscess which may complicate a silent perforation of an abdominal viscus, psoas abscess as a complication of colonic carcinoma or ileo-caecal Crohn's disease, and pericolic abscess resulting from diverticular disease or carcinoma. The abscess will require surgical drainage and concurrent or subsequent intestinal resection under appropriate antibiotic cover.

Septicaemia

Septicaemia includes patients with fever, constitutional disturbances and a positive blood culture without shock on the one hand, and those with circulatory collapse, oliguria, acidosis and secondary cardiac and electrolyte disturbance on the other. Septicaemia without shock is relatively benign, and if the focus of infection is drained and appropriate antibiotic therapy is instituted the prognosis is usually good. Septicaemic shock is a much more serious disorder and is probably due to the action of bacterial endotoxins. The precise pathogenesis of endotoxic shock is unknown, but the result is an increase in sympatho-adrenal activity with release of catecholamines, cortisol, glucogen, aldosterone and antidiuretic hormone. The principal functional impairment is on tissue oxygenation. Cell metabolism is disturbed and lactic acidosis develops. Acidosis alters vascular permeability and fluid leaks from the circulation into the interstitial spaces, a process which is further increased by release of histamine, kinins and prostaglandins. As a result of this fluid loss, the vascular compartment is depleted, venous return is impaired, myocardial depression occurs and a vicious circle develops which is often irreversible.

The organisms responsible for septicaemia in surgical patients depends on the underlying disease. Some of the more common sources of septicaemia are the biliary tract, large bowel, urinary tract, infected intravenous or central venous cannulas and gynaecological sepsis. Compromised hosts, for example renal transplant patients, are particularly susceptible. Probably the most frequent source of septicaemia after operation is the urinary tract, but the intestinal tract comes a close second. The common bacterial isolates from surgical patients with septic shock are *Escherichia coli, Pseudomonas aeruginosa, Klebsiella*, streptococci and staphylococci.

Tuberculosis

The tubercle bacillus is a non-sporing aerobic bacillus which is difficult to stain except by the Ziehl–Neelsen method. Culture is on Löwenstein–Jensen medium and takes up to 6 weeks. Tuberculosis is a chronic infection which is transmitted by droplet infection from patients with open pulmonary disease and less commonly by infected milk. Bovine tuberculosis is now uncommon in Europe due to tuberculin testing of herds and pasteurization of milk, but cases are still seen in the immigrant population from Africa, Latin America and India. Although the majority of infections involve the lung, almost any organ or tissue may be involved. The extrapulmonary sites of disease are the skin, joints, bones, lymph nodes, genitourinary system and bowel. The principal histopathological features of the disease are caseating necrosis with epithelioid and Langhans giant cells, infiltration by lymphocytes and fibroblasts, and surrounding fibrosis. There are two principal responses to the infecting organism: suppuration and fibrosis. Suppuration is commonly seen in tuberculous lymph nodes leading to formation of a cold abscess or in the lung causing cavitation. Fibrosis is the long-term result of infection when there has been healing, and is frequently observed in intestinal tuberculosis. The primary disease involves lymphatic tissue in the oropharynx, lungs and intestinal tract, which is followed either by healing or secondary lymphatic involvement with suppuration. Blood-stream infection is responsible for miliary tuberculosis, and for involvement of bone and the urinary tract. Detailed descriptions of tuberculosis are covered elsewhere. Tuberculous infection is associated with cell-mediated delayed hypersensitivity to tuberculoprotein. This hypersensitivity reaction can be used to determine evidence of past or present infection by observing the response to an intradermal injection of tuberculin PPD (purified protein derivative).

Actinomycosis

This is a rare chronic infection caused by *Actinomyces israelii*. It most commonly affects the lower jaw and is characterized by loculated abscesses, induration and sinuses. The organism is a normal commensal of the mouth. Infection usually follows trauma or dental extraction, but may also occur after human bites. The disease starts as an area of acute suppurative inflammation which persists to become chronic. Colonies of organisms occur in the pus as small greyish-yellow (sulphur) granules. Spread is by local penetration or by the blood stream which is responsible for metastatic (honeycomb) abscesses in the liver, lungs, bones, kidneys and brain. Cervico-facial actinomycosis (70 per cent) and ileo-caecal disease (20 per cent) are the principal sites of disease. The organism is usually sensitive to penicillin.

Sepsis in the compromised host

There are many patients receiving drugs such as steroids, azothioprine, and antimitotic agents for treatment of cancer, inflammatory bowel disease, collagen disorders and prevention of rejection after organ transplantation. Immunosuppressed patients are suceptible to microorganisms which are harmless to healthy individuals. Furthermore, antimicrobial agents are less effective in the absence of normal defence mechanisms. The common presentations include septicaemia, endocarditis, septic arthritis, encephalitis and respiratory, biliary or urinary infection. The organisms responsible for infection are listed in Table 30.4, the most important bacteria being staphylococci, aerobic Gram-negative bacteria and *Mycobacterium tuberculosis*. These patients are also susceptible to viral infections such as herpes zoster, cytomegalovirus and hepatitis B. Protozoal

Table 30.4 Common infections in the compromised host.

Bacteria	*Viruses*	*Protozoa*	*Fungi*
Staphylococcus aureus	*Herpes simplex*	Malaria (*Plasmodium sp.*)	*Candida sp.*
Staphylococcus albus	*Herpes zoster*	*Pneumocystis carinii*	*Aspergillus sp.*
Escherichia coli	*Cytomegalovirus*		
Klebsiella sp.	*Hepatitis B*		
Proteus sp.	*Polyoma virus*		
Pseudomonas aeruginosa	*Wart virus*		
Serratia sp.			
Acinetobacter sp.			
Enterobacter sp.			
Clostridium perfringens			
Mycobacterium tuberculosis			
Actinomycosis sp.			
Nocardia sp.			
Listeria monocytogenes			

infections, particularly *Pneumocystis carinii* and fungal overgrowth by candida, are also common.

Acquired sepsis

Principles of surgical prophylaxis

Under no circumstances should antimicrobial prophylaxis be considered a substitute for good surgical technique. There is an increased risk of surgical sepsis following prolonged operations if there has been inadequate haemostasis, if non-absorbable materials such as sutures are left in the wound, if operation has compromised the blood supply to an organ, and whenever open drains are used. When a hollow viscus containing bacteria such as the colon is opened, there is a greater risk of infection. Under these circumstances, the operation site should be isolated from the rest of the abdominal cavity with packs, the bowel should have been cleared of all visible intracolonic faecal material by efficient preoperative bowel preparation, and wound closure should only be performed after discarding contaminated instruments and changing into new gloves. Whenever possible closed suction drains should be used. If open drains are necessary, they must be brought out through a separate incision. There is no evidence that wound drapes reduce the incidence of postoperative sepsis.

Principles of control of hospital infection

Audit is an important means of maintaining a low incidence of postsurgical infection. Audit will improve surgical discipline and also provide early recognition of an outbreak of sepsis. If there is an epidemic of staphylococcal sepsis, elective operations should be stopped. Nasal swabs should be obtained from patients and staff to detect carriers. Carriers of staphylococci of the same phage type as those causing the outbreak should be treated and not allowed to return for duty until the staphylococcus has been eliminated. Patients with sepsis should also be isolated and barrier nursed.

Hygiene in the ward and in theatre are important. Hand-washing will reduce the risk of cros-infection in the ward and should include the use of skin disinfection after carrying out procedures such as endotracheal suction and emptying of infected urinary drainage bags. The patient should be adequately prepared for operation and shaving is best avoided where possible. Skin preparation should be with solutions of 0.5 per cent chlorhexidine in 70 per cent alcohol or 1 per cent povidone iodine. Surgeons should scrub with detergent solutions of chlorhexidine or iodine. Hats and masks should be worn to reduce dispersal of organisms, but measures to minimize the amount of movement and talking in theatre are also important. The theatres should be supplied with properly filtered air, and the pressure should be greater than that in adjacent rooms and corridors. The ventilation should achieve 20 changes of air per hour. Special operating enclosures with laminar air flow producing a turnover of 300 air changes per hour have been advised for orthopaedic implant surgery.

Principles of antimicrobial prophylaxis

The main requirement for successful antimicrobial prophylaxis is that a high level of antibiotic should be present in the tissues and circulation at the time at which bacteria contaminate the operation site. The antibiotic should be bactericidal and should be given in large doses, preferably by the intravenous route. It should be given immediately before operation in the anaesthetic room. A second dose given soon after the operation may be beneficial, but it is unnecessary to prolong the duration of antibiotic therapy any further. Systemic administration provides predictable serum levels and

Table 30.5 Choice of prophylactic antimicrobial agents.

Organism	*First choice*	*Alternatives*
AEROBES		
Gram-positive		
Staphylococcus aureus	Cloxacillin	Cefuroxime
Streptococcus pyogenes	Penicillin	Cefuroxime
Streptococcus faecalis	Ampicillin	
Streptococcus pneumoniae	Penicillin	Co-trimoxazole
Gram-negative		
Escherichia coli	Gentamicin	Cefuroxime
Proteus sp.	Gentamicin	Cefuroxime
Klebsiella sp.	Gentamicin	Cefuroxime
Pseudomonas sp.	Tobramycin	Cefuroxime
Enterobacter sp.	Gentamicin	Cefuroxime
Haemophilus influenzae	Ampicillin	Co-trimoxazole
ANAEROBES		
Gram-positive		
Peptostreptococcus sp.	Metronidazole	Clindamycin
Peptococcus sp.	Metronidazole	Clindamycin
Clostridium perfringens	Penicillin	Metronidazole
Gram-negative		
Bacteroides fragilis	Metronidazole	Clindamycin
Bacteroides melaninogenicus	Metronidazole	Penicillin

should be used in preference to topical or oral agents. Furthermore, systemic prophylaxis will minimize the risks of bacterial resistance, super-infection and antibiotic associated colitis. The choice of antibiotic is dictated by the organisms which typically cause infection following the surgical operation in question (Table 30.5). When the operation involves opening a viscus which has a normal bacterial flora, the organisms present will determine the likely pathogens and the choice of prophylactic antibiotic.

Further reading

Burdon DW. Principles of anti-microbial prophylaxis. *World Journal of Surgery* 1982, **6**: 262–7.

Eykyn SJ. The microbiology of post-operative bacteraemia. *World Journal of Surgery* 1982, **6**: 268–82.

Gorback SL. Intestinal micro-flora. *Gastroenterology* 1971, **66**: 1110–29.

Keighley MRB. Micro-organisms in the bile. *Annals of the Royal College of Surgeons* 1977, **59**: 328–34.

Keighley MRB, Burdon DW. *Anti-microbial Prophylaxis in Surgery*. Tunbridge Wells, Kent: Pitman Medical, 1979.

31

Healing and Repair

B Zederfeldt and F Rank

Introduction

Death of tissue incites a reparative process. While lower species can restore completely even complex tissues and organs, the reparative capacity in man is limited. Repair is complete only when injury is limited to epithelium. In injuries involving tissues other than epithelium, continuity and strength are restored by non-specific fibrous tissue. Such injuries therefore will give rise to a fibrous scar.

The reparative process is usually divided into three different phases: inflammation, fibroplasia and maturation. These phases are not completely separated, but gradually pass into each other so that, for example, inflammation may persist when fibroplasia is already under way.

Inflammation

The acute inflammatory reaction starts immediately after tissue injury and develops during the first 24 hours. Histologically, vascular stasis, interstitial oedema and leucocyte exudation are recognized, besides cell damage and blood coagulum.

The initial haemodynamic changes in the area of injury are those of active hyperaemia. After an initial transient constriction, arterioles relax. The increased blood flow results in capillary and venular stasis. Increased intravascular pressure is responsible for the passive escape of water and electrolytes early in the inflammatory reaction. This transudate is soon followed by exudation of plasma proteins. In a transient phase, leakage occurs through the endothelium of venules only. Increased venular permeability is caused by endogenous mediators, mainly histamine, stimulating endothelial cells to contract. Other cell-derived mediators are 5-hydroxytryptamine and prostaglandins. Plasma-derived mediators involve the so-called 'cascade system' composed of the clotting, fibrinolytic, kinin and complement systems. In a delayed, prolonged phase of active permeability, leakage occurs from both venules and capillaries. This leakage is mainly due to direct injury to the endothelium, and endogeneous mediators play a minor role. Exudation continues until the damaged endothelial cells recover or are replaced.

Polymorphonuclear leucocytes and monocytes appear in the injured tissue as a result of an active process, while escape of erythrocytes from the blood vessels is purely passive.

The neutrophil polymorphonuclear cells migrate through the venular walls mediated by chemotaxis. Chemotactic agents include products of the cascade system, injured tissue cells, microorganisms and partly denatured proteins. While some chemotactic agents also increase vascular permeability, this process, and leucocyte emigration, usually occur independently. Emigration of eosinophilic polymorphs is seen almost exclusively in acute atopic reactions and in parasitic infections. Basophil leucocytes are extremely rare in the inflammatory exudates.

Leucocytes and the protein-rich oedema constitute the inflammatory exudate.

Fibroplasia

Between 24 and 48 hours after injury there is a gradual decrease in the amount of polymorphonuclear leucocytes and concomitant appearance of cells from the mononuclear phagocyte system. When neutrophil polymorphonuclear cells are replaced by monocyte-derived macrophages, the cellular potentials for continuous resolution are preserved. The pluripotent macrophage is regarded as one of three cell types constituting the functional unit of cells in developing granulation tissue, the other two being the endothelial cell and the fibroblast. Probably influenced by a platelet factor, activated macrophages apparently initiate both endothelial budding and the migration and proliferation of fibroblasts from the adjacent connective tissue. Macrophages are also capable of stimulating fibroblasts to collagen formation. According to present knowledge then, platelets and especially macrophages are both the vanguards and the safeguards of initial vascularization and fibroplasia. The processes involved are not yet fully understood, but the search for 'wound hormones' apparently has found a basis.

From 3–5 days after injury fibrovascular proliferation predominates. New vascular channels are formed. Fibroblast proliferation increases and collagenous fibres are clearly visible from the third day. From the fifth day the cell content in the granulation tissue declines, and from the first week on, the histological picture is that of developing scar tissue containing mature fibroblasts and increasing amounts of extracellular collagenous material arranged in an irregular fashion. This material contains different types of collagen with composition somewhat different from that in the undamaged tissue.

Biochemically, the fibroplasia period is characterized by rapid increase in proteoglycan and collagen concentration, continuing to about 2 weeks after wounding.

When undisturbed, the acute inflammatory reaction following tissue injury thus proceeds to the formation of a fibrous scar which undergoes continuous remodelling for a very long time, probably decades.

Maturation

During the maturation phase, the collagen fibrils fuse to coarser fibres which are rearranged in such a way as to better withstand the stresses inflicted on the scar.

The maturation and rebuilding is not associated with increase of the amount of collagen in the wound area. Biochemically, however, collagen synthesis is increased over that in normal tissue. Obviously lysis of collagen balances synthesis during the maturation period.

The maturation phase is histologically also characterized by decreasing vascularization. Clinically, this is seen as transition from a red to a white scar.

Types of healing

When wound edges are brought together spontaneously or by mechanical means (sutures, tape) the bridging of the defect requires a minimal amount of new tissue and the scar will be small. This is the type of healing usually referred to as *primary healing*.

Secondary healing occurs when the wound edges cannot be brought together and consequently a larger defect must be filled by granulation tissue.

The healing process is principally the same in primary and secondary healing, but secondary healing takes a longer time, is to a higher degree disturbed by different factors, results in more scar tissue and leaves a larger surface covered by vulnerable epithelium. One characteristic feature of secondary healing is that the area finally covered by new epithelium is much smaller than the original defect. The granulation tissue develops contractile forces contributing to the closing of wound margins. Some of this capability is due to fibroblasts assuming several characteristics of smooth muscle cells. These myofibroblasts contain a contractile apparatus of massive bundles of cytoplasmatic fibrils with parallel orientation, and are otherwise morphologically characterized by multiple nuclear indentations.

Epithelialization does occur when granulation tissue fills the defect. Depressed or protuberant granulation tissue usually prevents growth of epithelium.

Large epithelial defects may be covered by grafts. This diminishes the negative influence of external factors and decreases the tendency to contraction.

Defects in tendons, nerves and vessels may likewise be bridged by grafted tissue. In these situations, the grafting means that possibilities for healing are created.

Wound strength

An important property of the scar is its strength. During the inflammatory phase the wound strength is only due to the coagulum and the mechanical support of the wound by sutures. During the fibroplasia period there is, however, a rapid increase of strength as a consequence of the bridging of the defect by granulation tissue, and sutures then play a successively decreasing role for the strength of the scar. Wounds in tissues with a small amount of collagen (e.g. intestine) have, just 10 days after surgery, a strength that is almost the same as that of the original tissue. At such time, however, wounds in tissues mainly consisting of fibrous tissue, such as skin, tendon and fascia, have attained only 5–10 per cent of the strength of the uninjured tissue. In this latter type of tissue, the strength of the scar increases during the maturation phase to finally reach almost, but not fully, the strength of the intact tissue.

Factors influencing healing

The normally developing healing process cannot be enhanced by any known factor.

Impairment of the process is, on the other hand, rather common and may occur during any of the three phases of healing—inflammation, fibroplasia and maturation.

Inflammation and fibroplasia

A normally developing inflammatory reaction is necessary for an undisturbed healing. Healing is as much impaired by an insufficient as by an exaggerated and/or prolonged inflammatory reaction. Insufficient inflammatory reaction may be a conseqence of iatrogenic measures such as immunosuppressive therapy or cortisone treatment. An exaggerated or prolonged inflammatory reaction occurs most often when bacterial contamination is marked, but can also be a consequence of a foreign body, such as devitalized tissue, suture materials or other foreign elements. A prolonged acute inflammatory reaction may resolve causing only delay in healing, but may also lead to formation of an abscess containing dead tissue, leucocytes and eventually bacteria. An abscess is delineated from the surrounding tissue by a collagenous membrane with tissues infiltrated by leucocytes and monocytes. Abscess formation invariably leads to a break of continuity, and repair after abscess formation consequently will be of the secondary healing type.

Changed inflammatory reaction may also influence healing, mainly the later phase of inflammation with prolonged infiltration of monocytes and macrophages often leading to increased fibroplasia. This is a type of reaction seen in chronic irritation and may be seen around non-resorbable suture materials.

The formation of granulation tissue during the fibroplasia period, and to a lesser extent the remodelling during the maturation phase, require an adequate supply of oxygen, amino acids and trace metals, as well as adequate removal of waste products from the area. Impaired circulation as well as different deficiency states, therefore, will influence the period of fibroplasia in a negative way.

Impaired circulation may be caused by local factors such as tightly tied sutures and arteriosclerotic narrowing of supplying vessels, or by more general factors such as shock. Such changes invariably lead to a lower oxygen tension with slower formation of granulation tissue and delayed collagen deposition in the extracellular space, resulting in delayed development of strength of the scar.

The occurence of haematoma or seroma in a wound causes delay of healing. The mechanisms include higher risk of infection, increased diffusion distances and the necessity for formation of more granulation tissue.

If the number of oxygen carriers is moderately reduced, oxygen tension in the tissue can be maintained by compensatory mechanisms. Therefore anaemia has to be pronounced before impairment of healing occurs.

While lack of specific amino acids seldom seem to cause impaired healing, malnutrition invariably is accompanied by a marked delay of healing. One mechanism is low oncotic pressure with resulting oedema, recognizable both clinically and histologically. The mode of action for impairment of healing seems to be increased diffusion distances with lowered oxygen tension. Malnutrition, however, also causes impaired host-resistance and for a given bacterial wound contamination, the rate of wound infection is markedly increased in a malnourished patient, again with delay in strength development.

The classical example of delayed healing due to a deficiency state is that of scurvy caused by C-avitaminosis. Vitamin C is necessary for transformation of procollagen to collagen fibres. In C-avitaminosis, therefore, procollagen accumulates in the wound area, but formation of collagen fibres is limited. An apparently mature scar may break if C-avitaminosis develops during healing. This is explained by continuing lysis of collagen while collagen synthesis is completely inhibited. The condition of C-avitaminosis is hardly seen nowadays, but there may be an influence of reduced concentration of vitamin C seen, for example, after major trauma or serious infections.

Zinc deficiency retards growth and repair. The mechanisms are not quite clear, but there seems to be an influence both on the inflammatory reaction and on the rate of fibroplasia in the zinc-deficient state.

Impaired healing in diabetes mellitus, uraemia and jaundice have complex causes where, however, impaired circulation is one factor of importance.

Iatrogenic impairment of healing is increasingly common. Glucocorticoid medication results in delayed healing, probably due to prolongation of the inflammatory phase eventually caused by lysosome stabilization since the effect can be reversed by treatment with vitamin A, a lysosome labilizer.

Delayed healing has to be anticipated in patients treated with immunosuppressive drugs, especially recognized clinically in wounds healing by second intention.

Cytostatic drugs cause delay of healing and strength development. The rapidly dividing cells in the granulation tissue are influenced by cytostatic drugs in the same manner as tumour cells. Vasoactive substances and substances blocking smooth muscle contraction may cause delayed healing, especially of wounds healing by second intention.

Finally, wounds in tissues treated by irradiation heal at a slow rate due in part to changes in vascularization of the tissue and in part to direct cellular effects of irradiation.

Impairment of maturation

Impairment of the maturation phase of the healing process is less conspicuous and less studied than that of inflammation and fibroplasia. However, such disturbances are not unusual.

The hypertrophic scar is characterized by a blue-red itching scar, often broad and protruding and hypersensitive to touch. Histologically, hypertrophic scars are characterized by immature granulation tissue with maintained amount of capillaries and presence of inflammatory cells long after the normal regression. The reasons for the lack of maturation of the granulation tissue are not known. However, tension over the granulation tissue may be of importance since compression of the wound, as well as long-lasting support of a wound, tend to give less of hypertrophic scar in sensitive areas. There are also racial differences in the frequency of hypertrophic scar formation. Such scars are more common in blacks than among white. In whites, wounds in certain areas, the regions over the sternum and the deltoid muscle, are especially apt to develop hypertrophic scars.

Another type of hypertrophic scar concerns increased production of collagen, the most spectacular being the keloid, genetically characteristic and apt to recurrence. Keloids are skin lesions, large, bulging and histologically hypocellular with dense fibrous tissue almost totally composed of irregular collagen bundles.

Hypertrophic scars are often seen after burn injuries. When these hypertrophic scars mature, a marked contraction process leads to deformations and/or contractures of joints.

The reasons for hypertrophic changes during scar evolution are obscure. As well as defects in activity systems, altered collagen synthesis and the presence of collagenase inhibitors have been considered. Eventually the changes are variants of fibromyosis elsewhere and represent non-neoplastic manifestations of defect macrophage fibroblast interaction.

Sinus formation and suture granuloma may develop in the scar region at any time. Sinus formation is due to an acute inflammation around buried sutures with abscess formation. Healing occurs only after removal of the suture material. Suture granuloma represents a more chronic inflammation around buried sutures resulting in fibrous tissue proliferation. A suture granuloma may be mistaken for an implantation metastasis. Sinus formation and suture granuloma are nowadays less common due to increasing use of synthetic resorbable suture materials.

Dystrophic calcifications and bone formation are occasionally seen in relation to scars in soft tissue. These changes may give tumour suspicion and be subjected to histological examination.

Knowledge about the wound healing process and the factors influencing it, is necessary for both surgeons and pathologists to allow evaluation of the normal healing process as well as healing subjected to different disturbances. It should be added that there are few occasions where difficulties arise in differential diagnosis between healing and other processes. Cellular granulation tissue by itself sometimes displays proliferative changes making conventional histological criteria of doubtful value for excluding sarcoma. The so-called 'pseudosarcomatous lesions' especially, may easily be misinterpreted. The pathologist must also be familiar with the changes caused by irradiation, both the cell pleomorphism and the obliterative vascular lesions.

Reparative processes in specialized tissues

Epithelial surfaces

Surface epithelia continue to proliferate throughout life, replacing exfoliated cells. The process is vital to maintenance of normal function. This capacity to regenerate is shared only by blood cells.

Minor injuries heal almost completely, but deeper defects leave scars which impair epithelial function. To assure epithelialization, surface levelling is necessary as is a basis of viable tissue. Sometimes epithelial repair might be difficult to distinguish from dysplasia or neoplastic proliferation. Most important, however, is that malignancy should always be considered when ulceration persists or fistulas develop.

Squamous epithelium is replaced from the basal cell layers. Regardless of location, type and severity of the injury, the process of repair involves cell migration, proliferation and differentiation. Within 24–48 hours an incised, sutured skin wound appears covered by an advancing sheet of cells. These cells are mobilized from enlarged basal cells derived from the thickened, sometimes inverted, epithelial edges. Epidermal spurs develop both at the site of incision and along the suture tracks. These spurs, as well as neighbouring pilo-sebaceous epithelial proliferations, disappear within two weeks. After one month, the surface is covered by differentiated epidermis. Scar epidermis, however, never regains normal rete ridges causing reduced area of dermal contact and subsequently increased vulnerability. Dermal elastic properties are never fully regained. Destroyed skin appendages are not restored.

Nodules in a scar should bring about suspicion of tumour metastasis or abscess, but most likely represent foreign body reaction to suture material or keratin or occasionally an epidermal keratinized implantation cyst. When infectious disease, ischemic lesions and irradiation dermatitis can be ruled out, a persistent ulceration always calls for a histological biopsy to exclude malignancy. Considerations put forward regarding the epidermis will apply also to the non-keratinized squamous epithelium of the oral cavity, the oesophagus and the anal region, as well as the genital tract. Because of less surface differentiation and the tendency to metaplasia, this epithelium, especially in the oesophagus and on the uterine cervix, sometimes shows reparative changes difficult to distinguish from dysplasia and neoplastic proliferation.

Transitional epithelium of the urinary tract easily matches squamous epithelium as regards the capacity for repair. It also provides the same diagnostic considerations.

Mucosal surfaces have a good regenerative capacity, best demonstrated by the continuous renewal of the endometrial surface. The basic scheme of repair is still that of migration, proliferation and differentiation.

The pseudostratified columnar epithelium of the respiratory tract is easily replaced. Problems arise when normal epithelium is replaced by excess mucus-secreting non-ciliated cells or by metaplastic squamous cells.

The mucosa of the gastrointestinal tract heals readily following surgical anastomoses. Also small ulcerations are easily restored. The major problems concern chronic and large gastric ulcers and ulcerative colitis, both of which probably have defective stroma–epithelial relations. Failure of re-epithelialization calls for histological biopsies, which often present difficulties of interpretation between dysplasia and adenocarcinoma. The wound edges show glandular derangement and always some cell and nuclear pleomorphism with basophilic cytoplasm, nuclear hyperchromasia and increased mitotic activity.

Stenosis in an anastomosis may be due either to defective healing or to tumour growth.

Serosa

The normal serosa consists of a single layer of mesodermally derived mesothelial cells on a supporting fibrous tissue without intervening basal membrane. The normal serosa provides gliding surface for intra-abdominal organs and allows transport of cells and fluid, but otherwise has no epithelial properties.

A healing process in the serosa may be induced by damage caused by inflammatory processes or by surgical procedures. The serosal lining has an extraordinary ability to restoration if not disturbed and complete covering of even large denuded areas is possible. However, in some instances a healing process causes dense adhesions. The reasons why this happens in some patients and not in others are obscure. It seems to be a fact, however, that marked inflammatory reaction with fibrin deposition tends to incite fibrous healing and adhesions.

Previously a special problem was talcum granuloma occurring when talcum deposited from surgeons gloves caused macrophage infiltration and fibrous tissue formation leading to granulomas. When they occur there might be questions of differential diagnosis between granuloma and carcinomatous nodules in the peritoneum.

Parenchymatous organs

Liver

The epithelial cells (hepatocytes and biliary epithelium) have a good capacity for regeneration. Minor cell injuries from toxic or inflammatory causes are easily repaired. However, when the stroma is concomitantly deranged, fibrous tissue increases. The fine reticular supporting framework is never fully restored, which makes it possible to identify histologically even minor lesions. The stimulus to fibrous tissue formation is not quite clear. It is, however, possible that activated macrophages (Kupfer cells) release fibroblast-stimulating substances.

The histological picture of cirrhosis is distinct and while it can give no indications as to cause, there should be no problems in differential diagnosis.

Trauma to the liver with ruptures of the parenchyma heals by fibrous tissue formation leaving a fibrous scar.

Injuries to the common duct are usually repaired without problems provided that some part of the circumference is preserved. If there is complete severance, an end-to-end anastomosis has a very high risk of stricture with serious clinical problems. The causes for the specially high incidence of strictures in this type of anastomosis are not clear. It may be speculated that the small canaliculi within the common duct wall, when disturbed by surgery and sutures, influence the granulation tissue in a negative way.

Kidney

Ruptures in the kidney parenchyma, following trauma, heal by fibrous scars.

More generally, fibrous scarring of the kidney may be the consequence of ischaemia or inflammatory processes. Such scarring may be associated with impaired renal function due to poor regenerative capacity of the glomerular apparatus and with anatomical alterations due to contraction. Again, there should be no problems in differential diagnosis.

Allotransplantation of kidneys has become a frequent procedure. If graft function deteriorates, problems arise in deciding if this is due to histoincompatibility mediated graft rejection or is a consequence of reparative processes related to ischaemia or infection.

Pancreas

Chronic pancreatitis, usually on the basis of alcohol abuse, is characterized by fibrous scarring often with calcium deposits. The endocrine part of the gland is rather well preserved functionally and histologically, at least in earlier stages of chronic pancreatitis.

The differential diagnosis against carcinoma of the pancreas may be difficult, especially as a carcinoma may cause pancreatitic changes distal to the tumour. Biopsies from the pancreas are difficult and, knowing the high rate of complications (e.g. fistulas), the surgeon tends to keep such biopsies rather superficial which may mean that tumour tissue is not included in the biopsy. The morphological picture of pancreatic biopsies is characterized by a reactive polymorphism which causes considerable difficulties for the pathologist. There is evidence that fine-needle biopsy is better than surgical biopsy from the pancreas in peroperative diagnosis.

Lungs

The lungs react with local fibrous scarring to many different injuries, for example, pulmonary infarcts, specific and non-specific pleuro-pneumonia etc.

More generalized lung fibrosis is a rather common clinical entity usually related to occupational inhaling of silica, coal or asbestos fibres. Fibrosis in these situations seems to be due to macrophages accumulating in response to these materials. When the macrophages are activated, they liberate substances stimulating fibroblasts to collagen deposition.

Mammary glands

Trauma to the breasts may result in haematoma or necrosis of adipose and fibrous tissue. Sequelae are often retracted scars clinically imitating malignant tumour.

Surgery, and even fine-needle biopsy, results in scar formation where both the clinical and the mammographic picture may be difficult to separate from that of malignancy. Here too excision biopsy and histology are necessary for definitive diagnosis.

Fibrocystic disease of the mammary gland involves increased fibrous tissue formation. The mechanism behind this is obscure, but may involve macrophage–fibroblast interactions.

Mesenchymal tissues

Bone and joints

Bone healing is similar to wound healing. With perfect adaptation and immobilization, fracture healing comes near to primary union. Under less favourable conditions, healing is of secondary union type with formation of granulation tissue, callus.

Cortical and medullary bone as well as periosteal tissue are involved in the reparative process. The occurrence of bone debris and often marked haematoma, strains the resolution process performed by osteoclasts and macrophages. Following resolution, granulation tissue fills the defect. This granulation tissue is specific by its content of proliferating osteoblasts inducing bone formation.

The external subperiosteal callus is the main source for bone formation and thus important for establishing continuity and stability. The internal endosteal callus is of major importance only in intracapsular fractures where periosteum is lacking. The original callus is subjected to a remodelling process extending over many months and resulting in almost complete restoration of bone structure and strength.

The fracture healing process requires optimal vascularization and immobilization. Impaired vascularization, and thereby decreased oxygen tension, delays and disturbs ossification. Signs of such disturbance are excess callus, increased formation of cartilage, non-calcified osteoid tissue or eventually only fibrous union (pseudo-arthrosis).

Delayed fracture healing is especially common in comminute fractures with extensive bone injury and in compound fractures with bacterial contamination.

A reparative process in bone similar to that of fracture healing may result from different types of bone injury or disease, for example, tumour. In case of bone biopsy, it is imperative to inform the pathologist about the clinical history and X-ray findings to allow correct interpretation.

Cartilage is hardly capable of intrinsic repair, and damage to articular surfaces at best results in repair by externally derived fibro-cartilage. This defective repair forms the basis for increased joint replacement by prosthesis of foreign materials. Tissue-compatibility of modern prosthetic materials is high and tissue reaction to implants are usually limited.

Tendon

The important characteristics of tendons are strength and gliding function, which ideally are both restored after injury.

Previously, re-establishment of strength could be obtained while restoration of gliding function was less successful. With the concept that tendons had no intrinsic capacity for repair, ingrowth from the peritendinous tissue was accepted and stimulated, for example, by excision of synovial membranes. Newer knowledge indicates, however, that tenocytes are capable of repair and that synovial fluid has nutritional value for the tendon. Therefore adhesions are not indispensable as was previously assumed. It should, therefore, be possible to re-establish strength with preserved gliding function.

Nervous tissue

Neurons are incapable of reproduction and nerve cell injuries in brain, cord and ganglia are followed by cell death and scar formation (gliosis). Peripheral nerves, however, repair injuries through a characteristic series of events if the lesion is not too close to the cell body. Following interuption of continuity, the nerve trunk retracts and axis cylinders and their myelin cover disintegrate distal to the lesion and are resolved by phagocytosis (Wallerian degeneration). Proximal to the lesion, the destruction stops at the nearest node of Ranvier. The cell body shows swelling and chromatolysis, preparing itself to replace the part of the axon lost peripherally.

Distally, Schwann cells proliferate and form endoneural tubes acting as pathways for regenerating nerve fibres from the proximal segment. After days to weeks, and at a speed of at maximum a few millimetres per day, these regenerating sprouts seek their way to establish end-organ connections. This journey is rather hazardous and unpredictable. The mechanisms involved are unknown, but probably growth-stimulating neurotropic factors are involved. Endoneural restoration, regulated by vascular and perineural barrier functions, is essential. The nerve cell potential for regeneration is thought to be at its maximum 2–3 weeks after injury. At this time, however, nerve cell sprouts have to pass through an unfriendly inflammatory environment and the endoneural tube undergoes fibrosis. Many nerve fibres therefore do not find their way, use wrong endoneural tubes or end up in microneurons. End organs degenerate if they are not re-innervated. Even meticulous surgery at this time often fails in achieving good and predictable results. The ideal time for nerve repair is currently under debate. At the time of re-establishment of nerve fascicles, a neuroma may develop in the area, either bridging the defect or appearing as a bulbous expansion at the end of an amputated nerve. The neuroma is a non-neoplastic proliferation of Schwann cells and fibroblasts with numerous intertwined nerve fibres in a dense collagenous matrix. Morton's neuroma, located at the interdigital plantar nerves near the head of the metatarsal bones, represents degenerative proliferation, mainly epi- and perineural. These circumscribed lesions may easily be mistaken for schwannoma or neurofibroma.

Muscle

Muscle cells are capable of hypertrophic and atrophic changes and may survive minor injuries. Despite a proliferative potential in smooth muscle cells, regenerative capacity in the true sense of the word is negligable. Devitalized skeletal and cardiac muscle, as well as smooth muscle, is replaced by connective tissue. For illustration it will be sufficient to mention Volkman's ischemic contracture of the forearm muscles, myocardial infarction and the changes in diseased or traumatized visceral and vascular walls.

Concluding remarks

The repair of injuries by fibrous tissue is in most instances beneficial, restoring continuity and strength of injured tissue. However, there are also negative effects of a healing process. Negative effects are obvious when healing occurs in unwanted situations, for example, intra-abdominal adhesions or adhesions between tendon and tendon sheet. Another negative effect of healing processes is due to the contraction that occurs in granulation tissue and which may cause stenosis of an anastomosis, cirrhosis of the liver, heart valvular disease, contractures in joints and, finally, narrowing of vessels as a result of an arteriosclerotic process which at least in part is related to healing.

As regards future research there are therefore two obvious main lines relating to possibilities to *increase the rate of repair*, and possibilities to *modify a healing process*. Some advances in the latter field have come during the last decade and it now seems possible that in the near future methods to modify healing will be found.

Further reading

Hunt TK, Dunphy JE (eds). *Fundamentals of Wound Management.* New York: Appleton-Century-Crofts, 1979.

Peacock EE, Van Winkle W. *Wound Repair.* Philadelphia, London, Toronto: WB Saunders, 1979.

Venge P (ed.) *The Inflammatory Process: an introduction to the study of cellular and humoral mechanisms.* Stockholm: Almqvist & Wiksell International, 1981.

32

Eyes

R J Cooling and A Garner

"For this beautiful organ is not only composed of a great variety of textures, but the transparency and ready examination of many of its parts in the living body admit of a great minuteness and accuracy of observation; and the various morbid changes can be seen going on much more distinctly than in any other part of the body."

James Wardrop, 1808

Introduction

An awareness of the eye and its diseases should not be confined to those who have made ophthalmology their speciality, for within the eye and its orbit is a microcosm of pathology. Apart from its own peculiar disorders, the eye and its adnexae can manifest an extraordinarily wide spectrum of systemic disease and it is sometimes in this setting that the diagnosis is first made. Sarcoidosis, for example, commonly affects ocular structures and may present as easily biopsied conjunctival nodules, and many of the metabolic storage diseases can be identified by study of subconjunctival fibroblasts. Moreover, because of the small size of the orbit, metastatic tumour deposits quickly produce signs and symptoms that may precede evidence of the primary lesion. In this chapter we have selected a number of disorders wherein a knowledge of the pathology is of particular importance, some of which may present in the first instance outside recognized eye departments.

Proptosis

As the signature of orbital disease, proptosis, or forward displacement of the globe, may be caused by a wide range of pathological processes which may originate within the orbital cavity, extend to involve the orbital tissues from adjacent structures or, most commonly, be the manifestation of systemic disease. The clinical investigation of a patient with proptosis must therefore aim to establish the location and extent of the lesion and to determine, in so far as is possible, its pathological nature. This informed approach depends upon an intimate knowledge of the likely diagnostic possibilities in any particular age group with due regard to the mode of presentation and progression of the disorder. It must be emphasized that the initial management, including diagnostic biopsy, is often of paramount importance in terms of visual preservation and possibly survival of the patient.

The following account considers just a few of the more common orbital disorders which may confront surgeons and pathologists in both general and specialist fields.

Dysthyroid eye disease

Thyroid dysfunction is undoubtedly the most frequent cause of proptosis and, while bilateral involvement is usual, unilateral exophthalmos is by no means uncommon. The essential changes concern the extraocular muscles which are the site of a chronic inflammatory reaction related to an autoallergic response to thyroglobulin, and possibly other endocrine factors, bound to receptors on the surface of these muscles. Consequent enlargement of the extraocular muscles embedded in oedematous connective tissue gives rise to proptosis, which may be non-axial, and restricted ocular movements, particularly elevation and abduction, signifying preferential involvement of the inferior and medial recti respectively. Engorgement of the muscles may also occur in the region of the orbital apex to produce optic nerve compression and visual loss. Ultimately, the eyes may be almost completely immobilized as the inflamed muscles undergo reparative fibrosis.

Dysthyroid eye disease as a cause of proptosis merits careful exclusion, particularly in the absence of overt thyroid dysfunction, in order to avoid unnecessary surgical exploration including diagnostic biopsy. Retraction of the upper lid and lid lag on downgaze are of considerable diagnostic importance and may be discovered in the apparently unaffected eye in unilateral cases. Biochemical tests of thyroid function, especially thyrotrophin releasing hormone (TRH) and serum T3 assay, and the detection of circulating autoantibodies to thyroglobulin, are of particular importance in patients with minimal evidence of generalized metabolic dysfunction. Laboratory studies must be correlated with the appearance on CAT scanning which optimally demonstrates extraocular muscle enlargement.

Although essentially a self-limiting disorder, the development of a progressive or so-called "malignant" phase (with markedly increased intraorbital pressure), necessitates urgent medical or surgical orbital decompression to prevent blindness from optic nerve damage or the effects of corneal exposure.

Vascular anomalies

Vascular maldevelopments constitute a frequent cause of unilateral proptosis in all but the elderly.

Capillary haemangiomas usually present within the first few weeks of life and behave as hamartomas, the majority undergoing spontaneous involution by the age of 10 years. This diffuse vascular lesion usually affects the anterior orbital tissues with involvement of the eyelids. During early infancy, a period of rapid growth may occur in which florid endothelial proliferation with few definitive capillaries may present a disturbing histological picture, although there is no risk of malignant transformation. In view of the known tendency to undergo spontaneous regression, active intervention should be delayed as long as possible unless the size of the mass threatens visual development. Partial surgical excision is more easily accomplished following the onset of involution.

Cavernous haemangiomas present in an older age group and are usually fairly discrete lesions with a well defined capsule, predominantly located within the extraocular muscle cone. This tumour, which is thought to arise from vasoformative cell rests, slowly expands over a number of years to present with relatively "silent" proptosis of insidious onset. On occasions, decreased vision may occur with impingement of the mass upon the posterior wall of the eyeball to produce choroidal and retinal folds, often associated with optic disc oedema. Largely sequestered from the systemic circulation, the tumour should be excised by a lateral orbitotomy approach at the time of presentation.

From recent clinical and radiological studies correlated with histopathological data, congenital orbital varices appear to be the most common vascular cause of proptosis. Congenital varices must be distinguished from varices secondary to an arteriovenous shunt located in the region of the cavernous sinus or within the orbit. Primary orbital varices present in childhood or early adult life and characteristically give rise to variable non-pulsatile proptosis, increasing with elevated central venous pressure. The lesion may be restricted to the deeper orbital tissues, but commonly involves the anterior orbit and is often accompanied by dilated veins in the lids and conjunctiva. Primary varices are subject to episodes of thrombophlebitis which may account for the development of phleboliths demonstrable on radiographic examination and virtually pathognomonic of this disorder. In addition, acute orbital haemorrhage may supervene and may necessitate immediate orbital decompression. In general, the indications for surgical intervention are cosmetic and any attempt to eradicate the lesion completely will inevitably result in damage to vital structures with visual loss.

Inflammatory disorders

Orbital cellulitis attributable to an infectious process is usually seen as a complication of paranasal sinus disease in childhood or suppurative lesions of the eyelids. Clinical evidence of orbital soft tissue involvement includes chemosis, proptosis and generalized limitation of ocular movement. In addition to the risk of visual loss, orbital cellulitis is a potentially life-threatening infection with the risk of spread to cause cavernous sinus thrombosis.

Initially, orbital inflammation accompanying sinus infection is confined by the periosteal lining of the orbital cavity and may be sterile. This may be followed by direct bacterial spread to produce a sub-periosteal abscess requiring drainage to prevent more widespread infection. Microbiological examination of the conjunctival sac, nasal discharge and blood cultures should be obtained (although the yield is often disappointing) and the use of intravenous broad-spectrum antibiotics instituted without delay. It should be noted that in immunosuppressed patients or following inadequate treatment with oral antibiotics, an orbital abscess may develop in an insidious manner masquerading as an orbital neoplasm.

Chronic paranasal sinus disease with impaired drainage may result in the accumulation of mucus leading to pressure atrophy of the bony wall. Such a mucocele of the frontal or ethmoidal sinus may extend into the orbit to cause proptosis and vertical displacement of the globe. Mucoceles are usually sterile and readily identifiable on plain X-ray.

A host of infectious organisms from bacteria to fungi and helminths can produce orbital swelling and on occasions biopsy allied to microbiological investigation may prove necessary to establish the diagnosis.

When the inflammatory process presents as a discrete swelling, suspicions of a neoplasm may be aroused. The term "pseudotumour" has been used in various ways to describe the whole gamut of such non-neoplastic disorders, inflammatory processes for which a cause cannot be identified, or lesions in which the essential cellular component is lymphocytic. Most authorities now confine the use of this term to idiopathic inflammatory lesions which typically present in adult life with proptosis of sub-acute onset, frequently accompanied by pain. Impaired ocular motility with a complaint of diplopia and erythematous lid-swelling are frequent accompaniments. However, the precise clinical presentation varies with the location of the inflammatory infiltrate, which can best be defined by axial and coronal CT scans. In general, definitive diagnosis of inflammatory pseudotumour requires incisional biopsy. Many of the lesions will then be seen to be composed of a mixture of leucocyte types and possibly be granulomatous; the presence of germinal lymphoid follicules is further evidence of an inflammatory process. In some cases, however, the cellular infiltrate is more or less confined to lymphoid tissue and distinction from malignant lymphoma on purely morphological grounds can be virtually impossible (Fig. 32.1). In such lesions, immunohistochemical staining for different antibody classes and light chains can be extremely useful; a monoclonal profile indicating a neoplastic process. Lesions which are clearly inflammatory will usually respond to a short course of high-dosage corticosteroids, whereas most of the pure lymphoid proliferations will ultimately require radiotherapy, including some that are shown to be polyclonal. It is also important to note that ostensibly idiopathic chronic inflammation can be an unusual expression of a more widespread disorder: dysthyroid disease and myasthenia gravis being examples wherein the true diagnosis may be overlooked initially.

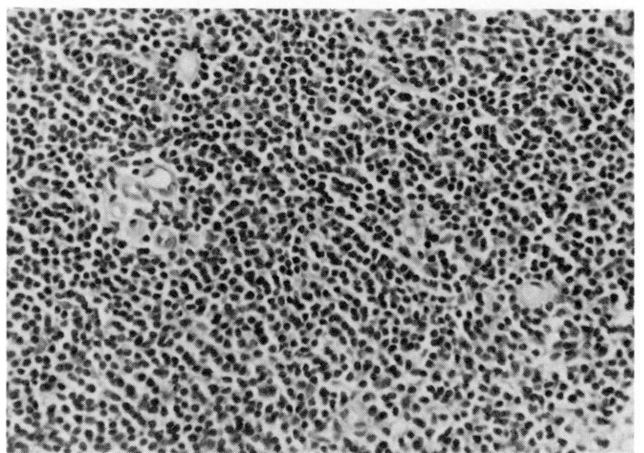

Fig. 32.1 Lymphoid pseudotumour of the orbit. The accumulation of solid masses of lymphocytes, as seen here, may be either hyperplastic (inflammatory) or neoplastic, and distinction an histological grounds can be extremely difficult. Biopsy diagnosis is facilitated by the application of immunolabelling techniques. (H & E × 455)

Neoplasia

The most frequent orbital neoplasms encountered in clinical practice are secondary in nature and are those in which the development of proptosis may precede clinical evidence of the primary lesion.

Direct spread from a carcinoma of the paranasal sinuses, from an intracranial meningioma, from epidermal carcinomas of the eyelids and from squamous carcinoma of the conjunctiva, are all well recognized causes of proptosis. As the most common intraocular malignant tumours, retinoblastoma or uveal melanoma may also produce proptosis from extraocular extension.

Metastatic carcinoma is not an uncommon cause of orbital neoplasia, carcinomas of the breast and bronchus being the predominant sources of blood-borne metastases. Biopsy may be appropriate when the existence or nature of the primary tumour is obscure.

In children, dermoid cysts are by far the commonest tumour, if that designation be allowed for a choristomatous lesion which possibly results from sequestration of skin during embryogenesis. This tumour typically presents as a painless and freely mobile mass located in the superotemporal quadrant of the orbit with displacement of the globe. The cyst usually possesses an attachment to the orbital bones and subsequently through a bony canal to the dura mater of the anterior cranial fossa. Complete excision of the lesion is the treatment of choice with avoidance of rupture of the cyst whose keratinous contents may incite a granulomatous inflammatory reaction.

Juvenile astrocytoma is the most common primary optic nerve tumour and is invariably benign. The patient usually presents in the first decade of life with proptosis followed by visual loss in cases where the tumour originates in the intraorbital optic nerve, but the reverse order holds in the case of intraorbital spread from the intracranial optic nerve or chiasm. Ophthalmoscopy may reveal oedema of the optic disc or optic atrophy. In a variable percentage of patients (12–38 per cent) the tumour develops in association with neurofibromatosis, although clinical evidence of this disorder often develops at a later date. Although the natural history is variable, this tumour is generally slow-growing, but on occasions a more rapid clinical course may develop from widespread mucinous accumulation within the tumour.

Astrocytic proliferation may remain confined within the optic nerve suggestive of a hamartomatous process, but in other tumours extension may occur into the subarachnoid space, whereupon reactive meningeal hyperplasia may develop and on biopsy be confused with a meningioma. In view of the uncertainty regarding the natural history of this tumour, the question of active surgical intervention remains controversial. Although rapid expansion may undoubtedly occur, there is no convincing evidence that this tumour is capable of longitudinal spread within the optic nerve with the risk of intracranial extension. However, other authorities consider that in cases of profound visual loss and active tumour growth, resection of the optic nerve from the optic chiasm via a transcranial approach may improve the ultimate prognosis.

Embryonal rhabdomyosarcoma is the principal malignant orbital tumour of childhood, notorious for a fulminating clinical onset often suggestive of an inflammatory process. The majority of such tumours develop from primitive mesenchymal cells with limited differentiation towards striated muscle. A palpable mass is usually evident and biopsy is essential for confirmation of the diagnosis, ultrastructural features providing a useful adjunct to conventional histopathology. Specific immunohistochemical marker studies may also be of value. Surgical management in the form of exenteration of the orbital contents has now largely been superseded by combined radiotherapy and chemotherapy with substantial improvement in the rate of survival.

The presentation of a space-occupying lesion in the lacrimal gland fossa poses an important diagnostic problem (Fig. 32.2). Epithelial neoplasms of the lacrimal gland must be recognized as early as possible and their likely pathological nature determined before resorting to any surgical intervention. Pleomorphic adenoma (benign mixed tumour) characteristically presents with an insidiously progressive and painless swelling in the absence of inflammatory signs. The duration of symptoms usually exceeds 12 months and radiography often reveals enlargement of the lacrimal fossa with no evidence of bony invasion. As befits a benign tumour, there is a surrounding capsule, but occasionally satellite groups of tumour cells may be seen extending into and even through the capsule. This probably accounts for a slight tendency to recur after resection, a risk that is considerably enhanced by rupture of the capsule during removal. Correspondingly, it is mandatory to avoid incisional biopsy with the potential risk of recurrence and the possibility of malignant change after repeated local recurrences. Benign mixed-cell tumours must therefore be treated by total excision of the lacrimal gland and adjacent tissues, including the periorbita, via a lateral orbitotomy approach. In contradistinction, malignant tumours of the lacrimal gland, predominantly adenoid cystic carcinoma arising *de novo*, present with a history of less than 12 months in which pain is an important diagnostic feature. However, it is important to note such features do not allow adequate distinction from inflammatory lesions in the region of the lacrimal gland, including dacryoadenitis and idiopathic inflammatory pseudotumour. Adenoid cystic carcinoma is a highly infiltrative tumour with a tendency to perineural and vascular invasion and carries a generally poor prognosis even with radical surgical excision.

Orbital meningiomas predominantly occur as direct extensions of an intracranial tumour in which reactive hyperostosis of the sphenoid may contribute to or account for the development of proptosis. Primary optic nerve meningiomas also occur, chiefly in middle-aged females, in which intradural expansion of the tumour gives rise to rapid visual deterioration followed by proptosis from extension through the dural sheath. The presence of shunt vessels on the optic disc is a helpful diagnostic feature of this tumour. Complete

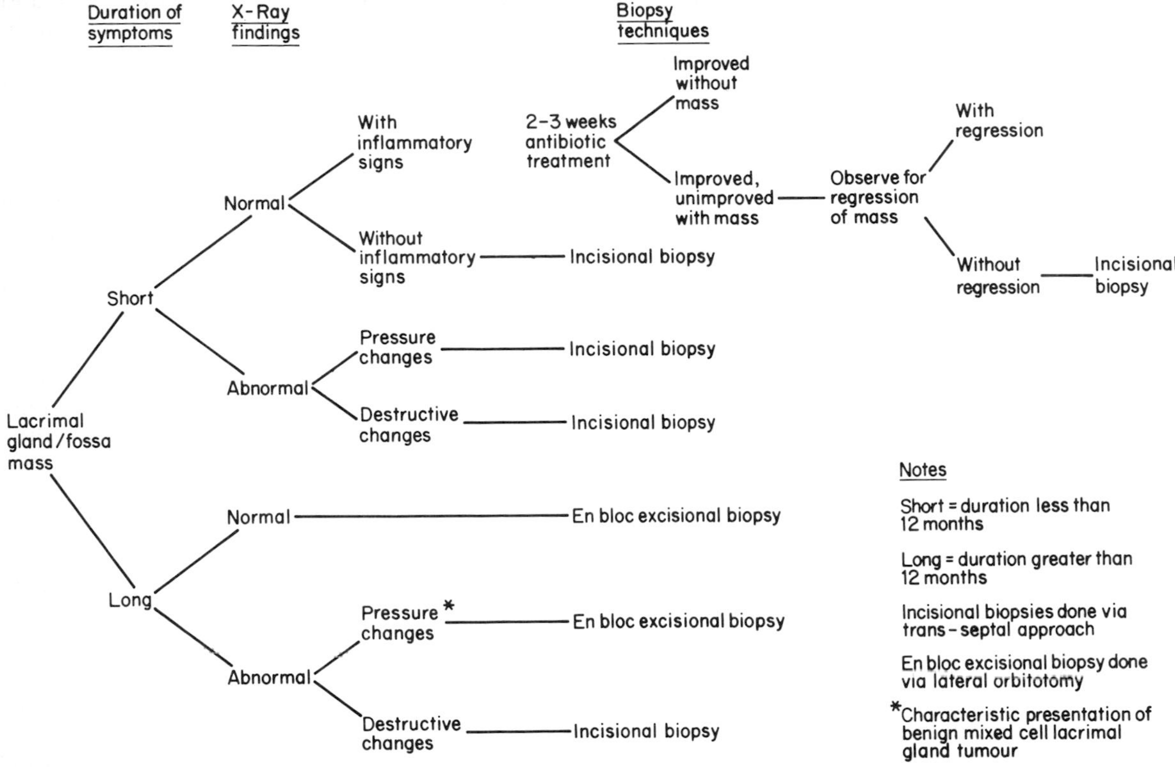

Fig. 32.2 Flowchart of management of lacrimal gland/fossa masses based on duration of symptoms and radiographic findings. (Reproduced from Wright, Stewart, and Krohel (1979) by permission of J.E. Wright and the Editor of the *Br J Ophthalmol.*)

excision of an optic nerve sheath meningioma cannot be accomplished without complete loss of vision and therefore in most instances surgical treatment is delayed until vision is already grossly impaired.

The orbital tissues may also be the site of a primary lymphoma usually arising within the superior orbit to produce painless displacement of the globe. The tumour often involves the subconjunctival tissues and appears as a fleshy pink mass. Biopsy is necessary to establish the diagnosis, although histological interpretation may be problematical and the future clinical behaviour of the lesion impossible to predict. In the more malignant lymphomas, cytological irregularity is seen but recognized of less malignant proliferations and is facilitated by the use of immunological techniques to confirm a monoclonal origin.

Biopsy

Diagnostic biopsy is indicated for lesions the nature of which is uncertain after the application of non-invasive investigative techniques. It is essential that the specimen submitted be of sufficient size to be representative of the whole; for instance, inflammatory tissue from the edge of a neoplasm has been known to be misinterpreted as an inflammatory pseudotumour and, as commented previously, biopsy of the optic nerve sheath alone can result in a diagnosis of meningioma rather than meningeal hyperplasia in association with a juvenile astrocytoma of the nerve. Squeeze artefact caused by forceps pressure should be avoided as much as possible, especially in the case of suspected lymphoproliferative disorders.

Fine-needle aspiration biopsy is favoured in some centres, particularly in the case of lymphoproliferative lesions but, in order to ensure that the sample is withdrawn from the appropriate site, radiological control is advisable.

Frozen sections have a limited role, the majority of surgeons preferring to await the more reliable findings of paraffin-embedded sections. Their principle value lies in determining the completeness of excision of malignant tumours where this is in doubt.

Leukocoria

Although, interestingly, the ominous significance of a cat's eye reflex eluded the great John Hunter, the development of a white pupillary reflex (leukocoria) in the first two years of life has long been recognized as the most common presenting feature of a retinoblastoma. This highly malignant and often congenital tumour is thought to originate from immature neuronal cells and may occur sporadically or be inherited as an autosomal dominant trait with incomplete penetrance. Although rare, retinoblastoma is the most common malignant intraocular tumour of childhood, responsible for approximately 1 per cent of all tumour deaths in the paediatric age group.

In most instances, the eye is of normal size with no evidence of inflammation, but with loss of fixation the development of a squint may be an early manifestation. Behind a clear lens, a creamy-white tumour mass encroaching on the vitreous cavity may be seen (endophytic growth). With increasing size the tumour becomes mottled in appearance with increased vascularity and engorged feeder vessels suggestive of an angiomatous lesion. A speckled appearance of the surface of the tumour resembling "cottage cheese" is of particular diagnostic importance and is due to focal deposition of calcium within areas of tumour necrosis. This feature may also be demonstrated by radiographic or ultrasound examination and in this age group is virtually pathognomonic of retinoblastoma. In other retinoblastomas, the tumour predominantly expands into the potential sub-retinal space (exophytic growth) giving rise to a progressive retinal detachment which may ultimately obscure the underlying tumour.

Retinoblastoma is a poorly cohesive tumour with minimal supporting stroma, facilitating dissemination of tumour cells throughout the eye. In large tumours, clusters of viable tumour cells may be seen within the vitreous and may ultimately migrate to the peripheral retinal surface to establish separate foci of tumour growth. Tumour seeding to the anterior segment may also occur with the formation of deposits on the iris and corneal endothelium and may accumulate in the anterior chamber to produce a pseudohypopyon. With increasing tumour volume, secondary glaucoma may ensue, resulting in overall expansion of the globe often accompanied by iris neovascularization from posterior segment ischaemia. Despite the existence of wide areas of necrosis identifiable in most tumours, ocular inflammation is an unusual clinical feature.

In its natural history, retinoblastoma often remains confined to the eye for a considerable period. As might be expected, the optic nerve is the principal route of extraocular spread. Although some resistance to tumour invasion is offered by the lamina cribrosa, cellular invasion of the retro-laminar nerve for 2 or 3 mm is a common finding (Fig. 32.3). Extension of tumour invasion to the point of entry and exit of the central retinal vessels at about 10 mm from the globe, allows access to the subarachnoid space with rapid dissemination to the basal meninges and spinal cord and an inevitable fatal outcome. It is therefore of crucial importance that a long section of optic nerve be excised at the time of enucleation and the nerve be subjected to careful histopathological scrutiny. Invasion of the retro-laminar nerve carries a 40–45 per cent mortality increasing to about 65 per cent with tumour extension to the line of resection.

Gross choroidal invasion on histopathological study is an adverse prognostic finding as the prelude to haematogenous spread and the development of osseous deposits. Extension into the orbital tissues through scleral emissary channels also carries a high mortality with potential invasion of the orbital bones and lymphatic spread to the preauricular and cervical glands.

A further histological finding of prognostic importance is the degree of differentiation; retinoblastomas showing evidence of photoreceptor cell differentiation in the form of rosettes and fleurettes having the most favourable prognosis despite reduced radiosensitivity.

In the majority of cases, the diagnosis of retinoblastoma can be readily established on clinical grounds. Although direct tumour biopsy is not feasible, cytological study of aspirated aqueous humour may be helpful. Detection of raised levels of aqueous lactic dehydrogenase and serum carcino-embryonic antigen may also be of value in the differentiation of retinoblastoma from various simulating conditions.

There are a number of non-lethal ocular conditions whose clinical appearances may closely resemble retinoblastoma and require careful differentiation to avoid unnecessary enucleation. The most common simulating disorders include

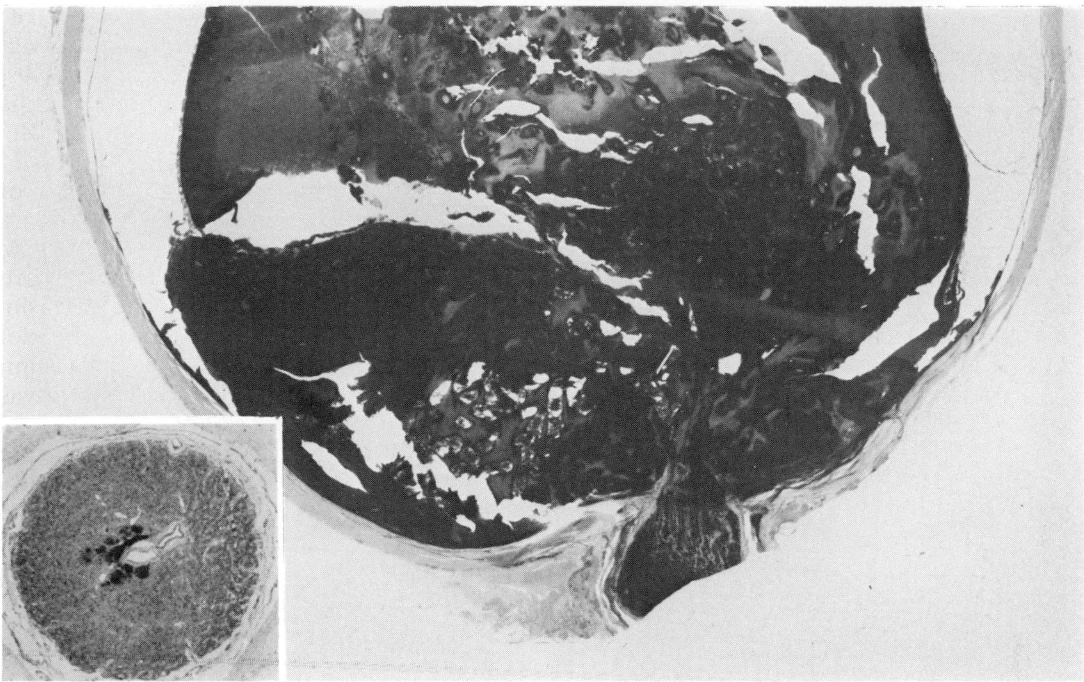

Fig. 32.3 Retinoblastoma. The posterior part of the eyeball is filled with tumour tissue which has also invaded the optic nerve. To check for complete removal in such cases it is useful to block the end of the optic nerve separately and cut transverse sections at the level of resection. (Inset shows tumour in the centre of the nerve at the resection level.) (H & E × 6. Inset × 15)

ocular toxocariasis, persistent hyperplastic primary vitreous and Coats' disease.

Infestation of the eye with the second-stage larva of *Toxocara canis* may give rise to an organized retinal granuloma or the development of an indolent endophthalmitis with a total serous retinal detachment, mimicking an exophytic retinoblastoma. Distinguishing clinical features include overt inflammatory changes and evidence of vitreoretinal traction. Aqueous cytology may reveal eosinophils and normal levels of lactate dehydrogenase.

Persistent hyperplastic primary vitreous is a unilateral developmental anomaly in which a vascularized retrolental mass with persistence of the hyaloid artery produces leukocoria evident from birth. Variable reduction in the size of the globe and traction on the ciliary processes are important diagnostic pointers.

Coats' disease is a unilateral retinal vascular disorder of unknown origin. Leakage of plasma constituents from telangiectatic retinal vessels may give rise to total exudative retinal detachment which may be difficult to differentiate from an exophytic retinoblastoma (Figs. 32.4a and 32.4b). The presence of sub-retinal lipid exudates and glistening cholesterol crystals facilitate accurate diagnosis.

Accurate staging of retinoblastoma at the time of presentation is essential and must include careful study of the fellow eye and exclusion of metastatic spread (see Table 32.1). For most unilateral retinoblastomas, prompt enucleation is the most appropriate treatment since the majority are moderately advanced at the time of presentation. Similarly, in bilateral cases the eye with the more advanced tumour usually requires enucleation. However, there are several alternative methods of treatment now available, the choice of which will depend upon the extent and laterality of the tumour. These methods are often used in combination and include external beam irradiation which also aims to sterilize the entire retina, the use of cobalt plaques, xenon photocoagulation and cryotherapy. As an adjunct to irradiation, chemotherapy may be useful in the management of orbital extension, selected bilateral tumours and metastatic disease. With modern treatment, the overall mortality rate has been reduced to approximately 20 per cent, largely confined to

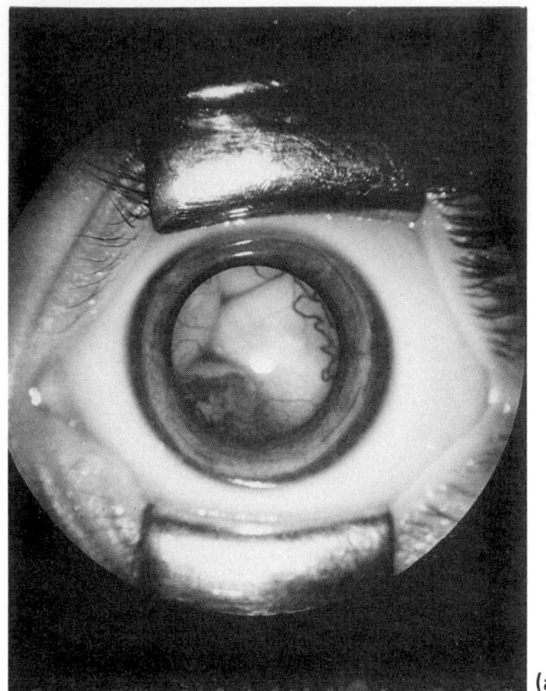

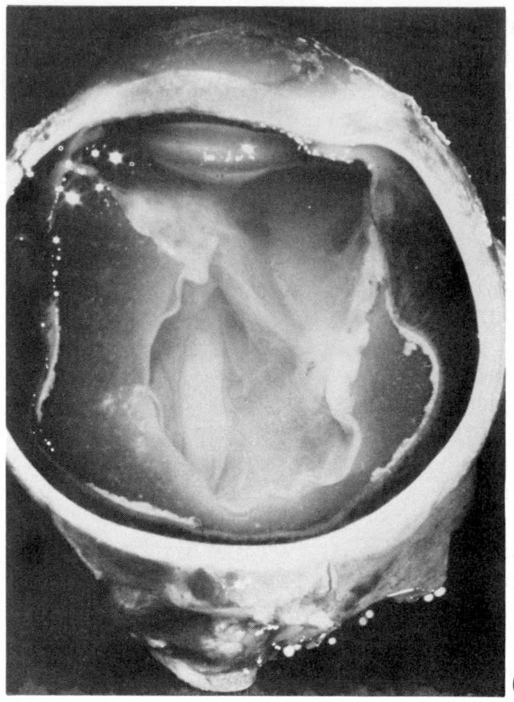

Fig. 32.4 Coats' disease (**a**) Leukocoria in an 18-month-old child. The retina is totally detached with telangiectatic retinal vessels, the appearances simulating an exophytic retinoblastoma. (**b**) Part of the globe has been removed to reveal a completely detached retina associated with serous sub-retinal exudate in which ch olesterol crystals are discernible. There is also some artefactual detachment of the choroid. (× 6)

Table 32.1 Modified Reese-Ellsworth classification of retinoblastoma.

Group	*Prognosis*	*Features*
I	Very favourable	Solitary or multiple tumours less than 6 mm diameter at or behind equator
II	Favourable	Solitary or multiple tumours 6–15 mm diameter at or behind equator
III	Doubtful	Pre-equatorial lesion Solitary tumour more than 15 mm diameter behind equator
IV	Unfavourable	Multiple tumours more than 15 mm diameter. Lesion extending anterior to ora serrata
V	Very unfavourable	Vitreous seeding Tumour involving more than half the retina
VI	Very unfavourable	Optic nerve invasion Extrascleral extension Residual orbital disease

patients with stage IV–VI disease. It is worth noting that, in patients with inherited retinoblastoma, there is an increased risk of second primary neoplasms, notably osteogenic sarcoma, which most commonly occurs in the irradiated field, but may arise spontaneously at other sites.

Raised pigmented fundus lesions

The presentation of a patient with an elevated pigmented lesion in the ocular fundus is a common clinical situation which not infrequently poses a difficult diagnostic problem. In the absence of a tissue diagnosis, the clinician must differentiate between a malignant melanoma of the choroid and a number of benign ocular conditions including other melanocytic lesions whose clinical appearances may closely resemble a melanoma. In the past, a disturbingly high proportion of eyes, enucleated because of a suspected choroidal melanoma, have been shown to contain a benign simulating lesion. However, with the availability of non-invasive diagnostic studies (including fluorescein angiography, diagnostic ultrasound and radio-isotope studies) and familiarity with the clinical features and behaviour of mimicking lesions, the incidence of erroneous enucleation has been substantially reduced.

Choroidal naevi are the most frequently encountered melanocytic fundus lesions with a reported incidence of 6 per cent in studies of autopsy eyes. Composed of dendritic, spindle-shaped or polyhedral melanocytes, naevi are located predominantly posterior to the equator of the globe and become clinically evident at or following puberty with the acquisition of pigment. The typical clinical appearance is that of a flat or slightly elevated greyish lesion with a maximum diameter rarely exceeding 7 mm. The majority of naevi occupy the outer choroid with the retention of an intact layer of capillary blood vessels between the lesion and the inner limiting (Bruch's) membrane of the choroid. With increasing size and thickness of the tumour, changes are frequently observed in the overlying retinal pigment epithelium manifested as pigment mottling or drusen bodies representing an accumulation of phagocytosed outer segment photoreceptor debris. Benign stationary choroidal naevi have also been shown to produce disturbances of the overlying sensory retina with loss of photoreceptors and an accompanying visual field defect.

Although of limited but variable growth potential and capable of periods of accelerated expansion, few choroidal naevi attain sufficient size or elevation to engender confusion with a malignant melanoma. However, suspicion of a melanoma or the rare possibility of malignant transformation of a choroidal naevus will be aroused by the presence of orange pigment on the surface of the tumour, associated sub-retinal fluid or documented expansion by serial fundus photography or diagnostic ultrasound. Such suspicious naevi must be closely monitored for increasing tumour volume, although this does not necessarily imply malignant change.

A distinctive type of naevus which usually arises in the optic nerve head and, exceptionally, in the choroid, is a melanocytoma or magnocellular naevus. Originally thought of as a malignant melanoma invading the optic nerve head, this lesion is entirely benign and often asymptomatic and, unlike malignant melanoma of the choroid, is frequently seen in non-Caucasians. The characteristic ophthalmoscopic appearance is of a jet black mass projecting above the surface of the optic disc, the intense pigmentation reflecting a histological profile of cells with abundant cytoplasm packed with melanin. Occasionally the tumour may infiltrate adjacent tissues, but the development of superimposed malignancy is virtually unknown.

Accounting for the majority of primary malignant intraocular tumours, choroidal melanoma is an extremely elusive neoplasm in which the natural history of any individual tumour is notoriously unpredictable. Intraocular melanomas, once regarded as occupying a privileged position, now appear to behave in a similar fashion to tumours of equivalent size arising elsewhere with respect to the overall mortality rate and metastatic potential. Furthermore, the precise histogenesis of malignant melanoma of the choroid is unknown, although it is widely believed that the majority originate from pre-existing naevi.

The presenting symptoms of a choroidal melanoma generally include a complaint of blurred vision or loss of visual field, but an increasing proportion are discovered in the course of a routine ophthalmic examination. Visual loss may be explained by direct involvement of the macula by the tumour or the presence of a serous retinal detachment involving the macula.

Choroidal melanoma usually presents as a well circumscribed globular mass, but approximately 5 per cent of tumours adopt a diffuse pattern of growth with extensive choroidal thickening and limited elevation. With continued expansion, erosion of Bruch's membrane occurs with the production of a collar-stud mass, a growth pattern which is almost pathognomonic of melanoma. This is in contrast to secondary choroidal tumours, for example carcinoma of the breast, which invariably develop as a placoid lesion. Ophthalmoscopically, the degree of pigmentation shows considerable variation, ranging from diffuse heavy pigmentation to an amelanotic appearance. Many choroidal melanomas show superficial orange pigmentation caused by the accumulation of lipofuscin within proliferating retinal pigment epithelial cells and macrophages overlying the tumour, a feature rarely seen in association with other choroidal tumours. Destruction of the capillary network of the choroid gives rise to early degeneration of the retinal pigment epithelium and breakdown of the blood-retinal barrier. This may allow serous exudate from choroidal vessels to collect beneath the neuroretina with consequent focal detachment. Ultimately, the majority of melanomas result in serous retinal detachment, typically commencing near the margin of the lesion and extending to involve the inferior retina. On occasions, the melanoma may directly spread into the sub-retinal space and possibly infiltrate the adjacent retina or vitreous cavity. Vitreous haemorrhage may also occur from dilated vascular channels or from areas of necrosis within the tumour. The existence of widespread necrosis characteristically induces a marked inflammatory response, which sometimes may be the initial manifestation of a choroidal melanoma.

Extraocular extension of choroidal melanoma predominantly occurs along trans-scleral vascular and nerve channels, often remaining undetected until the time of excision of the globe (Fig. 32.5).

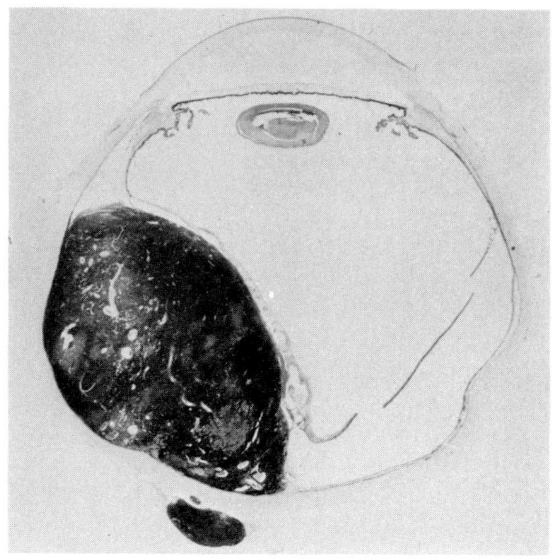

Fig. 32.5 Malignant melanoma of the choroid. The large pigmented intraocular tumour is associated with degeneration of the overlying retina and extraocular extension across the sclera. (H & E × 4)

Extrascleral extension is generally associated with cytologically more malignant tumours and is a frequent finding in diffuse choroidal melanomas. The latter tumours may also invade the optic nerve, which is otherwise an uncommon finding. Penetration of choroidal veins predisposes to distant metastasis, the liver being the prime site for secondary deposits.

In the presence of clear media, the majority of choroidal melanomas can be distinguished from simulating lesions on ophthalmoscopic examination. However, the greatest diagnostic difficulty is likely to be encountered in the differentiation of an enlarged choroidal naevus from a small choroidal melanoma. It is now recognized that there are no clinical features which can be considered pathognomonic of either lesion, but that certain clinical characteristics favour an expanding tumour with metastatic potential. These features include evidence of extensive pigment epithelial destruction overlying the lesion, multiple geographic patches of orange pigment and the presence of sub-retinal fluid surrounding the elevated lesion. Since the results of special diagnostic studies are also likely to prove equivocal, serial examination should be undertaken before resorting to definitive therapy.

A solitary haemangioma of the choroid may also cause diagnostic confusion. This hamartomatous lesion, which is not associated with the Sturge–Weber syndrome, appears as a red-orange sessile tumour and may resemble an amelanotic choroidal melanoma. Fibrous metaplasia of the overlying retinal pigment epithelium may develop, often accompanied by serous detachment of the retina. Treatment of this non-progressive lesion is generally directed towards management of the associated retinal detachment.

For many years, enucleation of the involved eye at the time of diagnosis has been the accepted method of treatment of choroidal melanoma. However, the validity of this approach, particularly in terms of patient survival, has recently been questioned and indeed it has been hypothesized that enucleation may actually increase the risk of metastatic spread. There has, therefore, been an increasing trend towards conservative management and the adoption of alternative methods of intervention to control or eradicate the tumour with preservation of useful vision and hopefully without an increased tumour-related mortality.

Broadly speaking, the management of choroidal melanoma is determined by the overall dimensions and location of the tumour, the apparent activity of the lesion, the status of the fellow eye and the age and general health of the patient.

As previously indicated, small melanomas of less than 10 mm diameter and 3 mm in thickness should be closely observed to document enlargement before resorting to active intervention. Many of these small melanomas appear to be biologically less active and are often asymptomatic with no accompanying visual loss. This conservative approach does not appear to materially affect the 10 per cent five-year mortality associated with small choroidal melanomas. However, in the event of documented enlargement of the tumour, active treatment should be undertaken since the tumour often undergoes an exponential growth phase with an increased metastatic potential.

For the management of enlarging small melanomas or medium-sized tumours (10–15 mm diameter and 5 mm in thickness) various methods of tumour eradication are currently available. These methods include the use of xenon arc or laser photocoagulation, local excision of the tumour and radiotherapy in the form of charged particle irradiation or the application of a radioactive plaque. Although the indications depend upon the characteristics of the individual tumour, the precise role of these alternative therapeutic approaches has not been established.

Enucleation remains the principal treatment for large choroidal melanomas with loss of central vision or in those tumours for which alternative methods of treatment cannot be employed and useful vision maintained. With the theoretical risk of tumour dissemination at the time of surgery, undue surgical manipulation must be avoided and the globe carefully inspected for evidence of extrascleral extension. Such orbital extension may be treated by local excision, exenteration of the orbital contents or postoperative radiotherapy.

The chief value of histopathological study of the enucleated specimen is in prognosis: lesions with a maximum diameter of more than 10 mm and showing an epithelioid cell morphology have a distinctly worse prognosis than smaller tumours composed of spindle cells. Since the morphology of uveal melanomas may vary from one part of the tumour to another, histological sections from multiple levels should be examined.

Although various clinical, histological, and immunological factors have been implicated, it is now generally acknowledged that tumour size, cell type and the presence of extrascleral spread, are the most important prognostic parameters in choroidal melanoma.

Further reading

Garner A, Klintworth GK. *Pathobiology of Ocular Disease*. New York: Marcel Dekker, 1982.

Henderson JW. *Orbital Tumours*. New York: Decker/Thieme–Stratton, 1980.

Shields JA. *Diagnosis and Management of Intraocular Tumours*. St Louis: C. V. Mosby, 1983.

Yanoff M, Fine BS. *Ocular Pathology*. Hagerstown, Maryland: Harper & Row, 1982.

33

Gynaecology

D Lowe and M D Cameron

Introduction

The intention of this chapter is to guide the general surgeon when he is confronted by a gynaecological problem and no gynaecological opinion is immediately available. This is most likely to happen when clinical examination reveals the presence of a pelvic or abdominal tumour, or at laparotomy when an unsuspected gynaecological disorder is found. The following conditions will be considered:

Ovarian tumours
Uterine tumours
Endometriosis
Pelvic Inflammatory Disease (Salpingitis)
Ectopic pregnancy

Ovarian tumours

There are several processes which may give rise to a localized or diffuse swelling of an ovary. Cystic Graafian follicles and corpora lutea form physiologically and may grow to easily visible ovarian masses. Up to 2.5 cm diameter, these structures are common and are regarded as being within the range of normality; above this size, follicular and luteal cysts are abnormal but usually are asymptomatic, involute spontaneously and have no malignant potential. Persistence and enlargement of the corpus luteum occurs in early pregnancy to form the corpus luteum of pregnancy, a unilateral plum-coloured nodule about 1.5–2.0 cm in diameter below the ovarian capsule. Recognition is important, as the corpus luteum of pregnancy provides the hormonal support for the developing embryo until placental function takes over at about the eighth gestational week. Excision may result in abortion. Severe abdominal bleeding from a ruptured follicle is a well known, but rare, complication of anticoagulant therapy.

Other non-neoplastic ovarian masses include inflammatory lesions such as tubo-ovarian abscesses and endometriosis, both of which will be considered later.

Classification of ovarian neoplasms

The classification of ovarian neoplasms is based on the developmental anatomy of the ovary, which results in a comprehensive and detailed list. The outline of the classification and the commoner ovarian tumours will be considered here.

Ovarian neoplasms most commonly arise from the surface epithelium, with or without stromal components; this *epithelial* group includes the cystadenomas and cystadenocarcinomas, endometrioid carcinomas and Brenner tumours. Development of tumours of *germ cells* is next in order of prevalence. Uncommonly, tumours arise from the *stromal cells* of the ovary, either from the endocrine cells of the sex cords, such as the granulosa and theca cell tumours, or from the less specialized ovarian fibrous tissue as fibromas and fibrosarcomas. Tumours of more than one element (*mixed tumours*) like gonadoblastoma may occur. Finally, the ovary may be host to tumours not specific to the ovary, such as metastatic carcinoma and lymphoma.

For the general surgeon an appreciation of the macroscopical differences between benign and malignant tumours (see Tables 33.1 and 33.2), of the frequency of bilaterality and of the appearances of the commoner tumours is important.

Epithelial neoplasms make up about 60 per cent of all ovarian tumours; about 30 per cent are serous neoplasms and 25 per cent are mucinous. The incidence of benign serous tumours exceeds their malignant counterparts by 3:1, while the ratio between benign and malignant mucinous tumours is greater, at over 4:1.

Table 33.1 Benign ovarian neoplasms.

	Frequency[1]	*Age*	*Laterality*[2]	*Appearance*
Serous cystadenoma	30	30–50	B	Unilocular thin-walled cyst containing serous clear fluid
Mucinous cystadenoma	25	30–50	U	Multilocular thick-walled cyst containing thick clear mucus
Teratoma (dermoid cyst)	20	15–40	B	Cystic tumour containing sebaceous material, hair and clear fluid. When small, usually multilocular. When large, one large cyst predominates
Brenner tumour[3]	22	40–70	U	Solid, white rubbery tumour mass
Fibroma, thecoma	10	50–70	U	Solid, white rubbery fibrous tumour mass

Notes
1 – frequency as percentage of all ovarian neoplasms
2 – B = high incidence of bilaterality of >20 per cent; U = usually unilateral
3 – most Brenner tumours are benign – less than 5% are malignant

Table 33.2 Malignant ovarian neoplasms.

	Frequency 1	*Frequency* 2	*Age*	*Laterality*	*Appearance*
Serous cystadenocarcinoma					
(a) borderline	2	10	30–60	B	Cystic tumour with solid areas
(b) frankly malignant	6	30	40–70	B	Solid tumour with cystic areas
Mucinous cystadenocarcinoma					
(a) borderline	2	10	40–70	B	Cystic tumour with solid areas
(b) frankly malignant	4	20	40–70	B	Solid tumour with cystic areas
Clear cell carcinoma	1	5	40–70	U	Usually solid with soft gelatinous areas
Endometrioid tumour	3	15	50–60	B	Solid tumour with cystic areas
Granulosa cell carcinoma	1	5	30–70	U	Solid, white, lobulated tumour
Dysgerminoma	<1	1	20–30	U	Solid, white, lobulated tumour

Notes
1 – frequency as percentage of all ovarian neoplasms
2 – frequency as percentage of all ovarian malignancies

Serous ovarian tumours

Serous neoplasms arise either from the surface epithelium over the ovary or from invaginations of it called *epithelial inclusion cysts*—small cystic spaces commonly found in healthy ovaries. *Serous cystadenomas* are usually thin-walled unilocular cysts of moderate size (10–20 cm) and contain thin clear straw-coloured fluid. The cysts may be smooth-surfaced or have papillary projections, which may be within the cyst cavity or, less often, arising from the outer surface. In benign tumours, these papillae are relatively thick and well formed; fine profuse papillae which shed fragments easily are more suggestive of borderline or frankly malignant tumours. Histologically, serous cystadenomas are lined by a single layer of columnar cells closely resembling the lining of the normal fallopian tube. In long-standing cysts, the lining epithelium may become so flattened by the internal pressure within the cyst that no specialized cells are identifiable, and a descriptive diagnosis of a benign simple cyst is made. Tumours with a prominent fibrous stromal element are termed serous cystadenofibromas or simply adenofibromas. Serous cystadenomas are bilateral in about 12 per cent of cases.

Serous cystadenocarcinomas account for only 8 per cent of all ovarian tumours, but are by far the commonest variety of ovarian carcinoma. The older the patient, the greater the prevalence of malignant serous tumours. The macroscopical appearance may resemble its benign counterpart, which might have malignant change present in only part of the cyst wall, but generally cystadenocarcinomas are more solid tumours with small irregular cystic spaces and soft luxuriant friable papillae within the cysts and on the surface of the ovary. There may be evidence of invasive growth into the adjacent pelvic tissues and, in late cases, peritoneal seedling spread and blood-stained ascites. A small percentage of serous carcinomas are completely solid, and at operation are extensively infiltrating and have widespread metastases. On histology the usual features of malignancy are present: cellular pleomorphism and hyperchromatism, multilayering of cells, increased mitotic rate, and an invasive growth pattern. In most cases the carcinomas are well differentiated, but predominantly solid tumours tend to be less so. The incidence of bilaterality is high, at 30 per cent or above.

A separate category is made of tumours which show all the above features of malignancy but without demonstrable stromal invasion. These are called low-grade or *borderline serous cystadenocarcinomas* and comprise 5–10 per cent of serous neoplasms. The distinction of this group from the frankly invasive carcinomas is clinically useful as they have a significantly better prognosis, but nevertheless are occasionally associated with peritoneal implants or more distant metastases. They have a 10-year survival of 75 per cent as against 20 per cent for invasive tumours, and a significant incidence of bilaterality of up to 26 per cent.

Mucinous ovarian tumours

Mucinous cystadenomas (the term pseudomucinous is obsolescent) are the second commonest group of ovarian neoplasms. The histogenesis is uncertain; origin from the surface epithelium with metaplasia into mucin-secreting cells is the most likely, but in 5 per cent of cases mucinous cystadenomas have teratomatous elements in their walls and it is possible that these represent a monomorphic development of a dermoid cyst.

Macroscopically, mucinous cystadenomas may have a single large cavity but are usually multilocular, and may reach enormous sizes. They are usually unilateral tumours. The cysts have thick fibrous walls and contain viscous clear fluid, though previous torsion and haemorrhage may change the colour to red, yellow or brown. Papilla formation is unusual; the morphological distinction between benign and malignant papillary growths is the same as for serous neoplasms. Histologically, mucinous cystadenomas show multiple cystic spaces lined by a single layer of tall columnar mucus-secreting cells which resemble endocervical epithelium. As with serous tumours, adenofibroma variants with a prominent fibrous stroma may be seen. Borderline mucinous cystadenocarcinomas show multilayered, disordered epithelium with obvious mitotic activity and shedding of cells into the cyst cavities, but with no apparent stromal invasion. *Mucinous cystadenocarcinomas* have similar features, but with infiltration of the fibrous stroma around the cysts.

Only about 15 per cent of mucinous cystadenocarcinomas of borderline malignancy are associated with peritoneal spread at the time of the original exploration. Mucinous carcinomas remain confined to the ovary for longer than serous carcinomas, but have a similar incidence of bilaterality.

The development of peritoneal seedlings from a borderline mucinous cystadenocarcinoma, or more rarely after rupture of a benign mucinous cystadenoma, may lead to the condition of myxomatous peritonitis or "pseudomyxoma peritonei". Gelatinous masses of tumour with copious mucin secretion cause a chronic peritonitis, fibrosis and intestinal obstruction. Interestingly, in myxomatous peritonitis associated with an ovarian tumour a mucocele of the appendix is usually seen as well, and surgical examination of the appendix is therefore important.

Endometrioid ovarian tumours

Though endometriosis of the ovary is quite common (see below), benign endometrioid neoplasms are rare. Endometrioid adenocarcinoma on the other hand is a common tumour which macroscopically resembles a malignant serous neoplasm. Histologically, these tumours are composed of epithelium which closely resembles adenocarcinoma of the endometrium, hence the name. The prognosis is significantly better than for malignant mucinous and serous tumours.

Germ cell tumours

The commonest germ cell neoplasm, and the third commonest type of ovarian tumour, is the benign dermoid cyst or cystic teratoma. These tumours are thought to arise from parthenogenetic fusion of two ova, producing an abortive development of organized adult tissues. The gross appearances are usually characteristic; the tumours are well demarcated rounded cysts with a smooth grey or yellowish external surface. Cut sections show yellow/brown greasy sebaceous material, which is fluid at body temperature but solidifies on cooling, and is mixed with hairs. The inner cyst wall shows developing or mature teeth in about one third of cases, below which bone, cartilage and fat may be found.

The histological appearances reflect the features seen macroscopically, with tissue elements representative of all three developmental germ layers. Cysts lined by keratinizing squamous epithelium, upper respiratory tract epithelium or gastrointestinal epithelium are common. The fibrous connective tissue encloses islands of cartilage, bone, muscle, fat, glandular and neural tissue.

The incidence of torsion of dermoid cysts is higher than for the other ovarian tumours. This is due to the smooth external surface, free mobility because adhesions are uncommon, and the development of a long pedicle. Rupture of a cyst occasionally occurs, the irritant sebaceous material producing a granulomatous peritonitis which may mimic disseminated malignancy. Bilateral tumours occur in about 20 per cent of cases.

Malignant behaviour in a teratoma is usually due to malignant change in an element of a previously benign dermoid cyst. About 2 per cent of dermoid cysts develop malignant tumours, most commonly invasive squamous carcinoma and rarely carcinoids, adenocarcinomas and sarcomas. Occasionally, in girls and young women, a teratoma may fail to develop fully mature adult tissues. These tumours are generally more solid, and are composed of a mixture of adult and embryonal tissues. The prognosis, which is generally grave, depends on the relative proportions of immature tissues present and is better when primitive neural tissue predominates.

Germ cell tumours other than teratomas are rare, accounting for only 2 per cent of the group. These are all malignant tumours, and comprise dysgerminomas, choriocarcinomas, yolk sac tumours and mixed forms. By the time of presentation their aggressive behaviour is usually apparent.

Sex cord stromal and other ovarian tumours

Sex cord stromal tumours account for about 10 per cent of ovarian tumours and include the majority of hormone-secreting tumours. Most are solid, pink or white nodular ovarian masses which are usually unilateral. Granulosa cell tumours are of low-grade malignancy, though the growth is often confined to the ovary at the time of excision. The histological appearances provide little indication of prognosis—clinical factors suggestive of a poor prognosis are a symptomatic or palpable abdominal mass, a solid tumour larger than 15 cm diameter, bilateral tumours or evidence of extra-ovarian spread at the time of laparotomy. Spread is typically local, though peritoneal dissemination may follow spontaneous rupture of a tumour, which occurs in about 5 per cent of cases. The prognosis is good, over 90 per cent of patients surviving 10 years. The comas and fibromas are benign tumours.

Because of the tendency of this group of tumours to secrete hormones, the endometrium may undergo hyperplasia, in some cases to such a degree that distinction from adenocarcinoma is very difficult; histological examination of endometrial curettings is therefore essential. Other complications include the association of ascites and hydrothorax with ovarian tumours (Meig's syndrome), usually fibromas and occasionally granulosa cell tumours.

Ovarian tumours other than those mentioned in the epithelial, germ cell and sex cord stromal groups are rare. The macroscopical appearance may provide a guide to their behaviour—for example haemorrhagic, necrotic tumours adherent to the surrounding structures are likely to be malignant—but in difficult cases definitive treatment may have to wait upon histological diagnosis.

Clinical features

Ovarian tumours of all kinds, like breast lumps, are notable for their absence of symptoms and, like breast lumps, are often first discovered on clinical examination (Fig. 33.1). Small cysts (less than 2.5 cm in diameter) found in young women usually have a physiological basis, being either follicular or luteal in origin and associated with temporary menstrual irregularity or early pregnancy. Such a cyst may be measured clinically or by ultrasound and observed over a period of time; its persistence or growth, especially if accompanied by pain, indicates the need for laparotomy.

Large ovarian tumours which can be felt abdominally and may be difficult to differentiate from ascites or fibroids require surgical exploration. Ascites causes dullness to percussion and visible fullness in the flanks, the centre remaining resonant, whereas with a cyst the flanks are resonant and the centre dull. If an ovarian cyst is suspected clinically, paracentesis must be avoided, but the cause and significance of ascites can be usefully determined by chemical and cytological examination.

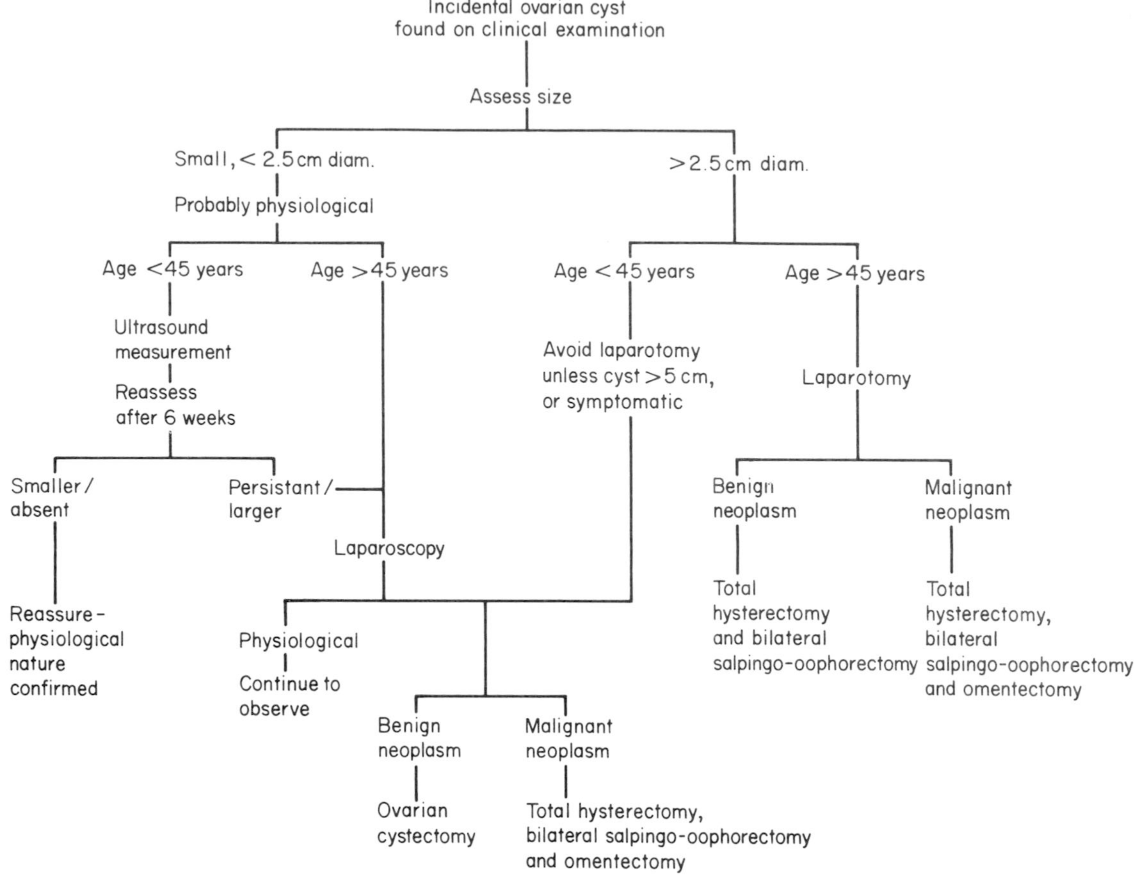

Fig. 33.1 Plan to indicate management of ovarian cysts.

Unexpected findings at laparotomy

Rules cannot be laid down with regard to the scale of surgery for different ovarian tumours. In each case the woman's age, her likely future fertility requirements, the pathology of the tumour and the symptoms it is causing must be considered; if the circumstances permit, detailed preoperative discussion with the patient is of the utmost importance. However, certain surgical guidelines can be recommended:

1. *Young women*—do not operate unless absolutely necessary; postoperative adhesions may lead to sterility. If a physiological cyst is incidentally found at operation, either leave it alone or enucleate it and repair the ovary. Do not remove any normal tissue and in particular avoid oophorectomy or salpingectomy unless the woman has previously been warned of this possibility.

2. *Menopausal women*—should usually have a total hysterectomy and bilateral salpingo-oophorectomy. It is axiomatic that what one ovary does today to the other ovary is likely to do tomorrow. The uterus at this age is functionless and may be a site for ovarian metastases.

3. *Women in the middle years* (aged 30–45)—malignancy requires total hysterectomy, bilateral salpingo-oophorectomy and omentectomy. Never operate on one ovary or tube without having inspected the other side first. Benign tumours can safely be treated by ovarian cystectomy, though oophorectomy may be necessary if the ovary is but a thin capsule stretched over the cyst. Frozen section is seldom helpful because of sampling difficulties.

Complications of ovarian tumours

When an ovarian cyst undergoes certain complications, the severity of pain and abdominal guarding may mask the presence of a tumour, which only becomes apparent at laparotomy. The commonest complication is haemorrhage, either into the cavity of a cyst or from its surface into the peritoneal cavity. Although such bleeding raises the possibility of malignancy, much more often one finds either a corpus luteum haematoma, endometriosis or, rarely, bleeding into a benign cystadenoma. The surgeon must be able to recognize these benign conditions in order to avoid serious mismanagement.

A corpus luteum in its active phase is an extremely vascular plum-coloured tumour up to 2.5 cm in diameter on the surface of the ovary. It is a very common cause of pain which occurs typically, but not necessarily, at mid-cycle (mittelschmerz), and if found at laparotomy may be enucleated from the ovary, which is then repaired. In the presence of early pregnancy, the corpus luteum persists and may form a palpable cyst up to 5 cm in diameter, usually demonstrable by ultrasound. Sufficient pain may be caused to raise the possibility of tubal pregnancy and lead to laparotomy, though the use of either ultrasound or laparoscopy should avoid this mistake. When a symptomless ovarian cyst is found in early pregnancy, periodic observation preferably by ultrasonic measurement is all that is initially required. Should the cyst then fail to diminish in size, thus indicating its pathological nature, laparotomy should be performed at about the fifteenth week. The risk of miscarriage after laparotomy is considered to be about 20 per cent.

An ovarian tumour may undergo torsion, the most common variety to do so being a benign teratoma. The severity of the pain is governed by the rapidity of onset of the torsion. Sometimes a history of attacks of pain of moderate severity for several years may be elicited, while other patients present with an "acute abdomen". The surgeon at operation should examine all the pelvic organs and especially the other ovary to exclude another cyst (20 per cent of benign teratomas are bilateral). Depending on the viability of the ovary, he may then decide whether to carry out ovarian cystectomy or salpingo-oophorectomy. Rupture of a pathological ovarian cyst is uncommon and should raise the question of malignancy as tumour infiltration of the capsule weakens its wall. Surgical treatment will depend on the nature of the cyst.

Ovarian carcinoma with widespread peritoneal metastases found at laparotomy

The surgeon confronted at laparotomy with disseminated ovarian carcinoma should attempt to remove as much of the tumour mass as possible. The problem in each case is likely to be different, but mobilization of the uterus, tubes and ovaries, followed by their removal, is usually possible. During this procedure the ureters, which may be surrounded by tumour, should not be endangered, and removal of the cervix, if technically hazardous, need not be too energetically pursued. Indeed, it has been argued that a sub-total hysterectomy lessens the risk of subsequent malignant infiltration of the vaginal vault. Hudson has recommended an extraperitoneal approach, including if necessary sigmoid resection, but this super-radical operation is not at present widely practised. The omentum should always be removed whether or not metastases are evident: seedling deposits, visible only histologically, may influence future treatment and omentectomy lessens the likelihood of subsequent ascites. The surgeon should explore and note the presence of metastases, paying particular attention to peritoneal surfaces, especially under the diaphragm. He should also inspect the liver and palpate the para-aortic glands.

Although the prognosis in ovarian cancer is very poor (in general a 5-year survival of only 20 per cent), an energetic surgical approach followed by chemotherapy and/or radiotherapy has improved both the quality and length of life of many women, though almost all will eventually die of the disease.

Uterine tumours

Fibroids

The general surgeon may encounter uterine fibroids (benign leiomyomata) on clinical examination or at laparotomy, when their presence should merely be noted. The finding of a fibroid at laparotomy is usually incidental to the purpose of the operation, and removal is unnecessary and unwise. Myomectomy is often associated with considerable bleeding which may only be controllable by hysterectomy. Unlike ovarian tumours, fibroids shrink in size after the menopause so that any pelvic tumour after this age must be considered to be ovarian and potentially malignant. Fibroids are sometimes single but usually are multiple. They arise within the wall of the uterus as tiny pale nodules and grow as round, rubbery, well defined masses. On cut surface the smooth-muscle bundles of which they are composed present a pale whorled appearance which bulges from the high tissue pressure of the tumour. Though all fibroids arise initially intramurally, growth may be predominantly in a submucosal or subserosal direction. Submucosal fibroids, which may cause menstrual disturbances, can only be identified by careful palpation of the uterus, for they are usually small and not evident on inspection at laparotomy; they are unlikely to come within the remit of the general surgeon. Intramural and subserosal fibroids may enlarge the uterus to 25 cm or more in diameter and cause symptoms of abdominal enlargement or pressure on adjacent structures, notably the bladder, resulting in urinary frequency or, occasionally, retention.

A fibroid may undergo infarction ("red degeneration"), especially during pregnancy, which causes severe abdominal pain and tenderness. The treatment of this condition is conservative as the pain will subside in a few days. Furthermore, the surgeon should never attempt myomectomy during pregnancy because of the risk of uncontrollable bleeding. Other degenerative changes may occur in fibroids, but are usually asymptomatic. Malignant change in a fibroid, or the occurrence of a leiomyosarcoma de novo, is rare.

Carcinoma of the body of the uterus

This occurs usually in women over the age of 50 years and manifests itself by post-menopausal bleeding. The uterus is very seldom enlarged unless the tumour is advanced or obstructs the cervical canal causing a pyometra. Diagnosis is made by uterine curettage. Endometrial adenocarcinomas are usually well differentiated tumours which remain confined to the inner aspect of the uterine wall until late in the disease.

Cervical carcinoma

This occurs in women of all ages and causes a blood-stained vaginal discharge, post-coital bleeding or, in late cases, urinary or rectal symptoms. The hope that routine cervical cytology would eliminate this disease has not been fulfilled, and death in young women from this cause is at present increasing. Carcinoma of the cervix cannot usually be diagnosed with confidence on palpation at vaginal or rectal examination for the normal cervix feels firm and is often irregular, especially in parous women. The passage of the Cusco speculum, which should not be outside the expertise of the general surgeon, reveals an ulcerated tumour and biopsy should be taken to confirm the diagnosis. Subsequent management, depending on the clinical stage of the tumour is by radiotherapy, gynaecological surgery or both.

Calcification in pelvic organs

Dystrophic calcification in fibroids which have undergone infarction may render them radio-opaque; they appear on plain pelvic X-ray as circular stippled areas. Other gynaecological causes of radio-opaque masses include calcification in elements of a benign cystic teratoma, especially bone and teeth; calcification in the wall of a serous cystadenoma of the ovary; and the presence of fetal parts. Very rarely in Great Britain, calcification may occur in tuberculous salpingitis.

Endometriosis

The ectopic endometrial tissue which characterizes this condition is usually found in the ovaries, pouch of Douglas or utero-sacral ligaments. The bowel, especially the recto-sigmoid, or caecum and appendix may be affected and, less often, the bladder, umbilicus or inguinal canal. Endometriosis may occasionally be found in abdominal scars after operations which involve opening the uterine cavity, and very rarely presents at sites outside the peritoneal cavity altogether.

Recognition of endometriosis macroscopically may be easy or very difficult. In early disease, superficial foci appear as tiny dark blue dots on the surface of organs. Later these develop a fibrous covering, producing a pale grey nodule through the wall of which the dark contents may still be visible. Later still, the continuing fibrosis distorts the tissue by contraction and conceals the presence of endometriosis below. At any site, but especially in the ovary, cyst formation may occur. When internal endometriosis (adenomyosis) develops within the myometrium, there may be diffuse uterine enlargement or development of a localized nodule. This latter closely resembles a leiomyoma, but cut section will often reveal tiny brown cystic areas.

Histologically, the diagnosis rests on the demonstration of both endometrial glands and their surrounding endometrial stroma. The presence of the glandular element alone, within say the bowel or bladder wall, strongly suggests a metastasis from a well differentiated endometrial adenocarcinoma. In about 20 per cent of cases endometriotic foci parallel the patient's periodic cycle. In late cases, because of the irritant nature of the cyst contents and the progressing fibrosis, distortion of the endometriotic foci may result in loss of the epithelial component; in such cases, only a presumptive diagnosis can be made. Treatment with hormone therapy induces decidual change in the stroma and degeneration of the glands, but has no effect on fibrosis. It is doubtful whether endometriosis has any malignant potential, but very rarely endometrioid carcinoma of the ovary has been found in close association with a focus of endometriosis.

The pathogenesis of endometriosis remains an enigma. The development of adenomyosis is easily explained by direct downgrowth of the endometrial glands and stroma from the uterine cavity, but the presence of endometriosis outside the uterus is more problematic. It has been shown that retrograde flow of endometrial tissue out of the fallopian tubes may occur in normal women during their menstrual period, and that this may implant within the abdominal cavity; however, new foci of endometriosis may arise in women with tubes completely blocked by a previous episode. Metaplasia of the peritoneal lining cells, which share a common coelomic ancestry with endometrial cells, has been postulated, but would not account for the existence of endometriosis at all the sites where it is found. The most recent suggestion is that it is the relatively unspecialized endometrial stromal cells, arising presumably from foci of uncommitted mesenchyme, which differentiate into endometrial glands.

Clinical features

Endometriosis is limited to the years of menstrual activity and is commonest in nulliparous women over the age of 30. The most important symptom is lower abdominal pain, which is worse premenstrually when the endometriotic glands become secretory and later haemorrhagic. Rupture of an endometriotic cyst (which because of its surrounding fibrosis, is rare) causes extreme pain and collapse. Other symptoms include dyspareunia, infertility and menstrual disorders. The characteristic finding on vaginal examination is of tender nodules in the pouch of Douglas and the diagnosis can most accurately be confirmed by laparoscopy.

At operation, the surgeon should be able to recognize endometriosis by the presence of endometrial cysts and fibrosis. The surrounding fibrous reaction produces dense adhesions which make dissection difficult and when the bowel is affected this may closely mimic carcinoma. The general surgeon should be conservative in his approach to this condition. After mobilization and inspection of the pelvic organs, all deposits of endometriosis are either excised or destroyed by diathermy, the uterus then being anteverted by shortening the round ligaments. Postoperative treatment with hormones may be beneficial, but of all treatments, pregnancy is the most efficacious. Women who are past the wish for childbearing are best treated by total hysterectomy and bilateral salpingo-oophorectomy.

Pelvic inflammatory disease

The general surgeon is likely to encounter pelvic inflammatory disease (PID) at operation when acute salpingitis has been mistaken for appendicitis or when a pelvic mass is found in a woman with severe pelvic pain.

The term pelvic inflammatory disease is rather woolly. It usually means salpingitis as the prime event, with extension of the inflammation to the ovaries and pelvic peritoneum in most cases.

Ascending infection is the commonest cause of PID. Sexually transmitted microorganisms are usually implicated but, more rarely, infection may follow the insertion of intrauterine contraceptive devices, septic abortion or puerperal sepsis. Blood-borne infections such as tuberculosis are carried from a primary focus elsewhere, and produce chronic salpingitis.

The most frequent isolated causative organisms are *Neisseria gonorrhoeae* and *Chlamydia trachomatis*. Anaerobic organisms like *Bacteroides fragilis* are also common, but will not be identified by conventional aerobic methods of specimen collection and culture. The techniques for chlamydia isolation are complicated and as yet provided only by specialized laboratories; however, serological tests using immunofluorescent antibodies are more widely available.

Acute PID from ascending infection begins as an endosalpingitis. The tube becomes hyperaemic and swollen due to oedema of its wall. Any adhesions at this stage are fine and fibrinous, and easily separated. The tube plicae become oedematous, congested and infiltrated with polymorphs, which also collect in the lumen as pus. As the inflammation progresses, the full thickness of the wall develops oedema and an inflammatory cell infiltrate.

Outflow of purulent material into the pelvic peritoneum results in a pelvic abscess which, if near to the appendix, may induce secondary appendicitis. Extension to the ovary may produce a tubo-ovarian abscess, rupture of which produces severe toxic effects and a high incidence of septicaemia.

Resolution of the acute inflammation may be complete or may progress to chronic PID, manifest as a pyosalpinx, hydrosalpinx or dense fibrosis of the tube wall. Pyosalpinx is the result of blockage of the tube lumen at the fimbrial and isthmic ends by fibrinous exudate and subsequent fibrosis, with accumulation of purulent material distending the tube into a fusiform or retort shape. The plicae become flattened from the pressure of intra-luminal pus and the stroma is infiltrated by chronic inflammatory cells. Acute exacerbations of the disease may superimpose oedema and a polymorph infiltrate over these appearances.

Phagocytosis of the cellular debris and resorption of the protein from the exudate of a pyosalpinx result in a hydrosalpinx, which is therefore seen late in the history of quiescent inflammation. Tubal distension may be marked or only slight. If the inflammation resolves into a hydrosalpinx before significant fibrosis develops, as is often the case, the tube wall is thin and translucent, and reveals the straw-coloured serous fluid within.

Chronic salpingitis may occasionally produce large amounts of fibrosis in the tube wall, with the formation of small cystic spaces in the lumen from the distorted and fused plicae. It is thought that this process may produce nodules of fibrous tissue enclosing gland-like spaces, the so-called "salpingitis isthmica nodosa", though other explanations for this have been suggested.

Granulomatous salpingitis is usually considered as a separate entity. The disease is most commonly secondary to tuberculous infection, but may be caused by other pathogens such as schistosomes and fungi. The macroscopical appearances are not specific, though miliary nodules are occasionally present and the fimbriae are usually less distorted than in post-gonococcal salpingitis.

In all of the above conditions, except mild acute salpingitis, the patency and function of the affected fallopian tube are compromised or lost completely.

Clinical features

Acute pelvic inflammatory disease

The woman usually presents with lower abdominal pain of sudden onset, malaise and rigors. A single episode of vomiting is common, but persistent nausea and other gastrointestinal symptoms are rare. A purulent vaginal discharge is likely to have preceded the illness.

On examination, fever of 39–40°C is usual. The abdomen is tender in both iliac fossae, where marked release tenderness and guarding are present; extreme tenderness of the pelvic organs makes their palpation difficult. A purulent vaginal discharge is seen coming from the external cervical os. Specimens of the discharge should be taken from the endocervix, vagina, urethra and rectum for bacterial culture with special attention to *N. gonorrhoeae*. However, even with the greatest care in transport, culture is often disappointingly unhelpful.

Acute salpingitis is treated conservatively, as the infection usually responds to antibiotics. However, diagnostic doubt demands laparoscopy or, if the surgeon is unfamiliar with this technique, laparotomy. No harm is done and no censure is attached to a surgeon who operates on a women with acute salpingitis. Indeed, it has been shown that permanent tubal damage causing sterility is less likely to follow salpingitis when surgical drainage is combined with chemotherapy. At such an operation, pus is expressed from the fimbrial ostia and any exudate in the pouch of Douglas is mopped out, a specimen being obtained for bacterial culture. Should the ostia be occluded, an opening is made to ensure drainage.

Chronic pelvic inflammatory disease

The recurrent lower abdominal pain and the presence of tender inflammatory masses which characterize this condition may lead the surgeon to exploratory laparotomy. The uterus, tubes and ovaries are mobilized by division of adhesions and the uterus stitched in an anteverted position by shortening the round ligaments. A pyosalpinx or tubo-ovarian abscess is opened and drained, but the tube should not be removed, even though future function appears hopeless; a specimen of the pus is taken for bacterial culture. Before the abdomen is closed, adequate drainage of the pelvis is ensured according to general surgical principles. Antibiotics are given in the postoperative period. Should the woman continue to have symptoms, the only satisfactory subsequent treatment may be hysterectomy and bilateral salpingectomy.

Ectopic pregnancy

By far the commonest site for an ectopic pregnancy is in the ampullary portion of the fallopian tube. Figures for prevalence are dependent on geography and social factors; about 1 in 200 pregnancies are ectopic, with a substantially higher incidence in Africa and South America. The prevalence of a second ectopic gestation in a patient who has suffered a previous ectopic is about 10 per cent.

Tubal ectopic pregnancy is caused by delay to the passage of the fertilized ovum—older ideas on factors which might increase the receptiveness of tubal mucosa have largely been abandoned. Fertilization usually takes place in the ampullary portion of the tube and the transit time between fertilization and endometrial implantation is about 48 hours. This may be prolonged because of physical obstruction to the passage of the conceptus; because conception occurs more distally at the fimbrial end of the tube or even within the abdominal cavity; or because the fertilized ovum is washed back into the tube by retrograde menstruation, in conceptions occurring late in a menstrual cycle.

Obstruction of the fallopian tube is the commonest cause of ectopic pregnancy. Evidence of previous episodes of salpingitis is present in about 50 per cent of cases, with obstruction to the lumen by distortion of plicae, or interstitial fibrosis reducing contractility. In some cases, spasm or irregular contractions of the myometrium and tubal muscularis may impede the progress of the ovum or conceptus.

Once established, implantation and nidation of an ectopic pregnancy proceeds in the same manner as a eutopic one. Developing villi penetrate the tubal wall and may extend to the serosal surface. Continued growth is restricted by the inability of the tube to mount an adequate decidual response and by the insubstantial muscle of the tube wall, which provides little support and is easily perforated.

The termination of an ectopic pregnancy may be by tubal abortion, rupture, spontaneous regression, secondary implantation of the conceptus elsewhere or lithopaedion formation. Erosion of large vessels by trophoblast usually results in profuse bleeding, which may be free into the abdominal cavity or between the leaves of the broad ligament to form a haematoma.

Changes are seen in the endometrium as a consequence of the hormonal changes of an ectopic pregnancy. An extremely florid secretory change may occur, the endometrial glands developing infolding, tufting, cellular atypia and increased mitotic activity, the *Aris–Stella* reaction. This picture is found in about 10 per cent of ectopics, but is also seen in eutopic pregnancies and patients taking oral contraceptives and is therefore not pathognomonic. Decidual change in the endometrium is usual. On the death of the ectopic embryo, the decidua degenerates and may slough in toto as a shaggy, soft decidual cast. Histologically, this contains no chorionic villi, which helps to distinguish the condition from abortion.

Diagnosis

Acute tubal rupture usually occurs when the implantation site is in the isthmus and causes little difficulty in diagnosis. The patient usually is a young woman who complains of sudden severe abdominal pain and is seen in a state of shock. She usually gives a history of a short period of amenorrhoea and may be found to have a little vaginal bleeding.

The sub-acute picture of tubal pregnancy poses a more difficult diagnostic problem. There is usually amenorrhoea of less than 6 weeks' duration, but there may be a history of prolonged bleeding punctuated by attacks of pain. Pain is the most important symptom and is characteristically severe and episodic. It is caused initially by distension of the tube and later by blood in the peritoneal cavity. In each attack the severe pain persists for about 30 minutes and then diminishes to a residual tenderness which is exacerbated by sudden movement. Even a small quantity of blood in the peritoneal cavity may cause vasovagal fainting, and if blood tracks up to irritate the diaphragm, pain is felt in the shoulder tip. Urinary and gastrointestinal symptoms are unusual, unless a pelvic haematocele is present. The blood passed per vaginam is initially dark in colour and comes from the implantation site in the tube; later, as the hormone levels diminish with the death of the embryo, bright red blood is passed with the endometrial decidua. On examination, the woman is shocked only when profuse intra-peritoneal bleeding has occurred; otherwise her condition is good. Pyrexia is unusual. Lower abdominal tenderness, especially release tenderness, is common and sometimes a mass of blood clot is palpable. On vaginal examination, dark blood may be seen escaping from the external cervical os. The uterus is normal or a little enlarged in size and extreme tenderness is elicited by movement of the cervix making palpation of any tubal swelling difficult.

The conditions which are most commonly confused with ectopic pregnancy are spontaneous abortion, salpingitis, appendicitis or complications of an ovarian cyst. The history is more helpful to the surgeon in reaching the correct diagnosis than are the physical signs. He should realize that it is a common condition and that the variability of the symptom sequence requires constant awareness of the condition. It should be remembered that the pregnancy test may be negative if the level of chorionic gonadotrophin is low because the ovum is already dead or because implantation was recent.

Laparoscopy, which is the one certain method of diagnosis, is used in difficult cases, but should be avoided if the woman is in a state of shock. Its widespread use has been a major help in the diagnosis of acute pelvic conditions.

Treatment

This consists of laparotomy, with concurrent blood transfusion if necessary. Through a small transverse suprapubic incision, blood in the pelvis is cleared away to allow inspection of the uterus, tubes and ovaries, and the site of the ectopic pregnancy is carefully identified. No organ is removed and no clamp is applied before such an inspection.

Subtotal salpingectomy is performed provided the other tube appears normal; the ovary should not be removed unless it is disrupted by haematoma. If the other tube is diseased or has already been removed, it may be possible to preserve the affected tube either by milking the conceptus through the abdominal ostium or by evacuation through a longitudinal incision in the tube. If this is not possible, resection of the affected segment of the tube may allow future restorative tubal surgery.

Further reading

Ovarian tumours

Serov SF, Scully RE, Sobin LH. *International histological classification of tumours. No. 9 Histological typing of ovarian tumours*. Geneva: World Health Organisation, 1973.

Fox H, Langley FA. *Tumours of the Ovary*. London: Heinemann, 1976.

Scully RE. Ovarian tumours: a review. *Am J Pathol* 1977; **87**:686–720.

Hart WR. Ovarian epithelial tumors of borderline malignancy (carcinomas of low malignant potential) *Hum Pathol* 1977; **8**:541–9.

Newman CE, Ford CHJ, Jordan JA. *Ovarian Cancer*. London: Pergamon Press, 1980.

Uterine tumours

Persaud V, Arjoon PD. Uterine leiomyoma. Incidence of degenerative change and a correlation of associated symptoms. *Obstet Gynecol* 1970; **35**:432–6.

Anderson MC. The aetiology and pathology of cancer of the cervix. *Clin Obstet Gynaecol* 1976; **3**:317–37.

Mazur MT, Kraus FT. Histogenesis of morphologic variations in tumours of the uterine wall. *Am J Surg Pathol* 1980; **4**:59–74.

Endometriosis

Ridley JH. The histogenesis of endometriosis. *Obstet Gynecol Surv* 1968; **23**:1–15.

Pratt JH, Shamblin WR. Spontaneous rupture of endometrial cysts of the ovary presenting as an acute abdominal emergency. *Am J Obstet Gynecol* 1970; **108**:56–62.

Chalmer JA. *Endometriosis*. London: Butterworth, 1975.

Salpingitis

Chow W, Patten V, Marshall JR. Bacteriology of acute pelvic inflammatory disease. *Am J Obstet Gynecol* 1979; **32**:362–5.

Ectopic pregnancy

Swollen K, Fall M. Ectopic pregnancy: recurrence, postoperative fertility and aspects of treatment based on 182 patients. *Acta Europaea Fertilitatis* 1972: **3**:147–57.

Westrom L, Bengtsson LP, Mrardh PA. Incidence, trends and risks of ectopic pregnancy in a population of women. *Br Med J* 1981; **282**:15–18.

34

Transplantation

P J Guillou and P R Millard

Introduction

Over the past 25 years transplantation has evolved into an important, and in many cases, definitive component of the treatment of end-stage renal failure. The 1100 renal allografts performed in the United Kingdom in 1982 attests to the almost commonplace nature of this surgical procedure. The lessons learned from clinical and experimental renal transplantation have now been extended to the use of grafts in the treatment of end-stage failure of other organs such as the liver, heart and pancreas.

It is of central importance in the management of the transplant patient to appreciate that although the commonest cause of graft failure is rejection, other processes may lead to the impairment of graft function. Some of these complications are amenable to surgical correction and their misdiagnosis as rejection with consquent increases in immunosuppression can lead to fatal infective illnesses. Following Medawar's observations, histological appearances have provided the basic evidence for rejection in experimental and clinical transplantation and no other way of demonstrating this phenomenon has attained such universal acceptance or reproducibility. In man, where allografts (Table 34.1) are invariably used, the features are modified by immunosuppression (Table 34.2). The increasing use of graft biopsy or fine-needle aspiration for the diagnosis of rejection, makes it of crucial importance to appreciate the significance of changes within transplanted organs. This knowledge leads to appropriate immunotherapeutic action which may even imply the withdrawal of immunosuppression and graft removal. The aim of this chapter is to describe and explain the clinical significance of these pathological changes in different organ grafts and some of the complications associated with transplantation. To understand these changes an appreciation of their underlying genetic and immunological basis is necessary.

Table 34.1 Graft nomenclature.

Graft	*Donor–recipient relationship*
Autograft	Same individual
Isograft	Same species and identical genotype e.g. identical twins
Allograft	Same species and different genotype e.g. cadaveric donor
Xenograft	Different species e.g. baboon → man

Table 34.2 Commonly used immunosuppressive agents for organ transplantation

Agent	*Mode of action*
Corticosteroids	Anti-inflammatory Lymphocytolytic Inhibit polymorph leukotaxis
Azathioprine	Suppress cellular and humoral response
Cyclophosphamide	Non-specific anti-proliferative effects on dividing lymphoid cells Synergism with steroids
Anti-lymphocyte Anti-thymocyte	Globulins (ALG) Lysis of circulating lymphocytes Inhibition of lymphocyte recirculation
Cyclosporin A	Selective effect on proliferating helper T-lymphocytes Inhibition of soluble messenger production (Interleukin-2)

Genetic and immunological basis of graft rejection

Genetic factors

The antigens (alloantigens) present on the surfaces of the cells of transplantable organs recognized as foreign by the recipient are, in all species, coded by a distinct set of genes, which in man occur on the short arm of the sixth chromosome (Fig. 34.1).

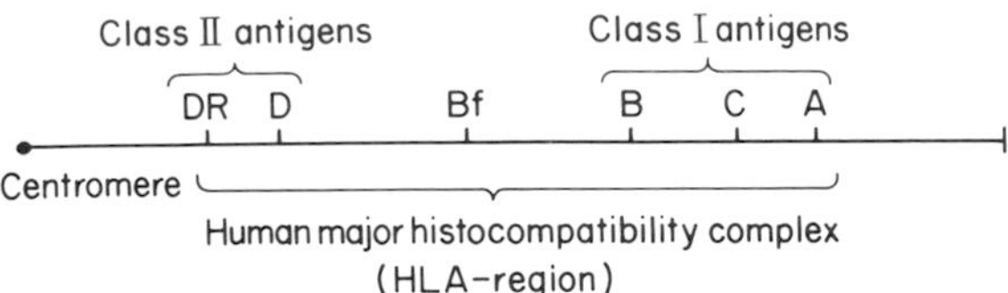

Fig. 34.1 Sites of HLA loci on the short arm of the sixth chromosome.

This complex of genes is known as the major histocompatibility complex (MHC), and the human antigens manufactured in response to the codes within these genes are known as the human lymphocytic antigens (HLA). Although first described, and in clinical practice detected, on lymphocytes, HLA antigens have a widespread tissue distribution and are found with a variable degree of expression on the cells of all organs. Several major loci have been identified within these gene complexes as coding for the HLA antigens of clinical importance in organ transplantation. These antigens are designated HLA-A,B,C,D and DR (D-related) (Fig. 34.1 and Table 34.3). Human lymphocytic antigens A,B and C are also known as serologically defined (class I) antigens because their presence on lymphocyte surfaces may be detected by complement-dependent cytotoxicity techniques. This is done by using antisera obtained from multiparous women or multiply-transfused individuals who have developed anti-HLA antibodies of known specificity. The practical importance of this is that such antisera enables tissue typing for these antigens to be performed within hours of receiving a blood or lymphocyte specimen from the donor or recipient. This contrasts with the procedure necessary to tissue type for the D-antigens (lymphocyte-defined or class II antigens). This involves a mixed-lymphocyte culture requiring lymphocytes from both donor and recipient plus specially typed homozygous cells and takes between 5 and 7 days to perform. Clearly, the use of D-typing for cadaveric donor–recipient pairs is impractical. However, more recently a further group of lymphocytic antigens known as DR-antigens have been described which are present on the surface of B-lymphocytes and vascular endothelium and which show a high degree of association, and may even be identical with, the corresponding D-antigen. DR-antigens are detected serologically using complement-dependent lymphocytotoxicity against B-lymphocytes. Although this is rather more time-consuming than typing for A,B and C antigens, in practical terms it probably represents a more convenient way of typing for D-antigens than does the use of mixed-lymphocyte cultures.

Every individual receives half the genetic material of each of his parents which is inherited as an immunogenetic package (haplotype) and is in turn always transmitted as such. The transmission of a maternal or paternal haplotype from each parent provides the offspring with four possible combinations of parental haplotypes (Fig. 34.2). The clinical importance of this arises in the case of living-related donor transplantation where immunogenetically identical and semi-identical siblings may donate an organ and expect a very high chance of success. Conversely, a significant risk of failure exists if the organ is donated by a sibling who possesses no immunogenetic identity whatsoever with the recipient and such a procedure is rarely undertaken. However, it remains one of the enigmas in transplantation surgery that the extrapolation of the principles of live-donor

Table 34.3 Properties of HLA antigens.

	Class I antigens (HLA-A,-B and -C)	*Class II antigens (HLA-D, and -DRw)*
Structure	Single chain glycoproteins (mol.wt 45 000) with beta-2 microglobulin	2-chain molecules (mol.wt 35 000 and 28 000)
Site	T- and B-lymphocytes Ubiquitious to varying degrees	B-lymphocytes Activated macrophages Dendritic cells Vascular endothelium
Functions	Target antigens for cytotoxic T-lymphocytes and antibodies	Stimulating antigens for lymphocyte proliferation. Part of antigen presenting system

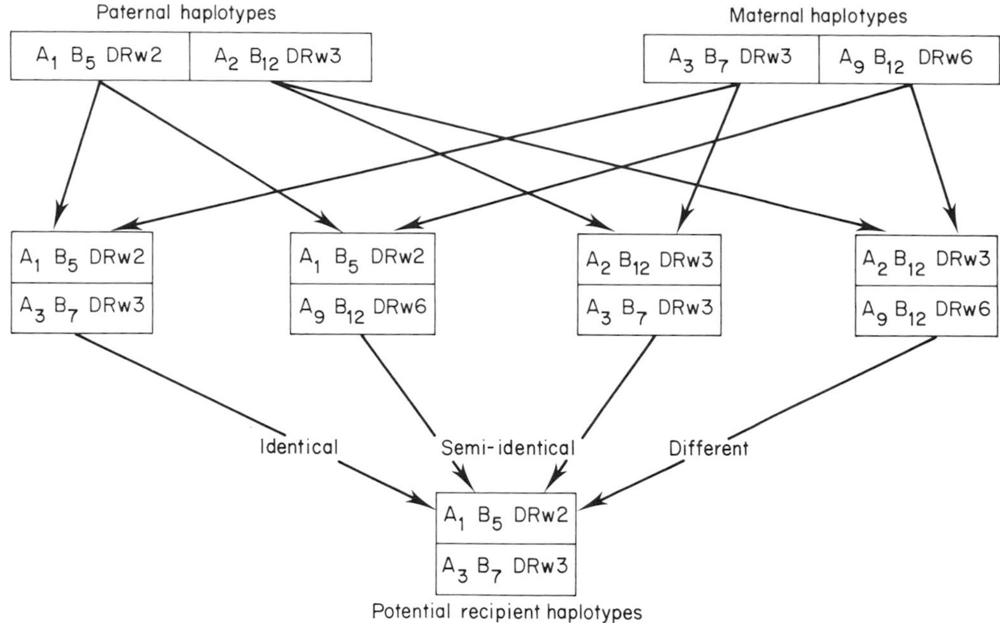

Fig. 34.2 Mode of inheritance of genes controlling HLA antigens. Application of familial transmission of human MHC genes to donor selection in live-related donor (sibling) transplantation. HLA-C antigens are not included since they do not exert a significant influence on the outcome of transplantation. The suffix 'w' after the DR-antigen denotes a number assigned at the various international workshops on tissue typing.

immunogenetics into cadaveric transplantation has not been straightforward. Statistically, the chances of success of a well-matched cadaveric renal allograft are greater than those of a poorly matched allograft, but acute rejection of the "full house" (i.e. all *recognizable* antigens)—matched cadaveric kidney—is a not unfamiliar experience. In contrast, most transplant centres have on record many cases of success with poorly matched kidneys. Thus, the degree of immunogenetic identity between the donor and recipient does not allow an accurate individual prognosis to be made, presumably because of non MHC-antigenic disparities and/or other organ-specific antigenic differences which are present. This has led some surgeons to place less emphasis on tissue typing as a rational basis for donor–recipient pairing, particularly in the context of immunosuppression with cyclosporin A (CyA). Nonetheless, recent evidence suggests that irrespective of the degree of HLA-A and B matching, considerable benefit accrues from matching for DR-antigens. It is possible that a combination of DR-matching and CyA therapy may produce excellent results. Since only about 12 DR-antigens exist, compared with totals of 17 A- and 29 B-antigens, this would considerably simplify the matching of donor–recipient pairs. However, although there is a demonstrable statistical advantage in HLA-matching in renal transplantation, this has not yet proven to be the case for transplantation of other organs.

Whole organ transplantation follows Landsteiner's laws of blood group ABO compatibility with the exception that Rhesus compatibility is not necessary. A blood group O donor is a universal donor and a blood group AB recipient may receive a kidney from a donor of any blood group. However, multiparous or multiply-transfused recipients may have developed anti-HLA antibodies and consequently it is vital that a direct cross-match between recipient serum and the donor's lymphocytes (which express surface HLA antigens) be negative. If the recipient's serum contains complement-dependent cytotoxic anti-donor HLA-A and B antibodies, hyperacute rejection will occur. Antibodies against DR-antigens do not cause hyperacute rejection. It is routine practice to screen the serum of all potential allograft recipients, particularly those who have had failed transplants or transfusions, for antibodies against the lymphocytes of a random pool of blood donors (usually 20, which is the minimum number of donors who will exhibit the majority of HLA antigens). Thus, if antibodies are found which react with the lymphocytes of 12 of 20 such blood donors, the recipient is described as possessing "60 per cent cytotoxic antibodies". Such patients are termed "sensitized" and the degree of sensitization, which may vary from time to time in any patient, may be described as "high" or "low" depending on the percentage of cytotoxic antibodies present. Sensitized recipients require very closely matched organs for transplantation and the avoidance of donor antigens with which they may have been previously transplanted. It has now been amply demonstrated that the graft survival rates of patients who have been previously transfused is significantly greater than those who have not had prior blood transfusions. However, this beneficial effect of blood transfusion must be weighed against the relative risk of causing sensitization of the potential recipient against HLA antigens. At present the relative risk of transfusion-induced anti-HLA antibody formation is about 10 per cent.

Immunological factors

The functional sub-unit of the immunological response is the lymphocyte but, as can be seen in Fig. 34.3, during the anti-allograft response, a number of cellular interactions conspire to produce the final sequence of events recognizable as rejection.

Sensitization of the lymphoid cells within the transplant may occur through direct contact between these host cells and the donor's endothelial cells. An alternative or associated explanation may be that any contact results in the release of soluble antigen and central sensitization of the

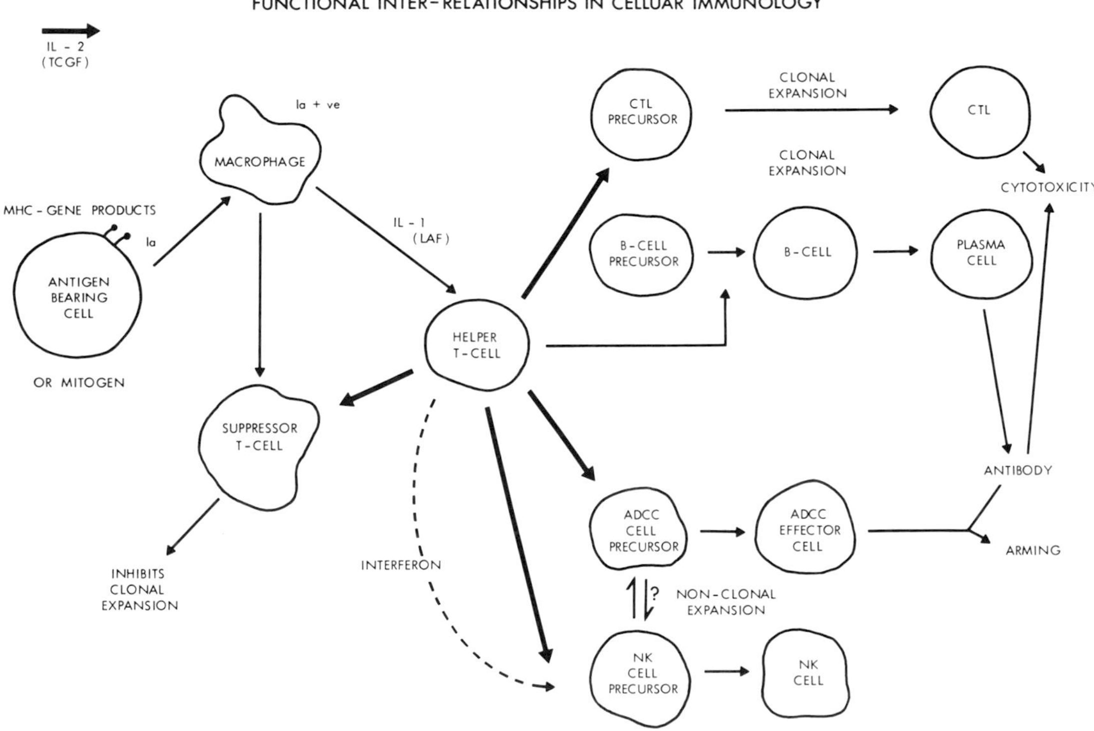

Fig. 34.3 Diagrammatic representation of cellular events during the allograft response. Soluble antigen is processed by activated D-antigen positive (Ia + ve) macrophages which produce a soluble factor, Interleukin-1 or lymphocyte activating factor, (LAF) which, in combination with antigen, stimulates helper T-cells. These in turn produce a second signal, Interleukin-2 (T-cell growth factor, TCGF) which influences the maturation of cytotoxic T-lymphocyte (CTL) precursors into mature effector CTL. Helper T-cells also have a direct effect on the induction of B-lymphocytes to produce specific antidonor antibody.

host. If this mechanism does occur, antigen release might also result from ischaemia and other factors damaging the endothelial cells or even other graft cells. In either circumstance the antigen is HLA-related. Currently, sensitization is attributed to passenger (dendritic) cells within the graft. These dendritic cells are characterized by class II antigen which can stimulate helper T-cells and so induce cytotoxic T-lymphocytes (CTL). Dendritic cells have been recognized in all organs, but in some species, particularly man, other structures especially endothelium also bear class II antigens. Passenger cells can be lost from grafts shortly after transplantation, but the endothelial cells persist as does their class II antigen. This state of affairs would explain the early very aggressive nature of rejection as well as the potential for long-term graft survival if donor and recipient bear identical class II antigens. Soluble antigens, processed by macrophages, stimulate the cytotoxic T-cell component of the immune response which represents the major effector mechanism for acute rejection (the first-set response of experimental animals). This maturation of CTL precursors into CTL is facilitated by soluble messengers from macrophages and by helper T-cells. T-cells also provide the necessary signals for B-cells to transform into plasma cells whose function is to produce antibodies against donor antigens. Classically, it is these antibodies demonstrated by immunofluorescence which are responsible for hyperacute and accelerated (2–5 days) rejection of allografts. The effector mechanisms which are currently considered responsible for chronic rejection consist of a mixture of antibody and cellular mechanisms, although this is at present rather more controversial.

During alloactivation, killer (K) cells bind specific antibody and may also contribute to the rejection process by the process of antibody-dependent cellular cytotoxicity (ADCC). In addition, natural killer cells (NK) are also stimulated. These cells are held to represent a host defence mechanism against lymphomas and their suppression may be partially responsible for the development of lymphomas during immunosuppession.

Once the host is sensitized and endothelial damage incurred, the complement and the clotting cascades will be initiated and thereby further damage is inflicted with fibrin and platelet deposition. These in turn will cause the release of vasoactive amines resulting in vasospasm, secondary ischaemia and further graft damage.

Influence of donor organ

The nature of the graft may also affect the host's rejection response. Cardiac grafts are rejected more avidly in some species, including man, than kidney grafts, and similar claims have been made for pancreatic grafts. In special circumstances the site of the transplant, the mass of transplanted tissue, the simultaneous transplantation of several organs, and the presence of pre-existing disease, for example renal failure, may also modify rejection.

General patterns of graft rejection

Hyperacute rejection

This occurs with restoration of the circulation to the organ. Widespread thrombosis and haemorrhagic necrosis are inevitable sequelae, and no mononuclear cells are seen. Neutrophil polymorphs may be evident.

Acute and accelerated acute rejection

Mononuclear cells and acute vascular lesions are the hallmark of these reactions. The mononuclear cells include various types of lymphocytes, plasma cells and macrophages and these infiltrate the graft via capillaries within 24–48 hours. They then diffuse into the parenchyma where they proliferate, as evidenced by the mitotic forms seen. Sex karyotyping and autoradiography studies have shown that these cells are of host origin. The cellular infiltrate is not necessarily progressive and can even partially abate. It is initially accompanied by increasing oedema. This may be due to severance of the organ's lymphatics, but may also be contributed to by the inevitable endothelial damage associated with ischaemia occuring prior to transplantation and with rejection. The cellular infiltrate in the later stages is found around and within the walls of arteries and veins, but not all vessels are involved or affected to the same degree (Fig. 34.4). Fibrinoid arterial and capillary necrosis, with and without thrombosis, and interstitial haemorrhage can accompany these changes and precipitate graft failure (Fig. 34.5). Vascular necrosis is never uniform throughout the graft or even in the affected vessels. Degeneration and necrosis of graft parenchyma is also found. This may directly be due to the rejection, but in part is undoubtedly secondary to the ischaemia from the vascular lesions. In recipients treated with cyclosporin A, foamy fenestrated macrophages may be evident.

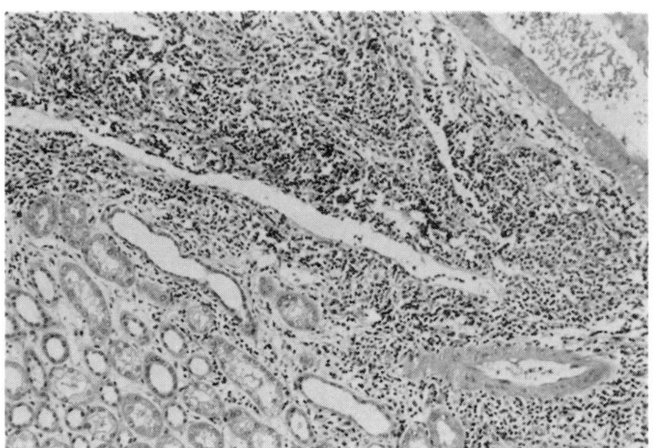

Fig. 34.4 Renal allograft biopsied as part of an investigation of impaired urinary output. Substantial numbers of mononuclear cells lie adjacent to interlobular arteries and veins and infiltrate the adjacent interstitial tissue. These cells are not evident in the walls of the arteries and there is no tubular necrosis or interstitial haemorrhage. The infiltrate should abate with increased immunosuppression and improved renal function follow. (HE × 160)

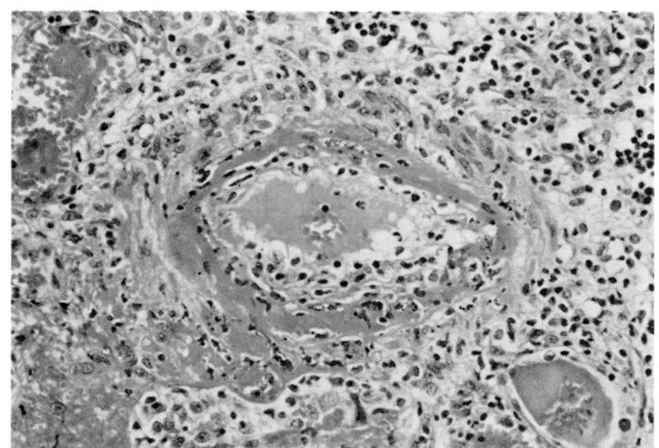

Fig. 34.5 Transverse section of interlobular artery in a renal allograft. Much of the media includes fibrinoid material with necrosis and small groups of neutrophil polymorphs. Mononuclear cells are present beneath parts of the intima and in the surrounding parenchyma where tubular atrophy (top right) and interstitial haemorrhage (bottom left) have occurred. These changes are characteristic of acute rejection, and are most unlikely to regress or repair with further immunosuppression. (HE × 350)

Chronic rejection

This is characterized by obliterative arterial lesions. A progressively worsening pattern occurs and within any graft there are a multiplicity of these changes which like those in acute rejection, are never uniform.

The arterial lumen is narrowed to a variable degree and, in contrast to atheroma, this is often concentric rather than the eccentric appearance characteristic of the latter condition (Fig. 34.6).

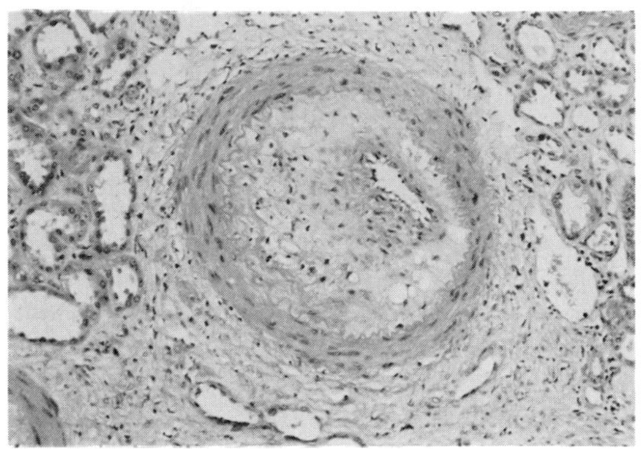

Fig. 34.6 Transverse section of an arcuate artery in a renal allograft. There is almost total obliteration of the lumen by cells and fibrous tissue. The internal elastic lamina is neither broken nor reduplicated and there are no infiltrating mononuclear cells. The appearance of this artery is characteristic of the late phase of chronic rejection. (HE × 180)

Cells cause the narrowing in its earlier stages, but later there is progressive fibrosis. Such cells include endothelial cells, smooth muscle cells and fibroblasts with platelets and fibrin enmeshed amongst them (Fig. 34.7). There can be mild to substantial infiltrates of mononuclear cells associated with some vessels. These cells are found in early lesions immediately beneath the endothelium which may be displaced (Fig. 34.8), but later in all parts of the vessel wall. Mononuclear cells, particularly in severely fibrotic vessels, can be absent. An additional feature in some vessels is single or multiple breaks in the internal elastic lamina (Fig. 34.8). There is never a marked increase in the elastic tissue analogous to that in hypertension or arteriosclerosis, nor are there cholesterol clefts, the hallmark of atheroma. The media can exhibit degenerative changes associated with fat-laden cells and focal fibrosis.

Vessels involved in these obliterative processes will produce ischaemia and when this is a gradual process the tissues supplied will undergo atrophy and gradual fibrosis. Since a scattering of mononuclear cells is sometimes observed, rejection and ischaemia probably both contribute to the fibrosis. In some grafts these chronic rejection changes will show superimposed acute rejection changes.

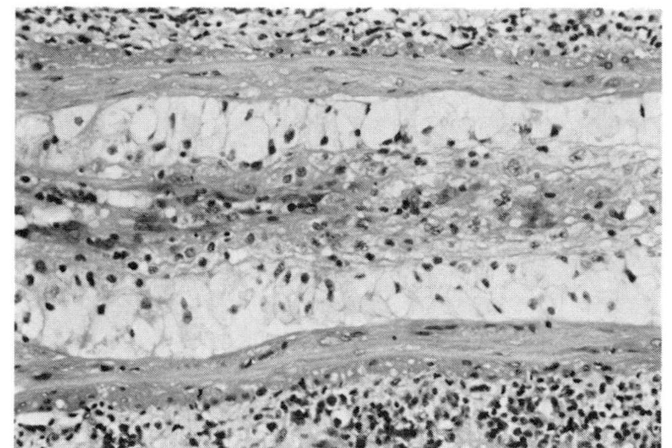

Fig. 34.7 Longitudinal section of an arcuate artery in a renal allograft. The lumen appears obliterated and there is substantial intimal thickening. The luminal portion of this includes mainly large and small mononuclear cells and the outer part large fat-ladened cells. Within the adventitia are substantial numbers of mononuclear cells. The arterial change is that of an early phase of chronic rejection and in this allograft this is accompanied by substantial cellular rejection. Increased immunosuppression would be unlikely to result in a dramatic improvement in renal function. (HE × 350)

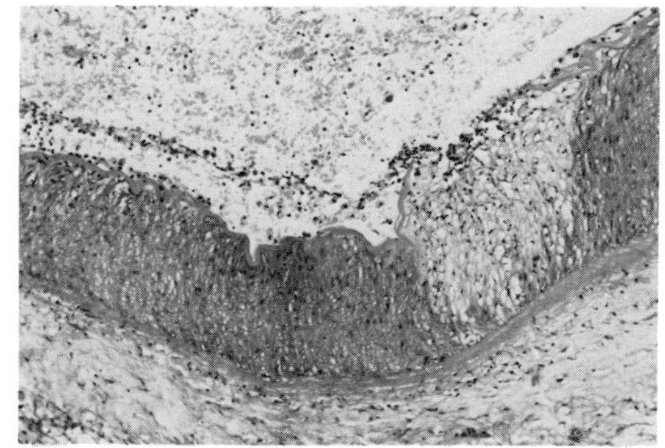

Fig. 34.8 Part of the wall of a hilar artery in a renal allograft. The intima has separated from the internal elastic lamina and between the two are mononuclear cells. The internal elastic lamina is fractured on the right side and the media beneath is degenerate and infiltrated by a few mononuclear cells. The changes indicate a poor outlook for the allograft, even with increased immunosuppression. (HE × 160)

Clinical transplants

Descriptions of human allografts are derived from graft biopsies, removed grafts and descriptions of autopsy specimens. Biopsies always raise the question of whether the specimen is representative or not. Many studies comparing biopsy and whole organ appearances indicate that they invariably are, especially if multiple levels of the tissue are examined. This procedure is most important because of the random and focal nature of rejection changes. Fibrinoid necrosis of vessels in renal allograft biopsies may only appear in one level and it is a finding of crucial prognostic and therapeutic importance. Grafts removed surgically and those obtained at autopsy while demonstrating rejection features will inevitably also include sequelae of other events. This will be particularly so with renal transplants, where a period of dialysis may have occurred prior to transplant nephrectomy and to pancreatic grafts which have been abandoned and supplemented by insulin. Comparative cardiac and liver transplants, lacking artificial means of replacement, may manifest changes of rejection more closely.

Renal and cardiac transplant biopsies undoubtedly have a place in patient management. Rejection can be recognized and attempts to halt this reaction instituted. Often, however, the changes indicate irreversible damage and result in graft destruction. If features could be identified before these changes had developed, hopefully the implementation of increased immunosuppression might halt the progression of rejection and improve graft survival. The urgent need for such a method is highlighted by the number of kidneys lost from rejection (Fig. 34.9). Recent progress towards this goal may come from fine-needle aspiration studies allied with monoclonal antibodies to T-cell sub-sets. This technique can be performed daily, whereas needle biopsies cannot. The preparation of these specimens is also straightforward and potentially the surgeon is offered information more quickly than from a formal biopsy.

Renal allografts

Rejection of renal allografts is the main reason for graft loss (Fig. 34.9) and an important underlying cause of patient death. Its clinical recognition has defied precise definition and no laboratory test or group of tests has received universal acceptance. Many centres rely upon biopsy appearances to recognize rejection, but the surgeon may also have

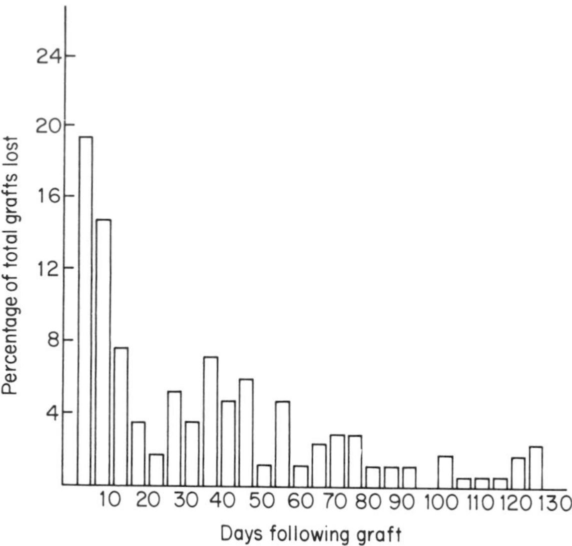

Fig. 34.9 Distribution of the day of rejection in 170 first cadaveric grafts. (Reproduced by kind permission of Dr B.A. Bradley, UK Transplant Service, Bristol.) Each block represents percentage of total lost during a 5-day period. Note the bimodality around 25–30-day point.

to decide for himself from the graft's macroscopic features.

Macroscopic appearances

These will be influenced by the type of rejection, the occurrence of repeated similar events during the life history of the graft and by factors unassociated with rejection. Kidneys from donors of all ages will hypertrophy and this will inevitably follow when one kidney replaces the function of two. Urinary tract infection is a complication after transplantation that can result in parenchymal infection of the graft and may also lead to papillary necrosis. Cortical scarring may also be a long-term result, but age changes and hypertension occurring in the donor or the recipient will have the same effect. In a graft with multiple renal arteries, a polar infarct may follow occlusion of a small artery and result in a large focal scar. If tumour is inadvertently transplanted within the kidney, nodules or diffuse infiltrates of this may be evident.

Hyperacute rejection follows within seconds of releasing the vascular clamps and the surgeon is faced with a uniformly flabby cyanotic graft. The anastomoses are patent and there is no improvement after intravenous heparin. Such a graft should be removed immediately. If it is left in situ, necrosis and widespread thrombosis will develop.

Acute and chronic rejection have no precise macroscopic counterparts. Both reactions are often complicated by infarction. Multiple small infarcts may have followed acute rejection, but in some allografts this reaction leads to an almost uniform cortical necrosis.

Nevertheless, three principal macroscopic forms of renal allografts can be distinguished and serve as a guideline to the surgeon.

A large pale kidney. This mimics that seen in some renal disorders. The graft has a uniform appearance and there are no other parenchymal changes. Oedema and a mononuclear cell infiltrate of variable intensity are the principal underlying features. In the absence of other irreversible factors contributing to renal dysfunction, this appearance can be regarded as potentially compatible with graft survival.

A large haemorrhagic kidney. The enlargement is uniform. The haemorrhage is both old and recent, occupying variably sized zones and is scattered haphazardly over the surface. There are comparable features in the parenchyma which is extremely friable. The pelvis and ureter include similar haemorrhage. Many vessels of all sizes include fibrinoid necrosis with and without obliterative vascular changes. Inevitable deterioration in renal function is the usual outcome even with increased immunosuppression.

A small scarred kidney. The size of these grafts approximates more closely to those of normal kidneys and may even be smaller. The kidney is pale. The scars are of variable depth and randomly distributed over the surface. The parenchyma will be similarly reduced and is tough with blurring of cortex and medulla. Deformities of the calyces and pelvis as well as narrowing of the ureteric and vascular anastomoses can occur. Changes of chronic rejection and fibrosis with or without glomerular lesions are found and they are generally associated with renal failure. The changes will be progressive and irreversible, but it is difficult to predict with any confidence the remaining life span to the graft. This type of graft is most often found in long-term recipients.

Biopsy appearances and microscopic features

Transplants from cadavers and live donors are most prone to rejection within the first 3 months after grafting (Fig. 34.9). Those from cadaver donors inevitably experience ischaemia prior to revascularization which can contribute to renal dysfunction and thereby make rejection more difficult to recognize at this time. Poor graft function associated with residual function from the recipient's own kidneys can also provide diagnostic difficulty at any stage. Renal allograft biopsy is thus indicated in the immediate postoperative period if the graft has failed to function or if the function is inadequate. Thereafter, biopsy forms part of the investigation of diminishing graft function and of patients subjected to increased immunosuppression but in whom there is no subsequent improvement in renal function.

Mononuclear cells occur in acute and chronic rejection and are invariably present in any biopsy (Fig. 34.4). If these are few and no vascular lesions are present, there will be no long-term deleterious effect. If renal function is impaired, however, an increase in immunosuppression may correct this, but without impaired renal function no change in immunosuppression is indicated.

Mononuclear cells adhering to the arterial endothelium or lying immediately beneath it may not be associated with good long-term graft function, particularly if these cells are in substantial numbers (Fig. 34.8). In these circumstances, the rejection process may progress even with increased immunosuppression and fibrinoid necrosis and obliterative lesions develop. A large proportion of cytotoxic/suppressor T-lymphocytes and lysozyme-positive macrophages also indicates a poor short-term prognosis for the graft.

Vascular changes of all types equate with a shortened life span for the graft and it is unusual for these to be reversed by increased immunosuppression. In particular fibrinoid necrosis, even if limited to a single vessel within a biopsy, is associated with an early onset of renal failure (Fig. 34.5). If this is found with interstitial haemorrhage and/or glomerular lesions, an even more rapid onset of renal failure develops and the graft will have ceased to function within one year and generally much sooner.

Obliterative vascular lesions (Figs. 34.6 and 34.7) will ultimately result in renal failure, but this often progresses slowly especially if unassociated with acute vascular changes and substantial numbers of mononuclear cells. The changes are patchy and focal and predominantly affect arcuate and interlobular vessels, but may also involve the large hilar vessels, sometimes exclusively. A similar spectrum of venous changes to those in the arteries occurs. Venous thrombosis and even mild obliterative changes are of little importance, probably because of the multitude of intrarenal venous anastomoses.

Tubules will manifest some degree of necrosis and regeneration in the early postoperative stages in most cadaver and even in some live donor grafts (Fig. 34.10). These changes are related to the ischaemic interval between removal of the donor organ and reperfusion, but no histological features have been correlated with the anuric or oliguric interval in the recipient. Tubular necrosis after the immediate postoperative interval accompanies acute rejection episodes, but may also complicate septicaemias and anastomotic complications. Atrophy and disappearance of tubules contribute substantially to the appearance of the small scarred kidney and to poor long-term renal function.

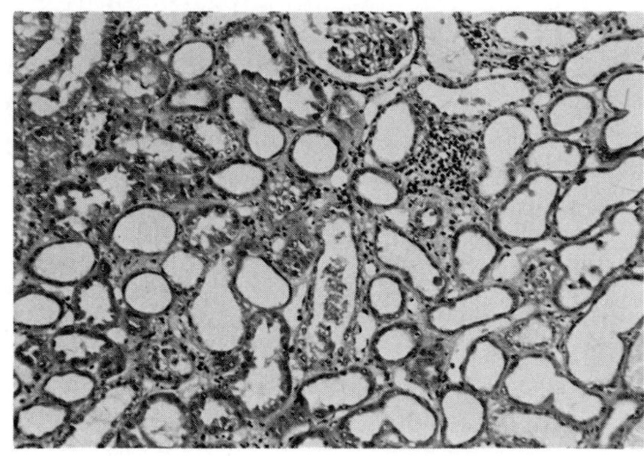

Fig. 34.10 Biopsy of a renal allograft with poor function. The majority of tubules have a very flattened epithelium and amongst some epithelial cells there is a pleomorphism of the nuclei. A few tubules (top left) are clearly proximal and all are separated by oedema. A small focus of mononuclear cells lies above a normal interlobular artery. The glomerulus includes no abnormality. There is no evidence of rejection and the features are those of recovering tubular necrosis. (HE × 350)

The interstitium of the graft can include oedema, haemorrhage and fibrosis. Oedema is manifest by separation of tubules (Fig. 34.10). The haemorrhage found in swollen haemorrhagic kidneys can be almost uniform. Because of the difficulty in adequately clearing this from the graft and also because it is most often associated with fibrinoid necrosis, haemorrhage is a bad prognostic finding. Fibrosis may develop in previous areas of haemorrhage, old infarcts or following tubular necrosis or loss. It will also develop in areas of ischaemia supplied by vessels with obliterative lesions and may be regarded as an end-stage change in the graft's life span.

Glomerular changes in allografts pose a difficult problem in interpretation. The glomerular thrombosis and necrosis of hyperacute and acute rejection are undoubtedly due to rejection. Mesangial increase, basement membrane thickening, focal and diffuse shrinkage and fibrosis of lobules and tufts, are other changes attributed to rejection, but ischaemia may also be an important contributory factor. These changes, in contrast to those of glomerulonephritis, never affect all the glomeruli uniformly and never show any consistent immunofluorescent localization of IgG, IgM or complement. Ultrastructurally, there is invariably widening of parts of the basement membrane associated with an accumulation of finely granular or even luscent material beneath the endothelium. An increase in mesangial matrix, often with sclerosis, accompanies these changes as does some fusion of epithelial cell foot processes.

Glomerulonephritis

Glomerulonephritis can develop in renal allografts and can manifest the same patterns found in the non-transplanted kidney. The uncertainty in making such a diagnosis arises because of the possibility of rejection simulating these changes as well as other factors including reflux, hypertension, viruses and some immunosuppressants. Glomeruli can only respond in a limited number of ways to any insult so that the effect of any of these different agents may be to mimic one another. The observation that glomerular immunoglobulin deposition can vary at different times in the life history of a graft and that in single examples of grafts differing patterns of glomerulonephritis can appear at varying intervals, are other reasons for caution before labelling a graft as involved by glomerulonephritis.

Donor kidneys harbouring glomerulonephritis have inadvertently been transplanted, but in most patients the disorder may develop spontaneously or may be transmitted from the host. The early report of glomerulonephritis in human renal isografts made it possible that recurrence in the graft would be a common cause of allograft failure. Fortunately, this fear has not been sustained. The true incidence of the complication remains unknown, but estimates vary between 5 and 48 per cent. In part, these extremes can be accounted for by the different authors' variations in terminology and by the amount of effort made to distinguish between de novo and recurrent glomerulonephritis. Strict similarity between light and electron microscopy appearances in host and grafted kidneys and between immunofluorescent and serological findings, are necessary to diagnose recurrent glomerulonephritis. However, if the recipient's kidneys are truly end-stage such a comparison may not be possible. Ultimate distinction between de novo and recurrent glomerulonephritis must await recognition of the antigens involved in glomerulonephritis. To date, only the antigens of cytomegalovirus, hepatitis B and ALG have been firmly identified with a very few examples of graft glomerulonephritis. In Table 34.4 an indication of the possibility of recurrent glomerulonephritis occurring, as well as the types of renal disorders that have been reported in renal allografts, are presented.

Table 34.4 Recurrent and de novo glomerulonephritis (GN) and other conditions diagnosed in renal allografts.

Commonly recurrent	Focal GN Mesangiocapillary (dense deposit type) GN IgA nephropathy Oxalosis Cystinosis
Uncertain frequency	Mesangiocapillary (Type 1) GN Anti-basement membrane disease (glomerular and tubular) Amyloid Diabetic glomerulopathy Progressive systemic sclerosis
Rarely recurrent	Membranous GN Idiopathic crescentic GN Henoch–Schonlein GN Haemolytic uraemic syndrome Malignant hypertension Renal Fanconi syndrome

Non-immunological causes of failure or impairment of renal allograft function

Most of the causes of renal graft failure or deteriorating function have few specific histological features and are detailed in Table 34.5. Some of these are amenable to surgical correction and biopsies are therefore invaluable in excluding rejection, so avoiding the disastrous consequences of over-immunosuppression. Biopsy of the revascularized kidney may reveal a pre-existing disorder in the donor organ such as glomerulonephritis or diabetic glomerulosclerosis. Although rare, failure of preservation may be diagnosed on biopsy when endothelial disruption and fibrin deposition in glomerular capillaries are seen.

Table 34.5 Non-immunological causes of renal allograft failure.

Abnormalities within the kidney prior to transplantation
(a) Glomerulonephritis
(b) Glomerulosclerosis (e.g. diabetes, hypertension)
(c) Infection
(d) Tumours
(e) Failure of preservation
(f) Acute tubular necrosis

Vascular complications
(a) Thrombosis – arterial
– venous
(b) Arterial stenosis – anastamotic
– atheromatous

External compression
(a) Lymphocele
(b) Abscess
(c) Haematoma

Ureteric complications
(a) Ureteric slough } associated with thrombosis
(b) Ureteric stenosis } of lower polar artery
(c) "Granuloma" of ureteroneocystostomy – role of fungi

"Spontaneous" rupture of kidney
(a) Associated with rejection and/or biopsy

Tubular changes associated with necrosis have been discussed.

Hepatic allografts

The major complication of liver transplantation has been leakage associated with the biliary anastomoses. Careful pre-implantation perfusion of the extrahepatic biliary tree has reduced these complications, particularly bile sludging, but leakage and fistulae with secondary infection still occur and contribute substantially to mortality.

Rejection can occur, but is not the problem encountered in renal transplantation. This is despite the rarity of close HLA matching and has been associated with less surface MHC antigen on hepatocytes than kidney cells and a greater resistance of liver cells than kidney cells to in vitro killing by allogeneic lymphocytes. The mass of the liver, its metabolic functions and alterations to Kuppfer cells during preservation, may also be involved. Rejection is manifest by alterations in liver function tests especially rises in serum bilirubin and alkaline phosphatase levels. The contribution of allograft biopsy in diagnosing rejection is less than that in renal transplantation. In part this is because interpretation is difficult, particularly if there are any complications in the extrahepatic biliary tree, but also the mild nature of the process make its recognition difficult. The drugs used in immunosuppression and the infections encountered by these patients will also induce not dissimilar changes.

Grafted livers removed at autopsy have been of normal size or enlarged. Their appearances have been modified by biliary fistulae producing bile stasis and local infections with adhesions and abscesses. Infarction of large areas complicated early grafts and was due to an inadequate anchorage of the liver and, sometimes, hepatic artery thrombosis. Microscopically, if rejection is present, mononuclear cells, vascular lesions and liver cell destruction are found together with some cholestasis and fibrosis. The cells first appear in portal tracts and later in sinusoids and around central veins. Obliterative vascular lesions occur and are common in the long-term grafts, but even in these are not invariably present. Fibrinoid necrosis of arteries is a very rare lesion. Destruction of the parenchyma is never uniform or severe and is mainly seen as scattered foci in the lobules and around central veins. The cholestasis is centrilobular and bile appears in liver and Kuppfer cells. Fibrosis has not progressed to cirrhosis and has been confined to the portal tracts. A lesion simulating primary biliary cirrhosis with destruction of duct walls and eventual disappearance of the ducts has rarely occurred, but in most grafts only bile plugging is found. The rarity of complement and immunoglobulin deposits, which are mainly IgG, in any of these lesions is evidence that the rejection is mainly cell-mediated, and will thus respond to pulse therapy with steroids.

Tumours have recurred or metastasized to the grafts in a few patients operated upon for malignancy, and recurrent hepatitis has also been a complication. Where the liver has been the seat of a metabolic disorder, this has been corrected and no evidence of the disease found in the transplant. To date, Wilson's disease, alpha-1-antitrypsin deficiency and Niemann–Pick disease, are examples in this category. It is claimed that primary biliary cirrhosis has recurred, but this is considered unproven even though mitochondrial antibodies persist.

Cardiac allografts

Rejection continues to be a major factor in the mortality from this form of transplantation. Ninety per cent of recipients will experience acute rejection episodes in the first 8–12 postoperatives weeks and all will receive greater amounts of immunosuppression than patients with other types of grafts. A greater endothelial and class II antigen positive cell complement than in other grafts and the substantial humoral response evoked might be the underlying cause. The penalty is a high rate of infection which is the major cause of death. Just over one third of the patients surviving the initial period will have severe obliterative vascular lesions in coronary arteries within 5 years, necessitating retransplantation or resulting in death. The effect of rejection upon the myocardium is to reduce its compliance and contractility, and on the vessels to induce parenchymal ischaemia. Involvement of the conduction system leads to arrhythmias. Although all of these effects can be associated with ECG changes these, like alterations in transaminase levels and changes in circulating T-cells, have shown no changes diagnostic for rejection nor produced changes heralding this reaction. Cardiac biopsies at weekly intervals during the initial 2 months after transplantation have demonstrated rejection which can precede functional changes. Such biopsies should be taken from several sites within the right ventricle. Occasional complications include periods of temporary arrhythmia and pneumothorax. Biopsy is useful to confirm rejection when this is clinically recognized and to assess the effectiveness of anti-rejection therapy.

Rejection contributes to generalized cardiac enlargement and right ventricular dilatation. When this is acute, congestion, oedema and focal haemorrhage occur and these are most marked subendocardially. Fibrosis may also be recognized in long-term grafts, and vessels within these may be markedly narrowed. Thrombus is not a feature either on the anastomoses or on the endocardium or within the coronary arteries. Fibrinous pericarditis and fibrous pericardial adhesions are invariably found.

Rejection changes occur throughout the transplanted heart with a sharp cut-off at places of contact between the donor and recipient organs. The myocardial and vascular features mirror those in human renal allografts, although deposits of immunoglobulin and complement are almost invariably seen. Possibly due to its vascularity, mononuclear cells infiltrate the conduction system in greater numbers than other parts of the heart. The valves manifest little change other than mild oedema. The obliterative vascular changes affect the muscular arteries and are most severe in the first portions of their intramyocardial branches. The concentric nature of these lesions and the absence of cholesterol clefts, differentiate them from atherosclerosis, but even with the most careful donor selection atheroma may have developed prior to transplantation.

Pancreatic allografts

The stimulus for clinical pancreatic transplantation is the cure of diabetes mellitus and amelioration or prevention of its invidious complications. Islet replacement alone is the ideal therapy, but it has proved impossible to date to transplant a sufficient number of viable islets. Auxillary segmental pancreatic grafts with or without duct obliteration are currently transplanted. Injection of a polymer is used to block the duct. In either circumstance, the pancreatic exocrine tissue will atrophy and fibrose making the transplant unsuitable for patients suffering from combined endocrine and exocrine failure. The long-term effects of this to the diabetic may not be so gloomy as is presently predicted, since similar fibrosis develops in chronic pancreatitis and is not invariably associated with diabetes. The exocrine function of the recipient's pancreas is unaffected by the auxillary graft. Such grafts have secreted insulin for periods of over a year and have possibly halted the progression of the recipient arteriopathy and renal lesions. Their use has mainly been confined to diabetics with severe complications and a preceding, concurrent or later renal transplant is usually necessary. Opinions have differed as to whether pancreatic tissue is more avidly rejected than other tissues, but clinical experience suggests that this is not so. Pancreatic rejection is difficult to recognize and can occur in the absence or presence of renal allograft rejection and vice versa. There are no specific diagnostic tests for this reaction but rises in amylase and blood sugar and falls in blood insulin and C-peptide levels occur. Substantial damage to beta-cells may have resulted before some of these changes are detected. The influence of tissue typing on pancreatic rejection awaits further study.

Descriptions of rejected grafts are either of autopsy specimens or of pancreases removed at a considerable time after the episode, since if the graft fails the patient is sustained with insulin. Grafts that have failed have often been associated with fistulae, abscesses and leakage of pancreatic juice further complicated by infection. Features of these events and fibrosis with acute inflammatory and mononuclear cell infiltrates are found, but islets may not always be affected. Vascular changes unassociated with inflammatory lesions have not been reported.

Systemic changes

The organ disorder, the treatment it necessitated and the complications arising from it will all produce tissue changes prior to transplantation. After transplantation all or some of these lesions may persist or recur and the administration of non-specific immunosuppression leads to infection and possibly tumours. It is therefore obvious that a wide range of organ changes can be anticipated in any transplant recipient. All of these cannot be discussed and mention will be made only of those which contribute to morbidity and mortality and are common to recipients of all types of graft.

Infection

Infection is the major cause of death in patients dying after transplantation and most patients will experience infection during their early postoperative period. Infective episodes, especially viral, have been cited as precipitating rejection, but conclusive proof is lacking. All immunosuppressive agents contribute towards infection, but high doses of steroids are particularly incriminated and splenectomy is associated with infection from capsular bacteria. Leucopenia results from azathioprine therapy, and a white cell count below 2000 per cm^3 is a potent risk factor.

A very wide variety of bacteria, fungi and viruses, as well as many protozoa, have been recognized at some time in many patients (Table 34.6). Frequently more than one species of organism is present and invariably at death many tissues are affected. As many as 50 per cent of the patients may have viral infections which are principally of the herpes groups and amongst which cytomegalovirus is the predominant organism. This and the other viruses are not usually fatal, but fulminant lethal cases do occur, especially when in combination with other microorganisms. Since many of the organisms are endogenous, it is important to screen the patient for potential reservoirs prior to transplantation.

Tumours

Unusual tumours and increased numbers of all tumours appear in transplant patients. Although the greatest experience of these has been amongst renal allograft recipients, recipients of all grafts have been affected, especially those with cardiac grafts. Tumour cells may be inadvertently transplanted with the graft or develop after transplantation. Grafts have also been performed in recipients with pre-existing tumours. Any of these circumstances can result in rapid tumour dissemination, but if either immunosuppression is reduced or stopped and/or the graft removed, regression and disappearance can follow. There is no satisfactory explanation for any of these findings and the contribution of sustained allogenic stimulation, immunosuppression, immunosuppressive agents and chronic infections, have all been implicated. The potential role of the herpes viruses is of current concern, but in other patients environmental factors are important. The Epstein–Barr virus has been associated with some lymphomas and the cytomegalovirus with Kaposi's sarcoma. Both of these viruses and tumours occur in transplant patients. Squamous cell carcinomas of the skin are common in people exposed to sunlight, but are even more frequent and aggressive amongst those who also have a transplant. They are also commoner than basal cell tumours in comparison with control populations. Environmental factors may initiate the tumour, but transplantation seems to stimulate its growth.

The transfer of tumour to the transplant recipient can be avoided by not using donors with any present or past malignancy. Donors with primary cerebral tumours are exceptions, but these tumours should be biopsied to rule out the possibility of metastasis. Recipients who have had a malignant neoplasm should not be transplanted for at least one year following tumour excision and during this period the patient must also be free of metastases. Fifty per cent of patients will develop metastases during this interval, but if the kidney or renal tract was the site of the primary and it was asymptomatic, recurrence after transplantation is unlikely.

Tumours may develop at any time after transplantation, but the risk increases with graft survival. Patients without cancer are twice as likely to reject their graft or develop infection as those with cancer. The overall incidence of tumours is 2–7 per cent with an 8 per cent incidence amongst cardiac patients, giving an incidence 100 times that of the general population. However, over a third of the tumours are low-grade, i.e. skin tumours and intraepithelial cervical cancer, and only 1 per cent of the afflicted patients die from their tumour.

Table 34.6 Examples of microorganisms complicating organ transplants with general, and some specific, aids to recognition.

General aids	*Microorganism*	*Specific aids*
BACTERIA		
Gram preparations	*Gram-positive*	
Blood and neutral	Staphlococci	
agar features	Listeria monocytogenes	
	Gram-negative	Sugar fermentation tests
	Escherichia coli	
	Enterobacter	
	Pseudomonas	
	Klebsiella	
	Proteus	
	Mycobacteria	Ziehl-Neelsen preparations
		Löwenstein's medium features
		Guinea pig inoculation
ACTINOMYCETES		
Gram preparations	Actinomyces	
Blood–brain–heart	Nocardia	
infusion agar features		
FUNGI		
Sabouraud's glucose	Aspergillus	PAS/Silver stained preparations
agar features	Candida	India ink preparations
	Cryptococcus	Giemsa preparations
	Histoplasma	
VIRUSES		
Tissue culture features	Herpes simplex	
Rising antibody titre	Herpes zoster	
Electron microscopy	Cytomegalovirus	Tissue inclusions
	Hepatitis B	Antigenaemia
PROTOZOA		
Rising antibody titre	Toxoplasma	Sabin–Feldman dye exclusion test
		Mouse inoculation
	Pneumocystis carinii	PAS/silver stained bronchial
		brushings/lung tissue
		Electron microscopy

Lymphomas, including Kaposi's sarcoma, constitute over one third of the tumours occurring in transplant recipients, but only a few of these are of the Hodgkin's type. In the general population, the incidence of lymphomas is 3–4 per cent and cerebral involvement is almost unknown. Amongst transplant recipients, however, 87 per cent of lymphomas are confined to the brain. The lymphoma is classified as immunoblastic and in the brain often occupies several different sites. Sex chromatin and HLA studies have shown that the malignant cells are of host origin. There may be an increased risk of this tumour when cyclosporin A is administered either in high dosage or in combination with other agents such as ALG.

When Kaposi's sarcoma has appeared it has been manifest both as the benign cutaneous form and as the malignant systemic form. The latter is an unusual finding outside Africa and the incidence of the sarcoma amongst all of the tumours in transplant patients is 3.2 per cent compared with 0.6 per cent for similar tumours in the USA.

Further reading

Bieber CP, Stinson EB, Shumway NE, Payne R, Kosek J. Cardiac transplantation in man. VII. Cardiac allograft pathology. *Circulation* 1970; **41**: 753–72.

Bradley BA, Selwood NH. The natural history of the transplantable kidneys. *Health Trends* 1983; **15**: 25–28.

Calne RY (ed.). *Clinical Organ Transplantation*, Oxford and Cambridge: Blackwell Scientific Publications, 1971.

Herbertson BM. The morphology of allograft reactions. In: *Immunological Aspects of Transplantation Surgery*. Ed. by RY Calne. Chapter 1, 4–38. Medical and Technical Publishing Co. Ltd, 1973.

Herbertson BM, Evans DB, Calne RY, Banerjee AK. Percutaneous needle biopsies of renal allografts: the relationship between morphological changes present in biopsies and subsequent allograft function. *Histopathology* 1977; **1**: 161–78.

Matas AJ, Sibley R, Mauer M, Sutherland DER, Simmons RL, Najarian JS. The value of needle renal allograft biopsy. I. A retrospective study of biopsies performed during putative rejection episodes. *Annals of Surgery* 1983; **197**: 226–37.

Morris PJ (ed.). *Tissue Transplantation. Clinical Surgery International*, Vol. 3. London and Edinburgh: Churchill Livingstone, 1982.

Penn I. Tumours arising in organ transplant recipients. *Advances in Cancer Research* 1978; **28**: 31–61.

Porter K A. Clinical renal transplantation. *International Review Experimental Pathology* 1972; **11**: 73–176.

35

Shock

O N Tubbs, H B Stoner and H Thompson

Introduction

Shock is essentially a functional disorder with few structural changes. The term is deeply engrained in surgical practice but it is difficult to define accurately and would be better avoided. Of the many available definitions of shock we will define it as "a condition due to loss of fluid in which the circulating blood volume is insufficient for the tissues which it perfuses; it is characterized by tachycardia, hypotension, a cold damp pale skin, rapid shallow breathing, a low output of urine and a metabolic acidosis". This limits the description to what is commonly called "surgical shock" and does not include septic shock, cardiogenic shock or psychogenic shock. It is, therefore, a potentially terminal state, which some have termed "necrobiosis", and which follows the body's defence against injury. The common causes of surgical shock are haemorrhage, multiple injuries and fluid loss from burns.

From the clinical point of view it is useful to think of two clinical phases in shock. The first phase is the direct response to fluid loss in which there are no morbid anatomical changes; the second phase, if the patient survives, may be regarded as the complications due to persisting fluid deprivation in which there are definite histological changes. Adequate and rapid treatment of the early stages, notably by the arrest of haemorrhage and the replacement of fluid, will reduce the incidence of complications.

Initial assessment

The blood pressure starts to fall after about 30 per cent of the blood volume has been lost. In the active phase of bleeding, the physical methods of assessing the blood volume by indicator dilution techniques are least accurate; three clinical methods of estimating blood loss are available:

1. Clinical estimate from the knowledge of injuries sustained.
2. A visual estimate of external blood loss.
3. Clinical estimate from the cardiovascular response.

The clinical estimate from the cardiovascular response is a rough guide to the amount of blood lost from the circulation. In a previously healthy adult, the pulse rate will increase after a blood loss of around 1 litre, but the blood pressure will not start to fall until about 1.5 litres are lost. Hence, a hypotensive patient who regains a normal blood pressure after a 1-litre infusion may be said to have been 2.5 litres deficient and is still 1.5 litres deficient. The visual estimate of external blood loss is self-explanatory; clearly this may be unreliable. The clinical estimate from the injuries sustained is a method popularized by Ruscoe Clarke. The blood loss is estimated according to the injury and its severity; the average blood loss into the tissues associated with various fractures etc. is known (Fig. 35.1). This method is particularly useful when

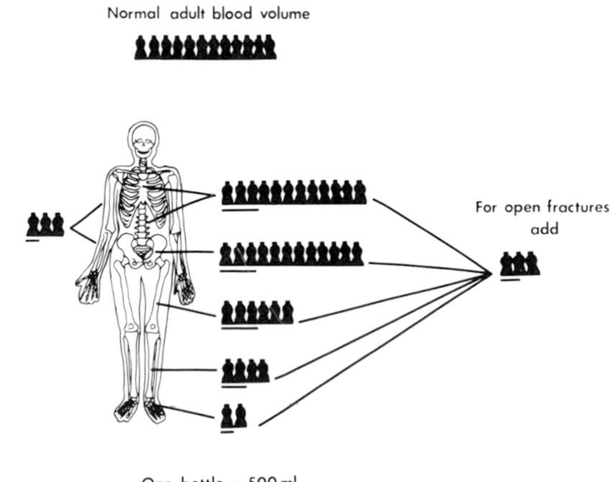

Fig. 35.1 Estimation of blood loss from a knowledge of the injuries sustained.

haemorrhage is complicated by tissue damage at the site of injury which may, by generating nociceptive afferent stimuli, interfere with normal homoeostatic responses to fluid loss.

At this stage the diagnosis is clinical. Shock may be taken as the failure of the body's defence against the injury. It is characrterized by a progressive reduction in oxygen transport and, in severe fluid loss, inevitably leads to death without, and sometimes with, vigorous treatment. With the latter, a proportion of severely injured patients may recover sufficiently to develop complications in the lungs, kidneys and elsewhere which may still prove fatal. To understand what is happening at this time it is necessary to look at the preceding events, when the body is still defending itself against the effects of injury.

Early neuroendocrine response to injury

The early general response to an injury is a neuroendocrine one and the main stimulus for it is loss of fluid from the vascular compartment. This loss may be whole blood, as in external or internal haemorrhage, or some fraction of the blood. After many injuries, the fluid lost into the tissues is close to plasma in its protein content. The presence of a higher than normal concentration of plasma protein in the interstitial fluid implies an increase in vascular permeability. There are two aspects to this change: very soon after an injury there is a local increase in venular permeability produced by endogenous mediators, followed by a further increase in permeability affecting a wide range of vessel types. This latter is quantitatively the more important, but its mechanisms are not fully understood. The two stages are well illustrated by burns. Although after burns the main fluid loss is similar to plasma, it is important to realize that there is also loss of erythrocytes, either through bleeding from the burn surface or from thermal damage to the red corpuscles. It should also be remembered that a local injury is not followed by any generalized change in vascular permeability in the uninjured parts of the body, except in the case of severe burns.

With this loss of circulating fluid there is a severity-related increase in the plasma concentrations of adrenaline and noradrenaline. The first is due to increased secretion by the adrenal medulla that will continue as long as there is a fluid deficit. The second is due to the increased activity of the sympathetic nervous system. The pharmacophysiological effect of this is a redistribution of the circulating blood volume from the "non-essential" organs such as skin to "essential" ones such as the brain and heart. This is manifest as a cold clammy skin. At this stage, fluid is being drawn into the vascular compartment from the interstitial space in the uninjured parts of the body.

Vasoconstriction, together with this redistribution of fluid, acccounts for the maintenance of the systolic blood pressure at clinically acceptable levels after considerable blood or plasma loss. Considerably more fluid input is needed to restore normovolaemia than might be expected from the degree of hypotension.

Metabolic changes

With the greater output of adrenaline and the increased sympathetic activity, there are striking metabolic changes which can be summarized as the mobilization of the stores of glycogen and fat. In this process, liver glycogen is broken down to glucose and released into the circulation. Glycogenolysis also occurs in muscle leading to the production of lactate which is carried in the blood stream to the liver to be converted to glucose in the Cori cycle. Gluconeogenesis and the release of glucose from the liver into the circulation continues after trauma, despite high concentrations of glucose in the plasma. Transient glycosuria is frequently found after severe injury. The vasopressin released from the posterior lobe of the pituitary at this stage is also involved in promoting liver glycogenolysis. Glycogenolysis liberates the water stored with the glycogen and thus helps combat the hypovolaemia. Some think that the increase in plasma osmolality brought about by high glucose concentrations also helps the inward movement of fluid from the extravascular space.

As a result, there are positive relationships between the severity of injury and the plasma lactate and glucose concentrations over the whole range of severity of injury, as measured by Baker's Injury Severity Score. Although lipolysis is increased by injury, the relationship between the plasma concentration of the non-esterified fatty acids (NEFA) produced and the severity of the injury is only a partial one. The concentration of NEFA in the plasma rises as the severity of the injury is increased from minor to moderate, but there is no further increase after severe injury. The NEFA concentration in the plasma after severe injuries is often quite low, although experimental work indicates that lipolysis would continue under these conditions. Since the transfer of NEFA from adipocyte to plasma depends on the presence of the carrier albumin, these relationships are thought to be due to decreased blood flow through the fat depots after severe injury.

Part of the circulating NEFA is taken up by the liver and converted to ketone bodies. These are released from the liver into the circulation to be extracted and oxidized elsewhere. There is a close relationship between the plasma concentrations of NEFA and ketone bodies in normal and injured man. It is this relationship which gives the illusion of two groups of injured patients, one with a high and the other with a low concentration of plasma ketone bodies, whereas the real separation is by severity, in which patients with very severe injuries have low NEFA and therefore low ketone body concentrations.

At this early stage after the injury the plasma contains adequate amounts of both fat and carbohydrate. However, after severe injury, despite the hyperglycaemia, fat is the preferred substrate for oxidation in the body. The total energy expenditure by these patients is very variable.

Activation of hypothalamus

There are widespread changes in the endocrine system of the injured patient. The hypothalamus is stimulated by the afferent information reaching it from many parts of the body and from within itself. One result is activation of the neurones which produce the hypothalamic releasing hormones which pass down in the pituitary portal system to the anterior hypophysis. An important hormone of this type is the corticotrophin releasing hormone which stimulates the release of adrenocorticotrophic hormone (ACTH) and β-endorphin. This leads in turn to the release of cortisol from the adrenal cortex. The cortisol concentration in the plasma rises in keeping with the severity of injury, at least up to injuries of moderate severity (Injury Severity Score <12). With more severe injuries the plasma cortisol concentration does not rise further but tends to fall. As there seems to be no shortage of ACTH in these severely injured patients, the most likely explanation for this difference in response is a fall in the circulation through the adrenal cortex. It is also of interest that the cortisol concentration in the plasma of injured patients is never very high, certainly not as high as when the gland is maximally stimulated by exogenous ACTH.

Important changes occur in the posterior lobe of the pituitary as a result of stimulation of the paraventricular and supraoptic nuclei of the hypothalamus which leads to the release of vasopressin and neurophysin from the posterior lobe.

In man, other seemingly less important changes in hormones occur as, for example, the increased secretion of growth hormone and prolactin. The functional role of these hormones in the response to injury is not known.

From the time of John Hunter, the changes provoked in the body by injury have been thought to be defensive. Of course, when Hunter put forward this idea knowledge of the changes occurring in the body was very much less than today; nevertheless it is still possible to develop an argument in favour of the Hunterian view. At the same time, Hunter's hypothesis cannot be considered as proved, particularly for the patient receiving full modern treatment.

Accepting an element of defence in the neuroendocrine response of the early period after injury, this can fail in two circumstances: the trauma may be overwhelming or the treatment may be insufficiently vigorous so that changes such as hypotension and vasoconstriction persist for long periods. As will be shown later, these changes can lead to structural changes. In both cases the essential feature of failure is the decline of oxygen transport leading to progressive organ failure. When the trauma is overwhelming, this is reflected in the very high, rising plasma lactate concentrations and by a shift in redox state in the direction of reduction in the cytoplasm and mitochondria. As these changes get worse and the flow through the tissues deteriorates, death will ultimately occur from respiratory failure. This course of events will be seen in the patient who is being ineffectually treated. In those patients a number of contributory factors can be identified.

Although some features of the response, particularly the stimulation of the endocrine system, may be set in motion by nociceptive afferent impulses, these same impulses may also inhibit homoeostatic cardiovascular and thermoregulatory reflexes in ways that at first sight would appear to be deleterious.

Toxic factors may also be invoked and at this stage the most important ones are probably particulate, the small clots of "sludged" blood, fat emboli and the like which will be filtered off by the lungs leading to vascular damage and interstitial pulmonary oedema.

Once these metabolic changes have begun they seem to run their course irrespective of treatment. After a severe injury, hyperglycaemia, for instance, will persist for 24 hours. Rapid, early restoration of the circulating fluid volume will, however, influence those changes, such as a continuously increasing plasma lactate concentration, which are related to tissue hypoxia. It would also be expected to improve matters where the changes are due to poor tissue perfusion. For this reason the early diagnosis and assessment of the amount of fluid lost is important.

Monitoring the pulse rate, blood pressure and trends in central venous pressure will indicate whether fluid replacement is sufficient, except in myocardial trauma, if it is remembered that there has been redistribution of fluid from the extravascular to the intravascular system; time must be allowed for the reversal to occur.

Early haematological changes

Many of the changes in the blood cells occur relatively early and are a direct result of untreated blood loss. Stored platelets and leucocytes are released into the blood. Rouleaux may form in the general circulation and microthrombi ("sludged" blood) will be produced as blood passes through areas of tissue damage, thus embarassing the circulation further.

Injury leads to extensive changes in the proteolytic enzyme cascades of the plasma with the activation of the coagulation, fibrinolysis, kinin and complement systems. Hageman factor is important here, but both intrinsic and extrinsic clotting mechanisms are activated as well as both the classical and alternative pathways of complement. Changes in the protease inhibitors in the plasma also occur in injured patients and may play an important part. After serious injuries, the overall effect is a decrease in the availability of these substances and for some factors a positive relationship between their depletion and the severity of injury has been demonstrated. After severe injuries, therapeutic replacement of some of these factors may be required.

Early treatment

In the very early phase, arrest of haemorrhage, fluid replacement and early treatment of coexisting injuries (to bones and abdominal organs, etc.) are all prime requirements. Whole blood is the logical replacement fluid for blood loss, but even this has been questioned. It has been argued that blood would flow better with an haematocrit below normal. Although O-negative blood can be used at once for very severe haemorrhage, in most patients, as cross-matched blood is not instantly available, other fluids are used initially which will incidentally lower the haematocrit and may improve the flow. The three categories of fluid readily available are:

1. Plasma and plasma fractions.
2. Colloidal plasma substitutes.
3. Electrolyte solutions (commonly called "crystalloids").

All have their advantages and disadvantages. Fresh frozen plasma and reconstituted plasma are relatively expensive and may occasionally contain hepatitis virus, but are very similar to the plasma which has been lost. Plasma protein fraction is expensive but exerts the appropriate colloid osmotic pressure.

Many colloidal plasma substitutes have been used in the past. At present there are three main classes depending upon whether they are based on polyglucose (dextran), hydroxyethylstarch or gelatin.

Several dextran preparations of different molecular weight are available. While modern dextran preparations do not cause the allergic reactions and impairment of haemostasis encountered with the early samples, both Dextran 70 and Dextran 40 are more viscous (× 4) than the plasma proteins and for this reason may impair renal function. The combination of rapid glomerular filtration of low molecular weight dextran and tubular reabsorption of water may lead to a high concentration of dextran in the tubules. Dextran 40 is contraindicated in dehydrated patients. The higher dextrans persist longer in the circulation than Dextran 40 which is rapidly eliminated.

Hydroxyethylstarch behaves like Dextran 70 and has similar effects on haemostasis. Many advantages have been claimed for the modern gelatin plasma substitutes such as Haemaccel (polygeline) and Plasmagel. These preparations are pharmacologically inert and are without effect on haemostasis or renal function. The molecular weight of the gelatin preparations is less than Dextran 70 and they are more rapidly eliminated from the circulation. The most rapidly eliminated are of course the various electrolyte solutions—0.9 per cent NaCl, Ringer-lactate solution, Hartmann's solution—which are also used. Rapid elimination is not always a disadvantage. If a lot of plasma substitute has to be given rapidly it is useful if some has been eliminated when cross-matched blood becomes available and can be given without danger of over-transfusion.

Transfusion techniques and the fluids to be used are still being actively investigated. Among the newer topics here are the use of patients' own blood recovered and suitably filtered from the abdominal cavity in auto-transfusion, the use of frozen red cells, the use of concentrated red cells diluted with either colloid or electrolyte solutions, the use of artificial oxygen carrying emulsions (fluoro-carbons), and the redistribution of body fluids with "medical anti-shock" trousers.

A working plan is to use a litre of colloid initially; if the systolic blood pressure is restored to normal it is safe to wait until cross-matched blood is available, if the systolic blood pressure is still low, O-negative blood is given until cross-matched blood is available. For shock in burns there are a number of published formulae for achieving fluid replacement.

If the systolic blood pressure has been restored to normal it does *not* mean that the blood volume has been restored to normal; it can still be about 30 per cent deficient, i.e. if the normal blood volume is 5 litres, it may still be 1.5 litres deficient.

In major trauma the loss of blood will have been rapid and the fluid should be replaced rapidly, usually as quickly as possible via several cannulae if necessary. When several cannulae are being used it may be an advantage to use veins in such a way that the incoming fluid is delivered above and below the diaphragm. The more rapid the replacement, the less organ damage is likely to occur. Transfusions are often given rather slowly in elderly patients for fear of overloading the circulation. This fear must be balanced against the very real danger of permanent damage to organs, especially the brain, if poor perfusion is allowed to continue for more than a short time. It should be remembered that in the elderly a systolic blood pressure of, say, 120 mm Hg may be well below their normal "working pressure".

Some way of evaluating the success of the fluid replacement is needed. In addition to measuring the pulse rate, systolic blood pressure and urine output, the central venous pressure is the best indicator for most purposes. A further step in this type of monitoring is the use of the Swan–Ganz catheter floated into the pulmonary artery. With this one can measure the pulmonary artery wedge pressure and, by thermodilution, the cardiac output.

Treatment of metabolic changes

The metabolic changes outlined above are mainly those due to glycogenolysis and lipolysis. Both these processes may be thought of as defensive and, at worst, are not harmful to the patient. There is little need either to counteract or to enhance the processes. It should be recognized that hyperglycaemia and glycosuria are natural sequels to severe trauma and do not need treatment. Indeed, measurement of plasma lactate and glucose concentrations may give some indication of the severity of injury.

There is no need to use steroids for their hormonal effect. In moderately severe injuries sufficient ACTH is released and the plasma cortisol level rises with the severity of injury. In very severe injuries the plasma cortisol does not rise concomitantly, but it is doubtful if the administration of pharmacological doses of steroids has any beneficial effect. Glucocorticoids should only be given in replacement doses and then only when there is evidence of insufficiency.

Complications

The treatment of the acute phase of hypovolaemic shock is relatively easy. The recognition, prevention and treatment of the complications is more difficult. Indeed there are those who doubt that these complications are the direct result of hypovolaemia and believe that they can be caused by treatment. Whatever the cause it is undoubted that many organs undergo pathological change many hours after hypovolaemia.

Late haematological changes

Acute phase response protein reactions, for example hyperfibrinogenaemia, will induce rouleaux formation and increased viscosity of the plasma and whole blood. Release of thromboplastin from damaged cells and hypoxic endothelium may be associated with the formation of thrombin which promotes aggregation of platelets and intravascular formation of fibrin. Aggregated platelets also release adenosine diphosphate which causes further platelet aggregation. Other mechanisms aggravate the situation such as neutrophil pavementation, release of enzymes which activate the kinin system, and production of prostaglandins.

Occasionally, the increased fibrinolysis may become pathological following disseminated intravascular coagulation (DIC), usually more than 24 hours after injury. This condition can be diagnosed by identifying increased concentrations of fibrin degradation products in the serum. The treatment of this complication, which presents as a steady bleeding from many sites, involves the infusion of fresh frozen plasma or platelet concentrates; heparin may be required in selected cases following discussion with the haematologist.

Pulmonary complications

Nowadays, pulmonary complications are among the most important of those which can occur in the injured patient and are frequently life-threatening.

Early pulmonary changes

In discussing those pulmonary changes which appear shortly after an accident it is important to decide the role of any direct injury to the chest. Pulmonary contusion following direct trauma to the rib cage and underlying lung is perhaps the commonest cause of post-traumatic pulmonary insufficiency. The extent of these changes will vary with the amount of initial damage, but they can increase and become extensive. At autopsy, extravascular blood will be found in the lung along with interstitial and alveolar oedema, in addition to evidence of direct damage.

Pulmonary insufficiency and increased shunting may also be caused by fat emboli soon after peripheral injuries. Since microscopic fat emboli are probably of universal occurrence after injuries such as fractures, minor degrees of this must be relatively common. It is, however, uncommon to see gross lung changes and the other manifestations of fat emboli, unconsciousness, petechiae in the skin, conjunctivae and retina, and a fall in the concentration of platelets.

Pulmonary oedema may also occur as a complication of head injury. This is a serious, but relatively rare, complication which is due to pulmonary hypertension secondary to damage to the brain stem.

Delayed pulmonary changes

The main complication under this heading is the adult respiratory distress syndrome (ARDS). There are many synonyms for this condition but this is the commonest. This is a serious condition with a very poor prognosis.

The pathogenesis of ARDS is not clear. Vascular permeability in the lung is increased giving rise to a protein-rich fluid which accumulates first in the interstitial spaces of the lung and, later, when the lymphatics are no longer able to handle the increased volume, spills over into the alveoli. Later there will be fibrosis. The reasons for the increased permeability are not known. In part, the condition is iatrogenic and nowadays, with more moderate fluid replacement and the wider use of blood filters, the incidence is less than during the Vietnam War in which this condition came to be recognized. Anything, such as the early treatment of wounds and fractures, which decreases the amount of particulate matter being filtered off by the lungs will reduce the incidence of this condition. Nevertheless, the early changes in the lungs are probably not entirely mechanical. The generation of pharmacologically active compounds such as the degradation products of fibrin, rupture of mast cells, changes in the distribution of prostaglandins and their metabolites, changes in complement and the clearance by the lung of circulating substances with pharmacological activities, may all be more important. It is unlikely that any single factor is responsible. With the recognition of this condition and improvements in the treatment of shock, ARDS is probably now most frequently seen as a complication of sepsis.

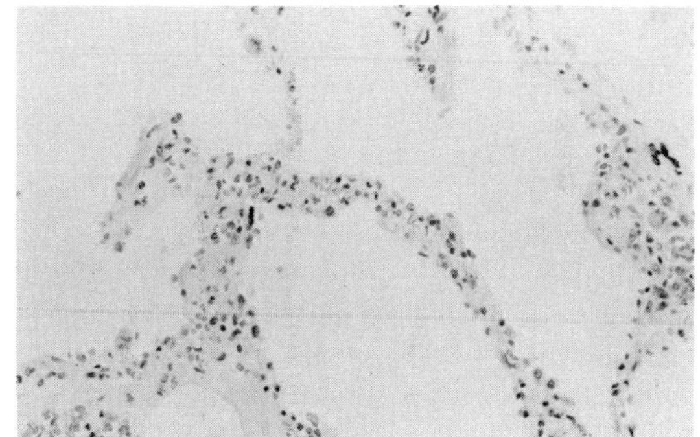

Fig. 35.2 Interstitial pulmonary oedema in ARDS.

Prevention of ARDS following shock is not wholly possible, but there are factors which can be eliminated. Transfusion is the essential treatment for shock and since blood contains micro-thrombi and aggregated cells, micro-embolization can be prevented by filtering the blood. Oxygen toxicity to the lungs is only manifest after administration of at least 40 per cent oxygen for several days; if possible the concentration of oxygen should be kept below this level. Fluid and blood over-transfusion can be avoided if the central venous pressure is monitored. The two contentious subjects are whether one can prevent infection or even ARDS itself. There are some factors in infection which can be eliminated; it has been shown that pulmonary infection with some organisms such as *Pseudomonas aeroginosa* can be prevented by steps to minimize the risk of cross-infection by the wearing of gloves for patient care, increasing the space between beds etc. Opinions vary as to whether prophylactic antibiotics are effective; certainly antibiotics should be used once infection is established, but the use of prophylactic antibiotics as a routine has not resulted in any dramatic change in the rate of pulmonary infection after shock. The use of parenteral glucocorticoids in this connection has been debated for years. There is no doubt that methylprednisolone and dexamethasone give effective prophylaxis in many other conditions, such as the prevention of pulmonary oedema in cardiac surgery and the prevention of cerebral oedema in neurosurgery, but the steroid is given before the trauma. More recently there has been some evidence that methylprednisolone is useful in pulmonary contusion, but it remains to be shown that steroids are useful prophylaxis against ARDS.

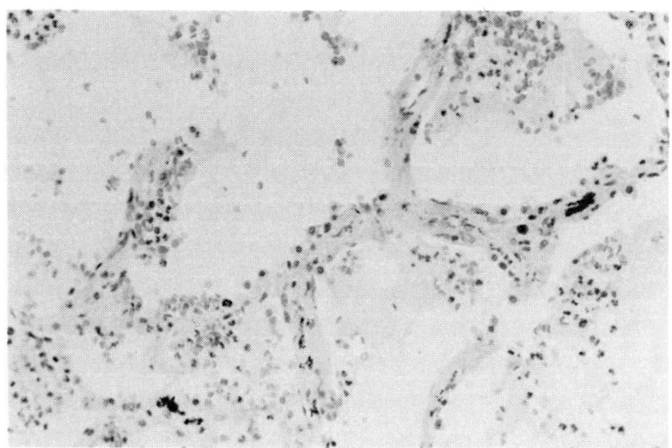

Fig. 35.3 Interstitial pulmonary oedema and leucocytic infiltration in ARDS.

The diagnosis of ARDS is relatively simple. By its nature it usually presents as a decreased and decreasing arterial PO_2. It may be diagnosed early with a high index of suspicion by measuring the PaO_2. Later, the full clinical picture will be manifest as hypoxia, dyspnoea, disorientation, pulmonary opacification on the radiograph and a high pulmonary artery wedge pressure.

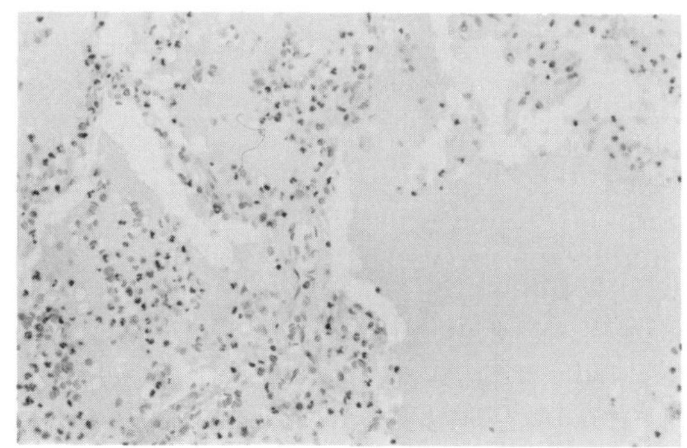

Fig. 35.4 Pulmonary oedema and leucocytic infiltration in ARDS.

Treatment is mainly supportive. Diuretics may relieve some of the pulmonary oedema while artificial ventilation with positive end expiratory pressure (PEEP) may help to express oedema fluid from alveoli but not from the interstitial spaces. PEEP has the further advantage of improving the matching of ventilation with perfusion such that it causes a rise in PaO_2 for a given inspired oxygen concentration. Oxygen itself is valuable and should be used to maintain an acceptable PaO_2 of about 10 kPa (75 mm Hg). Unfortunately, oxygen can also cause the pulmonary damage which will reduce the transfer of oxygen to capillary blood. A downward spiral may occur in which a higher oxygen concentration is needed to maintain the PaO_2, but the increased oxygen is further toxic to the lung. Antibiotics may be useful. There is no evidence yet to suggest that steroids, such as methylprednisolone, have any beneficial effect once ARDS is established.

In those patients who die with this condition, the lungs may be heavy, dark red to blue in colour with foci of collapse. Histologically (*see* Fig. 35.2),

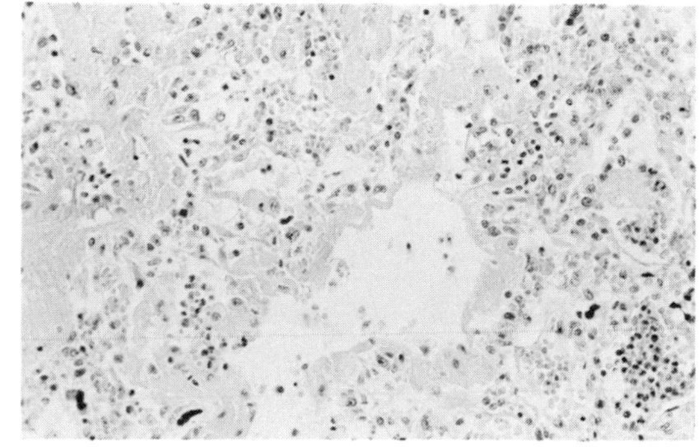

Fig. 35.5 Hyaline membranes, pneumocytes and leucocytes in ARDS.

there may be a variety of changes which indicate interstitial, intra-alveolar and septal oedema, congestion of the alveolar walls and endothelial cell proliferation. The alveoli contain red blood corpuscles, neutrophil polymorphs, macrophages, amorphous pulmonary oedema fluid and strands of fibrin. Microthrombi representing evidence of disseminated intravascular coagulation occur in the pulmonary arterioles and capillaries (*see* Fig. 35.6), according to Riede (1979), in 60 per cent of

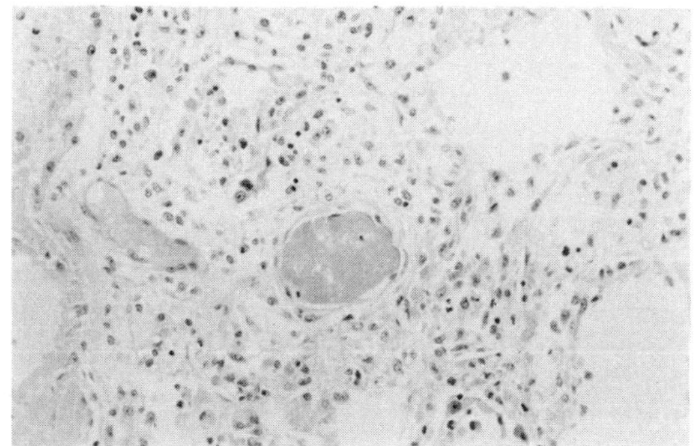

Fig. 35.6 Microthrombi due to disseminated intravascular coagulation in ARDS.

autopsy material and are usually associated with intra-alveolar haemorrhage and giant endothelial cells. Fat embolism is an important feature in many cases. Hyaline membranes develop in the alveoli, alveolar ducts and respiratory bronchioles in a significant proportion of cases. When death occurs after 48 hours, there may be evidence of interstitial fibrosis and intra-alveolar fibrosis (*see* Fig. 35.7). Electron microscope studies show degenerative changes in Type 1 pneumocytes in the early stages, followed by proliferation of the

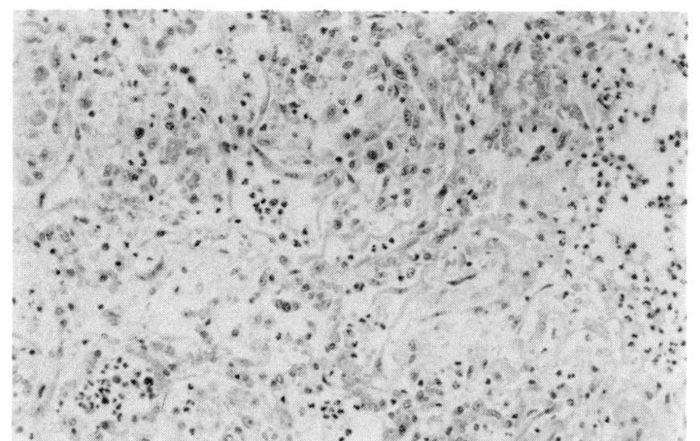

Fig. 35.7 Later stage of ARDS with early intra-alveolar and interstitial fibrosis.

cuboidal Type 2 granular pneumocytes which line the alveolar walls. Plasma cells, histiocytes and lymphocytes accumulate in the chronic stage. Progressive fibrosing alveolitis may be encountered in patients surviving ARDS and dying from other causes at a later stage.

The gross and histological features of this syndrome are not specific and can occur in a wide variety of conditions, for example bronchopneumonia, pulmonary embolism, myocardial infarction, inhalation of gastric contents, pancreatitis, paraquat overdose etc. The pathogenesis is equally diverse and includes fat embolism, disseminated intravascular coagulation, blast injury, oxygen toxicity, inhalation of smoke and other products of combustion (cadmium fumes, hydrogen cyanide), aspirated gastric contents, complicating infection, renal failure etc.

Dysfunction of other organs

The kidneys, brain, heart and other organs may be affected, and where there are histological changes these are mainly due to failure of the autoregulation of the blood flow through these organs. Under normal circumstances the blood flow through these organs remains fairly constant despite changes in arterial blood pressure, provided that the pressure is above a certain critical level. These critical pressures are quite low—60 mmHg for liver, 30 mmHg for brain. However, if the pressure remains in the vicinity of the critical pressure for any length of time, autoregulation will fail and the blood flow through the organ will decrease. There is, therefore, a limit to the time during which an organ can withstand hypotension.

It might be thought that with a low critical pressure of 30 mmHg, the brain would be well protected, except possibly in the very terminal stages. This is not the case if there is accompanying head injury, for such trauma has been shown to impair autoregulation. Under these conditions the perfusion pressure may be dangerously reduced by anything which raises the intracranial pressure. Such falls in cerebral perfusion pressure may lead to ischaemic brain damage, with necrosis of neurones particularly evident in the so-called "watershed zones" between two adjacent arterial territories, for example between anterior and middle cerebral arteries. These changes are especially likely in elderly patients with antecedent cardiovascular problems. Another lesion in younger patients that almost comes into this category is the infarction of the enlarged anterior pituitary of pregnancy associated with large haemorrhage occurring during or shortly after labour.

Functional renal insufficiency can occur at an early stage due to renal vasoconstriction. There may not be any renal tubular necrosis and, although enzymatic studies show cytochemical changes in the tubular epithelial cells in a proportion of cases, the condition is reversible. The danger of these renal changes can be reduced by ensuring adequate fluid replacement at an early stage.

In the later and more serious form of post-traumatic renal failure, tubular necrosis may be found. It can affect both proximal and distal tubules and the extent of the damage is very variable. Rupture of the basement membrane may occur and tubulo-venous haemorrhage or herniation of a disrupted tubule into the lumen of an adjacent vein may be encountered. Eosinophilic hyaline casts and brown casts which give a positive reaction with benzidine appear in the tubules. The basis of the casts is Tamm–Horsfall mucoprotein. Myoglobin casts may also occur in association with muscle damage, for example in "crush syndrome". Later, chronic inflammatory cellular infiltration of the interstitial tissues will develop according to the severity and duration of the necrosis. Tubular necrosis never involves all the nephrons. Although tubular necrosis may be the main histological change, its role in this renal failure is obscure and the pathogenesis cannot be completely explained.

Nowadays, with adequate early treatment, renal failure is relatively uncommon except in association with sepsis. The mechanism in this case is not understood. Glomerular microthrombosis, which is sometimes seen in injury or burns and which may be very extensive, could be involved in this form of renal failure.

Splanchnic vasoconstriction can lead to ischaemic colitis or ischaemic enteritis characterized by haemorrhagic infarction or ischaemic necrosis in the mucosa which leads to haemorrhage and ulceration. Thrombosis of the submucosal and subserosal veins or thrombosis of capillaries within the mucosa can be demonstrated in the majority of cases.

Infarction or intestinal necrosis in a segment of intestine involving all layers represents a more serious development which can be complicated by perforation, peritonitis, clostridial proliferation, endotoxic shock or Gram-negative septicaemia. Full-thickness infarction is characterized by necrosis and leucocytic infiltration of the muscularis propria accompanied by thrombosis of submucous and subserous veins.

It is worth pointing out that the changes in the human gut are usually much less striking than those found during haemorrhagic shock in the dog. Although "irreversible haemorrhagic shock" in the dog, the Wiggers Model, has often been used in experimental studies on haemorrhage, the value of this model is limited. It fails as a model on many scores, but mainly because of the sudden reduction in the blood pressure to very low levels and because profuse haemorrhage from the gut can continue after the restoration of the blood to the circulation at the end of the bleeding period of that technique.

During recovery from severe shock due to massive gastrointestinal haemorrhage, occasional patients develop jaundice associated with ischaemic centrilobular necrosis. Recovery is rapid if the patient survives and no specific treatment is required.

Patients with established coronary artery disease who develop surgical shock due to trauma, haemorrhage or surgical operation run the risk of coronary thrombosis, myocardial infarction, heart failure or dysrhythmia. The state of shock may be corrected, but the patient can die from an infarct. Foci of myocardial necrosis can also occur in severe surgical shock, although systemic fat embolism and disseminated intravascular coagulation may be involved in the pathogenesis.

The role of the autopsy

Most civilian patients who die after trauma come to autopsy for medico-legal reasons. Since the cause of death, for many of these purposes, is often obvious, such autopsies are often incomplete. This is unfortunate and detailed examinations should be carried out whenever possible. In addition to amplifying our still very incomplete knowledge of events after injury, they will help the surgeon resolve difficulties in diagnosis and assessment which may have occurred during the management of the patient. Autopsy may, for instance, reveal unsuspected sites of haemorrhage, fractures and other lesions as well as underlying pathology which may have been present before the accident. The autopsy is an essential part of surgical audit.

Further reading

Barton RN (ed.) Trauma and its metabolic problems. *Brit med Bull* 1985. **41** No. 3.

Davies JWL. *Physiological Responses to Burning Injury*. London: Academic Press, 1982.
Hasleton PS. Adult respiratory distress syndrome—a review. *Histopathology* 1983; **7**:307–32.
Hunt AC (ed.) *Pathology of Injury*. London: Harvey Miller and Medcalf, 1972.
Riede UN, Mittermayer C, Friedburg H, Wybitul K, Sandritter W, et al. Morphological development of human shock lung. *Pathology Research and Practice* 1979; **165**: 264–86.
Sevitt S, Stoner HB (eds). The pathology of trauma. *J Clin Path* 1970; **23** Suppl. (Roy Coll Path) **4**.
Tubbs ON. *Pathology of Blood Loss in Multiple Injuries*. Slide Tape. London: Royal College of Surgeons, 1978.

Index